The Study of Abnormal Behavior

The Study of Abnormal Behavior

SELECTED READINGS / Third Edition

Melvin Zax and George Stricker

Macmillan Publishing Co., Inc.
New York

Macmillan Publishing Co., Inc.,
866 Third Avenue,
New York, New York 10022

Collier-Macmillan Canada, Ltd.

Library of Congress Cataloging in Publication Data

Zax, Melvin, ed.
The study of abnormal behavior.
Includes bibliographies.
1. Psychiatry—Addresses, essays, lectures. I. Stricker, George, joint ed. II. Title. [DNLM: 1. Psychopathology—Collected works. 2. Psychotherapy—Collected works. WM100 Z41s 1974]
RC458.Z3 1974 616.8'9'008 72-13975
ISBN 0-02-431410-2

Printing: 2 3 4 5 6 7 8 Year: 4 5 6 7 8 9 0

Preface

The instructive merits of primary source materials and their motivating appeal to students are unchallenged. To place a reasonable selection of such material in a convenient format begets a favored teaching aid—the book of readings. Obviously, no single collection of source writing can satisfy all needs, but a book that supplies the kind of close view of empirical literature that is missing from most textbooks can prove at once useful and illuminating.

In selecting from the literature of abnormal behavior, we sought to compile articles that reflect the breadth of research in the area. Simultaneously, we attempted to avoid imbalance among the various theoretical positions. It was our further aim to balance the theoretical and the empirical, and thus our choices range from the very well known to younger, less established researchers and pathfinders. The overriding criterion for every choice was that it represent a significant contribution to student understanding of its particular area. Some important but overly sophisticated papers regretfully had to be eliminated.

In this third edition of readings for abnormal psychology, many new materials have been introduced. Of the forty-four selections presented, twenty-five were not in the second edition. New selections have been introduced to update topics presented earlier and to introduce new topics that are currently having a significant impact on abnormal psychology. Among the latter are exciting new research approaches to understanding schizophrenia, new ways of conceptualizing psychoneurosis, new treatment approaches including group methods, increased emphasis on addiction problems, and additional materials on community psychology. As in previous editions, each chapter has been edited to eliminate the need for highly technical knowledge on the part of the reader, and is introduced with a statement intended both to place the paper in an appropriate context and to highlight its major points.

The book is organized into four major units, each with an introductory section explaining chapter divisions. The first unit covers significant theoretical problems of current concern in the study of abnormal behavior. We hope the student will derive an adequate background of the content of the field from the selections and progress to the second unit with a working appreciation of the many problems involved. The next section offers a variety of approaches to psychopathology, the core of any consideration of abnormal psychology. The third section represents a separate and extensive treatment of psychotherapy, reinforcing its intimate relationship with psychopathology. The final section of the book is devoted to recent issues and trends in community psychology.

Acknowledgments are more directly appreciated in a book of readings than in any other work, and we wish to express our gratitude to the authors and publishers who were kind enough to allow us to reprint their works. Specific acknowledgments are included on the first page of each article. Special thanks are due Hannah Ehrenfeld, Dale Grossman, and Melody Nichols who helped prepare and assemble the manuscript. As ever, our wives, Joanne Zax and Joan Stricker, must be acknowledged for their support and encouragement.

M. Z.
G. S.

Contents

Section I

General Issues in Abnormal Psychology

Section II

Psychopathology

Section IV

Recent Issues and Trends

Section I

General Issues in Abnormal Psychology

As in all fields there are numerous general issues of far-reaching consequence that workers in abnormal psychology have found reason to debate over the years. This section includes a sampling of these. Some have only become prominent in recent years, while others have been the cause of concern over a much longer period. It will be noted further that while in some cases the questions raised seem specifically relevant to the domain of abnormal psychology, in other cases their generality takes them well beyond the subject matter of this area. If the editors have made good choices, the reader should be left with many more questions than answers after a careful and thoughtful reading of the material in this section. Definitive answers are not easily provided in these speculative realms, and there was no intention to provide anything more than a sampling of a variety of representative views.

1 Models for the Understanding of Abnormal Behavior

Traditionally, the diagnosis and treatment of abnormal behavior have been conceptualized within a framework known as the medical model. Recently a number of different approaches have developed, all of which have criticized the medical model, although each for a different reason. One principal component of the medical model is the disease or illness concept of abnormal behavior. This views such behavior as the result of the presence of some internal, sickness-producing agent, and is similar to the germ theory of physical disorder. This conception leads to the widely used term mental illness, as though such behavior were an illness produced in a manner similar to other physical illnesses. This section includes a number of papers critical of the illness formulation, although from different points of view, and a reformulation and defense of the illness model. Another component of the medical model views the therapist as a removed, passive individual to whom patients come for treatment. This aspect also has been critically questioned, and questions of this nature are explored in an article that is also relevant to Section IV of the book concerned with developments in community psychology.

MAGGIE SCARF

Normality Is a Square Circle or a Four-Sided Triangle

It has been traditional to view "abnormal" behavior as an indication of mental illness. In this paper Maggie Scarf introduces the ideas of Dr. Thomas Szasz, whose theoretical position represents a radical departure from more traditional approaches to understanding abnormal behavior. Szasz allows that behavior

---

From *The New York Times Magazine*, **6** (October 3, 1971).
Reprinted by permission of Brandt & Brandt.

occasionally displays peculiarities that make it appear abnormal, but he does not feel that it is appropriate to label this behavior "mental illness." To do so implies that the behavior is caused by some damage to the brain, can be diagnosed without any value judgments, and can be treated medically by the physician. Dr. Szasz prefers to see these behaviors as deviations from social, ethical, and legal codes that result in problems of living for the troubled individual. They are not the direct result of neural malfunctioning, can only be diagnosed by the application of value judgments, and must be treated in a social context rather than a medical context. The implications of this point of view are far-reaching and enormous. It follows from this argument that the individual cannot be called a patient, should not be treated in a hospital, and need not be treated by a physician. In fact, he should not be "treated" at all, because his problems are not medical, but are problems of adjustment in society. The legal implications of this approach are that mental illness cannot be used as a defense in a court of law, since the defendant is not actually ill, and that individuals are committed to institutions for the convenience of society rather than because of their inherent illness. A strict adherence to the implications of Dr. Szasz' views would necessitate a drastic reorganization of our approach to phenomena currently referred to as mental illness.

At New York State University's Upstate Medical Center, a routine diagnostic interview is in progress. The patient, a dowdy woman in her late fifties, had been referred for psychiatric evaluation after complaining persistently of a mysterious "pulling in her head." In a flat voice she unfolds a life story so filled with disaster, loss and sudden death that it seems more the stuff of theater than medicine. From time to time, as she answers the questions of the young resident in psychiatry, she cries briefly; and yet for the most part she speaks in a curiously emotionless tone, as though telling someone else's story. The senior psychiatrist on the case, Dr. Thomas Szasz, sits quietly to one side, jotting on a yellow note pad. There are some 12 students in the consultation room, all juniors in the medical school: their expressions range from slight embarrassment to stern scientific interest.

"Well, what is your diagnosis?" Szasz asks, turning to them after the patient has been escorted from the room. He is a compact, curly-haired man in his early 50's, with a sharply intelligent face; his eyes are bright with mockery. Uncertain, the students look at him without answering.

"Come now," he prods ironically. "You are the *doctors* and she is the *patient*, so that means there must be an *illness*. Otherwise we wouldn't all be here, would we?"

"I think," ventures a young man with a sprouting blond beard, "that she's in a chronic depression."

"Oh, a depression," says the older man, nodding. "And you?" he asks, turning to the next student, whose appearance is almost anachronistically clean-cut. "What do you think?"

"I think that potentially it's a case of involutional melancholia. But for right now, I guess I'd concur in a diagnosis of chronic, severe depression."

Szasz looks at him with interest: "And then how would you go about treating this 'condition'?"

There is a pause. "Er... isn't there a drug called Elavil that's good for depression?"

The psychiatrist blinks several times, parodying extreme amazement: "So you would treat this 'sickness' she's got with *drugs*?" There are several uncomfortable, uncomprehending laughs from around the room. "But what, exactly, are you treating? Is feeling miserable—and needing someone to talk things over with—a form of medical *illness*?" Szasz gets to his feet, walks over to a blackboard and picks up a piece of chalk.

"I don't understand—we're just trying to arrive at a diagnosis," protests the student, his voice confused.

"Of what?" demands Szasz. "Has she got an illness called depression, or has she got a lot of problems and troubles which make her unhappy?" He turns and writes in large block letters: "DEPRESSION." And underneath that: "UNHAPPY HUMAN BEING." "Tell me," he says, facing the class, "does the psychiatric term say more than the simple descriptive phrase? Does it do anything other than turn a 'person' with problems into a 'patient' with a sickness?" He puts down the chalk so hard that a cloud of dust rises. There is a low muttering among the students as he returns to his seat.

"But if this woman comes in complaining of a 'pulling in her head,' and we can't give a name to what's wrong with her, how can we go about treating her?" asks someone indignantly.

Szasz turns to him with one of his elaborately astonished expressions: "What do you call 'treatment'? Suppose someone is sad because he's poor and I give him money, and then he feels happy; is that 'treatment'?"

The student hesitates: "Well, yes, in a way."

Szasz laughs. "So then whatever makes a person feel better is 'medical therapy'; the term is infinitely elastic. But then, what *isn't* medicine?"

The group looks at him as if he were a minister who had suddenly started blaspheming in church: "Are you saying that psychiatry isn't?" asks someone in a voice tart with offense. "And if so, then why should we be wasting four weeks of our time on this service?"

Szasz cocks his head to one side comically: "You're asking *me?*" he demands. There is a moment's stunned silence; then everyone breaks into roars of laughter. In the wake of it come the questions—angry, confused, belligerent, intrigued. And the problem of diagnosing the patient becomes superceded for a time by Szasz's far more passionate and pressing concern—diagnosing what is wrong with the current practice of psychiatry.

Thomas Szasz is a psychiatrist and psychoanalyst in private practice, a professor of psychiatry at the Upstate Medical Center of the State University of New York in Syracuse and probably the most controversial figure in his profession today. For more than a decade he has mounted a virtually single-handed and doggedly persistent attack on the view of mental illness as a "disease" to be "diagnosed" by medically trained psychiatrists, "treated" and, one hopes, "cured." While mental-health organizations have been winning public acceptance of such propositions as "Mental illness is like any other illness," Szasz has infuriated many of his psychiatric colleagues by asserting that it simply does not exist. The concept of mental illness, he insists, is a metaphor run amuck. It is a mythical construct which, in common with most myths, serves covert social purposes. For one thing, it provides "reasons" and "explanations" why an individual may behave in ways that are different, disturbing, incomprehensible (i.e., because he has a "mental disease"); for another, it furnishes an acceptable, even humanitarian-appearing mode of controlling such behavior (the distressing person comes to be defined as "ill" and this justifies locking him up in a mental hospital until he is "well").

And yet, Szasz maintains, there is no such thing as a "sick mind" which can be cured by medicine, any more than a "sick economy" or a "sick society" can be. While the behavior and problems defined as "mental illness" certainly exist—people do become confused, guilty, excessively anxious, unhappy, unwilling or unable to play the game of social living—but these represent problems in adjusting and communicating or what he terms "problems in living." They are not disease entities, nor indeed symptoms of any disease.

At present, vast numbers of people in this country are incarcerated in psychiatric hospitals for the care and treatment of their mental disorders: there are about half a million people in mental institutions, 90 per cent of them on an involuntary basis. Nevertheless, according to Dr. Szasz, a diagnosis or finding of "mental disease" is an imposed *social* definition placed upon individuals who are either threatening to the community (the criminal, the deviant), or are disturbing or frightening people around them (the person who claims to "hear God's voice" or to be the Virgin Mary), or who are merely burdensome (old people comprise approximately 40 per cent of the population of American public mental-health hospitals). Calling these people "mentally ill" is, says Szasz, a strategic tagging process facilitating their shipment out of the social order; it is a moral and political, not a medical, act.

Szasz is the author of more than 150 articles and seven books, including "The Myth of Mental Illness," published in 1961 and now in its 12th hard-cover and seventh paperback printing. He is also a witty and moving speaker, whose unusual views—and verbal gymnastics—attract large audiences where-ever he lectures. Szasz has been called everything from a crank and a paranoid to a prophet and passionate humanitarian. In reviewing "Law, Liberty and Psychiatry," Szasz's third book, the late Manfred Guttmacher, an eminent forensic psychiatrist, complained: "A bird that fouls its nest courts criticism. Dr. Szasz doubtless enjoys the contention which he is creating." Of the most recent Szasz book, "The Manufacture of Madness," Mr. David J. Vail has said: "There is something in it to offend practically everyone." Nevertheless, Vail, who is director of mental health programs for the State of Minnesota, concedes in the same article: "Szasz is like dry martinis. Szaszophiles, like dry-martini *aficionados*, may have their preference as to the potency. But they are hooked, and after that they find it virtually impossible to go back to the sweet stuff...."

Szasz has hammered away at virtually every basic assumption of accepted psychiatric thought—and most vehemently at the practice of involuntary therapy. "One of my main concerns," he explains, "is trying to make clear the important distinction between voluntary and involuntary psychiatric interventions. I'm wholly in favor of the former, which I'd compare to the religious worship of one's own choosing. I'm unalterably opposed to the latter, which I'd consider similar to forced conversions or inquisitorial practices. You know, at this moment thousands of American citizens are being forced to submit to psychiatric 'therapies' against their will: to loss of liberty, to lifelong stigmatization, to extremely toxic drugs like Thorazine, to the brain-damaging assaults of electroshock, and until recently, even to such incredible barbarities as lobotomy. I submit that this is nothing less than a crime against humanity."

Seated in his office, a long narrow room lined at one side with windows, Szasz is friendly, voluble, erudite. He is dressed in the expected gray suit and a striped tie; his black hair, very faintly tinged with gray, is cut short. "It's absolutely essential," he says earnestly, "that we look not at what psychiatrists *say* they do; but at what they actually do. They are not concerned with mental illnesses and their treatments. In practice, they deal with personal, social and ethical problems in living.

"As far as I'm concerned the concept of illness should be restricted to disorders of the body—things like diabetes, organic brain damage, cancer. Because, as the most simple-minded of observations ought to make clear, what is called 'mentally ill' is in fact behavior which is disapproved of by the speaker." Szasz speaks rapidly, his low-pitched voice intense.

"In our society the words 'good' and 'bad' are swiftly becoming obscured by notions about mental health and mental illness. And what is 'mental health' anyway? Ask six different psychiatrists what 'normal' means; you'll get six totally different answers. And if you asked me, I'd say normality is either a four-sided triangle or a square circle.

"So how do psychiatrists decide who is, and who isn't, 'healthy'? Well, Disraeli was once asked to define an agreeable gentleman, and he said: 'A gentleman who agrees with me.' In the same way, a normal person is one whose beliefs and conduct coincide with those of the examining psychiatrist. If the psychiatrist happens to think that homosexuality or suicidal inclinations are 'mental illness,' then by definition that person must be mentally ill. And yet what underlies this 'scientific diagnosis' is that the doctor *disapproves* of homosexuality; that he thinks trying to commit suicide is *bad*." Szasz shrugs, pauses. He turns and takes a sip from a steaming cup of tea which sits on a round table next to his chair.

"Take the Calley trial for instance," he resumes. "Why raise the insanity issue in a case like that? Many people seemed to assume that he must have a 'mental disease' to have perpetrated such a massacre; but such things have been going on for centuries; they're as old as history. Calley performed a perfectly simple act: murder. It was bad, not mentally ill."

The psychiatrist smiles slightly. "We seem to have mystified aggression in the same way that the Victorians mystified sex. Man is a predator; everyone knows that. But after World War II, perhaps in face of the horror of the Nazis, everyone began massively denying that fundamentally we are beasts and that the only things which keep men from murder are moral inhibitions or other people—that is, the sanctions of law. Look, for thousands of years people understood perfectly well why it was that Cain killed Abel. But now, of course, you couldn't have Cain stand trial without an insanity plea. Everybody would insist that he must be crazy because of what he did: He killed his brother!"

"But what," I inquire, "about cases which appear utterly bizarre; for example, one cited by an English psychiatrist in which a young man killed his mother, cut off her head and cooked it in the oven. Wouldn't you call *that* mental illness?"

"Why call it that?"

"Because the deed is grotesque. One doesn't understand what the motivations can have been; it's incomprehensible."

He gives me a pained look: "You've certainly just defined what 'mental illness' is. What cannot be comprehended about someone else is 'mental illness.' Now I don't know any more than you do why the man committed such a horrible act—he himself is the only one who knows. The explanation that it was because of a 'sickness' seems to satisfy you, to calm your intellectual disquietude. But as far as I'm concerned, it's exactly the same as attributing the 'cause' of his deed to witchcraft.

"The very essence of my work—what I've tried to point out over and over again—is that we have replaced a theological outlook on life with a therapeutic one. Psychiatry in this country *is* a form of religion. Just as we all recognize that there is a religion called Catholicism with a church in Rome, and a religion called Anglicanism with its church based in England, so we should all realize that there's an American church at the National Institute of Mental Health, and the name of the religion is Mental Health. The cardinals are people like Dr. Karl Menninger, Judge David Bazelon—all of the evangelists of the mental-health movement—and they're pontificating not about how many angels can stand on the head of a pin, but about how many human acts are caused by 'mental diseases' which require 'treatment.'

"I think men like Menninger and Bazelon, who want to raise the question of insanity every time some poor jerk steals $5 have been unwilling to commit themselves in simple understandable terms about what's good and what's evil. They claim that all crime is sickness and don't want to punish legally; they only want to punish psychiatrically.

"When someone is acquitted by reason of insanity," Szasz adds ironically, "he only gets a nonpunishing punishment; they call it 'treatment.' But as most criminals are aware, such an acquittal can result in their being locked up in a mad-house forever. In my opinion, 'treatment,' in a free society, can only be that intervention to which a person submits voluntarily. If he's incarcerated in a hospital that's punishment, no matter what his benefactors may care to call it."

"Then do you believe," I ask, "as some experts on law and psychiatry have recently suggested, that the insanity defense should be abolished?"

Szasz smiles disingenuously: "If there is no insanity, how can there be an insanity defense? Of course I think it should be abolished. I think societies should have a limited set of rules about what behavior is permissible, that these should apply to absolutely everybody, and that they should be enforced with savage consistency. *No* people who are merely 'suspected' of being dangerous or different or potentially antisocial should be committed to mental institutions. *All* people who break the law should be punished. But isn't what I'm saying simply—excuse the expression—what 'law and order' is supposed to be about? Punishing lawbreakers? Right now we've got two sets of law and order—legal order and psychiatric order."

"But don't you think," I ask, "that society has the right and the duty to care for those individuals adjudged to be 'dangerous to themselves or others'?"

The psychiatrist laughs. 'I think the idea of 'helping' people by imprisoning them and doing terrible things to them is a religious concept, as the idea of 'saving' witches by torture and burning once was. As far as 'dangerousness to self' is concerned, I believe, as did John Stuart Mill, that a man's body and soul are his own, not the state's. And furthermore, that each individual has the 'right,' if you will, to do with his body as he pleases—so long as he doesn't harm someone else, or infringe on someone else's right.

"As far as 'dangerousness to others' goes, most psychiatrists working with hospitalized patients would admit this is pure fantasy—like those tales about Jews roasting Christian children and eating them for Passover. Both claims only justify seeking out and persecuting a class of scapegoats. There have in fact been statistical studies made which show that mental patients are much more law-abiding than the normal population. They're de-energized, cut off for the most part, less engaged in the real world. But, of course," Szasz takes a sip of tea, "dangerousness is often not the issue."

He puts down the cup with a clatter. "Actually, what gets diagnosed as 'mental illness' is usually just behavior that other people don't want to tolerate. Say, for instance, a man goes walking around saying people are laughing at him and talking about him. Well, either those close to him will stand for it, or they'll try to cast him out of the social framework. Let's imagine that he's old and poor—most of those diagnosed 'mentally ill' are—and that his children don't want him. How do they get rid of him? By having him examined, and found to be suffering from 'senile psychosis'—instead of from children who don't want him. Then he'll be thrown into a New York State mental hospital where he'll be locked up and drugged, and have a far shorter life expectancy.

"This is the way that the mentally healthy help the 'sick' person; he receives 'therapy.' And, of course, it disposes of the problem in a rather convenient way."

The publication, 10 years ago, of "The Myth of Mental Illness" provoked a furious reaction in psychiatric circles and a major cataclysm at the Upstate Medical Center. In the shock waves which followed, the chairman of the psychiatry department resigned and many of Szasz's younger followers were, as he puts it, "purged" from the faculty. Far from being chastised, however, Szasz has mounted an increasingly virulent campaign against many accepted psychiatric practices; he has even questioned the motives and ethics of psychiatrists as a professional group. In his 1963 book, "Law, Liberty and Psychiatry," he writes: "Offensive as the analogy may be, I suggest that, quite often, husbands and wives who commit their mates act like the bosses of crime syndicates. They hire henchmen—psychiatrists—to dispose of their adversaries." And in a later book, "Ideology and Insanity," he characterized the whole of legal psychiatry and involuntary mental care as a "pseudomedical form of social control."

Addressing the convention of the American Trial Lawyers Association in Miami Beach a year ago, Szasz declared: "More than the practice of any other medical specialty, many psychiatric practices make use of, and indeed rest on, force and fraud," and he went on to suggest that lawyers who succeeded in "freeing" involuntary mental patients ought to bring suit for false imprisonment, seeking heavy damages against the doctors involved.

Curiously enough, such provocative statements no longer arouse widespread reactions (the Miami speech evoked only a few protesting letters); they fall into a well of official silence. No professional colleague has mounted a serious counterattack against Szasz's accusations. Either he is simply ignored or—and this is coming to be far more common—he is conceded privately to be raising some important points.

If "mental illness is a myth," says Dr. Alan D. Miller, Commissioner of the New York State Department of Mental Hygiene, "then it's a myth that patients all over the world act as if they believe in. If you visit a psychiatric ward anywhere, you'll see similarities in words, gestures, dress. Of course Szasz has a very legitimate point when he suggests that 'mental illness' is by no means a unified thing; the phrase is a catch-all and is misleading.

"There are, nevertheless, various categories of mental disturbance and they are quite tangible and real. One of the ways we deduce their presence is that someone starts behaving very differently. Admittedly, a psychiatrist's data may be more impressionistic than that of the internist who can point to a diseased organ. But the fact that you can't X-ray it or dissect it doesn't exclude the existence of an illness.

"Most people who have schizophrenia complain about it. Something funny is happening to them, and it's frightening. They start behaving in ways that make it impossible for them to cope, terrorizing not only those around them, but themselves. I think if we emptied the wards of all of the hospitals in Manhattan tomorrow it would be—cruel. Actually, most of the complaints we receive are not about our having committed someone unjustly; 99 out of 100 are because we've refused to admit a person whom we haven't thought needed hospitalization."

Yet despite wide areas of disagreement, Dr. Miller believes Szasz has played an important role as a reformer. "By taking an extreme position," Miller says, "and even questioning the ethics of people who considered themselves decent, hard-working doctors, he's managed to shock us all into some serious self-examination. That's upsetting; it's painful. But the effect has been to move the entire spectrum of the way people think about involuntary hospitalization. In New York State, for example, we're making a conscious move toward more open hospitals, with patients permitted to come and go freely. We're concentrating on short-term hospitalization and trying not to produce new chronic patients. In fact, the population of our public psychiatric hospitals has gone down 40 to 50 per cent in the last decade.

"Also, very largely in response to the kinds of issues Dr. Szasz, among others, has been raising, the state has set up a mental-health information service. This agency gets in touch with every new patient, voluntary and involuntary, to make sure that he and his family know his legal rights; it continues in touch throughout his stay and serves on his behalf in the courts."

Since psychiatrists are empowered by our mental-hygiene laws to certify people, to detain them and to judge whether or not they are competent to stand trial, they are empowered, as one psychiatrist recently observed, "to condemn or absolve in our own ways."

Bruce Ennis, a young staff attorney with the New York Civil Liberties Union says: "Szasz was early in recognizing this as a clear civil-rights issue. He's a social philosopher, and two generations ahead of his time.

"The decision to commit someone usually revolves around a finding of 'dangerousness to self or others.' I think it's intellectually dishonest to lock up people who, for example, are suicidal but sane. Our presents laws imply that anyone who attempts suicide must be mentally ill. But of course many suicidal people are either just physically sick, or have lost someone they don't want to go on living without, or simply have crummy jobs, horrible lives. They can't by any stretch of the imagination be called crazy.

"As far as 'dangerousness to others' goes," continues Ennis, whose present practice is limited to test-case litigation on behalf of involuntarily committed mental patients, "why is it that we're willing to confine people if they're dangerous insane and not if they're dangerous but sane? We know that 85 per cent of all ex-convicts will commit more crimes in the future, and that ghetto residents and teen-age males are far more likely to commit crime than the average member of the population. We also know, from recent studies, that mental patients are statistically *less* dangerous than the average guy. So if what we're really worried about is danger, why don't we, first, lock up all former convicts, and then lock up all ghetto residents, and then why don't we lock up all teen-age males?" He laughs briefly. "Then if we're still worried, we can try mental patients.

"The question Szasz has been asking," Ennis adds, "is: If a person hasn't broken a law, what right has society to lock him up? What Szasz has done is to make it respectable for lawyers to challenge the myriad psychiatric assumptions that are the foundations of our current mental-hygiene laws."

Last May, in what might seem like a fresh bid for unpopularity, Szasz put on display at the annual meeting of the American Psychiatric Association a paper entitled "The Ethics of Addiction." Its argument was that "dangerous" drugs, heroin, for example, should be available to adults in the same mildly regulated manner that alcohol is now, and that other drugs, such as marijuana, ought to be simply sold over the counter like aspirin and cigarettes. The decision as to whether to use or take drugs, asserted Szasz, should be a personal choice and an individual responsibility; the state should not respond in any way, either by calling the drug user "sick" and forcing treatment upon him, or by calling him "criminal" and imprisoning him.

"Clearly," he wrote, "the argument that marijuana—or heroin, or methadone, or morphine—is prohibited because it is addictive or dangerous cannot be supported by facts. For one thing, there are many drugs—from insulin to penicillin—that are neither addictive nor dangerous but are nevertheless prohibitied: they can be obtained only through a physician's prescription. For another there are many things—from dynamite to guns—that are much more dangerous than narcotics (especially to others!) but are not prohibited. As everyone knows, it is still possible, in the United States, to walk into a store and walk out with a shotgun. We enjoy this right not because we do not think guns are dangerous, but because we believe even more strongly that civil liberties are precious."

The reality of our situation, he suggested, is that our society is coming to value medical paternalism more highly than individual freedoms: "Our so-called drug-abuse problem is an integral part of our present social ethic which accepts 'protections' and repressions justified by appeals to health similar to those that medieval societies accepted when they were justified by appeals to faith. . . .

"Sooner or later," he concluded, "we shall have to confront the basic moral and political issues underlying the problem of addiction. . . . In a conflict between the individual and the state, where should the former's autonomy and the latter's right to intervene begin? . . . As American citizens, do we, and should we, have the right to take narcotics and other drugs? Further, if we take drugs and conduct ourselves as law-abiding citizens, do we, or should we, have the right to remain unmolested by the Government? Lastly, if we take drugs and break the law, do we, and should we, have the right to be treated as persons accused of crime, rather than as patients accused of mental illness?"

Szasz's paper will soon be reprinted in Psychiatric News, the journal of the American Psychiatric Association. Questioning him about the stand he has taken I ask: "Do you really think that the Government should abandon all attempts to protect its citizens, and that anyone should be able to take any drug—even to commit suicide—just as he pleases?"

"No," answers Szasz, "not as he pleases, but only without harming anyone else. A distinction certainly ought to be made between shooting oneself or blowing oneself up in a crowded airplane. If the latter attempt failed, I would insist that such a person be tried for attempted murder.

"I do think, however, that we should worry less about preventing suicides, and more about preventing homicides. We should worry less about people abusing their bodies by ingesting harmful drugs (the toxic effects of these drugs will be punishment enough) and more about people abusing other people through reckless driving, theft, assault, stigmatization and all of the countless other ways human beings have devised for injuring one another."

"But don't you think," I protest, "that if drugs became freely available to adults in the manner which you suggest, that addiction among children would rise?"

Szasz shakes his head. "I don't know what would happen immediately, but I'm convinced there would be a reasonable adjustment to it, as there has been to alcohol. I doubt, personally, that the drugs would be significantly more available to minors: they would only be more visible, and therefore more easily subject to parental control. In other words, the responsibility would be where it belongs: on the parents and their children.

"What do you think would happen if a child brought a bottle of gin into school and got drunk? Do you think the liquor store would be blamed as the pusher? Or would the parents and the child himself be blamed? Practically every home in America has liquor in it; yet you don't hear about that being brought to school. Whereas marijuana, dexedrine and heroin—things they are certainly *not* finding at home—frequently find their way into the school."

"But do you think the Government should prohibit nothing?" I persist. "What about such substances as cyclamates, which have been linked to cancer; shouldn't the state remove them from the market by fiat?"

"Absolutely not," Szasz replies. "No more than cigarettes, which have been linked to lung cancer, or ice cream and butter, which have been linked to coronary artery disease, or alcohol, which has been linked to all kinds of ills, including death on the highway."

"Do you then believe," I ask, "that the Government should exercise *no* protective public-health measures, like vaccination and fluoridation of the water?"

Szasz smiles, like a student who has just been asked the very question he is prepared to answer: "The Government should control those things which cannot be controlled by the individual, such as sewage, the level of radioactive waste, the labeling of poisons. In this sense, I suppose I would be against fluoridation of the water, because it imposes on an entire population something which is presumed to be beneficial for only a small proportion of it—that is, growing children. Certainly 70-year-old women don't need it, and God knows what it does to them.

"I've no objection to the Government's advertising fluorides. And let them *offer* vaccines, as they did with polio. Beyond that, why don't we leave it up to the person himself, what he needs or wants in his own body?

"In other words," he adds, "let's distinguish between genuine protection by a decent government of an enlightened citizenry—enlightened through warmth—and the tyrannizing of a cowed, infantilized society by the paternalistic despotism of a corrupt government." He leans back in his chair confidently.

O. HOBART MOWRER

"Sin," the Lesser of Two Evils

In this paper, Mowrer objects to the conception of abnormal behavior as a product of mental illness. His major objection is that this formulation allows no moral dimensions to such behavior. To consider an individual as sick removes any responsibility for his behavior from him, and makes any moral judgment of his actions inappropriate. In searching for an alternative to the illness model, Dr. Mowrer leans heavily on theology and arrives at sin as an alternative to illness in understanding abnormal behavior. If an individual's behavior is seen as sinful, it places responsibility for that behavior on the individual himself, instead of excusing him by saying that it was

---

Reprinted from the *American Psychologist*, **15**, (1960), 301–304, with the permission of the American Psychological Association and Dr. Mowrer.

the product of illness and thus beyond his control. Mowrer's attempt to restore responsibility for his behavior to the individual is very much in keeping with an emphasis on existentialist thought that is prevalent currently in some areas of psychology, although his emphasis on sin and moral values is somewhat atypical. The implications of this approach for psychotherapy are drastic. Rather than have the individual learn to accept his behavior, he must reject it as sinful, and the therapist's job is not to promote understanding in a nonevaluative atmosphere, but to blame the patient in a guilt-arousing atmosphere. It is only through the experience of guilt and the rejection of sinful behavior that an individual can find personal peace.

Following the presentation of a paper on "Constructive Aspects of the Concept of Sin in Psychotherapy" at the 1959 APA convention in Cincinnati, I have repeatedly been asked by psychologists and psychiatrists: "But *why* must you use that awful word 'sin,' instead of some more neutral term such as 'wrongdoing,' 'irresponsibility,' or 'immorality'?" And even a religious layman has reproached me on the grounds that "Sin is such a *strong* word." Its *strength*, surely, is an asset, not a liability; for in the face of failure which has resulted from our erstwhile use of feebler concepts, we have very heavy work for it to do. Besides, sin (in contrast to its more neutral equivalents) is such a handy *little* word that it would be a pity to let it entirely disappear from usage. With Humpty-Dumpty, we ought to expect words to be "well-behaved" and to mean what *we* want them to!

A few years ago I was invited to teach in the summer session at one of our great Pacific Coast universities; and toward the end of the term, a student in my class on Personality Theory said to me one day: "Did you know that near the beginning of this course you created a kind of scandal on this campus?" Then he explained that I had once used the word "sin" without saying "so-called" or making a joke about it. This, the student said, was virtually unheard-of in a psychology professor and had occasioned considerable dismay and perplexity. I did not even recall the incident; but the more I have thought about the reaction it produced, the more frequently I have found myself using the term—with, I hope, something more than mere perversity.

Traditionally, sin has been thought of as whatever causes one to go to Hell; and since Hell, as a place of other-worldly retribution and torment, has conveniently dropped out of most religious as well as secular thought, the concept of sin might indeed seem antiquated and absurd. But, as I observed in the Cincinnati paper, Hell is still very much with us in those states of mind and being which we call neurosis and psychosis; and I have come increasingly, at least in my own mind, to identify anything that carries us toward these forms of perdition as *sin*. Irresponsibility, wrongdoing, immorality, sin: what do the terms matter if we can thus understand more accurately the nature of psychopathology and gain greater practical control over its ramified forms and manifestations?

But now the fat is in the fire! Have we not been taught on high authority that personality disorder is not one's own "fault," that the neurotic is *not* "responsible" for his suffering, that he has done nothing wrong, committed no "sin?" "Mental illness," according to a poster which was widely circulated a few years ago, "is no disgrace. It might happen to anyone." And behind all this, of course, was the Freudian hypothesis that neurosis stems from a "too severe superego," which is the product of a too strenuous socialization of the individual at the hands of harsh, unloving parents and an irrational society. The trouble lay, supposedly, not in anything wrong or "sinful" which the individual has himself *done*, but in things he merely *wants* to do but cannot, because of *repression.*

The neurotic was thus not sinful but *sick*, the helpless, innocent victim of "the sins of the fathers," and could be rescued only by a specialized, esoteric form of *treatment.* Anna Russell catches the spirit of this doctrine well when she sings, in "Psychiatric Folksong,"

> At three I had a feeling of
>   Ambivalence toward my brothers,
> And so it follows naturally
>   I poisoned all my lovers.
> But now I'm happy; I have learned
>   The lesson this has taught;
> That everything I do that's wrong
>   Is someone else's fault.

Freud saw all this not only as a great scientific discovery but also as a strategic gain for the profession which had thus far treated him so indifferently. It was, one may conjecture, a sort of gift, an offering or service which would place medicine in such debt to him that it could no longer ignore or reject him. In his *Autobiography* Freud (1935) puts it thus:

> My medical conscience felt pleased at my having arrived at this conclusion [that neurosis has a sexual basis]. I hoped that I had filled up a gap in medical science, which, in dealing with a function of such great biological importance, had failed to take into account any injuries beyond those caused by infection or by gross anatomical lesions. The medical aspect of the matter was, moreover, supported by the fact that sexuality was not something purely mental. It had a somatic side as well . . . (p. 45).

In his book on *The Problem of Lay Analysis*, Freud (1927) later took a somewhat different position (see also Chapter 9 of the third volume of Jones' biography of Freud, 1957); but by this time his Big Idea had been let loose in the world and was no longer entirely under his control.

Psychologists were, as we know, among the first of the outlying professional groups to "take up" psychoanalysis. By being analyzed, we not only learned—in an intimate, personal way—about this new and revolutionary science; we also (or so we imagined) were qualifying ourselves for the practice of analysis as a form of therapy. Now we are beginning to see how illusory this all was. We accepted psychoanalytic theory long before it had been adequately tested and thus embraced as "science" a set of presuppositions which we are now painfully having to repudiate. But, more than this, in accepting the premise that the neurotically disturbed person is basically *sick*, we surrendered our professional independence and authenticity. Now, to the extent that we have subscribed to the doctrine of mental *illness* (and tried to take part in its "treatment"), we have laid ourselves open to some really very embarrassing charges from our friends in psychiatry.

In 1954 the American Psychiatric Association, with the approval of the American Medical Association and the American Psychoanalytic Association, published a resolution on "relations between medicine and psychology," which it reissued (during the supposed "moratorium") in 1957. This document needs no extensive review in these pages; but a few sentences may be quoted to indicate what a powerful fulcrum the sickness conception of neurosis provides for the aggrandizement of medicine.

> For centuries the Western world has placed on the medical profession responsibility for the diagnosis and treatment of illness. Medical practice acts have been designed to protect the public from unqualified practitioners and to define the special responsibilities assumed by those who practice the healing art. . . . Psychiatry is the medical specialty concerned with illness that has chiefly mental symptoms. . . . Psychotherapy is a form of medical treatment and does not form the basis for a separate profession. . . . When members of these [other] professions contribute to the diagnosis and treatment of illness, their professional contributions must be coordinated under medical responsibility (pp. 1–2).

So long as we subscribe to the view that neurosis is a bona fide "illness," without moral implications or dimensions, our position will, of necessity, continue to be an awkward one. And it is here I suggest that, as between the concept of sin (however unsatisfactory it may in some ways be) and that of sickness, sin is indeed the lesser of two evils. We have tried the sickness horn of this dilemma and impaled ourselves upon it. Perhaps, despite our erstwhile protestations, we shall yet find sin more congenial.

We psychologists do not, I believe, object *in principle* to the type of authority which psychiatrists wish to exercise, or to our being subject to other medical controls, if they were truly functional. But authority and power ought to go with demonstrated competence, which medicine clearly has in the physical realm but, equally clearly, does not have in "psychiatry." Despite some pretentious affirmations to the contrary, the fact is that psychoanalysis, on which modern "dynamic" psychiatry is largely based, is in a state of virtual collapse and imminent demise. And the tranquilizers and other forms of so-called chemotherapy are admittedly only ameliorative, not basically curative. So now, to the extent that we have accepted the "illness" postulate and thus been lured under the penumbra of medicine, we are in the ungraceful maneuver of "getting out."[1]

But the question remains: Where do we *go*, what do we *do*, now? Some believe that our best policy is to become frankly agnostic for the time being, to admit that we know next to nothing about either the cause or correction of psychopathology and therefore ought to concentrate on *research*. This is certainly a safe policy, and it may also be the wisest one. But since this matter of man's total adjustment and psychosocial survival does not quickly yield up its innermost secrets to conventional types of scientific inquiry, I believe it will do no harm for us at the same time to be thinking about some frankly ideological matters.

For several decades we psychologists looked upon the whole matter of sin and moral accountability as a great incubus and acclaimed our liberation from it as epoch-making. But at length we have discovered that to be "free" in this sense, i.e., to have the excuse of being "sick" rather than *sinful*, is to court the danger of also becoming *lost*. This danger is, I believe, betokened by the widespread interest in Existentialism which we are presently witnessing. In becoming amoral, ethically neutral, and "free," we have cut the very roots of our being; lost our deepest sense of self-hood and identity; and, with neurotics themselves, find ourselves asking: Who *am* I? What is my *destiny*? What does living (existence) *mean*?

In reaction to the state of near-limbo into which we have drifted, we have become suddenly aware, once again, of the problem of *values* and of their centrality in the human enterprise. This trend is clearly apparent in the programs at our recent professional meetings, in journal articles, and, to some extent already, in our elementary textbooks. Something very basic is obviously happening to psychologists and their "self-image."

In this process of moving away from our erstwhile medical "entanglements," it would be a very natural thing for us to form a closer and friendlier relationship than we have previously had with religion and theology. And something of this sort is unquestionably occuring. At the APA Annual Convention in 1956 there was, for the first time in our history I believe, a symposium on religion and mental health; and each ensuing year has seen other clear indications of a developing rapprochement.

However, here too there is a difficulty—of a most surprising kind. At the very time that psychologists are becoming distrustful of the sickness approach to personality disturbance and are beginning to look with more benign interest and respect toward certain moral and religious precepts, religionists themselves

[1] Thoughtful psychiatrists are also beginning to question the legitimacy of the disease concept in this area. In an article entitled "The Myth of Mental Illness" which appeared after this paper went to press, Thomas S. Szasz (1960) is particularly outspoken on this score. He says: "... the notion of mental illness has outlived whatever usefulness it might have had and ... now functions merely as a convenient myth. . . . mental illness is a myth, whose function it is to disguise and thus render more palatable the bitter pill of moral conflicts in human relations" (p. 118). Szasz' entire article deserves careful attention.

are being caught up in and bedazzled by the same preposterous system of thought as that from which we psychologists are just recovering. It would be possible to document this development at length; but reference to such recent "theological" works as Richard V. McCann's *Delinquency—Sickness or Sin?* (1957) and Carl Michalson's *Faith for Personal Crises* (1958, see especially Chapter 3) will suffice.

We have already alluded to Anna Russell's "Psychiatric Folksong" and, in addition, should call attention to Katie Lee's 12-inch LP recording "Songs of Couch and Consultation." That entertainment and literary people are broadly rejecting psychoanalytic froth for the more solid substance of moral accountability is indicated by many current novels and plays. It is not without significance that Arthur Miller's *Death of a Salesman*, written in the philosophical vein of Hawthorne's great novel *The Scarlet Letter*, has, for example, been received so well.

How very strange and inverted our present situation therefore is! Traditionally clergymen have worried about the world's entertainments and entertainers and, for a time at least, about psychology and psychologists. Now, ironically, the entertainers and psychologists are *worrying about the clergymen*. Eventually, of course, clergymen will return to a sounder, less fantastic position; but in the meantime, we psychologists can perhaps play a socially useful and, also, scientifically productive role if we pursue, with all seriousness and candor, our discovery of the essentially moral nature of human existence and of that "living death" which we call psychopathology. This, of course, is not the place to go deeply into the substantive aspects of the problem; but one illustration of the fruitfulness of such exploration may be cited.

In reconsidering the possibility that sin must, after all, be taken seriously, many psychologists seem perplexed as to what attitude one should take *toward the sinner*. "Nonjudgmental," "nonpunitive," "nondirective," "warm," "accepting," "ethically neutral": these words have been so very generally used to form the supposedly proper therapeutic imago that reintroduction of the concept of sin throws us badly off balance. *Our* attitudes, as would-be therapists or helping persons, toward the neurotic (sinner) are apparently less important than his attitude *toward himself*; and, as we know, it is usually—in the most general sense—a rejecting one. Therefore, we have reasoned, the way to get the neurotic to accept and love himself is for us to love and accept *him*, an inference which flows equally from the Freudian assumption that the patient is not really guilty or sinful but only fancies himself so and from the view of Rogers that we are all inherently good and are corrupted by our experiences with the external, everyday world.

But what is here generally overlooked, it seems, is that recove (constructive change, redemption) is most assuredly attained, not by hel a person reject and rise above his sins, but by helping him *accept ther* is the paradox which we have not at all understood and which is the v of the problem. Just so long as a person lives under the shado unacknowledged, and unexpiated guilt, he *cannot* (if he has any character at all) "accept himself"; and all *our* efforts to reassure and accept him will avail nothing. He will continue to hate himself and to suffer the inevitable consequences of self-hatred. But the moment he (with or without "assistance") begins to accept his guilt and his sinfulness, the possibility of radical reformation opens up; and with this, the individual may legitimately, though not without pain and effort, pass from deep, pervasive self-rejection and self-torture to a new freedom, of self-respect and peace.

Thus we arrive, not only at a new (really very old) conception of the nature of "neurosis" which may change our entire approach to this problem, but also at an understanding of one of the most fundamental fallacies of Freudian psychoanalysis and many kindred efforts at psychotherapy. Freud observed, quite accurately, that the neurotic tortures himself; and he conjectured that this type of suffering arose from the irrationality and overseverity of the superego. But at once there was an empirical as well as logical difficulty which Freud (unlike some of his followers) faithfully acknowledged. In the *New Introductory Lectures on Psychoanalysis* (1933), he said:

> The superego [paradoxically] seems to have made a one-sided selection [as between the loving and the punitive attitudes of the parents], and to have chosen only the harshness and severity of the parents, their preventive and punitive functions, while their loving care is not taken up and continued by it. If the parents have really ruled with a rod of iron, we easily understand the child developing a severe superego, but, contrary to our expectations, experience shows that the superego may reflect the same relentless harshness even when the up-bringing has been gentle and kind (p. 90).

And then Freud adds, candidly: "We ourselves do not feel that we have fully understood it." In this we can fully agree. For the only way to resolve the paradox of self-hatred and self-punishment is to assume, not that it represents merely an "introjection" of the attitudes of others, but that the self-hatred is realistically justified and will persist until the individual, by radically altered attitude *and action*, honestly and realistically comes to feel that he now deserves something better. As long as one remains, in old-fashioned religious phraseology, hard-of-heart and unrepentant, just so long will one's conscience hold him in the vise-like grip of "neurotic" rigidity and suffering. But if, at length, an individual confesses his past stupidities and errors and makes what poor attempts he can at restitution, then the superego (like the parents of an earlier day—and society in general) forgives and relaxes its stern hold; and the individual once again is free, "well" (Mowrer, 1959).

But here we too, like Freud, encounter a difficulty. There is some evidence that human beings do not change radically unless they first acknowledge their sins; but we also know how hard it is for one to make such an acknowledgment unless he has *already changed*. In other words, the full realization of deep worthlessness is a severe ego "insult"; and one must have some new source of strength, it seems, to endure it. This is a mystery (or is it a mistaken observation?) which traditional theology has tried to resolve in various ways —without complete success. Can we psychologists do better?

References

American Psychiatric Association. (1954). Committee on Relations Between Psychiatry and Psychology. Resolution on relations of medicine and psychology. *Amer. Psychiat. Ass. Mail Pouch*, October.

Freud, S. (1927). *The Problem of Lay Analysis.* New York: Brentano.

Freud, S. (1933). *New Introductory Lectures on Psychoanalysis.* New York: Norton.

Freud, S. (1935). *Autobiography.* New York: Norton.

Jones, E. (1957). *The Life and Work of Sigmund Freud.* Vol. 3. New York: Basic Books.

McCann, R. V. (1957). *Delinquency: Sickness or Sin?* New York: Harper.

Michalson, C. (1958). *Faith for Personal Crises.* London: Epworth.

Mowrer, O. H. (1959). Changing conceptions of the unconscious. *J. Nerv. Ment. Dis.*, **129**, 222–234.

Szasz, T. S. (1960). The myth of mental illness. *Amer. Psychologist*, **15**, 113–118.

DAVID P. AUSUBEL

Personality Disorder Is Disease

Dr. Ausubel prepared this paper as a rejoinder to the views of Drs. Szasz and Mowrer, and as a defense of the term disease in viewing abnormal behavior. He does express agreement with two of the principal positions taken by Szasz and Mowrer. He agrees that it is not necessary for the handling of behavior disorders to be restricted to physicians, or to be controlled by the medical profession. He also objects to a distant, nonjudgmental approach to the treatment of these problems. However, Dr. Ausubel maintains that these two approaches can be rejected without discarding the concept of disease. He views disease as a marked deviation of any sort from usual standards, and sees merit in viewing disordered behavior in this manner. By doing so, it should be clear that disease is used as a description rather than an explanation of abnormal behavior.

Reprinted from the *American Psychologist*, **16** (1961), 69–74, with the permission of the American Psychological Association and Dr. Ausubel.

In two recent articles in the *American Psychologist*, Szasz (1960) and Mowrer (1960) have argued the case for discarding the concept of mental illness. The essence of Mowrer's position is that since medical science lacks "demonstrated competence . . . in psychiatry," psychology would be wise to "get out" from "under the penumbra of medicine," and to regard the behavior disorders as manifestations of sin rather than of disease (p. 302). Szasz' position, as we shall see shortly, is somewhat more complex than Mowrer's, but agrees with the latter in emphasizing the moral as opposed to the psychopathological basis of abnormal behavior.

For a long time now, clinical psychology has both repudiated the relevance of moral judgment and accountability for assessing behavioral acts and choices, and has chafed under medical (psychiatric) control and authority in diagnosing and treating the personality disorders. One can readily appreciate, therefore, Mowrer's eagerness to sever the historical and professional ties that bind clinical psychology to medicine, even if this means denying that psychological disturbances constitute a form of illness, and even if psychology's close working relationship with psychiatry must be replaced by a new rapprochement with sin and theology, as "the lesser of two evils" (pp. 302–303). One can also sympathize with Mowrer's and Szasz' dissatisfaction with prevailing amoral and nonjudgmental trends in clinical psychology and with their entirely commendable efforts to restore moral judgment and accountability to a respectable place among the criteria used in evaluating human behavior, both normal and abnormal.

Opposition to these two trends in the handling of the behavior disorders (i.e., to medical control and to nonjudgmental therapeutic attitudes), however, does not necessarily imply abandonment of the concept of mental illness. There is no inconsistency whatsoever in maintaining, on the one hand, that more purposeful human activity has a moral aspect the reality of which psychologists cannot afford to ignore (Ausubel, 1952, p. 462), that man is morally accountable for the majority of his misdeeds (Ausubel, 1952, p. 469), and that psychological rather than medical training and sophistication are basic to competence in the personality disorders (Ausubel, 1956, p. 101), and affirming, on the other hand, that the latter disorders are genuine manifestations of illness. In recent years psychology has been steadily moving away from the formerly fashionable stance of ethical neutrality in the behavioral sciences; and in spite of strident medical claims regarding superior professional qualifications and preclusive legal responsibility for treating psychiatric patients, and notwithstanding the nominally restrictive provisions of medical practice acts, clinical psychologists have been assuming an increasingly more important, independent, and responsible role in treating the mentally ill population of the United States.

It would be instructive at this point to examine the tactics of certain other medically allied professions in freeing themselves from medical control and in acquiring independent, legally recognized professional status. In no instance have they resorted to the devious stratagem of denying that they were treating diseases, in the hope of mollifying medical opposition and legitimizing their own professional activities. They took the position instead that simply because a given condition is defined as a disease, its treatment need not necessarily be turned over to doctors of medicine if other equally competent professional specialists were available. That this position is legally and politically tenable is demonstrated by the fact that an impressively large number of recognized diseases are legally treated today by both medical *and* nonmedical specialists (e.g., diseases of the mouth, face, jaws, teeth, eyes, and feet). And there are few convincing reasons for believing that psychiatrists wield that much more political power than physicians, maxillofacial surgeons, ophthalmologists, and orthopedic surgeons, that they could be successful where these latter specialists have failed, in legally restricting practice in their particular area of competence to holders of the medical degree. Hence, even if psychologists were not currently managing to hold their own vis-à-vis psychiatrists, it would be far less dangerous and much more forthright to press for the necessary ameliorative legislation than to seek cover behind an outmoded and thoroughly discredited conception of the behavior disorders.

The Szasz-Mowrer Position

Szasz' (1960) contention that the concept of mental illness "now functions merely as a convenient myth" (p. 118) is grounded on four unsubstantiated and logically untenable propositions, which can be fairly summarized as follows:

1. Only symptoms resulting from demonstrable physical lesions qualify as legitimate manifestations of disease. Brain pathology is a type of physical lesion, but its symptoms properly speaking, are neurological rather than psychological in nature. Under no circumstances, therefore, can mental symptoms be considered a form of illness.

2. A basic dichotomy exists between *mental* symptoms, on the one hand, which are subjective in nature, dependent on subjective judgment and personal involvement of the observer, and referable to cultural-ethical norms, and *physical* symptoms, on the other hand, which are allegedly objective in nature, ascertainable without personal involvement of the observer, and independent of cultural norms and ethical standards. Only symptoms possessing the latter set of characteristics are genuinely reflective of illness and amenable to medical treatment.

3. Mental symptoms are merely expressions of problems of living and, hence, cannot be regarded as manifestations of a pathological condition. The concept of mental illness is misleading and demonological because it seeks to explain psychological disturbance in particular and human disharmony in general in terms of a metaphorical but nonexistent disease entity, instead of attributing them to inherent difficulties in coming to grips with elusive problems of choice and responsibility.

4. Personality disorders, therefore, can be more fruitfully conceptualized as products of moral conflict, confusion, and aberration. Mowrer (1960) extends this latter proposition to include the dictum that psychiatric symptoms are primarily reflective of unacknowledged sin, and that individuals manifesting these symptoms are responsible for and deserve their suffering, both because of their original transgressions and because they refuse to avow and expiate their guilt (pp. 301, 304).

Widespread adoption of the Szasz-Mowrer view of the personality disorders would, in my opinion, turn back the psychiatric clock twenty-five hundred years. The most significant and perhaps the only real advance registered by mankind in evolving a rational and humane method of handling behavioral aberrations has been in substituting a concept of disease for the demonological and retributional doctrines regarding their nature and etiology that flourished until comparatively recent times. Conceptualized as illness, the symptoms of personality disorders can be interpreted in the light of underlying stresses and resistances, both genic and environmental, and can be evaluated in relation to *specifiable* quantitative and qualitative norms of appropriately adaptive behavior, both cross-culturally and within a particular cultural context. It would behoove us, therefore, before we abandon the concept of mental illness and return to the medieval doctrine of unexpiated sin or adopt Szasz' ambiguous criterion of difficulty in ethical choice and responsibility, to subject the foregoing propositions to careful and detailed study.

Mental symptoms and brain pathology

Although I agree with Szasz in rejecting the doctrine that ultimately some neuroanatomic or neurophysiologic defect will be discovered in *all* cases of personality disorder, I disagree with his reasons for not accepting this proposition. Notwithstanding Szasz' straw man presentation of their position, the proponents of the extreme somatic view do not really assert that the *particular nature* of a patient's disordered beliefs can be correlated with "certain definite lesions in the nervous system" (Szasz, 1960, p. 113). They hold rather that normal cognitive and behavioral functioning depends on the anatomic and physiologic integrity of certain key areas of the brain, and that impairment of this substrate integrity, therefore, provides a physical basis for disturbed ideation and behavior, but does not explain, except in a very gross way, the particular kinds of symptoms involved. In fact, they are generally inclined to attribute the *specific* character of the patient's symptoms to the nature of his pre-illness personality structure, the substrate integrity of which is impaired by the lesion or metabolic defect in question.

Nevertheless, even though this type of reasoning plausibly accounts for the psychological symptoms found in general paresis, various toxic deleria, and other comparable conditions, it is an extremely improbable explanation of *all* instances of personality disorder. Unlike the tissues of any other organ, brain tissue possesses the unique property of making possible awareness of and adjustment to the world of sensory, social, and symbolic stimulation. Hence by virtue of this unique relationship of the nervous system to the environment, diseases of behavior and personality may reflect abnormalities in personal and social adjustment, quite apart from any structural or metabolic disturbance in the underlying neural substrate. I would conclude, therefore, that although brain pathology is probably not the most important cause of behavior disorder, it is undoubtedly responsible for the incidence of *some* psychological abnormalities *as well as* for various neurological signs and symptoms.

But even if we completely accepted Szasz' view that brain pathology does not account for any symptoms of personality disorder, it would still be unnecessary to accept his assertion that to qualify as a genuine manifestation of disease a given symptom must be caused by a physical lesion. Adoption of such a criterion would be arbitrary and inconsistent both with medical and lay connotations of the term "disease," which in current usage is generally regarded as including any marked deviation, physical, mental, or behavioral, from normally desirable standards of structural and functional integrity.

Mental versus physical symptoms

Szasz contends that since the analogy between physical and mental symptoms is patently fallacious, the postulated parallelism between physical and mental disease is logically untenable. This line of reasoning is based on the assumption that the two categories of symptoms can be sharply dichotomized with respect to such basic dimensions as objectivity-subjectivity, the relevance of cultural norms, and the need for personal involvement of the observer. In my opinion, the existence of such a dichotomy cannot be empirically demonstrated in convincing fashion.

Practically all symptoms of bodily disease involve some elements of subjective judgment—both on the part of the patient and of the physician. Pain is perhaps the most important and commonly used criterion of physical illness. Yet, any evaluation of its reported locus, intensity, character, and duration is dependent upon the patient's subjective appraisal of his own sensations and on the physician's assessment of the latter's pain threshold, intelligence, and personality structure. It is also a medical commonplace that the severity of pain in most instances of bodily illness may be mitigated by the administration of a placebo. Furthermore, in taking a meaningful history the physician must not only serve as a participant observer but also as a skilled interpreter of human behavior. It is the rare patient who does not react psychologically to the signs of physical illness; and hence physicians are constantly called upon to decide, for example, to what extent precordial pain and reported tightness in the chest are manifestations of coronary insufficiency, of fear of cardiac disease and impending death, or of combinations of both conditions. Even such allegedly objective signs as pulse rate, BMR, blood pressure, and blood cholesterol have their subjective and relativistic aspects. Pulse rate and blood pressure are notoriously susceptible to emotional influences, and BMR and blood cholesterol fluctuate widely from one cultural environment to another

(Dreyfuss & Czaczkes, 1959). And anyone who believes that ethical norms have no relevance for physical illness has obviously failed to consider the problems confronting Catholic patients and/or physicians when issues of contraception, abortion, and preferential saving of the mother's as against the fetus' life must be faced in the context of various obstetrical emergencies and medical contraindications to pregnancy.

It should now be clear, therefore, that symptoms not only do not need a physical basis to qualify as manifestations of illness, but also that the evaluation of *all* symptoms, physical as well as mental, is dependent in large measure on subjective judgment, emotional factors, cultural-ethical norms, and personal involvement on the part of the observer. These considerations alone render no longer tenable Szasz' contention (1960, p. 114) that there is an inherent contradiction between using cultural and ethical norms as criteria of mental disease, on the one hand, and of employing medical measures of treatment on the other. But even if the postulated dichotomy between mental and physical symptoms were valid, the use of physical measures in treating subjective and relativistic psychological symptoms would still be warranted. Once we accept the proposition that impairment of the neural substrate of personality can result in behavior disorder, it is logically consistent to accept the corollary proposition that other kinds of manipulation of the same neural substrate can conceivably have therapeutic effects, irrespective of whether the underlying cause of the mental symptoms is physical or psychological.

Mental illness and problems of living

"The phenomena now called mental illness," argues Szasz (1960), can be regarded more forthrightly and simply as "expressions of man's struggle with the problem of how he should live" (p. 117). This statement undoubtedly oversimplifies the nature of personality disorders; but even if it were adequately inclusive it would not be inconsistent with the position that these disorders are a manifestation of illness. There is no valid reason why a particular symptom cannot both reflect a problem in living *and* constitute a manifestation of disease. The notion of mental illness, conceived in this way, would not "obscure the everyday fact that life for most people is a continuous struggle . . . for a 'place in the sun,' 'peace of mind,' or some other human value" (p. 118). It is quite true, as Szasz points out, that "human relations are inherently fraught with difficulties" (p. 117), and that most people manage to cope with such difficulties without becoming mentally ill. But conceding this fact hardly precludes the possibility that some individuals, either because of the magnitude of the stress involved, or because of genically or environmentally induced susceptibility to ordinary degrees of stress, respond to the problems of living with behavior that is either seriously distorted or sufficiently unadaptive to prevent normal interpersonal relations and vocational functioning. The latter outcome—gross deviation from a designated range of desirable behavioral variability—conforms to the generally understood meaning of mental illness.

The plausibility of subsuming abnormal behavioral reactions to stress under the general rubric of disease is further enhanced by the fact that these reactions include the same three principal categories of symptoms found in physical illness. Depression and catastrophic impairment of self-esteem, for example, are manifestations of personality disorder which are symptomologically comparable to edema in cardiac failure or to heart murmurs in valvular disease. They are indicative of underlying pathology but are neither adaptive nor adjustive. Symptoms such as hypomanic overactivity and compulsive striving toward unrealistically high achievement goals, on the other hand, are both adaptive and adjustive, and constitute a type of compensatory response to basic feelings of inadequacy, which is not unlike cardiac hypertrophy in hypertensive heart disease or elevated white blood cell count in acute infections. And finally, distortive psychological defenses that have some adjustive value but are generally maladaptive (e.g., phobias, delusions, autistic fantasies) are analogous to the pathological situation found in conditions like pneumonia, in which the excessive outpouring of serum and phagocytes in defensive response to pathogenic bacteria literally causes the patient to drown in his own fluids.

Within the context of this same general proposition, Szasz repudiates the concept of mental illness as demonological in nature, i.e., as the "true heir to religious myths in general and to the belief in witchcraft in particular" (p. 118) because it allegedly employs a reified abstraction ("a deformity of personality") to account in causal terms both for "human disharmony" and for symptoms of behavior disorder (p. 114). But again he appears to be demolishing a straw man. Modern students of personality disorder do not regard mental illness as a cause of human disharmony, but as a co-manifestation with it of inherent difficulties in personal adjustment and interpersonal relations; and in so far as I can accurately interpret the literature, psychopathologists do not conceive of mental illness as a cause of particular behavioral symptoms but as a generic term under which these symptoms can be subsumed.

Mental illness and moral responsibility

Szasz' final reason for regarding mental illness as a myth is really a corollary of his previously considered more general proposition that mental symptoms are essentially reflective of problems of living and hence do not legitimately qualify as manifestations of disease. It focuses on difficulties of ethical choice and responsibility as the particular life problems most likely to be productive of personality disorder. Mowrer (1960) further extends this corollary by asserting that neurotic and psychotic individuals are responsible for their suffering (p. 301), and that unacknowledged and unexpiated sin, in turn, is the basic cause of this suffering (p. 304). As previously suggested, however, one can plausibly accept the proposition that psychiatrists and clinical psychologists have erred in trying to divorce behavioral evaluation from ethical considerations, in conducting psychotherapy in an amoral setting, and in confusing the psychological explanation of unethical behavior with absolution from accountability for same, *without* necessarily endorsing the view that personality disorders are basically a reflection of sin, and that victims of these disorders are less ill than responsible for their symptoms (Ausubel, 1952, pp. 392–397, 465–471).

In the first place, it is possible in most instances (although admittedly difficult in some) to distinguish quite unambiguously between mental illness and ordinary cases of immorality. The vast majority of persons who are guilty of moral lapses knowingly violate their own ethical precepts for expediential reasons—despite being volitionally capable at the time, both of choosing the more moral alternative and of exercising the necessary inhibitory control (Ausubel, 1952, pp. 465–471). Such persons, also, usually do not exhibit any signs of behavior disorder. At crucial choice points in facing the problems of living they simply choose the opportunistic instead of the moral alternative. They are not mentally ill, but they are clearly accountable for their misconduct. Hence, since personality disorder and immorality are neither coextensive nor mutually exclusive conditions, the concept of mental illness need not necessarily obscure the issue of moral accountability.

Second, guilt may be a contributory factor in behavior disorder, but is by no means the only or principal cause thereof. Feelings of guilt may give rise to anxiety and depression; but in the absence of catastrophic impairment of self-esteem induced by *other* factors, these symptoms tend to be transitory and peripheral in nature (Ausubel, 1952, pp. 362–363). Repression of guilt, is more a consequence than a cause of anxiety. Guilt is repressed in order to avoid the anxiety producing trauma to self-esteem that would otherwise result if it were acknowledged. Repression per se enters the causal picture in anxiety only secondarily—by obviating "the possibility of punishment, confession, expiation, and other guilt reduction mechanisms" (Ausubel, 1952, p. 456). Furthermore, in most types of personality disorder other than anxiety, depression, and various complications of anxiety such as phobias, obsessions, and compulsion, guilt feelings are either not particularly prominent (schizophrenic reactions), or are conspicuously absent (e.g., classical cases of inadequate or aggressive, antisocial psychopathy).

Third, it is just as unreasonable to hold an individual responsible for symptoms of behavior disorder as to deem him accountable for symptoms of physical illness. He is no more culpable for his inability to cope with sociopsychological stress than he would be for his inability to resist the spread of infectious organisms. In those instances where warranted guilt feelings *do* contribute to personality disorder, the patient is accountable for the misdeeds underlying his guilt, but is hardly responsible for the symptoms brought on by the guilt feelings or for unlawful acts committed during his illness. Acknowledgment of guilt may be therapeutically beneficial under these circumstances, but punishment for the original misconduct should obviously be deferred until after recovery.

Lastly, even if it were true that all personality disorder is a reflection of sin and that people are accountable for their behavioral symptoms, it would still be unnecessary to deny that these symptoms are manifestations of disease. Illness is no less real because the victim happens to be culpable for his illness. A glutton with hypertensive heart disease undoubtedly aggravates his condition by overeating, and is culpable in part for the often fatal symptoms of his disease, but what reasonable person would claim that for this reason he is not really ill?

Conclusions

Four propositions in support of the argument for discarding the concept of mental illness were carefully examined, and the following conclusions were reached:

First, although brain pathology is probably not the major cause of personality disorder, it does account for *some* psychological symptoms by impairing the neural substrate of personality. In any case, however, a symptom need not reflect a physical lesion in order to qualify as a genuine manifestation of disease.

Second, Szasz' postulated dichotomy between mental and physical symptoms is untenable because the assessment of *all* symptoms is dependent to some extent on subjective judgment, emotional factors, cultural-ethical norms, and personal involvement of the observer. Furthermore, the use of medical measures in treating behavior disorders—irrespective of whether the underlying causes are neural or psychological—is defensible on the grounds that if inadvertent impairment of the neural substrate of personality can have distortive effects on behavior, directed manipulation of the same substrate may have therapeutic effects.

Third, there is no inherent contradiction in regarding mental symptoms both as expressions of problems in living *and* as manifestations of illness. The latter situation results when individuals are for various reasons unable to cope with such problems, and react with seriously distorted or maladaptive behavior. The three principal categories of behavioral symptoms—manifestations of impaired functioning, adaptive compensation, and defensive overreaction—are also found in bodily disease. The concept of mental illness has never been advanced as a demonological cause of human disharmony, but only as a co-manifestation with it of certain inescapable difficulties and hazards in personal and social adjustment. The same concept is also generally accepted as a generic term for all behavioral symptoms rather than as a reified cause of these symptoms.

Fourth, the view that personality disorder is less a manifestation of illness than of sin, i.e., of culpable inadequacy in meeting problems of ethical choice and responsibility, and that victims of behavior disorder are therefore morally accountable for their symptoms, is neither logically nor empirically tenable. In most instances immoral behavior and mental illness are clearly distinguishable conditions. Guilt is only a secondary etiological factor in anxiety and depression, and in other personality disorders is either not prominent or conspicuously absent. The issue of culpability for symptoms is largely irrelevant in handling the behavior disorders, and in any case does not detract from the reality of the illness.

In general, it is both unnecessary and potentially dangerous to discard the concept of mental illness on the grounds that only in this way can clinical psychology escape from the professional domination of medicine. Dentists, podiatrists, optometrists, and osteopaths have managed to acquire an independent professional status without rejecting the concept of disease. It is equally unnecessary and dangerous to substitute the doctrine of sin for illness in order to counteract prevailing amoral and nonjudgmental trends in psychotherapy. The hypothesis of repressed guilt does not adequately explain most kinds and instances of personality disorder, and the concept of mental illness does not preclude judgments of moral accountability where warranted. Definition of behavior disorder in terms of sin or of difficulties associated with ethical choice and responsibility would substitute theological disputation and philosophical wrangling about values for specifiable quantitative and qualitative criteria of disease.

References

AUSUBEL, D. P. (1952). *Ego Development and the Personality Disorders.* New York: Grune & Stratton, Inc.

AUSUBEL, D. P. (1956). Relationships between psychology and psychiatry: the hidden issues. *Amer. Psychologist*, **11**, 99–105.

DREYFUSS, F., & CZACZKES, J. W. (1959). Blood cholesterol and uric acid of healthy medical students under the stress of an examination. *AMA Arch. Intern. Med.*, **103**, 708.

MOWRER, O. H. (1960). "Sin," the lesser of two evils. *Amer. Psychologist*, **15**, 301–304.

SZASZ, T. S. (1960). The myth of mental illness. *Amer. Psychologist*, **15**, 113–118.

BERNARD L. BLOOM

The "Medical Model," Miasma Theory, and Community Mental Health

This paper by Dr. Bloom points up the similarity between the thinking and practices in the community mental health field today and in the early public health model. Both seem to operate on the basis of "miasma" theory, which lacked validity as a theory but which nevertheless prescribed practices useful for the prevention of physical illness. Another point of similarity between the public health and community mental health movement is that both eschew the "medical model," which has come under close scrutiny in recent years. It has been attacked as a theory of how illness is caused and as a way of practicing, although rarely both ways by the same people. The prevention-oriented and community-oriented person in the mental health field has found that the medical model, with its emphasis on waiting for people with fully developed illness to appeal for his help, is extremely limiting. His concern has been with preventing full-blown illness as it is viewed traditionally and to ameliorate or prevent many problems that have not been widely regarded as mental health problems either by professionals or even by the afflicted persons. This has forced the worker to adopt a more active role that brings him out of office practice and into key parts of the community where his influence can be felt by a significant proportion of individuals needing his service. Some of the specific programs described in Section IV will reflect this reaction against the medical model.

Questions about the appropriateness of the so-called medical model in the field of the emotional disorders have long been voiced by professionals of many disciplines. The components of the medical model which have been especially singled out for comment by mental health practitioners include: (1) the belief that one is dealing with diseases or disease syndromes, each with a specific etiology, a disease-specific cure, and ultimately a disease-specific

Reprinted from Community *Mental Health Journal*, **1** (1965), 333–338, with the permission of Behavioral Publications, Inc. and Dr. Bloom.

prevention; (2) the belief that the cause, as well as the appropriate prevention and treatment of emotional disorders, will ultimately be found in the biology of the organism, as opposed to its psychology or sociology; and (3) the belief that definitive treatment of emotional disorders takes place almost exclusively in the dyad between practioner-patient. Perhaps the only characteristic of the medical model with which there appears to be general agreement, at least by the profession of psychology, is that one's formal training has not been completed until the title of "Doctor" has been earned.

The medical model grew out of and received its major impetus during the past century as a consequence of the extraordinary successes of germ theory and the doctrine of contagion in the field of the infectious diseases, and from the equally striking successes in the treatment and prevention of nutritional disorders. In view of its characteristics as well as its historical development, this model should, perhaps more properly, be called the biological model. It is not surprising that the model has been applied to the field of the chronic diseases, including the emotional disorders. Yet there appears to be little convincing evidence that the model is appropriate for the emotional disorders. Since emotional disorders are still mainly conditions of unknown etiology and meaningful diagnostic nomenclature continues to be the object of considerable research and speculation, it seems therefore premature to most mental health professionals to give major emphasis for the amelioration of these disorders to the dyadic treatment model or to any other single treatment approach.

With the rapid current growth of the field of community mental health, particularly with its emphasis upon primary prevention, questions about the appropriateness of the biological model are being raised anew. Less is known about community dis-ease than about individual dis-ease. Techniques of prevention and treatment, imperfectly understood in the case of the individual, are even more tentative in the case of communities. Study of the community and of techniques for inducing community change so clearly involves the social sciences and group action that the unilateral emphasis on the patient-practitioner interaction seems foolhardy.

In this paper some beliefs and practices in the field of mental health in general, and in the field of community mental health in particular, will be considered in order to induce information about the apparent model being followed. In arguing inductively—that is, from the practice to the theory—it will be suggested: (1) that the biological model as defined above is not actually a major philosophical influence in the field of community mental health, and (2) that the model which is apparently employed is strikingly similar to the notions of miasma theory.

Miasma theory preceded germ theory as the major explanatory concept in the understanding of disease processes. It held that soil polluted with waste products of any kind gave off a "miasma" into the air, which caused many major infectious diseases of the day. This theory, which dated from the writings of Hippocrates, suggested that these "poisonous substances" rose up from the earth and were spread through the winds. People living near swamps, and thus particularly vulnerable to marsh gases, were thought to develop fever from these gases—a fever which came to be known as malaria (bad air). The doctrine of miasma, which will be further elaborated below, was preeminent until the end of the nineteenth century, by which time germ theory had become established as the prevailing explanation of the infectious diseases. The major differences between miasma theory and germ theory have implications for an analysis of current thought regarding the theory and practice of community mental health.

While miasma theory has been generally discredited, it possessed great utility at the time it was being applied. Many of the current concepts in community mental health appear to share this potential usefulness. In suggesting that these concepts are similar to miasma theory, no criticism of current practice is intended. Indeed, there is reason to believe that miasma theory provides a quite proper model to be followed.

The Taxonomy of Disease

The biological model holds that there are a large number, perhaps an unlimited number, of discrete, uniquely caused diseases. Diseases are, therefore, essentially independent of each other. Miasma theory, on the other hand, suggests that there are very few diseases, perhaps as few as one, and the disease states are quite interdependent and even interchangeable. Florence Nightingale, who is reputed to have founded the nursing profession as a protest against germ theory, and who was a confirmed miasmatist throughout her lifetime, wrote,

> I was brought up . . . to believe that small-pox, for instance, was a thing of which there was once a first specimen in the world, which went on propagating itself, in a perpetual chain of descent. . . . Since then I have seen with my own eyes and smelt with my nose small-pox growing up in first specimens, either in close rooms or in overcrowded wards where it could not by any possibility have been "caught" but must have begun. Nay more, I have seen diseases begin, grow up, and pass into one another. I have seen, for instance, with a little overcrowding continued fever grow up; and with a little more, typhus, and all in the same ward or hut [Cope, 1958, pp. 14–15].

Thus, different names were assigned to what was thought to be the same disorder as a function of its severity, much as in the South Pacific different names are assigned to the same fish as a function of its size.

There can be little question but that general thought in the field of mental health follows the miasma theory quite closely. While there is no single generally accepted theory of psychopathology, one commonly espoused point of view postulates that differences between normal and abnormal, between neurosis and psychosis are essentially quantitative in character—that a psychosis was once a neurosis. No psychiatric nomenclature suggests that each mental disorder is uniquely caused, however elaborate or sophisticated the nomenclature. Most proposals for the quantitative reporting of psychiatric hospitalizations take the position that there is only one emotional disorder. That is to say, in most suggested statistical reporting systems, a patient cannot be listed as being admitted for the first time for a condition different from the condition for which he was previously admitted. There has been no recognition of the logical possibility that within the same individual two or more different independent emotional disorders can arise, each requiring a first admission into a treatment facility.

Diagnosis and Treatment

The biological model contends that etiology and treatment are disease-specific. Accordingly, the establishment of a diagnosis is generally necessary before appropriate treatment can be instituted. Since, according to miasma theory, diagnosis was essentially irrelevant, there was no particular relationship postulated between treatment and prior diagnosis. Actually, miasma theory offered little specific direction regarding treatment. It was primarily a theory aimed at the prevention of disease. Treatment was seen as making the patient as comfortable as possible and relying on the patient's own restitutive potential. That is, while the biological model views treatment as doing something to the patient, miasma theory proposed that treatment consisted of arranging optimal conditions for the patient to help himself. While the physician is thus the key treatment figure, according to the contemporary medical model, a century ago miasma theory accorded primary treatment responsibility to the nursing profession.

Most thinking in the field of mental health takes positions quite similar to miasma theory, both on the issue of diagnosis and on the relationship of diagnosis to rational treatment. While the hope is frequently expressed that a diagnostic system will ultimately be developed which will yield diagnosis-specific treatment procedures, many mental health practitioners doubt that this state of affairs can or will ever come to pass. Certainly, treatment for emotional disorders today can hardly be considered to be diagnosis-specific. And even the most physiologically oriented practitioner is aware that a major consideration in the successful treatment of mental disorders is to involve the patient actively in his own behalf. This situation is even more cogent when the patient is the community, that is, when community change is desired. To a considerable extent, then, current mental health practice seeks to utilize the same techniques as the bedside nurse of the last century, namely, to create a milieu which will facilitate natural forces bringing about restitution or change whether in the patient or in the community.

In the context of a discussion of the relationship between treatment of a disorder and one's understanding of its history or cause, it may be perhaps useful to note that the term "cause" as applied to diseases has two distinguishable meanings (Cassel, 1964). The onset of a disease is "caused," and a patient's lack of recovery from the disease is "caused," but there is no reason to believe that these two "causes" are identical. Understanding the first set of causes can help in the prevention of a particular disorder but may not be useful in treating an existing case. The practices of the miasmatists fell in this category. Alternatively, understanding the second set of causes can help in the treatment of a disorder, but not necessarily in its prevention. This occurs in the case, for example, of applying the known relationship between insulin metabolism and diabetes. The disease can be treated but not prevented. Questions can be raised not only about the extent of our valid knowledge of techniques for the treatment of emotional disorders, but also about the extent to which these techniques or their underlying theory can be appropriately applied in the task of primary prevention.

Prevention and the Doctrine of Contagion

The doctrine of contagion, without its biological implications, long predated miasma theory. All evil was considered contagious by early peoples, including misfortune, uncleanliness, wickedness, and disease (Singer, 1918). It was a habit of ancient literature, wrote Greenwood (1953),

> to speak of seeds of pestilence, of victims struck down by the contagion, passing it on, infecting others. But there is no hint in the Greek or Roman writers that this notion of seeds was more than a metaphor, that arrows or particles might not have been substituted for seeds [p. 502].

With the development of miasma theory even the metaphorical use of the term "contagion" was rejected. The real triumph of the concept occurred subsequently when its essentially biological nature was finally recognized. With an understanding of the agent of disease transmission, a considerably more sophisticated view of disease prevention could develop.

Medico-biological theory now views disease as developing out of the interaction of host, agent, and environment. An appropriate modification of any one of these three factors can result in the prevention of disease. Not only has this three-factor theory been useful in the field of traditional diseases, but also the model is being effectively exploited in such related fields as accident prevention—the automobile driver is viewed as the host, the automobile as the agent, and the road and weather as examples of the relevant environment. Prevention of disease has been found feasible either by influencing the host, as by immunization against smallpox; or by direct action on the agent, as by the proper use of soap and water in the prevention of syphilis; or by modification of the environment, as by spraying mosquito-infested areas in the prevention of malaria and yellow fever. There is thus a relatively rich armamentarium of techniques available to the contemporary practitioner to control the development of infectious diseases.

In contrast, the miasmatist had but a single major avenue open to him to prevent disease. In the absence of the theory of contagion, and as as a direct consequence of miasma theory itself, the major technique for disease prevention was to attempt to modify the environment by removing the sources of the miasma. The early miasmatists declared war on all refuse quite indiscriminately. Accumulated manure was considered just as dangerous as a cesspool which was contaminating a supply of drinking water. The public health movement had its beginnings with the early environmental and sanitary engineers who sought to prevent disease by removing and preventing the accumulation of filth. Indeed, physicians played a relatively small role in disease prevention, and the medical profession was not always represented on early national health boards. Secondary to modification of the environment, miasmatists sought, by public education, to alert the potential victims of disease—that is, the host—to the dangers of the environment in which they lived.

Except in a metaphorical sense, the concept of contagion plays little significant role in the considerations of mental health practitioners. Accordingly, theories in the field of primary prevention are relatively limited. Even today proposals about the prevention of mental disorder are mainly hypotheses to be tested, rather than established principles. These proposals include both direct environmental modification as well as certain attempts to improve individuals' resistance to deleterious psychic forces around them. In a manner of speaking, current concepts of primary prevention in the field of mental disorders appear to be designed to remove existing accumulations of psychic sewage and to develop improved-techniques to prevent their further accretion, both in the individual and in the community. Representing the first category, modification of the environment, are such activities as mental health education, community organization, and administrative consultation. In the second category, modification of the host, are such activities as anticipatory guidance, crisis intervention, and case-centered or consultee-centered agency consultation. Thus, the theory of prevention underlying community mental health practice appears to be patterned after the model first proposed by the miasmatists.

Miasma Theory as a Community Mental Health Model

It may be discouraging to contemplate the fact that current concepts in community mental health closely follow a set of earlier ideas which have been shown to be without scientific validity. But it must not be supposed that miasma theory was methodologically unscientific or irrational or capricious. The sanitation movement was an entirely rational application of the then prevailing theory of disease. It was an attempt to deal with an extremely serious health situation and played a vital and stable role in the provision of health services of a century ago, particularly during the industrial revolution in Europe and the United States which, among other things, resulted in extreme overcrowding and uncleanliness in urban areas. There was an immense amount of sickness in the poorer crowded sections of most large cities (a situation not unlike estimates of mental disorders today); and it was felt that beyond any doubt, disease—particularly the communicable diseases—was due to the lack of drainage, water supply, and the means for removing refuse from houses and streets. Rene Dubois (1961) wrote:

> To a group of public-minded citizens guided by the physician Southwood Smith and the engineer Edwin Chadwick, it appeared that, since disease always accompanied want, dirt, and pollution, health could be restored only by bringing back to the multitudes pure air, pure water, pure food, and pleasant surroundings. This simple concept was synthesized in the movement "The Health of Towns Association," the prototype of the present-day voluntary health associations throughout the world. Its aim was to "substitute health for disease, cleanliness for filth, order for disorder, . . . order for palliation, . . . enlightened self-interest for ignorant selfishness, and bring home to the poorest, . . . in purity and abundance, the simple blessings which ignorance and negligence have long combined to spoil—*Air, Water, Light!*" [pp. 127–8].

Scientists of a century ago were as concerned about the evaluation of their theory and practice as are mental health scientists today. For example, Lilienfeld (1958) has noted that an association was observed between elevation of residence and cholera mortality in London in 1848–49. With increasing elevation, there was decreasing cholera mortality. Cholera mortality was reported as 102 deaths per 10,000 inhabitants in homes located less than 20 feet above sea level, 65 deaths per 10,000 inhabitants in homes between 20–40 feet above sea level, with the mortality rate declining in a curvilinear fashion until at elevations of over 340 feet above sea level the mortality rate was 7 per 100,000. While this statistical association can now be understood in terms of the relationship of the purity of the water supply to the elevation of the pump, it was consistent with miasma theory as well, and was interpreted as confirmatory evidence for it.

It must also not be assumed that miasma theory, because it was ultimately discredited as theory, was not effective in practice. Shryock (1949), in commenting on the miasmatist's effectiveness in disease prevention in contrast to disease treatment, noted:

> The conviction that the quickest way to improve the health of the poor was through sanitation received statistical verification during the 1850's when various British towns showed marked mortality declines following the establishment of sanitary controls. . . . At the same time that sanitation promised so much, direct medical care of the poor seemed to promise little. . . . It is no wonder that lay reformers . . . had more confidence in what mathematics could do for the poor than they had in medicine [p. 41].

Under the leadership of Max von Pettenkofer, Munich began a city-wide cleanup and beautification program. Clean water was brought in from the surrounding mountains, and city sewage was diluted. As a consequence, typhoid mortality fell from 72 per million in 1880 to 14 per million in 1898. The incidence and mortality of yellow fever was significantly decreased in large Spanish cities following the anti-filth campaigns. Mortality from tuberculosis fell from a high of 500 per 100,000 in 1845 to 200 per 100,000 in 1900. Earlier, again as a direct consequence of the striving for cleanliness, maternal mortality had already been reduced from 24 per 1000 live births in 1750 to 3.5 per 1000 live births in 1800. Infant mortality rates had shown a parallel decrease. In addition, the sanitation movement resulted in major decreases in the morbidity and mortality associated with typhus and cholera. These successes, it should be remembered, occurred as a result of programs instituted by people who did not believe in contagion, let alone in the germ theory of disease, and occurred in the total absence of any disease-specific therapeutic or preventive techniques. While, as was already mentioned, miasma theory offered little direction for treatment, its contribution to disease prevention was no less than extraordinary.

Some future historian may look back at our beginning efforts in the prevention and early treatment of mental disorders with some of the same amused compassion that we feel in considering miasma theory of a century ago. But miasma theory and the practical programs which it generated have probably done more to raise the general level of health in the world than have the programs instituted as a consequence of germ theory. To quote again from Dubois (1961),

> It is easy to see how the appearance of the new antibacterial drugs on the medical scene gave rise to the illusion that the age-old problem of infection had finally been solved. A few diseases almost universally fatal could now be cured. . . . The course of other infectious processes could be interrupted with incredible rapidity. . . . It is obvious that these triumphs . . . are changing the very pattern of disease in the Western world, but there is no reason to believe that they spell the *conquest* of microbial diseases. While it is true that the mortality of many of these afflictions is at an all-time low, the amount of disease that they cause remains very high. Drugs are far more effective in the dramatic acute conditions which are relatively rare than in the countless chronic ailments that account for so much misery in everyday life. Furthermore, as we have seen, the decrease in mortality caused by infection began almost a century ago and has continued ever since at a fairly constant rate irrespective of the use of any specific therapy. The effect of antibacterial drugs is but a ripple on the wave which has been wearing down the mortality caused by infection in our communities [pp. 136–7].

The model introduced by the practices of the miasmatists should be carefully considered by professionals entering the field of community mental health. Its successes were outstanding, albeit for the wrong reasons. As was previously noted, the field of public health was begun by miasmatists. While the practice of community mental health involves interaction with programs in welfare, in education, as well as in general health, it represents, in part, the application of basic public health concepts to the mental disorders. These concepts, introduced so usefully more than a century ago, include: (1) an emphasis upon primary prevention rather than on treatment or rehabilitation; (2) an emphasis on the total community rather than on the individual; and (3) the recognition that progress is made by working with and through community agencies, that is, that communities are organized and that this community organization is a powerful and relevant force in the service of improving a community's emotional well-being.

In a sense, miasma theory suffered from being insufficiently precise. Imbedded within its borders was a small but important island of validity. Until the reasons for their effectiveness were properly understood, miasmatists were concerned about much which, in retrospect, was not within their proper scope of interest. This phenomenon has probably characterized many other theories as well. Certainly the contemporary community mental health professional is being attacked for his involvement in areas such as poverty, urban renewal, and social disequilibrium, which people consider outside the direct scope of mental health. Yet, as one examines the current state of knowledge in the field and the array of hypotheses available to anyone particularly interested in the prevention of emotional disorders, the miasma model seems entirely appropriate. It may be that the theories which lie behind the practice of community mental health—and this paper has sought to show how similar these theories actually are to those of the miasmatists—may one day also be considered naive. But in return for results equivalent to those obtained by the sanitarians and engineers in the prevention of infectious diseases, we might willingly pay the price.

References

ASSEL, J. (1964). Social science theory as source of hypotheses in epidemiological research. *Amer. J. Publ. Hlth.*, **54**, 1482–1488.

COPE, Z. (1958). *Florence Nightingale and the Doctors.* Philadelphia: Lippincott.

DUBOIS, R. (1961). *The Mirage of Health.* New York: Doubleday.

GREENWOOD, M. (1953). Miasma and contagion. In E. A. Underwood (ed.), *Science, Medicine and History.* Vol. II. London: Oxford University Press.

LILIENFELD, A. M. (1958). Epidemiological methods and inferences in studies of noninfectious diseases. *Publ. Hlth. Rep.*, **72**, 51–60.

SHRYOCK, R. H. (1949). In the 1840's. In I. Galdston (ed.), *Social Medicine: Its Derivations and Objectives.* New York: Commonwealth Fund.

SINGER, C. (1918–1919). Discussion. *Proc. Royal Soc. Med.*, **12**, 71–72.

2 Problems in the Diagnosis of Abnormal Behavior

Although some highly humanistic psychologists completely eschew the need for diagnosis, most clinicians agree that the diagnostic procedure is a critical first step in the understanding and treatment of abnormal behavior. However, a number of issues have been raised, both about the diagnostic categories that have been employed and about the system by which we arrive at diagnoses. The papers in this section deal with such issues.

WILLIAM G. SMITH

A Model for Psychiatric Diagnosis

In this research project Smith combines computer technology with a sophisticated mathematical approach to test whether some of the problems with diagnosis might be due to imprecision in the categories. He found that this was not so, the diagnostic categories being conceptually clear and adequate. Therefore, any problems of unreliability that arise with diagnosis must originate in the application of the terms rather than in the categories themselves. In the course of presenting the study, Smith clearly defines and outlines many psychiatric symptoms and diagnostic classifications. This article has been abridged by eliminating portions that detail the Bayesian mathematics that underlie the study. The interested reader is referred back to the original article for this information.

Reprinted from the *Archives of General Psychiatry*, **14** (1966), 521–529, with the permission of the American Medical Association and Dr. Smith.

The advance of any science requires a widely shared and explicit definition of the phenomena which it studies. For effective clinical intervention and research psychiatry needs a reliable classification system to facilitate communication among its professionals. At present there is a commonly held impression, backed by a number of studies (1–8), that the current psychiatric categories do not adequately meet this criterion of reliability. Some have advocated a totally new nosologic system, while others have reacted to this situation by downgrading the importance of diagnostic labels. Even if a new diagnostic system were devised and judged to be adequate, it would take years for it to gain widespread acceptance and use. Such a strategy also implies that the accumulated observations and traditions of clinicians for the past century have little value. While attempts to construct better diagnostic systems are not to be discouraged, an alternate plan might involve refinement of the present classification scheme, thus building upon past experience and perhaps evolving a clearer understanding and more precise use of the terms employed. The present project is an attempt to follow this alternate strategy.

A frequent technique employed to solve complex problems involves the selection of an appropriate model of the real world situation. By manipulating the model in various ways the consequences of a great many approaches can be traced without requiring lengthy and expensive trial and error experiments in real life. Modern computer technology has greatly enhanced the possibility of testing such complex models in a relatively economic way. This investigation has selected Bayes' theorem of conditional probability and has utilized the speed and flexibility of the digital computer as an appropriate model for representing the process of psychiatric diagnosis. By applying this model a test was made of the consensus among professionals in the mental health field in their use of the conventional nosologic nomenclature. In other words, the question was asked whether there was enough conceptual agreement among psychiatric personnel to warrant use of the current diagnostic scheme if it were applied in a systematic manner.

The Model and Method

In arriving at a medical diagnosis the physician first makes a survey of his patient for symptoms and signs indicative of pathology. He then tries to match the particular constellation of findings in his patient with certain clusters of phenomena found repeatedly by others and which go by the name of syndromes or diseases. Often this proves to be a complex process because many symptoms are found in a variety of diseases. It then becomes a task for the diagnostician to make a differential diagnosis, i.e., to somehow assign different operational weights to each of the symptoms so that it will reflect the likelihood of a patient's belonging to one of the possible syndromes under consideration. In other words, the final diagnosis is the most likely or most probable diagnosis, given a particular group of findings. Diagnosis can be viewed as the process of matching clusters of observable symptoms with clusters of symptoms found by other physicians over a long period of time. This in effect is what a "conditional probability model" does. It differentially weights each meaningful symptom for each syndrome or disorder so that the most likely diagnosis will be assigned to any particular pattern of symptoms actually found. Thus, in the simplest case, "distorted conceptualization" is more characteristic of schizophrenia than of passive-aggressive personality disorder, while "obstructionism" is more likely to be associated with passive-aggressive disorder than with schizophrenia. Hence, if "distorted conceptualization" is present in a patient, while "obstructionism" is not observed, the diagnosis of schizophrenia is more likely. The "conditional probability model" merely carries out a similar process of reasoning with many symptoms and many disorders in a systematic way. It asks: what is the chance of having disorder A *on the condition* that this particular set of symptoms is present.

Symptom, as defined here, means a commonly used description of psychopathology. Forty-one *symptoms* were selected for this study. They are listed with their operational definitions in Table 1. It was intended that each *symptom* refer to an element of psychopathology that could be separately described about an individual and that required a minimum of inference from observable or reported behavior. The *symptoms* selected were also meant to cover a wide range of phenomena relevant to psychopathology. A *pattern* here means any group of *symptoms*. A *disorder* means a diagnostic category. Thirty-eight *disorders* were selected from the APA *Diagnostic and Statistical Manual* (9) as representative of the range of psychiatric syndromes (Table 2).

Fourteen fully trained diagnosticians of varying orientations (11 psychiatrists and three doctors of clinical psychology) provided the basic data for this investigation. For each *disorder* each judge was asked to consider his idea of a typical patient representing that *disorder*. He then sorted all 41 *symptoms* into four categories according to the degree to which he thought they were characteristic of the *disorder* under consideration. If a *symptom* was

TABLE 1 *Symptoms of psychopathology*

1. *Mental deficiency*: low native intelligence or ability to reason: potential unaffected by learning and culture
2. *Defect in abstract reasoning*: the ability to separate out similarities and differences, or to generalize from presented data in solving a simple problem in reasoning is impaired: inability to grasp meanings and distinctions in spite of adequate native intelligence
3. *Memory impairment*: subject has defects in various memory functions, e.g., ability to learn, recall, or recognize
4. *Concentration impairment*: defective attention span or organized inattention is evident
5. *Distorted conceptualization*: subject evidences bizarre, autistic thinking and symbolization
6. *Delusions*: false beliefs; not culturally shared; include paranoid
7. *Hallucinations*: perceptual experience without adequate stimuli
8. *Dissociation*: evidence of fugue, depersonalization feelings, stupor, amnesia, dream state, somnambulism
9. *Obsessive-compulsiveness*: useless and often morbid repetitive thoughts, impulses, and actions
10. *Phobia*: classic fear of a neutral object, person, or place not usually expected to incite fear

11. *Excitement*: general increase in activity: verbal, motor, thought, e.g., pressure of speech, hyperactivity, purposeless expenditure of energy; elation or irritability included
12. *Depression*: sadness, discouragement, hopelessness; general decrease in activity: verbal, motor, thought; self-recrimination; depressed mood
13. *Anxiety*: objective signs and subjective experience of tension; vague fear and worry
14. *Hostile Affect*: anger, resentment, vindictive feelings, hate; difficulty adjusting the issues at the origin of this affect
15. *Cyclothymia*: wide swings in quantity or quality of mood; mood changes out of proportion to existing stimuli; affect unsuited to thought content, or lack of affective resonance accompanying thought
16. *Withdrawnness*: lack of social contact; preoccupation with fantasy; aloofness; eccentricity
17. *Impulsivity*: impulse control impaired regarding any affect, e.g., hostility, sexuality, discouragement, etc.; low frustration tolerance
18. *Passivity*: evidences inactivity that does not change markedly with perception of a problem or stress; low initiative level; indecisiveness
19. *Dependency*: subject evidences helplessness; whining clinging behavior; hypersensitivity
20. *Hostile aggressiveness*: fighting, destructiveness, temper tantrums, pouting, stubbornness, procrastination, obstructionism, inefficiency
21. *Suspiciousness*: high rate of nonselective distrust; envy, jealousy, overcaution
22. *Responsibility defect*: evidence that subject is callous, hedonistic, narcissistic, undependable; exhibits behavior that transgresses social sanctions and expectations frequently
23. *Histrionic behavior*: evidence that the subject is overdramatic, exaggerating, is sexually provocative in mannerisms; affectation
24. *Sexual maladaptation*: sexual assault, mutilation, sexual deviation (fetishism, transvestism, homosexuality, promiscuity)
25. *Self-appraisal disturbance*: Subject displays lack of confidence, feelings of inferiority or of being unable to deal with a situation; feeling grandiose; unrealistic self-evaluation
26. *Subjective discomfort*: concern that current health is low or inadequate due to emotional symptoms: feeling that problems interfere with duties, goals, well-being, happiness, etc.
27. *Inadequate family role*: chronic pattern of behaviors not in support of familial goals, e.g., inability to act as an adequate father, son, etc.
28. *Inadequate vocational role*: poor performance or achievement vocationally compared with ability in that role
29. *Skin*: rashes, urticaria, pruritus, etc.
30. *Musculoskeletal*: backache, muscle cramps, myalgias, etc.
31. *Respiratory*: hyperventilation, asthma, sighing, etc.
32. *Cardiovascular*: paroxysmal tachycardia, palpitations, pericardial distress, hypertension
33. *Gastrointestinal*: peptic ulcer symptoms, spastic colon, gastritis, pylorospasm, heartburn, nausea, vomiting
34. *Genitourinary*: chronic dysuria, frequency, dysmennorrhea, dyspareunia
35. *Headache*: chronic or cyclic
36. *Body weight disturbance*: obesity, underweight
37. *Psychaesthenia*: generalized complaints of weakness, fatigue, and nonspecific somatic complaints
38. *Sleep disturbance*: disturbances in starting, maintaining, or stopping sleep; include excessive sleeping and early awakening
39. *Disorder of special organs*: anesthesia, hyperaesthesia, blindness, deafness, paralysis, impotence, frigidity—without physical-mechanical cause
40. *Generalized motor disturbance*: seizures, tremors, posturing, spasms, tone disturbance (distinguish from musculoskeletal complaints)
41. *Drug or alcohol abuse*: excessive and/or destructive use of a pharmacologically active substance; include both habituation and addiction

---

The *symptom* identification numbers in this table will be used throughout this report.

TABLE 2 *The psychiatric disorders*

1. Acute brain syndrome
2. Chronic brain syndrome
3. Mental deficiency
4. Involutional psychotic reaction
5. Manic-depressive reaction, manic type
6. Manic-depressive reaction, depressed type
7. Psychotic depressive reaction
8. Acute schizophrenic reaction
9. Chronic schizophrenic reaction
10. Borderline schizophrenia
11. Paranoia
12. Paranoid state
13. Psychophysiologic skin reaction
14. Psychophysiologic musculoskeletal reaction
15. Psychophysiologic respiratory reaction
16. Psychophysiologic cardiovascular reaction
17. Psychophysiologic gastrointestinal reaction
18. Psychophysiologic genitourinary reaction
19. Anxiety reaction
20. Dissociative reaction
21. Conversion reaction
22. Phobic reaction
23. Obsessive-compulsive reaction
24. Psychoneurotic depressive reaction
25. Inadequate personality disorder
26. Schizoid personality disorder
27. Cyclothymic personality disorder
28. Paranoid personality
29. Emotionally unstable personality
30. Passive-aggressive personality
31. Compulsive personality
32. Antisocial reaction
33. Dyssocial reaction
34. Sexual deviation
35. Alcoholism
36. Drug addiction
37. Adult situational reaction
38. Adjustment reaction of adolescence

The *disorder* identification numbers in this table will be used throughout this report.

judged to be very characteristic (nearly always present) it was given a rating of 3 (high). A moderately characteristic *symptom* was rated 2; a slightly characteristic *symptom* was rated 1. If a *symptom* was viewed as *not* characteristic (or very atypical) for a *disorder* it was rated zero. This was done in turn for all 38 Disorders by each of the 14 judges.

From the pool of these ratings, the conditional probabilities of each *symptom* for each *disorder* were derived. Thus, if the *symptom* "anxiety" was judged to be moderately characteristic of the *disorder* "schizophrenia" by 12 out of 14 judges it was given a conditional probability of 12/14 or 0.86, i.e., the probability of the symptom "anxiety" being present *on the condition* that "schizophrenia" was the *disorder* under consideration is 86%. A sample of conditional probabilities, those for acute schizophrenia, is presented in Table 3.

After deriving the conditional probabilities for each *symptom* in each *disorder* (Table 3), the Baysean formula was applied to each *pattern* of each judge to test the conceptual agreement between his idea of the *disorder* and the symptom-pattern for that *disorder* from the entire pool of judges.

This procedure was carried out by the programmed computer for each of the 38 diagnostic stereotypes rated by each of the 14 diagnosticians. A total of 532 diagnostic classifications were made.

Finally a crossvalidity study was undertaken with 30 hospitalized psychiatric patients. A psychiatrist evaluated each of them via a diagnostic interview. He then rated each patient on the 41 operationally defined *symptoms*. In addition he formulated a clinical diagnosis. The clinical diagnosis was compared with the computer-derived diagnosis (based on the *symptom* ratings) as a check on the model's accuracy.

Findings

Of the 532 original diagnoses, 456 were confirmed by the conditional probability computer program. This yields a consensus rate of 86%. Of the 76 disagreements, 58% showed agreement between the initial clinical and second computer diagnoses. In other words, first or second diagnoses were "correct" in 93% of the cases. Table 4 summarizes by *disorders* the agreement between initial diagnoses by the individual judges and the computer diagnoses derived from the entire pool. There was virtually complete conceptual agreement on 56% of the *disorders*. On only four of the 38 *disorders* did consensus drop below 75% agreement among judges, viz., borderline schizophrenia, paranoid state, emotionally unstable personality, and dyssocial reaction.

In the crossvalidity study on 30 clinically evaluated patients, the programmed diagnosis agreed with the clinical diagnosis in 87% of the cases on the first computer diagnosis and 97% of the time if both first and second computer diagnoses were allowed. When symptoms were simply rated as either present or absent, instead of using the 4–degree range (not present, mild, moderate, marked), the clinical judgment-computer concordance dropped to 60% on first diagnosis and to 80% agreement on either first or second

TABLE 3 *Conditional probabilities of symptoms, given a disorder (Example: disorder 8, acute schizophrenia)*

Symptom	Rating			
	Atypical	Mildly characteristic	Moderately characteristic	Very characteristic
1	1.00	0.00	0.00	0.00
2	0.07	0.00	0.29	0.64
3	0.57	0.21	0.21	0.00
4	0.07	0.14	0.21	0.57
5	0.00	0.00	0.00	1.00
6	0.00	0.00	0.07	0.93
7	0.00	0.00	0.21	0.79
8	0.21	0.07	0.21	0.51
9	0.36	0.50	0.14	0.00
10	0.57	0.21	0.21	0.00
11	0.14	0.21	0.29	0.36
12	0.36	0.36	0.29	0.00
13	0.07	0.14	0.43	0.36
14	0.14	0.50	0.29	0.07
15	0.64	0.07	0.29	0.00
16	0.00	0.14	0.43	0.43
17	0.14	0.36	0.36	0.14
18	0.43	0.50	0.00	0.07
19	0.71	0.14	0.14	0.00
20	0.07	0.43	0.43	0.07
21	0.07	0.14	0.64	0.14
22	0.57	0.07	0.21	0.14
23	0.64	0.36	0.00	0.00
24	0.36	0.43	0.14	0.07
25	0.00	0.50	0.27	0.21
26	0.36	0.36	0.21	0.07
27	0.21	0.14	0.43	0.21
28	0.21	0.14	0.43	0.21
29	1.00	0.00	0.00	0.00
30	1.00	0.00	0.00	0.00
31	0.93	0.07	0.00	0.00
32	1.00	0.00	0.00	0.00
33	1.00	0.00	0.00	0.00
34	1.00	0.00	0.00	0.00
35	1.00	0.00	0.00	0.00
36	0.71	0.14	0.14	0.00
37	0.36	0.57	0.07	0.00
38	0.14	0.36	0.36	0.14
39	0.93	0.00	0.07	0.00
40	0.64	0.14	0.21	0.00
41	0.71	0.29	0.00	0.00

TABLE 4 *Agreement between clinically described stereotypes and computer programmed diagnoses (Baysean conditional probability model)**

Disorder	First diagnosis: clinical-computer agreements	First computer diagnosis: disagreements (Disorder No.)	Second diagnosis when first incorrect (Disorder No.)
1. Acute brain syndrome	13	2	$\underline{1}$
2. Chronic brain syndrome	11	3,3,3	$\underline{2}$,27,$\underline{2}$
3. Mental deficiency	14		
4. Involutional	12	10,24	$\underline{4}$,23
5. Manic-depressive, manic	11	8,31,33	$\underline{5}$,$\underline{5}$,27
6. Manic-depressive, depressive	11	4,6,7	$\underline{6}$,7,$\underline{6}$
7. Psychotic depressive	11	4,6,6	$\underline{7}$,$\underline{7}$,$\underline{7}$
8. Acute schizophrenia	14		
9. Chronic schizophrenia	14		
10. Borderline schizophrenia	10	9,9,27,31	10,8,11,23
11. Paranoia	11	4,13,28	2,21,11
12. Paranoid state	7	4,11,11,11,11,11,13	2,$\underline{12}$,$\underline{12}$,$\underline{12}$,$\underline{12}$,$\underline{12}$,31
13. Skin reaction	12	4,37	10,$\underline{13}$
14. Musculoskeletal	13	5	$\underline{14}$
15. Respiratory	12	4,14	10,15
16. Cardiovascular	10	4,15,17,29	10,$\underline{16}$,30,$\underline{16}$
17. Gastrointestinal	13	4	10
18. Genitourinary	13	4	10
19. Anxiety reaction	11	16,23,37	37,16,23
20. Dissociative reaction	12	19,23	4,31
21. Conversion	14		
22. Phobic	14		
23. Obsessive-compulsive	11	20,31,31	$\underline{23}$,$\underline{23}$,$\underline{23}$
24. Neurotic depressive	14		
25. Inadequate personality	13	33	32
26. Schizoid	14		
27. Cyclothymic	14		
28. Paranoid	14		
29. Emotionally unstable	8	25,30,32,33,33,38	$\underline{29}$,32,$\underline{29}$,$\underline{29}$,32,31
30. Passive-aggressive	13	25	36
31. Compulsive-personal	13	10	31
32. Antisocial	11	33,33,33	$\underline{32}$,34,$\underline{32}$
33. Dysocial	8	29,31,31,32,32,34	25,29,$\underline{33}$,23,$\underline{33}$,$\underline{33}$
34. Sexual deviation	13	31	23
35. Alcoholism	12	36,36	$\underline{35}$,$\underline{35}$
36. Drug addiction	12	35,35	$\underline{36}$,$\underline{36}$
37. Adult situational	11	23,30,38	13,23,37
38. Adolescent adjustment	11	23,30,37	31,23,$\underline{38}$

* N for any one *disorder* = 14;
Line under second diagnosis indicates "agreement."
Percent "correct" first diagnoses = 86%.
"Correct" first or second diagnoses = 93%.

TABLE 5 *A sample scheme for teaching psychiatric diagnosis based on conditional probabilities*

Organic	Presence of defects in abstraction, memory impairment, and concentration disturbance
Psychotic	A pathgnomonic symptom from the "psychotic cluster," or at least one highly probable and one moderately probable symptom from this cluster
Psychophysiologic	No "psychotic" symptoms: one symptom from the "psychophysiologic cluster" plus "anxiety"
Neurotic	Not more than one symptom from the "psychotic cluster" plus one highly probable "neurotic cluster" symptom and one or more from the "ubiquitous cluster"
Personality disorder	Not more than one symptom from the "psychotic cluster" plus two or more symptoms from the "personality cluster"; none from the "sociopathic cluster"
Sociopathy	Not more than one symptom from the "psychotic cluster" plus at least one from the "sociopathic cluster"; symptoms from the "personality cluster" do not detract

This diagnostic scheme is purely *qualitative* and does not comment on the severity of the disorder.

diagnosis. With regard to the *main* diagnostic classes (viz., organic disorder, psychosis, neurosis, psychophysiologic disorder, personality disorder, and sociopathy) agreement still reached 87% even when the choice of rating for a *symptom* was reduced to "probably present" versus "probably absent."

Certain symptoms were highly associated with particular diagnostic classes, while others played a role in a variety of different disorders. For instance, "delusion" was found to be exclusively associated with the psychotic disorders, while "anxiety" was present throughout the range of *disorders.* From the set of conditional probabilities between *disorders* and *symptoms* five clusters of *symptoms* were selected which might form the basis for a set of heuristic rules in teaching diagnostic techniques (Table 5). A few symptoms, such as, "depression" (No. 12) and "anxiety" were ubiquitous, i.e., they were highly associated with disorders of nearly every main diagnostic type.

Comment

The high degree of agreement between clinical judgment and the computerized conditional probability model lends support to the idea that there is a substantial diagnostic consensus among professionals dealing with psychiatric disorder. The low degree of agreement actually achieved in other studies must be due to sources of variance other than conceptual disagreement. Such sources probably include imprecise definitions of the original observable phenomena, lack of completeness in the types of symptoms surveyed or an absence of precise and explicit rules for integrating the various bits of basic information into higher order classifications. Habits of selective attention and inattention on the part of various clinicians or special emphasis they may give to particular systems may also contribute to diagnostic differences.

Rather low concordance was reached on several disorders. Paranoid state and paranoia might be collapsed into paranoid reaction. Obsessive-compulsive neurosis and compulsive personality could be reduced to compulsive reaction. Unless it is more exactly defined "emotionally unstable personality" ought to be dropped. Borderline schizophrenic reaction could be subsumed under the category of chronic schizophrenia. Antisocial and dyssocial reactions might be joined under antisocial reaction alone.

Epidemiologic investigations of psychiatric disorder in general populations and studies evaluating the need for facilities or effectiveness of treatment in large programs of community psychiatry both require accurate, reliable, and economic methods of psychiatric assessment. If the use of this computer program can be based on gross judgments by minimally trained personnel, it may offer a practical technique for such undertakings. Such a goal may be attainable if the *symptom* ratings are derived from data gathered through the use of a structured interviewing technique (10, 11). The method may contribute to other research programs which require the use of standardized and comparable diagnostic decisions.

In teaching medical diagnosis a number of diseases are classified by combining salient symptoms according to some hierarchical scheme. For instance, in rheumatic fever, some symptoms are designated as major symptoms while others are considered minor. Certain combinations of major and minor symptoms are taken as indicators for the presence of the disease. The use of conditional probabilities might afford an analogous method for teaching psychiatric diagnosis. For example, the diagnosis of "psychophysiologic reaction" can be made if one of the symptoms from the psychophysiologic cluster is present along with "anxiety." The particular symptom from the psychophysiologic cluster gives the specific diagnostic classification. Similar reasoning might be applied to the other diagnostic categories as suggested in Table 5.

The main point to be taken from these charts is that reliable diagnostic categories can be attained using the traditional psychiatric nosology, *provided* the basic phenomena of psychopathology are operationally defined and combined in some systematic way. A scheme built on a model of conditional probability offers one such systematic method to integrate a complex variety of clinical observations. It does this by assigning specific weights to each symptom so that the most likely diagnosis is achieved. If such a scheme were employed fairly widely in describing patients, research projects might be more comparable. It might also improve the meaning of communications between clinicians involved in making therapeutic decisions.

Using a conditional probability model the reliability of diagnosis is limited only by the consistency with which the operational symptom categories can be measured in actual cases. How feasible this may be employing persons with varying degrees of training must be elaborated by further research.

Summary

A method for making diagnostic classifications of persons with psychiatric disorders based upon a conditional probability decision model is described in detail. The model revealed an 86% rate of conceptual agreement among 14 trained diagnosticians over a range of 38 traditional psychiatric disorders. It also achieved 87% agreement with clinical evaluations on 30 psychiatric patients. This degree of concordance was viewed as sufficient to warrant further exploration with this technique in researches which deal with a high volume of cases that must be classified in a standardized manner. Possible usefulness in investigations of psychiatric epidemiology and in evaluation of the effectiveness of large programs in community psychiatry was suggested. Conditional probability schemes were also seen as applicable in teaching diagnostic technique to professionals in training. The reliability of psychiatric diagnosis using a computerized Baysean model is limited only by the consistency of the operationally defined measurements on which it is based.

References

1. Ash, P. (1949). The reliability of psychiatric diagnoses. *J. Abnorm. Soc. Psychol.*, **44**, 272–276.
2. Beck, A. T. (1962). Reliability of psychiatric diagnoses: I. A critique of systematic studies. *Amer. J. Psychiat.*, **119**, 210–216.
3. Beck, A. T., et al. (1962). Reliability of psychiatric diagnoses: II. A study of clinical judgments and ratings. *Amer. J. Psychiat.*, **119**, 351–357.
4. Hoch, J. H., & Zubin, J. (1953). *Current Problems in Psychiatric Diagnosis.* New York: Grune & Stratton, Inc.
5. Hunt, A. W., Wittson, C. L., & Hunt, E. B. (1953). A theoretical and practical analysis of the diagnostic process. In Hoch, P. H., & Zubin, J. (eds.), *Current Problems in Psychiatric Diagnosis.* New York: Grune & Stratton, Inc.
6. Sandler, M. G., Peltus, C., & Quade, D. (to be published). A study of psychiatric diagnosis. *J. Nerv. Ment. Dis.*
7. Schmidt, H. O., & Fonda, C. P. (1956). The reliability of psychiatric diagnosis, *J. Abnorm. Soc. Psychol.*, **52**, 262–267.
8. Wallinga, J. V. (1956). Variability of psychiatric diagnosis. *U.S. Armed Forces Med. J.*, **7**, 1305–1312.
9. American Psychiatric Association. (1952). *Diagnostic and Statistical Manual—Mental Disorders.* Washington, D.C.: the Association.
10. Leighton, D. C., et al. (1963). *The Character of Danger*. New York: Basic Books, Inc.
11. Spitzer, R. L., et al. (1965). Mental status schedule. *Arch. Gen. Psychiat.*, **12**, 448–455.

FREDERICK H. KANFER and GEORGE SASLOW

Behavioral Analysis: An Alternative to Diagnostic Classification

Kanfer and Saslow reject systems of classification based on the cause or the prognosis of a syndrome. They also reject a system based on symptoms on the basis that it has little relationship to therapy and is unreliable. Instead, they offer behavioral analysis as an alternative to diagnosis. Behavioral analysis is a technique that grows out of the behavior modification approach to therapy, an approach that emphasizes the applicability of laws of learning to clinical phenomena. It is most strikingly different from traditional diagnosis in that it is an attempt to arrive at a unique diagnostic assessment for each individual, instead of grouping individuals according to common features. It is also remarkably different from traditional approaches in being action oriented instead of descriptive. It is tied in specifically with a treatment plan, and organizes an individual's behavior in such a manner as to clarify antecedent conditions, current behavioral patterns, and areas and techniques of possible therapeutic intervention. On the other hand, this great detail sacrifices the efficiency of a descriptive system, and seems to represent an excellent organizational scheme for a case history instead of a simple act of descriptive classification.

During the past decade attacks on conventional psychiatric diagnosis have been so widespread that many clinicians now use diagnostic labels sparingly and apologetically. The continued adherence to the nosological terms of the traditional classificatory scheme suggests some utility of the present categorization of behavior disorders, despite its apparently low reliability (1, 21); its limited prognostic value (7, 26); and its multiple feebly related assumption supports. In a recent study of this problem, the symptom patterns of carefully diagnosed paranoid schizophrenics were compared. Katz et al. (12) found considerable divergence among patients with the same diagnosis and concluded that "diagnostic systems which are more circumscribed in their intent, for example, based on manifest behavior alone, rather than systems which attempt

Reprinted from the *Archives of General Psychiatry*, **12** (1965), 529–538, with the permission of the American Medical Association and Dr. Kanfer.

to comprehend etiology, symptom patterns and prognosis, may be more directly applicable to current problems in psychiatric research" (p. 202).

We propose here to examine some sources of dissatisfaction with the present approach to diagnosis, to describe a framework for a behavioral analysis of individual patients which implies both suggestions for treatment and outcome criteria for the single case, and to indicate the conditions for collecting the data for such an analysis.

I. Problems in Current Diagnostic Systems

Numerous criticisms deal with the internal consistency, the explicitness, the precision, and the reliability of psychiatric classifications. It seems to us that the more important fault lies in our lack of sufficient knowledge to categorize behavior along those pertinent dimensions which permit prediction of responses to social stresses, life crises, or psychiatric treatment. This limitation obviates anything but a crude and tentative approximation to a taxonomy of effective individual behaviors.

Zigler and Phillips (28), in discussing the requirement for an adequate system of classification, suggest that an etiologically-oriented closed system of diagnosis is premature. Instead, they believe that an empirical attack is needed, using "symptoms broadly defined as meaningful and discernible behaviors, as the basis of the classificatory system" (p. 616). But symptoms as a class of responses are defined after all only by their nuisance value to the patient's social environment or to himself as a social being. They are also notoriously unreliable in predicting the patient's particular etiological history or his response to treatment. An alternate approach lies in an attempt to identify classes of dependent variables in human behavior which would allow inferences about the particular controlling factors, the social stimuli, the physiological stimuli, and the reinforcing stimuli, of which they are a function. In the present early stage of the art of psychological prognostication, it appears most reasonable to develop a program of analysis which is closely related to subsequent treatment. A classification scheme which implies a program for behavioral change is one which has not only utility but the potential for experimental validation.

The task of assessment and prognosis can therefore be reduced to efforts which answer the following three questions: (*a*) which specific behavior patterns require change in their frequency of occurrence, their intensity, their duration or in the conditions under which they occur, (*b*) what are the best practical means which can produce the desired changes in this individual (manipulation of the environment, of the behavior, or the self-attitudes of the patient), and (*c*) what factors are currently maintaining it and what are the conditions under which this behavior was acquired. The investigation of the history of the problematic behavior is mainly of academic interest, except as it contributes information about the probable efficacy of a specific treatment method.

Expectations of current diagnostic systems

In traditional medicine, a diagnostic statement about a patient has often been viewed as an essential prerequisite to treatment because a diagnosis suggests that the physician has some knowledge of the origin and future course of the illness. Further, in medicine diagnosis frequently brings together the accumulated knowledge about the pathological process which leads to the manifestation of the symptoms, and the experiences which others have had in the past in treating patients with such a disease process. Modern medicine recognizes that any particular disease need not have a single cause or even a small number of antecedent conditions. Nevertheless, the diagnostic label attempts to define at least the necessary conditions which are most relevant in considering a treatment program. Some diagnostic classification system is also invaluable as a basis for many social decisions involving entire populations. For example, planning for treatment facilities, research efforts and educational programs take into account the distribution frequencies of specified syndromes in the general population.

Ledley and Lusted (14) give an excellent conception of the traditional model in medicine by their analysis of the reasoning underlying it. The authors differentiate between a disease complex and a symptom complex. While the former describes known pathological processes and their correlated signs, the latter represents particular signs present in a particular patient. The bridge between disease and symptom complexes is provided by available medical knowledge and the final diagnosis is tantamount to labeling the disease complex. However, the current gaps in medical knowledge necessitate the use of probability statements when relating disease to symptoms, admitting that there is some possibility for error in the diagnosis. Once the diagnosis is established, decisions about treatment still depend on many other factors including social, moral, and economic conditions. Ledley and Lusted (14) thus separate the clinical diagnosis into a two-step process. A statistical procedure is suggested to facilitate the primary or diagnostic labeling process. However, the choice of treatment depends not only on the diagnosis proper. Treatment decisions are also influenced by the moral, ethical, social, and economic conditions of the individual patient, his family and the society in which he lives. The proper assignment of the weight to be given to each of these values must in the last analysis be left to the physician's judgment (Ledley and Lusted, 14).

The Ledley and Lusted model presumes available methods for the observation of relevant behavior (the symptom complex), and some scientific knowledge relating it to known antecedents or correlates (the disease process). Contemporary theories of behavior pathology do not yet provide adequate guidelines for the observer to suggest what is to be observed. In fact, Szasz (25) has expressed the view that the medical model may be totally inadequate because psychiatry should be concerned with problems of living and not with diseases of the brain or other biological organs. Szasz (25) argues that "mental illness is a myth, whose function it is to disguise and thus render more potable the bitter pill of moral conflict in human relations" (p. 118).

The attack against use of the medical model in psychiatry comes from many quarters. Scheflen (23) describes a model of somatic psychiatry which is very similar to the traditional medical model of disease. A pathological process results in onset of an illness; the symptoms are correlated with a pathological state and represent our evidence of "mental disease." Treatment consists of removal of the pathogen, and the state of health is restored. Scheflen suggests that this traditional medical model is used in psychiatry not on the basis of its adequacy but because of its emotional appeal.

The limitations of the somatic model have been discussed even in some areas of medicine for which the model seems most appropriate. For example, in the nomenclature for diagnosis of disease of the heart and blood vessels, the criteria committee of the New York Heart Association (17) suggests the use of multiple criteria for cardiovascular diseases, including a statement of the patient's functional capacity. The committee suggests that the functional capacity be ". . . estimated by appraising the patient's ability to perform physical activity" (p. 80), and decided largely by inference from his history. Further (17), ". . . (it) should not be influenced by the character of the structural lesion or by an opinion as to treatment or prognosis" (p. 81). This approach makes it clear that a comprehensive assessment of a patient, regardless of the physical disease which he suffers, must also take into account his social effectiveness and the particular ways in which physiological, anatomical, and psychological factors interact to produce a particular behavior pattern in an individual patient.

Multiple diagnosis

A widely used practical solution and circumvention of the difficulty inherent in the application of the medical model to psychiatric diagnosis is offered by Noyes and Kolb (18). They suggest that the clinician construct a diagnostic formulation consisting of three parts: (1) A *genetic* diagnosis incorporating the constitutional, somatic, and historical-traumatic factors representing the primary sources or determinants of the mental illness; (2) A *dynamic* diagnosis which describes the mechanisms and techniques unconsciously used by the individual to manage anxiety, enhance self-esteem, i.e., that traces the psychopathological processes; and (3) A *clinical* diagnosis which conveys useful connotations concerning the reaction syndrome, the probable course of the disorder, and the methods of treatment which will most probably prove beneficial. Noyes' and Kolb's multiple criteria (18) can be arranged along three simpler dimensions of diagnosis which may have some practical value to the clinician: (1) etiological, (2) behavioral, and (3) predictive. The kind of information which is conveyed by each type of diagnostic label is somewhat different and specifically adapted to the purpose for which the diagnosis is used. The triple-label approach attempts to counter the criticism aimed at use of any single classificatory system. Confusion in a single system is due in part to the fact that a diagnostic formulation intended to describe current behavior, for example, may be found useless in an attempt to predict the response to specific treatment, or to postdict the patient's personal history and development, or to permit collection of frequency data on hospital populations.

Classification by etiology

The Kraepelinian system and portions of the 1952 APA classification emphasize etiological factors. They share the assumption that common etiological factors lead to similar symptoms and respond to similar treatment. This dimension of diagnosis is considerably more fruitful when dealing with behavior disorders which are mainly under control of some biological condition. When a patient is known to suffer from excessive intake of alcohol his hallucinatory behavior, lack of motor coordination, poor judgment, and other behavioral evidence of disorganization can often be related directly to some antecedent condition such as the toxic effect of alcohol on the central nervous system, liver, etc. For these cases, classification by etiology also has some implications for prognosis and treatment. Acute hallucinations and other disorganized behavior due to alcohol usually clear up when the alcohol level in the blood stream falls. Similar examples can be drawn from any class of behavior disorders in which a change in behavior is associated primarily or exclusively with a single, *particular* antecedent factor. Under these conditions this factor can be called a pathogen and the situation closely approximates the condition described by the traditional medical model.

Utilization of this dimension as a basis for psychiatric diagnosis, however, has many problems apart from the rarity with which a specified condition can be shown to have a direct "causal" relationship to a pathogen. Among the current areas of ignorance in the fields of psychology and psychiatry, the etiology of most common disturbances probably takes first place. No specific family environment, no dramatic traumatic experience, or known constitutional abnormality has yet been found which results in the same pattern of disordered behavior. While current research efforts have aimed at investigating family patterns of schizophrenic patients, and several studies suggest a relationship between the mother's behavior and a schizophrenic process in the child (10), it is not at all clear why the presence of these same factors in other families fails to yield a similar incidence of schizophrenia. Further, patients may exhibit behavior diagnosed as schizophrenic when there is no evidence of the postulated mother-child relationship.

In a recent paper Meehl (16) postulates schizophrenia as a neurological disease, with learned content and a dispositional basis. With this array of interactive etiological factors, it is clear that the etiological dimension for classification would at best result in an extremely cumbersome system, at worst in a useless one.

Classification by symptoms

A clinical diagnosis often is a summarizing statement about the way in which a person behaves. On the assumption that a variety of behaviors are correlated and consistent in any given individual, it becomes more economical to assign the individual to a class of persons than to list and categorize all of his behaviors. The utility of such a system rests heavily on the availability of empirical evidence concerning correlations among various behaviors (response-response relationships), and the further assumption that the frequency of occurrence of such behaviors is relatively independent of specific stimulus conditions and of specific reinforcement. There are two major limitations to such a system. The first is that diagnosis by symptoms, as we have indicated in an earlier section, is often misleading because it implies common etiological factors. Freedman (7) gives an excellent illustration of the differences both in probable antecedent factors and subsequent treatment response among three cases diagnosed as schizophrenics. Freedman's patients were diagnosed by at least two psychiatrists, and one would expect that the traditional approach should result in whatever treatment of schizophrenia is practiced in the locale where the patients are seen. The first patient eventually gave increasing evidence of an endocrinopathy, and when this was recognized and treated, the psychotic symptoms went into remission. The second case had a definite history of seizures and appropriate anticonvulsant medication was effective in relieving his symptoms. In the third case, treatment directed at an uncovering analysis of the patient's adaptive techniques resulted in considerable improvement in the patient's behavior and subsequent relief from psychotic episodes. Freedman (7) suggests that schizophrenia is not a disease entity in the sense that it has a unique etiology, pathogenesis, etc., but that it represents the evocation of a final common pathway in the same sense as do headache, epilepsy, sore throat, or indeed any other symptom complex. It is further suggested that the term "schizophrenia has outlived its usefulness and should be discarded" (p. 5). Opler (19, 20) has further shown the importance of cultural factors in the divergence of symptoms observed in patients collectively labeled as schizophrenic.

Descriptive classification is not always this deceptive, however. Assessment of intellectual performance sometimes results in a diagnostic statement which has predictive value for the patient's behavior in school or on a job. To date, there seem to be very few general statements about individual characteristics, which have as much predictive utility as the IQ.

A second limitation is that the current approach to diagnosis by symptoms tends to center on a group of behaviors which is often irrelevant with regard to the patient's total life pattern. These behaviors may be of interest only because they are popularly associated with deviancy and disorder. For example, occasional mild delusions interfere little or not at all with the social or occupational effectiveness of many ambulatory patients. Nevertheless, admission of their occurrence is often sufficient for a diagnosis of psychosis. Refinement of such an approach beyond current usage appears possible, as shown for example by Lorr et al. (15) but this does not remove the above limitations.

Utilization of a symptom-descriptive approach frequently focuses attention on by-products of larger behavior patterns, and results in attempted treatment of behaviors (symptoms) which may be simple consequences of other important aspects of the patient's life. Emphasis on the patient's subjective complaints, moods and feelings tends to encourage use of a syndrome-oriented classification. It also results frequently in efforts to change the feelings, anxieties, and moods (or at least the patient's report about them), rather than to investigate the life conditions, interpersonal reactions, and environmental factors which produce and maintain these habitual response patterns.

Classification by prognosis

To date, the least effort has been devoted to construction of a classification system which assigns patients to the same category on the basis of their similar response to specific treatments. The proper question raised for such a classification system consists of the manner in which a patient will react to treatments, regardless of his current behavior, or his past history. The numerous studies attempting to establish prognostic signs from projective personality tests or somatic tests represent efforts to categorize the patients on this dimension.

Windle (26) has called attention to the low degree of predictability afforded by personality (projective) test scores, and has pointed out the difficulties encountered in evaluating research in this area due to the inadequate description of the population sampled and of the improvement criteria. In a later review Fulkerson and Barry (8) came to the similar conclusion that psychological test performance is a poor predictor of outcome in mental illness. They suggest that demographic variables such as severity, duration, acuteness of onset, degree of precipitating stress, etc., appear to have stronger relationships to outcome than test data. The lack of reliable relationships between diagnostic categories, test data, demographic variables, or other measures taken on the patient on the one hand, and duration of illness, response to specific treatment, or degree of recovery, on the other hand, precludes the construction of a simple empiric framework for a diagnostic-prognostic classification system based only on an array of symptoms.

None of the currently used dimensions for diagnosis is directly related to methods of modification of a patient's behavior, attitudes, response patterns, and interpersonal actions. Since the etiological model clearly stresses causative factors, it is much more compatible with a personality theory which strongly emphasizes genetic-developmental factors. The classification by symptoms facilitates social-administrative decisions about patients by providing some basis for judging the degree of deviation from social and ethical norms. Such a classification is compatible with a personality theory founded on the normal curve hypothesis and concerned with characterization by comparison with a fictitious average. The prognostic-predictive approach appears to have the most direct practical applicability. If continued research were to support certain early findings, it would be indeed comforting to be able to predict outcome of mental illness from a patient's premorbid social competence score (28), or from the patient's score on an ego-strength scale (4), or from many of the other signs and single variables which have been shown to have some predictive powers It is unfortunate that these powers are frequently dissipated in cross validation. As Fulkerson and Barry have indicated (8), single predictors have not yet shown much success.

II. A Functional (Behavioral-Analytic) Approach

The growing literature on behavior modification procedures derived from learning theory (3, 6, 11, 13, 27) suggests that an effective diagnostic procedure would be one in which the eventual therapeutic methods can be directly related to the information obtained from a continuing assessment of the patient's current behaviors and their controlling stimuli. Ferster (6) has said ". . . a functional analysis of behavior has the advantage that it specifies the causes of behavior in the form of explicit environmental events which can be objectively identified and which are potentially manipulable" (p. 3). Such a diagnostic undertaking makes the assumption that a description of the problematic behavior, its controlling factors, and the means by which it can be changed are the most appropriate "explanations." It further makes the assumption that a diagnostic evaluation is never complete. It implies that additional information about the circumstances of the patient's life pattern, relationships among his behaviors, and controlling stimuli in his social milieu and his private experience is obtained continuously until it proves sufficient to effect a noticeable change in the patient's behavior, thus resolving "the problem." In a functional approach it is necessary to continue evaluation of the patient's life pattern and its controlling factors, concurrent with attempted manipulation of these variables by reinforcement, direct intervention, or other means until the resultant change in the patient's behavior permits restoration of more efficient life experiences.

The present approach shares with some psychological theories the assumption that psychotherapy is *not* an effort aimed at removal of intrapsychic conflicts, nor at a change in the personality structure by therapeutic interactions of intense nonverbal nature, (e.g., transference, self-actualization, etc.). We adopt the assumption instead that the job of psychological treatment involves the utilization of a variety of methods to devise a program which controls the patient's environment, his behavior, and the consequences of his behavior in such a way that the presenting problem is resolved. We hypothesize that the essential ingredients of a psychotherapeutic endeavor usually involve two separate stages: (1) a change in the perceptual discriminations of a patient, i.e., in his approach to perceiving, classifying, and organizing sensory events, including perception of himself, and (2) changes in the response patterns which he has established in relation to social objects and to himself over the years (11). In addition, the clinician's task may involve direct intervention in the patient's environmental circumstances, modification of the behavior of other people significant in his life, and control of reinforcing stimuli which are available either through self-administration, or by contingency upon the behavior of others. These latter procedures complement the verbal interactions of traditional psychotherapy. They require that the clinician, at the invitation of the patient or his family, participate more fully in planning the total life pattern of the patient outside the clinician's office.

It is necessary to indicate what the theoretical view here presented does *not* espouse in order to understand the differences from other procedures. It does *not* rest upon the assumption that (*a*) insight is a sine qua non of psychotherapy, (*b*) changes in thoughts or ideas inevitably lead to ultimate changes in actions, (*c*) verbal therapeutic sessions serve as replications of and equivalents for actual life situations, and (*d*) a symptom can be removed only by uprooting its cause or origin. In the absence of these assumptions it becomes unnecessary to conceptualize behavior disorder in etiological terms, in psychodynamic terms, or in terms of a specifiable disease process. While psychotherapy by verbal means may be sufficient in some instances, the combination of behavior modification in life situations as well as in verbal interactions serves to extend the armamentarium of the therapist. Therefore verbal psychotherapy is seen as an *adjunct* in the implementation of therapeutic behavior changes in the patient's total life pattern, not as an end in itself, nor as the sole vehicle for increasing psychological effectiveness.

In embracing this view of behavior modification, there is a further commitment to a constant interplay between assessment and therapeutic strategies. An initial diagnostic formulation seeks to ascertain the major variables which can be directly controlled or modified during treatment. During successive treatment stages additional information is collected about the patient's behavior repertoire, his reinforcement history, the pertinent controlling stimuli in his social and physical environment, and the sociological limitations within which both patient and therapist have to operate. Therefore, the initial formulation will constantly be enlarged or changed, resulting either in confirmation of the previous therapeutic strategy or in its change.

A guide to a functional analysis of individual behavior

In order to help the clinician in the collection and organization of information for a behavioral analysis, we have constructed an outline which aims to provide a working model of the patient's behavior at a relatively low level of abstraction. A series of questions are so organized as to yield immediate implications for treatment. This outline has been found useful both in clinical practice and in teaching. Following is a brief summary of the categories in the outline.

> 1. Analysis of a Problem Situation:[1] The patient's major complaints are categorized into classes of behavioral excesses and deficits. For each excess or deficit the dimensions of frequency, intensity, duration, appropriateness of form, and stimulus conditions are described. In content, the response classes represent the major targets of the therapeutic intervention. As an additional indispensable feature, the behavioral assets of the patient are listed for utilization in a therapy program.

[1] For each patient a detailed analysis is required. For example, a list of behavorial excesses may include specific aggressive acts, hallucinatory behaviors, crying, submission to others in social situations, etc. It is recognized that some behaviors can be viewed as excesses or deficits depending on the vantage point from which the imbalance is observed. For instance, excessive withdrawal and deficient social responsiveness, or excessive social autonomy (nonconformity) and deficient self-inhibitory behavior may be complementary. The particular view taken is of consequence because of its impact on a treatment plan. Regarding certain behavior as excessively aggressive, to be reduced by constraints, clearly differs from regarding the same behavior as a deficit in self-control, subject to increase by training and treatment.

2. Clarification of the Problem Situation: Here we consider the people and circumstances which tend to maintain the problem behaviors, and the consequences of these behaviors to the patient and to others in his environment. Attention is given also to the consequences of changes in these behaviors which may result from psychiatric intervention.

3. Motivational Analysis: Since reinforcing stimuli are idiosyncratic and depend for their effect on a number of unique parameters for each person, a hierarchy of particular persons, events, and objects which serve as reinforcers is established for each patient. Included in this hierarchy are those reinforcing events which facilitate approach behaviors as well as those which, because of their aversiveness, prompt avoidance responses. This information has as its purpose to lay plans for utilization of various reinforcers in prescription of a specific behavior therapy program for the patient, and to permit utilization of appropriate reinforcing behaviors by the therapist and significant others in the patient's social environment.

4. Developmental Analysis: Questions are asked about the patient's biological equipment, his sociocultural experiences, and his characteristic behavioral development. They are phrased in such a way as (*a*) to evoke descriptions of his habitual behavior at various chronological stages of his life, (*b*) to relate specific new stimulus conditions to noticeable changes from his habitual behavior, and (*c*) to relate such altered behavior and other residuals of biological and sociocultural events to the present problem.

5. Analysis of Self-Control: This section examines both the methods and the degree of self-control exercised by the patient in his daily life. Persons, events, or institutions which have successfully reinforced self-controlling behaviors are considered. The deficits or excesses of self-control are evaluated in relation to their importance as therapeutic targets and to their utilization in a therapeutic program.

6. Analysis of Social Relationships: Examination of the patient's social network is carried out to evaluate the significance of people in the patient's environment who have some influence over the problematic behaviors, or who in turn are influenced by the patient for his own satisfactions. These interpersonal relationships are reviewed in order to plan the potential participation of significant others in a treatment program, based on the principles of behavior modification. The review also helps the therapist to consider the range of actual social relationships in which the patient needs to function.

7. Analysis of the Social-Cultural-Physical Environment: In this section we add to the preceding analysis of the patient's behavior as an individual, consideration of the norms in his natural environment. Agreements and discrepancies between the patient's idiosyncratic life patterns and the norms in his environment are defined so that the importance of these factors can be decided in formulating treatment goals which allow as explicitly for the patient's needs as for the pressures of his social environment.

The preceding outline has its purpose to achieve definition of a patient's problem in a manner which suggests specific treatment operations, or that none are feasible, and specific behaviors as targets for modification. Therefore, the formulation is *action oriented*. It can be used as a guide for the initial collection of information, as a device for organising available data, or as a design for treatment.

The formulation of a treatment plan follows from this type of analysis because knowledge of the reinforcing conditions suggests the motivational controls at the disposal of the clinician for the modification of the patient's behavior. The analysis of specific problem behaviors also provides a series of goals for psychotherapy or other treatment, and for the evaluation of treatment progress. Knowledge of the patient's biological, social, and cultural conditions should help to determine what resources can be used, and what limitations must be considered in a treatment plan.

The various categories attempt to call attention to important variables affecting the patient's *current* behavior. Therefore, they aim to elicit descriptions of low-level abstraction. Answers to these specific questions are best phrased by describing classes of events reported by the patient, observed by others, or by critical incidents described by an informant. The analysis does not exclude description of the patient's habitual verbal-symbolic behaviors. However, in using verbal behaviors as the basis for this analysis, one should be catious not to "explain" verbal processes in terms of postulated internal mechanisms without adequate supportive evidence, nor should inference be made about nonobserved processes or events without corroborative evidence. The analysis includes many items which are not known or not applicable for a given patient. Lack of information on some items does not necessarily indicate incompleteness of the analysis. These lacks must be noted nevertheless because they often contribute to the better understanding of what the patient needs to learn to become an autonomous person. Just as important is an inventory of his existing socially effective behavioral repertoire which can be put in the service of any treatment procedure.

This analysis is consistent with our earlier formulations of the principles of comprehensive medicine (9, 22) which emphasized the joint operation of biological, social and psychological factors in psychiatric disorders. The language and orientation of the proposed approach are rooted in contemporary learning theory. The conceptual framework is consonant with the view that the course of psychiatric disorders can be modified by systematic application of scientific principles from the fields of psychology and medicine to the patient's habitual mode of living.

This approach is not a substitute for assignment of the patient to traditional diagnostic categories. Such labeling may be desirable for statistical, administrative, or research purposes. But the current analysis is intended to replace other diagnostic formulations purporting to serve as a basis for making decisions about specific therapeutic interventions.

III. Methods of Data Collection for a Functional Analysis

Traditional diagnostic approaches have utilized as the main sources of information the patient's verbal report, his nonverbal behavior during an interview, and his performance on psychological tests. These observations are sufficient if one regards behavior problems only as a property of the patient's particular pattern of associations or his personality structure. A mental disorder would be expected to reveal itself by stylistic characteristics in the patient's behavior repertoire. However, if one views behavior disorders as sets of response patterns which are learned under particular conditions and maintained by definable environmental and internal stimuli, an assessment of the patient's behavior output is insufficient unless it also describes the conditions under which it occurs. This view requires an expansion of the clinician's sources of observations to include the stimulation fields in which the patient lives, and the variations of patient behavior as a function of exposure to these various stimulational variables. Therefore, the resourceful clinician need not limit himself to test findings, interview observations in the clinician's office, or referral histories alone in the formulation of the specific case. Nor need he regard himself as hopelessly handicapped when the patient has little observational or communicative skill in verbally reconstructing his life experiences for the clinician. Regardless of the patient's communicative skills the data must consist of a description of the patient's behavior *in relationship* to varying environmental conditions.

A behavioral analysis excludes no data relating to a patient's past or present experiences as irrelevant. However, the relative merit of any information (as, e.g., growing up in a broken home or having had homosexual experiences) lies in its relation to the independent variables which can be identified as controlling the current problematic behavior. The observation that a patient has hallucinated on occasions may be important only if it has bearing on his present problem. If looked upon in isolation, a report about hallucinations may be misleading, resulting in emphasis on classification rather than treatment.

In the *psychiatric interview* a behavioral-analytic approach opposes acceptance of the content of the verbal self-report as equivalent to actual events or experiences. However, verbal reports provide information concerning the patient's verbal construction of his environment and of his person, his recall of past experiences, and his fantasies about them. While these self-descriptions do not represent data about events which actually occur internally, they do represent current behaviors of the patient and indicate the verbal chains and repertoires which the patient has built up. Therefore, the verbal behavior may be useful for description of a patient's thinking processes. To make the most of such an approach, variations on traditional interview procedures may be obtained by such techniques as role playing, discussion, and interpretation of current life events, or controlled free association. Since there is little experimental evidence of specific relationships between the patient's verbal statements and his nonverbal behavioral acts, the verbal report alone remains insufficient for a complete analysis and for prediction of his daily behavior. Further, it is well known that a person responds to environmental conditions and to internal cues which he cannot describe adequately. Therefore, any verbal report may miss or mask the most important aspects of a behavioral analysis, i.e., the description of the relationship between antecedent conditions and subsequent behavior.

In addition to the use of the clinician's own person as a controlled stimulus object in interview situations, *observations of interaction with significant others* can be used for the analysis of variations in frequency of various behaviors as a function of the person with whom the patient interacts. For example, use of prescribed standard roles for nurses and attendants, utilization of members of the patient's family or his friends, may be made to obtain data relevant to the patient's habitual interpersonal response pattern. Such observations are especially useful if in a later interview the patient is asked to describe and discuss the observed sessions. Confrontations with tape recordings for comparisons between the patient's report and the actual session as witnessed by the observer may provide information about the patient's perception of himself and others as well as his habitual behavior toward peers, authority figures, and other significant people in his life.

Except in working with children or family units, insufficient use has been made of material obtained from *other informants* in interviews about the patient. These reports can aid the observer to recognize behavioral domains in which the patient's report deviates from or agrees with the descriptions provided by others. Such information is also useful for contrasting the patient's reports about his presumptive effects on another person with the stated effects by that person. If a patient's interpersonal problems extend to areas in which social contacts are not clearly defined, contributions by informants other than the patient are essential.

It must be noted that verbal reports by other informants may be no more congruent with actual events than the patient's own reports and need to be equally related to the informant's own credibility. If such crucial figures as parents, spouses, employers can be so interviewed, they also provide the clinician with some information about those people with whom the patient must interact repeatedly and with whom interpersonal problems may have developed.

Some observation of the patient's daily *work behavior* represents an excellent source of information, if it can be made available. Observation of the patient by the clinician or his staff may be preferable to descriptions by peers or supervisors. Work observations are especially important for patients whose complaints include difficulties in their daily work activity or who describe work situations as contributing factors to their problem. While freer use of this technique may be hampered by cultural attitudes toward psychiatric treatment in the marginally adjusted, such observations may be freely accessible in hospital situations or in sheltered work situations. With use of behavior rating scales or other simple measurement devices, brief samples of patient behaviors in work situations can be obtained by minimally trained observers.

The patient himself may be asked to provide samples of his own behavior by using tape recorders for the recording of segments of interactions in his family, at work, or in other situations during his everyday life. A television monitoring system for the patient's behavior is an excellent technique from a theoretical viewpoint but it is extremely cumbersome and expensive. Use of recordings for diagnostic and therapeutic purposes has been reported by some investigators (2, 5, 24). Playback of the recordings and a recording of the patient's reactions to the playback can be used further in interviews to clarify the patient's behavior toward others and his reaction to himself as a social stimulus.

Psychological tests represent problems to be solved under specified interactional conditions. Between the highly standardized intelligence tests and the unstructured and ambiguous projective tests lies a dimension of structure along which more and more responsibility for providing appropriate responses falls on the patient. By comparison with interview procedures, most psychological tests provide a relatively greater standardization of stimulus conditions. But, in addition to the specific answers given on intelligence tests or on projective tests these tests also provide a behavioral sample of the patient's reaction to a problem situation in a relatively stressful interpersonal setting. Therefore, psychological tests can provide not only quantitative scores but they can also be treated as a miniature life experience, yielding information about the patient's interpersonal behavior and variations in his behavior as a function of the nature of the stimulus conditions.

In this section we have mentioned only some of the numerous life situations which can be evaluated in order to provide information about the patient. Criteria for their use lies in economy, accessibility to the clinician, and relevance to the patient's problem. While it is more convenient to gather data from a patient in an office, it may be necessary for the clinician to have first-hand information about the actual conditions under which the patient lives and works. Such familiarity may be obtained either by utilization of informants or by the clinician's entry into the home, the job situation, or the social environment in which the patient lives. Under all these conditions the clinician is effective only if it is possible for him to maintain a nonparticipating, objective, and observational role with no untoward consequences for the patient or the treatment relationship.

The methods of data collecting for a functional analysis described here differ from traditional psychiatric approaches only in that they require inclusion of the physical and social stimulus field in which the patient actually operates. Only a full appraisal of the patient's living and working conditions and his way of life allow a description of the actual problems which the patient faces and the specification of steps to be taken for altering the problematic situation.

Summary

Current psychiatric classification falls short of providing a satisfactory basis for the understanding and treatment of maladaptive behavior. Diagnostic schemas now in use are based on etiology, symptom description, or prognosis. While each of these approaches has a limited utility, no unified schema is available which permits prediction of response to treatment or future course of the disorder from the assignment of the patient to a specific category.

This paper suggests a behavior-analytic approach which is based on contemporary learning theory, as an alternative to assignment of the patient to a conventional diagnostic category. It includes the summary of an outline which can serve as a guide for the collection of information and formulation of the problem, including the biological, social, and behavioral conditions which are determining the patient's behavior. The outline aims toward integration of information about a patient for formulation of an action plan which would modify the patient's problematic behavior. Emphasis is given to the particular variables affecting the *individual* patient rather than determination of the similarity of the patient's history or his symptoms to known pathological groups.

The last section of the paper deals with methods useful for collection of information necessary to complete such a behavioral analysis.

This paper was written in conjunction with Research grant MH 06921-03 from the National Institutes of Mental Health, United States Public Health Service.

References

1. Ash, P. (1949). Reliability of psychiatric diagnosis. *J. Abnorm. Soc. Psychol.*, **44**, 272–277.
2. Bach, G. (1963). In Alexander S. (ed.), Fight promoter for battle of sexes. *Life*, **54**, 102–108 (May 17).
3. Bandura, A. (1961). Psychotherapy as learning process. *Psychol. Bull.*, **58**, 143–159.
4. Barron, F. (1953). Ego-strength scale which predicts response to psychotherapy. *J. Consult. Psychol.*, **17**, 235–241.
5. Cameron, D. E., et al. (1964). Automation of psychotherapy. *Compr. Psychiat.*, **5**, 1–14.
6. Ferster, C. B. (1965). Classification of behavioral pathology. In Ullmann, L. P., and Krasner, L. (eds.), *Behavior Modification Research.* New York: Holt, Rinehart & Winston.
7. Freedman, D. A. (1958). Various etiologies of schizophrenic syndrome. *Dis. Nerv. Syst.*, **19**, 1–6.
8. Fulkerson, S. E., & Barry, J. R. (1961). Methodology and research on prognostic use of psychological tests. *Psychol. Bull.*, **58**, 177–204.
9. Guze, S. B., Matarazzo, J. D., & Saslow, G. (1953). Formulation of principles of comprehensive medicine with special reference to learning theory. *J. Clin. Psychol.*, **9**, 127–136.
10. Jackson, D. D. A. (1960). *Etiology of Schizophrenia.* New York: Basic Books, Inc.
11. Kanfer, F. H. (1961). Comments on learning in psychotherapy. *Psychol. Rep.*, **9**, 681–699.
12. Katz, M. M., Cole, J. O., & Lowery, H. A. (1964). Non-specificity of diagnosis of paranoid schizophrenia. *Arch. Gen. Psychiat.*, **11**, 197–202.
13. Krasner, L. (1962). Therapist as social reinforcement machine. In Strupp, H., and Luborsky, L. (eds.), *Research in Psychotherapy.* Washington, D.C.: American Psychological Association.
14. Ledley, R. S., & Lusted, L. B. (1959). Reasoning foundations of medical diagnosis. *Science*, **130**, 9–21.
15. Lorr, M., Klett, C. J., & McNair, D. M. (1963). *Syndromes of Psychosis.* New York: Macmillan.
16. Meehl, P. E. (1962). Schizotaxia, schizotypy, schizophrenia. *Amer. Psychol.*, **17**, 827–838.
17. New York Heart Association. (1953). *Nomenclature and criteria for diagnosis of disease of the heart and blood vessels.* New York: New York Heart Association.
18. Noyes, A. P., & Kolb, L. C. (1963). *Modern Clinical Psychiatry.* Philadelphia: W. B. Saunders & Co.

19. OPLER, M. K. (1957). Schizophrenia and culture. *Sci. Amer.*, **197**, 103–112.

20. OPLER, M. K. (1963). Need for new diagnostic categories in psychiatry. *J. Nat. Med. Assoc.*, **55**, 133–137.

21. ROTTER, J. B. (1954). *Social Learning and Clinical Psychology*. New York: Prentice-Hall.

22. SASLOW, G. (1952). On concept of comprehensive medicine. *Bull. Menninger Clin.*, **16**, 57–65.

23. SCHEFLEN, A. E. (1958). Analysis of thought model which persists in psychiatry. *Psychosom. Med.*, **20**, 235–241.

24. SLACK, C. W. (1960). Experimenter-subject psychotherapy—A new method of introducing intensive office treatment for unreachable cases. *Ment. Hyg.*, **44**, 238–256.

25. SZASZ, T. S. (1960). Myth of mental illness. *Amer. Psychol.*, **15**, 113–118.

26. WINDLE, C. (1952). Psychological tests in psychopathological prognosis. *Psychol. Bull.*, **49**, 451–482.

27. WOLPE, J. (1958). *Psychotherapy in Reciprocal Inhibition.* Stanford, Calif.: Stanford University Press.

28. ZIGLER, E., & PHILLIPS, L. (1961). Psychiatric diagnosis: Critique. *J. Abnor. Soc. Psychol.*, **63**, 607–618.

D. L. ROSENHAN

On Being Sane in Insane Places

In the article that follows Dr. Rosenhan provides a fascinating summary of the observations of a group of people (mostly professionals) who feigned psychotic symptoms to gain admission to several mental hospitals. The experiences of this group point up many of the problems and dangers of a diagnostic scheme in which a label carries with it a train of adverse consequences for the person to whom it is applied. The article also illustrates many of the worst features of the average mental institution.

If sanity and insanity exist, how shall we know them?

The question is neither capricious nor itself insane. However much we may be personally convinced that we can tell the normal from the abnormal, the evidence is simply not compelling. It is commonplace, for example, to read about murder trials wherein eminent psychiatrists for the defense are contradicted by equally eminent psychiatrists for the prosecution on the matter of the defendant's sanity. More generally, there are a great deal of conflicting data on the reliability, utility, and meaning of such terms as "sanity,"

Reprinted from *Science*, **179** (1973), 250–258 with the permission of the American Association for the Advancement of Science and Dr. Rosenhan.

"insanity," "mental illness," and "schizophrenia" (1). Finally, as early as 1934, Benedict suggested that normality and abnormality are not universal (2). What is viewed as normal in one culture may be seen as quite aberrant in another. Thus, notions of normality and abnormality may not be quite as accurate as people believe they are.

To raise questions regarding normality and abnormality is in no way to question the fact that some behaviors are deviant or odd. Murder is deviant. So, too, are hallucinations. Nor does raising such questions deny the existence of the personal anguish that is often associated with "mental illness." Anxiety and depression exist. Psychological suffering exists. But normality and abnormality, sanity and insanity, and the diagnoses that flow from them may be less substantive than many believe them to be.

At its heart, the question of whether the sane can be distinguished from the insane (and whether degrees of insanity can be distinguished from each other) is a simple matter: do the salient characteristics that lead to diagnoses reside in the patients themselves or in the environments and contexts in which observers find them? From Bleuler, through Kretchmer, through the formulators of the recently revised *Diagnostic and Statistical Manual* of the American Psychiatric Association, the belief has been strong that patients present symptoms, that those symptoms can be categorized, and, implicitly, that the sane are distinguishable from the insane. More recently, however, this belief has been questioned. Based in part on theoretical and anthropological considerations, but also on philosophical, legal, and therapeutic ones, the view has grown that psychological categorization of mental illness is useless at best and downright harmful, misleading, and pejorative at worst. Psychiatric diagnoses, in this view, are in the minds of the observers and are not valid summaries of characteristics displayed by the observed (3–5).

Gains can be made in deciding which of these is more nearly accurate by getting normal people (that is, people who do not have, and have never suffered, symptoms of serious psychiatric disorders) admitted to psychiatric hospitals and then determining whether they were discovered to be sane and, if so, how. If the sanity of such pseudo-patients were always detected, there would be prima facie evidence that a sane individual can be distinguished from the insane context in which he is found. Normality (and presumably abnormality) is distinct enough that it can be recognized wherever it occurs, for it is carried within the person. If, on the other hand, the sanity of the pseudopatients were never discovered, serious difficulties would arise for those who support traditional modes of psychiatric diagnosis. Given that the hospital staff was not incompetent, that the pseudopatient had been behaving as sanely as he had been outside of the hospital, and that it had never been previously suggested that he belonged in a psychiatric hospital, such an unlikely outcome would support the view that psychiatric diagnosis betrays little about the patient but much about the environment in which an observer finds him.

This article describes such an experiment. Eight sane people gained secret admission to 12 different hospitals (6). Their diagnostic experiences constitute the data of the first part of this article; the remainder is devoted to a description of their experiences in psychiatric institutions. Too few psychiatrists and psychologists, even those who have worked in such hospitals, know what the experience is like. They rarely talk about it with former patients, perhaps because they distrust information coming from the previously insane. Those who have worked in psychiatric hospitals are likely to have adapted so thoroughly to the settings that they are insensitive to the impact of that experience. And while there have been occasional reports of researchers who submitted themselves to psychiatric hospitalization (7), these researchers have commonly remained in the hospitals for short periods of time, often with the knowledge of the hospital staff. It is difficult to know the extent to which they were treated like patients or like research colleagues. Nevertheless, their reports about the inside of the psychiatric hospital have been valuable. This article extends those efforts.

Pseudopatients and Their Settings

The eight pseudopatients were a varied group. One was a psychology graduate student in his 20's. The remaining seven were older and "established." Among them were three psychologists, a pediatrician, a psychiatrist, a painter, and a housewife. Three pseudopatients were women, five were men. All of them employed pseudonyms, lest their alleged diagnoses embarrass them later. Those who were in mental health professions alleged another occupation in order to avoid the special attentions that might be accorded by staff, as a matter of courtesy or caution, to ailing colleagues (8). With the exception of myself (I was the first pseudopatient and my presence was known to the hospital administrator and chief psychologist and, so far as I can tell, to them alone), the presence of pseudopatients and the nature of the research program was not known to the hospital staffs (9).

The settings were similarly varied. In order to generalize the findings, admission into a variety of hospitals was sought. The 12 hospitals in the sample were located in five different states on the East and West coasts. Some were old and shabby, some were quite new. Some were research-oriented, others not. Some had good staff-patient ratios, others were quite understaffed. Only one was a strictly private hospital. All of the others were supported by state or federal funds or, in one instance, by university funds.

After calling the hospital for an appointment, the pseudopatient arrived at the admissions office complaining that he had been hearing voices. Asked what the voices said, he replied that they were often unclear, but as far as he could tell they said "empty," "hollow," and "thud." The voices were unfamiliar and were of the same sex as the pseudopatient. The choice of these symptoms was occasioned by their apparent similarity to existential symptoms. Such symptoms are alleged to arise from painful concerns about the perceived meaninglessness of one's life. It is as if the hallucinating person were saying,

"My life is empty and hollow." The choice of these symptoms was also determined by the *absence* of a single report of existential psychoses in the literature.

Beyond alleging the symptoms and falsifying name, vocation, and employment, no further alterations of person, history, or circumstances were made. The significant events of the pseudopatient's life history were presented as they had actually occurred. Relationships with parents and siblings, with spouse and children, with people at work and in school, consistent with the aforementioned exceptions, were described as they were or had been. Frustrations and upsets were described along with joys and satisfactions. These facts are important to remember. If anything, they strongly biased the subsequent results in favor of detecting sanity, since none of their histories or current behaviors were seriously pathological in any way.

Immediately upon admission to the psychiatric ward, the pseudopatient ceased simulating *any* symptoms of abnormality. In some cases, there was a brief period of mild nervousness and anxiety, since none of the pseudopatients really believed that they would be admitted so easily. Indeed, their shared fear was that they would be immediately exposed as frauds and greatly embarrassed. Moreover, many of them had never visited a psychiatric ward; even those who had, nevertheless had some genuine fears about what might happen to them. Their nervousness, then, was quite appropriate to the novelty of the hospital setting, and it abated rapidly.

Apart from that short-lived nervousness, the pseudopatient behaved on the ward as he "normally" behaved. The pseudopatient spoke to patients and staff as he might ordinarily. Because there is uncommonly little to do on a psychiatric ward, he attempted to engage others in conversation. When asked by staff how he was feeling, he indicated that he was fine, that he no longer experienced symptoms. He responded to instructions from attendants, to calls for medication (which was not swallowed), and to dining-hall instructions. Beyond such activities as were available to him on the admissions ward, he spent his time writing down his observations about the ward, its patients, and the staff. Initially these notes were written "secretly," but as it soon became clear that no one much cared, they were subsequently written on standard tablets of paper in such public places as the dayroom. No secret was made of these activities.

The pseudopatient, very much as a true psychiatric patient, entered a hospital with no foreknowledge of when he would be discharged. Each was told that he would have to get out by his own devices, essentially by convincing the staff that he was sane. The psychological stresses associated with hospitalization were considerable, and all but one of the pseudopatients desired to be discharged almost immediately after being admitted. They were, therefore, motivated not only to behave sanely, but to be paragons of cooperation. That their behavior was in no way disruptive is confirmed by nursing reports, which have been obtained on most of the patients. These reports uniformly indicate that the patients were "friendly," "cooperative," and "exhibited no abnormal indications."

The Normal Are Not Detectably Sane

Despite their public "show" of sanity, the pseudopatients were never detected. Admitted, except in one case, with a diagnosis of schizophrenia (10), each was discharged with a diagnosis of schizophrenia "in remission." The label "in remission" should in no way be dismissed as a formality, for at no time during any hospitalization had any question been raised about any pseudopatient's simulation. Nor are there any indications in the hospital records that the pseudopatient's status was suspect. Rather, the evidence is strong that, once labeled schizophrenic, the pseudopatient was stuck with that label. If the pseudopatient was to be discharged, he must naturally be "in remission"; but he was not sane, nor, in the institution's view, had he ever been sane.

The uniform failure to recognize sanity cannot be attributed to the quality of the hospitals, for, although there were considerable variations among them, several are considered excellent. Nor can it be alleged that there was simply not enough time to observe the pseudopatients. Length of hospitalization ranged from 7 to 52 days, with an average of 19 days. The pseudopatients were not, in fact, carefully observed, but this failure clearly speaks more to traditions within psychiatric hospitals than to lack of opportunity.

Finally, it cannot be said that the failure to recognize the pseudopatients' sanity was due to the fact that they were not behaving sanely. While there was clearly some tension present in all of them, their daily visitors could detect no serious behavioral consequences—nor, indeed, could other patients. It was quite common for the patients to "detect" the pseudopatients' sanity. During the first three hospitalizations, when accurate counts were kept, 35 of a total of 118 patients on the admissions ward voiced their suspicions, some vigorously. "You're not crazy. You're a journalist, or a professor [referring to the continual note-taking]. You're checking up on the hospital." While most of the patients were reassured by the pseudopatient's insistence that he had been sick before he came in but was fine now, some continued to believe that the pseudopatient was sane throughout his hospitalization (11). The fact that the patients often recognized normality when staff did not raises important questions.

Failure to detect sanity during the course of hospitalization may be due to the fact that physicians operate with a strong bias toward what statisticians call the type 2 error (5). This is to say that physicians are more inclined to call a healthy person sick (a false positive, type 2) than a sick person healthy (a false negative, type 1). The reasons for this are not hard to find: it is clearly more dangerous to misdiagnose illness than health. Better to err on the side of caution, to suspect illness even among the healthy.

But what holds for medicine does not hold equally well for psychiatry. Medical illnesses, while unfortunate, are not commonly pejorative. Psychiatric diagnoses, on the contrary, carry with them personal, legal, and social stigmas (12). It was therefore important to see whether the tendency toward diagnosing the sane insane could be reversed. The following experiment was arranged at a research and teaching hospital whose staff had heard these findings but doubted that such an error could occur in their hospital. The staff was informed that at some time during the following 3 months, one or more pseudopatients would attempt to be admitted into the psychiatric hospital. Each staff member was asked to rate each patient who presented himself at admissions or on the ward according to the likelihood that the patient was a pseudopatient. A 10-point scale was used, with a 1 and 2 reflecting high confidence that the patient was a pseudopatient.

Judgments were obtained on 193 patients who were admitted for psychiatric treatment. All staff who had had sustained contact with or primary responsibility for the patient—attendants, nurses, psychiatrists, physicians, and psychologists—were asked to make judgments. Forty-one patients were alleged, with high confidence, to be pseudopatients by at least one member of the staff. Twenty-three were considered suspect by at least one psychiatrist. Nineteen were suspected by one psychiatrist *and* one other staff member. Actually, no genuine pseudopatient (at least from my group) presented himself during this period.

The experiment is instructive. It indicates that the tendency to designate sane people as insane can be reversed when the stakes (in this case, prestige and diagnostic acumen) are high. But what can be said of the 19 people who were suspected of being "sane" by one psychiatrist and another staff member? Were these people truly "sane," or was it rather the case that in the course of avoiding the type 2 error the staff tended to make more errors of the first sort—calling the crazy "sane"? There is no way of knowing. But one thing is certain: any diagnostic process that lends itself so readily to massive errors of this sort cannot be a very reliable one.

The Stickiness of Psychodiagnostic Labels

Beyond the tendency to call the healthy sick—a tendency that accounts better for diagnostic behavior on admission than it does for such behavior after a lengthy period of exposure—the data speak to the massive role of labeling in psychiatric assessment. Having once been labeled schizophrenic, there is nothing the pseudopatient can do to overcome the tag. The tag profoundly colors others' perceptions of him and his behavior.

From one viewpoint, these data are hardly surprising, for it has long been known that elements are given meaning by the context in which they occur. Gestalt psychology made this point vigorously, and Asch (13) demonstrated that there are "central" personality traits (such as "warm" versus "cold") which are so powerful that they markedly color the meaning of other information in forming an impression of a given personality (14). "Insane," "schizophrenic," "manic-depressive," and "crazy" are probably among the most powerful of such central traits. Once a person is designated abnormal, all of his other behaviors and characteristics are colored by that label. Indeed, that label is so powerful that many of the pseudopatients' normal behaviors were overlooked entirely or profoundly misinterpreted. Some examples may clarify this issue.

Earlier I indicated that there were no changes in the pseudopatient's personal history and current status beyond those of name, employment, and, where necessary, vocation. Otherwise, a veridical description of personal history and circumstances was offered. Those circumstances were not psychotic. How were they made consonant with the diagnosis of psychosis? Or were those diagnoses modified in such a way as to bring them into accord with the circumstances of the pseudopatient's life, as described by him?

As far as I can determine, diagnoses were in no way affected by the relative health of the circumstances of a pseudopatient's life. Rather, the reverse occurred: the perception of his circumstances was shaped entirely by the diagnosis. A clear example of such translation is found in the case of a pseudopatient who had had a close relationship with his mother but was rather remote from his father during his early childhood. During adolescence and beyond, however, his father became a close friend, while his relationship with his mother cooled. His present relationship with his wife was characteristically close and warm. Apart from occasional angry exchanges, friction was minimal. The children had rarely been spanked. Surely there is nothing especially pathological about such a history. Indeed, many readers may see a similar pattern in their own experiences, with no markedly deleterious consequences. Observe, however, how such a history was translated in the psychopathological context, this from the case summary prepared after the patient was discharged.

> This white 39-year-old male . . . manifests a long history of considerable ambivalence in close relationships, which begins in early childhood. A warm relationship with his mother cools during his adolescence. A distant relationship to his father is described as becoming very intense. Affective stability is absent. His attempts to control emotionality with his wife and children are punctuated by angry outbursts and, in the case of the children, spankings. And while he says that he has several good friends, one senses considerable ambivalence embedded in those relationships also. . . .

The facts of the case were unintentionally distorted by the staff to achieve consistency with a popular theory of the dynamics of a schizophrenic reaction (15). Nothing of an ambivalent nature had been described in relations with parents, spouse, or friends. To the extent that ambivalence could be inferred, it was probably not greater than is found in all human relationships. It is true the pseudopatient's relationships with his parents changed over time, but in the ordinary context that would hardly be remarkable—indeed, it might very well be expected. Clearly, the meaning ascribed to his verbalizations (that is, ambivalence, affective instability) was determined by the diagnosis: schizophrenia. An entirely different meaning would have been ascribed if it were known that the man was "normal."

All pseudopatients took extensive notes publicly. Under ordinary circumstances, such behavior would have raised questions in the minds of observers, as, in fact, it did among patients. Indeed, it seemed so certain that the notes would elicit suspicion that elaborate precautions were taken to remove them from the ward each day. But the precautions proved needless. The closest any staff member came to questioning these notes occurred when one pseudopatient asked his physician what kind of medication he was receiving and began to write down the response. "You needn't write it," he was told gently. "If you havc trouble remembering, just ask me again."

If no questions were asked of the pseudopatients, how was their writing interpreted? Nursing records for three patients indicate that the writing was seen as an aspect of their pathological behavior. "Patient engages in writing behavior" was the daily nursing comment on one of the pseudopatients who was never questioned about his writing. Given that the patient is in the hospital, he must be psychologically disturbed. And given that he is disturbed, continuous writing must be a behavioral manifestation of that disturbance, perhaps a subset of the compulsive behaviors that are sometimes correlated with schizophrenia.

One tacit characteristic of psychiatric diagnosis is that it locates the sources of aberration within the individual and only rarely within the complex of stimuli that surrounds him. Consequently, behaviors that are stimulated by the environment are commonly misattributed to the patient's disorder. For example, one kindly nurse found a pseudopatient pacing the long hospital corridors. "Nervous, Mr. X?" she asked. "No, bored," he said.

The notes kept by pseudopatients are full of patient behaviors that were misinterpreted by well-intentioned staff. Often enough, a patient would go "berserk" because he had, wittingly or unwittingly, been mistreated by, say, an attendant. A nurse coming upon the scene would rarely inquire even cursorily into the environmental stimuli of the patient's behavior. Rather, she assumed that his upset derived from his pathology, not from his present interactions with other staff members. Occasionally, the staff might assume that the patient's family (especially when they had recently visited) or other patients had stimulated the outburst. But never were the staff found to assume that one of themselves or the structure of the hospital had anything to do with a patient's behavior. One psychiatrist pointed to a group of patients who were sitting outside the cafeteria entrance half an hour before lunchtime. To a group of young residents he indicated that such behavior was characteristic of the oral-acquisitive nature of the syndrome. It seemed not to occur to him that there were very few things to anticipate in a psychiatric hospital besides eating.

A psychiatric label has a life and an influence of its own. Once the impression has been formed that the patient is schizophrenic, the expectation is that he will continue to be schizophrenic. When a sufficient amount of time has passed, during which the patient has done nothing bizarre, he is considered to be in remission and available for discharge. But the label endures beyond discharge, with the unconfirmed expectation that he will behave as a schizophrenic again. Such labels, conferred by mental health professionals, are as influential on the patient as they are on his relatives and friends, and it should not surprise anyone that the diagnosis acts on all of them as a self-fulfilling prophecy. Eventually, the patient himself accepts the diagnosis, with all of its surplus meanings and expectations, and behaves accordingly (5).

The inferences to be made from these matters are quite simple. Much as Zigler and Phillips have demonstrated that there is enormous overlap in the symptoms presented by patients who have been variously diagnosed (16), so there is enormous overlap in the behaviors of the sane and the insane. The sane are not "sane" all of the time. We lose our tempers "for no good reason." We are occasionally depressed or anxious, again for no good reason. And we may find it difficult to get along with one or another person—again for no reason that we can specify. Similarly, the insane are not always insane. Indeed, it was the impression of the pseudopatients while living with them that they were sane for long periods of time—that the bizarre behaviors upon which their diagnoses were allegedly predicated constituted only a small fraction of their total behavior. If it makes no sense to label ourselves permanently depressed on the basis of an occasional depression, then it takes better evidence than is presently available to label all patients insane or schizophrenic on the basis of bizarre behaviors or cognitions. It seems more useful, as Mischel (17) has pointed out, to limit our discussions to *behaviors*, the stimuli that provoke them, and their correlates.

It is not known why powerful impressions of personality traits, such as "crazy" or "insane," arise. Conceivably, when the origins of and stimuli that give rise to a behavior are remote or unknown, or when the behavior strikes us as immutable, trait labels regarding the *behaver* arise. When, on the other hand, the origins and stimuli are known and available, discourse is limited to the behavior itself. Thus, I may hallucinate because I am sleeping, or I may hallucinate because I have ingested a peculiar drug. These are termed sleep-induced hallucinations, or dreams, and drug-induced hallucinations, respectively. But when the stimuli to my hallucinations are unknown, that is called craziness, or schizophrenia—as if that inference were somehow as illuminating as the others.

The Experience of Psychiatric Hospitalization

The term "mental illness" is of recent origin. It was coined by people who were humane in their inclinations and who wanted very much to raise the station of (and the public's sympathies toward) the psychologically disturbed from that of witches and "crazies" to one that was akin to the physically ill. And they were at least partially successful, for the treatment of the mentally ill *has* improved considerably over the years. But while treatment has improved, it is doubtful that people really regard the mentally ill in the same way that they view the physically ill. A broken leg is something one recovers from, but mental illness allegedly endures forever (18). A broken leg does not threaten the observer, but a crazy schizophrenic? There is by now a host of evidence that attitudes toward the mentally ill are characterized by fear, hostility, aloofness, suspicion, and dread (19). The mentally ill are society's lepers.

That such attitudes infect the general population is perhaps not surprising, only upsetting. But that they affect the professionals—attendants, nurses, physicians, psychologists, and social workers—who treat and deal with the mentally ill is more disconcerting, both because such attitudes are self-evidently pernicious and because they are unwitting. Most mental health professionals would insist that they are sympathetic toward the mentally ill, that they are neither avoidant nor hostile. But it is more likely that an exquisite ambivalence characterizes their relations with psychiatric patients, such that their avowed impulses are only part of their entire attitude. Negative attitudes are there too and can easily be detected. Such attitudes should not surprise us. They are the natural offspring of the labels patients wear and the places in which they are found.

Consider the structure of the typical psychiatric hospital. Staff and patients are strictly segregated. Staff have their own living space, including their dining facilities, bathrooms, and assembly places. The glassed quarters that contain the professional staff, which the pseudopatients came to call "the cage," sit out on every dayroom. The staff emerge primarily for caretaking purposes—to give medication, to conduct a therapy or group meeting, to instruct or reprimand a patient. Otherwise, staff keep to themselves, almost as if the disorder that afflicts their charges is somehow catching.

So much is patient-staff segregation the rule that, for four public hospitals in which an attempt was made to measure the degree to which staff and patients mingle, it was necessary to use "time out of the staff cage" as the operational measure. While it was not the case that all time spent out of the cage was spent mingling with patients (attendants, for example, would occasionally emerge to watch television in the dayroom), it was the only way in which one could gather reliable data on time for measuring.

The average amount of time spent by attendants outside of the cage was 11.3 percent (range, 3 to 52 percent). This figure does not represent only time spent mingling with patients, but also includes time spent on such chores as folding laundry, supervising patients while they shave, directing ward clean-up, and sending patients to off-ward activities. It was the relatively rare attendant who spent time talking with patients or playing games with them. It proved impossible to obtain a "percent mingling time" for nurses, since the amount of time they spent out of the cage was too brief. Rather, we counted instances of emergence from the cage. On the average, daytime nurses emerged from the cage 11.5 times per shift, including instances when they left the ward entirely (range, 4 to 39 times). Late afternoon and night nurses were even less available, emerging on the average 9.4 times per shift (range, 4 to 41 times). Data on early morning nurses, who arrived usually after midnight and departed at 8 a.m., are not available because patients were asleep during most of this period.

Physicians, especially psychiatrists, were even less available. They were rarely seen on the wards. Quite commonly, they would be seen only when they arrived and departed, with the remaining time being spent in their offices or in the cage. On the average, physicians emerged on the ward 6.7 times per day (range, 1 to 17 times). It proved difficult to make an accurate estimate in this regard, since physicians often maintained hours that allowed them to come and go at different times.

The hierarchical organization of the psychiatric hospital has been commented on before (20), but the latent meaning of that kind of organization is worth noting again. Those with the most power have least to do with patients, and those with the least power are most involved with them. Recall, however, that the acquisition of role-appropriate behaviors occurs mainly through the observation of others, with the most powerful having the most influence. Consequently, it is understandable that attendants not only spend more time with patients than do any other members of the staff—that is required by their station in the hierarchy—but also, insofar as they learn from their superiors' behavior, spend as little time with patients as they can. Attendants are seen mainly in the cage, which is where the models, the action, and the power are.

I turn now to a different set of studies, these dealing with staff response to patient-initiated contact. It has long been known that the amount of time a person spends with you can be an index of your significance to him. If he initiates and maintains eye contact, there is reason to believe that he is considering your requests and needs. If he pauses to chat or actually stops and talks, there is added reason to infer that he is individuating you. In four hospitals, the pseudopatient approached the staff member with a request which took the following form: "Pardon me, Mr. [or Dr. or Mrs.] X, could you tell me when I will be eligible for grounds privileges?" (or ". . . when I will be presented at the staff meeting?" or ". . . when I am likely to be discharged?"). While the content of the question varied according to the appropriateness of the target and the pseudopatient's (apparent) current needs the form was always a courteous and relevant request for information. Care was taken never to approach a particular member of the staff more than once a day, lest the staff member become suspicious or irritated. In examining these data, remember that the behavior of the pseudopatients was neither bizarre nor disruptive. One could indeed engage in good conversation with them.

The data for these experiments are shown in Table 1, separately for physicians (column 1) and for nurses and attendants (column 2). Minor differences between these four institutions were overwhelmed by the degree to which staff avoided continuing contacts that patients had initiated. By far, their most common response consisted of either a brief response to the question, offered while they were "on the move" and with head averted, or no response at all.

The encounter frequently took the following bizarre form: (pseudopatient)

TABLE 1 *Self-initiated contact by pseudopatients with psychiatrists and nurses and attendants, compared to contact with other groups*

Contact	Psychiatric hospitals		University campus (nonmedical)	University medical center Physicians		
	(1) Psychiatrists	(2) Nurses and attendants	(3) Faculty	(4) "Looking for a psychiatrist"	(5) "Looking for an internist"	(6) No additional comment
Responses						
Moves on, head averted (%)	71	88	0	0	0	0
Makes eye contact (%)	23	10	0	11	0	0
Pauses and chats (%)	2	2	0	11	0	10
Stops and talks (%)	4	0.5	100	78	100	90
Mean number of questions answered (out of 6)	*	*	6	3.8	4.8	4.5
Respondents (No.)	13	47	14	18	15	10
Attempts (No.)	185	1283	14	18	15	10

* Not applicable.

"Pardon me, Dr. X. Could you tell me when I am eligible for grounds privileges?" (physician) "Good morning, Dave. How are you today?" (Moves off without waiting for a response.)

It is instructive to compare these data with data recently obtained at Stanford University. It has been alleged that large and eminent universities are characterized by faculty who are so busy that they have not time for students. For this comparison, a young lady approached individual faculty members who seemed to be walking purposefully to some meeting or teaching engagement and asked them the following six questions.

1. "Pardon me, could you direct me to Encina Hall?" (at the medical school: ". . . to the Clinical Research Center?").
2. "Do you know where Fish Annex is?" (there is no Fish Annex at Stanford).
3. "Do you teach here?"
4. "How does one apply for admission to the college?" (at the medical school: ". . . to the medical school?").
5. "Is it difficult to get in?"
6. "Is there financial aid?"

Without exception, as can be seen in Table 1 (column 3), all of the questions were answered. No matter how rushed they were, all respondents not only maintained eye contact, but stopped to talk. Indeed, many of the respondents went out of their way to direct or take the questioner to the office she was seeking, to try to locate "Fish Annex," or to discuss with her the possibilities of being admitted to the university.

Similar data, also shown in Table 1 (columns 4, 5, and 6), were obtained in the hospital. Here too, the young lady came prepared with six questions. After the first question, however, she remarked to 18 of her respondents (column 4), "I'm looking for a psychiatrist," and to 15 others (column 5), "I'm looking for an internist." Ten other respondents received no inserted comment (column 6). The general degree of cooperative responses is considerably higher for these university groups than it was for pseudopatients in psychiatric hospitals. Even so, differences are apparent within the medical school setting. Once having indicated that she was looking for a psychiatrist, the degree of cooperation elicited was less than when she sought an internist.

Powerlessness and Depersonalization

Eye contact and verbal contact reflect concern and individuation; their absence, avoidance and depersonalization. The data I have presented do not do justice to the rich daily encounters that grew up around matters of depersonalization and avoidance. I have records of patients who were beaten by staff for the sin of having initiated verbal contact. During my own experience, for example, one patient was beaten in the presence of other patients for having approached an attendant and told him, "I like you." Occasionally, punishment meted out to patients for misdemeanors seemed so excessive that it could not be justified by the most radical interpretations of psychiatric canon. Nevertheless, they appeared to go unquestioned. Tempers were often short. A patient who had not heard a call for medication would be roundly excoriated, and the morning attendants would often wake patients with, "Come on, you m-----f-----s, out of bed!"

Neither anecdotal nor "hard" data can convey the overwhelming sense of powerlessness which invades the individual as he is continually exposed to the depersonalization of the psychiatric hospital. It hardly matters *which* psychiatric hospital—the excellent public ones and the very plush private hospital were better than the rural and shabby ones in this regard, but, again, the features that psychiatric hospitals had in common overwhelmed by far their apparent differences.

Powerlessness was evident everywhere. The patient is deprived of many of his legal rights by dint of his psychiatric commitment (21). He is shorn of credibility by virtue of his psychiatric label. His freedom of movement is restricted. He cannot initiate contact with the staff, but may only respond to such overtures as they make. Personal privacy is minimal. Patient quarters and possessions can be entered and examined by any staff member, for whatever reason. His personal history and anguish is available to any staff member (often including the "grey lady" and "candy striper" volunteer) who chooses to read his folder, regardless of their therapeutic relationship to him. His personal hygiene and waste evacuation are often monitored. The water closets may have no doors.

At times, depersonalization reached such proportions that pseudopatients had the sense that they were invisible, or at least unworthy of account. Upon being admitted, I and other pseudopatients took the initial physical examinations in a semipublic room, where staff members went about their own business as if we were not there.

On the ward, attendants delivered verbal and occasionally serious physical abuse to patients in the presence of other observing patients, some of whom (the pseudopatients) were writing it all down. Abusive behavior, on the other hand, terminated quite abruptly when other staff members were known to be coming. Staff are credible witnesses. Patients are not.

A nurse unbuttoned her uniform to adjust her brassiere in the presence of an entire ward of viewing men. One did not have the sense that she was being seductive. Rather, she didn't notice us. A group of staff persons might point to a patient in the dayroom and discuss him animatedly, as if he were not there.

One illuminating instance of depersonalization and invisibility occurred with regard to medications. All told, the pseudopatients were administered nearly 2100 pills, including Elavil, Stelazine, Compazine, and Thorazine, to name but a few. (That such a variety of medications should have been administered to patients presenting identical symptoms is itself worthy of note.) Only two were swallowed. The rest were either pocketed or deposited in the toilet. The pseudopatients were not alone in this. Although I have no precise records on how many patients rejected their medications, the pseudopatients frequently found the medications of other patients in the toilet before they deposited their own. As long as they were cooperative, their behavior and the pseudopatients' own in this matter, as in other important matters, went unnoticed throughout.

Reactions to such depersonalization among pseudopatients were intense. Although they had come to the hospital as participant observers and were fully aware that they did not "belong," they nevertheless found themselves caught up in and fighting the process of depersonalization. Some examples: a graduate student in psychology asked his wife to bring his textbooks to the hospital so he could "catch up on his homework"—this despite the elaborate precautions taken to conceal his professional association. The same student, who had trained for quite some time to get into the hospital, and who had looked forward to the experience, "remembered" some drag races that he had wanted to see on the weekend and insisted that he be discharged by that time. Another pseudopatient attempted a romance with a nurse. Subsequently, he informed the staff that he was applying for admission to graduate school in psychology and was very likely to be admitted, since a graduate professor was one of his regular hospital visitors. The same person began to engage in psychotherapy with other patients—all of this as a way of becoming a person in an impersonal environment.

The Sources of Depersonalization

What are the origins of depersonalization? I have already mentioned two. First are attitudes held by all of us toward the mentally ill—including those who treat them—attitudes characterized by fear, distrust, and horrible expectations on the one hand, and benevolent intentions on the other. Our ambivalence leads, in this instance as in others, to avoidance.

Second, and not entirely separate, the hierarchical structure of the psychiatric hospital facilitates depersonalization. Those who are at the top have least to do with patients, and their behavior inspires the rest of the staff. Average daily contact with psychiatrists, psychologists, residents, and physicians combined ranged from 3.9 to 25.1 minutes, with an overall mean of 6.8 (six pseudopatients over a total of 129 days of hospitalization). Included in this average are time spent in the admissions interview, ward meetings in the presence of a senior staff member, group and individual psychotherapy contacts, case presentation conferences, and discharge meetings. Clearly, patients do not spend much time in interpersonal contact with doctoral staff. And doctoral staff serve as models for nurses and attendants.

There are probably other sources. Psychiatric installations are presently in serious financial straits. Staff shortages are pervasive, staff time at a premium. Something has to give, and that something is patient contact. Yet, while financial stresses are realities, too much can be made of them. I have the impression that the psychological forces that result in depersonalization are much stronger than the fiscal ones and that the addition of more staff would not correspondingly improve patient care in this regard. The incidence of staff meetings and the enormous amount of record-keeping on patients, for example, have not been as substantially reduced as has patient contact. Priorities exist, even during hard times. Patient contact is not a significant priority in the traditional psychiatric hospital, and fiscal pressures do not account for this. Avoidance and depersonalization may.

Heavy reliance upon psychotropic medication tacitly contributes to depersonalization by convincing staff that treatment is indeed being conducted and that further patient contact may not be necessary. Even here, however, caution needs to be exercised in understanding the role of psychotropic drugs. If patients were powerful rather than powerless, if they were viewed as interesting individuals rather than diagnostic entities, if they were socially significant rather than social lepers, if their anguish truly and wholly compelled our sympathies and concerns, would we not *seek* contact with them, despite the availability of medications? Perhaps for the pleasure of it all?

The Consequences of Labeling and Depersonalization

Whenever the ratio of what is known to what needs to be known approaches zero, we tend to invent "knowledge" and assume that we understand more than we actually do. We seem unable to acknowledge that we simply don't know. The needs for diagnosis and remediation of behavioral and emotional problems are enormous. But rather than acknowledge that we are just embarking on understanding, we continue to label patients "schizophrenic," "manic-depressive," and "insane," as if in those words we had captured the essence of understanding. The facts of the matter are that we have known for a long time that diagnoses are often not useful or reliable, but we have nevertheless continued to use them. We now know that we cannot distinguish insanity from sanity. It is depressing to consider how that information will be used.

Not merely depressing, but frightening. How many people, one wonders, are sane but not recognized as such in our psychiatric institutions? How many have been needlessly stripped of their privileges of citizenship, from the right to vote and drive to that of handling their own accounts? How many have feigned insanity in order to avoid the criminal consequences of their behavior, and, conversely, how many would rather stand trial than live interminably in a psychiatric hospital—but are wrongly thought to be mentally ill? How many have been stigmatized by well-intentioned, but nevertheless erroneous, diagnoses? On the last point, recall again that a "type 2 error" in psychiatric diagnosis does not have the same consequences it does in medical diagnosis. A diagnosis of cancer that has been found to be in error is cause for celebration. But psychiatric diagnoses are rarely found to be in error. The label sticks, a mark of inadequacy forever.

Finally, how many patients might be "sane" outside the psychiatric hospital but seem insane in it—not because craziness resides in them, as it were, but because they are responding to a bizarre setting, one that may be unique to institutions which harbor nether people? Goffman (4) calls the process of socialization to such institutions "mortification"—an apt metaphor that includes the processes of depersonalization that have been described here. And while it is impossible to know whether the pseudopatients' responses to these processes are characteristic of all inmates—they were, after all, not real patients—it is difficult to believe that these processes of socialization to a psychiatric hospital provide useful attitudes or habits of response for living in the "real world."

Summary and Conclusions

It is clear that we cannot distinguish the sane from the insane in psychiatric hospitals. The hospital itself imposes a special environment in which the meanings of behavior can easily be misunderstood. The consequences to patients hospitalized in such an environment—the powerlessness, depersonalization, segregation, mortification, and self-labeling—seem undoubtedly countertherapeutic.

I do not, even now, understand this problem well enough to perceive solutions. But two matters seem to have some promise. The first concerns the proliferation of community mental health facilities, of crisis intervention centers, of the human potential movement, and of behavior therapies that, for all of their own problems, tend to avoid psychiatric labels, to focus on specific problems and behaviors, and to retain the individual in a relatively nonpejorative environment. Clearly, to the extent that we refrain from sending the distressed to insane places, our impressions of them are less likely to be distorted. (The risk of distorted perceptions, it seems to me, is always present, since we are much more sensitive to an individual's behaviors and verbalizations than we are to the subtle contextual stimuli that often promote them. At issue here is a matter of magnitude. And, as I have shown, the magnitude of distortion is exceedingly high in the extreme context that is a psychiatric hospital.)

The second matter that might prove promising speaks to the need to increase the sensitivity of mental health workers and researchers to the *Catch 22* position of psychiatric patients. Simply reading materials in this area will be of help to some such workers and researchers. For others, directly experiencing the impact of psychiatric hospitalization will be of enormous use. Clearly, further research into the social psychology of such total institutions will both facilitate treatment and deepen understanding.

I and the other pseudopatients in the psychiatric setting had distinctly negative reactions. We do not pretend to describe the subjective experiences of true patients. Theirs may be different from ours, particularly with the passage of time and the necessary process of adaptation to one's environment. But we can and do speak to the relatively more objective indices of treatment within the hospital. It could be a mistake, and a very unfortunate one, to consider that what happened to us derived from malice or stupidity on the part of the staff. Quite the contrary, our overwhelming impression of them was of people who really cared, who were committed and who were uncommonly intelligent. Where they failed, as they sometimes did painfully, it would be more accurate to attribute those failures to the environment in which they, too, found themselves than to personal callousness. Their perceptions and behavior were controlled by the situation, rather than being motivated by a malicious disposition. In a more benign environment, one that was less attached to global diagnosis, their behaviors and judgments might have been more benign and effective.

References and Notes

1. P. Ash, *J. Abnorm. Soc. Psychol.* **44**, 272 (1949); A. T. Beck, *Amer. J. Psychiat.* **119**, 210 (1962); A. T. Boisen, *Psychiatry* **2**, 233 (1938); N. Kreitman, *J. Ment. Sci.* **107**, 876 (1961); N. Kreitman, P. Sainsbury, J. Morrisey, J. Towers, J. Scrivener, ibid., p. 887; H. O. Schmidt and C. P. Fonda, *J. Abnorm. Soc. Psychol.* **52**, 262 (1956); W. Seeman, *J. Nerv. Ment. Dis.* **118**, 541 (1953). For an analysis of these artifacts and summaries of the disputes, see J. Zubin, *Annu. Rev. Psychol.* **18**, 373 (1967); L. Phillips and J. G. Draguns, ibid., **22**, 447 (1971).
2. R. Benedict, *J. Gen. Psychol.* **10**, 59 (1934).
3. See in this regard H. Becker, *Outsiders: Studies in the Sociology of Deviance* (Free Press, New York, 1963); B. M. Braginsky, D. D. Braginsky, K. Ring, *Methods of Madness: The*

Mental Hospital as a Last Resort (Holt, Rinehart & Winston, New York, 1969); G. M. CROCETTI and P. V. LEMKAU, *Amer. Sociol. Rev.* **30**, 577 (1965); E. GOFFMAN, *Behavior in Public Places* (Free Press, New York, 1964); R. D. LAING, *The Divided Self: A Study of Sanity and Madness* (Quadrangle, Chicago, 1960); D. L. PHILLIPS, *Amer. Sociol. Rev.* **28**, 963 (1963); T. R. SARBIN, *Psychol. Today* **6**, 18 (1972); E. SCHUR, *Amer. J. Sociol.* **75**, 309 (1969); T. SZASZ, *Law, Liberty and Psychiatry* (Macmillan, New York, 1963); *The Myth of Mental Illness: Foundations of a Theory of Mental Illness* (Hoeber Harper, New York, 1963). For a critique of some of these views, see W. R. GOVE, *Amer. Sociol. Rev.* **35**, 873 (1970).

4. E. GOFFMAN, *Asylums* (Doubleday, Garden City, N.Y., 1961).
5. T. J. SCHEFF, *Being Mentally Ill: A Sociological Theory* (Aldine, Chicago, 1966).
6. Data from a ninth pseudopatient are not incorporated in this report because although his sanity went undetected, he falsified aspects of his personal history, including his marital status and parental relationships. His experimental behaviors therefore were not identical to those of the other pseudopatients.
7. A. BARRY, *Bellevue Is a State of Mind* (Harcourt Brace Jovanovich, New York, 1971); I. BELKNAP, *Human Problems of a State Mental Hospital* (McGraw-Hill, New York, 1956); W. CAUDILL, F. C. REDLICH, H. R. GILMORE, E. B. BRODY, *Amer. J. Orthopsychiat.* **22**, 314 (1952); A. R. GOLDMAN, R. H. BOHR, T. A. STEINBERG, *Prof. Psychol.* **1**, 427 (1970); unauthored, *Roche Report* **1** (No. 13), 8 (1971).
8. Beyond the personal difficulties that the pseudopatient is likely to experience in the hospital, there are legal and social ones that, combined, require considerable attention before entry. For example, once admitted to a psychiatric institution, it is difficult, if not impossible, to be discharged on short notice, state law to the contrary notwithstanding. I was not sensitive to these difficulties at the outset of the project, nor to the personal and situational emergencies that can arise, but later a writ of habeas corpus was prepared for each of the entering pseudopatients and an attorney was kept "on call" during every hospitalization. I am grateful to John Kaplan and Robert Bartels for legal advice and assistance in these matters.
9. However distasteful such concealment is, it was a necessary first step to examining these questions. Without concealment, there would have been no way to know how valid these experiences were; nor was there any way of knowing whether whatever detections occurred were a tribute to the diagnostic acumen of the staff or to the hospital's rumor network. Obviously, since my concerns are general ones that cut across individual hospitals and staffs, I have respected their anonymity and have eliminated clues that might lead to their identification.
10. Interestingly, of the 12 admissions, 11 were diagnosed as schizophrenic and one, with the identical symptomatology, as manic-depressive psychosis. This diagnosis has a more favorable prognosis, and it was given by the only private hospital in our sample. On the relations between social class and psychiatric diagnosis, see A. deB. HOLLINGSHEAD and F. C. REDLICH, *Social Class and Mental Illness: A Community Study* (Wiley, New York, 1958).
11. It is possible, of course, that patients have quite broad latitudes in diagnosis and therefore are inclined to call many people sane, even those whose behavior is patently aberrant. However, although we have no hard data on this matter, it was our distinct impression that this was not the case. In many instances, patients not only singled us out for attention, but came to imitate our behaviors and styles.
12. J. CUMMING and E. CUMMING, *Community Ment. Health* **1**, 135 (1965); A. FARINA and K. RING, *J. Abnorm. Psychol.* **70**, 47 (1965); H. E. FREEMAN and O. G. SIMMONS, *The Mental Patient Comes Home* (Wiley, New York, 1963); W. J. JOHANNSEN, *Ment. Hygiene* **53**, 218 (1969); A. S. LINSKY, *Soc. Psychiat.* **5**, 166 (1970).
13. S. E. ASCH, *J. Abnorm. Soc. Psychol.* **41**, 258 (1946); *Social Psychology* (Prentice-Hall, New York, 1952).
14. See also I. N. MENSH and J. WISHNER, *J. Personality* **16**, 188 (1947); J. WISHNER, *Psychol. Rev.* **67**, 96 (1960); J. S. BRUNER and R. TAGIURI, in *Handbook of Social Psychology*, G. LINDZEY, Ed. (Addison-Wesley, Cambridge, Mass., 1954), vol. 2, pp. 634–654; J. S. BRUNER, D. SHAPIRO, R. TAGIURI, in *Person Perception and Interpersonal Behavior*, R. TAGIURI and L. PETRULLO, eds. (Stanford Univ. Press, Stanford, Calif., 1958), pp. 277–288.

15. For an example of a similar self-fulfilling prophecy, in this instance dealing with the "central" trait of intelligence, see R. ROSENTHAL and L. JACOBSON, *Pygmalion in the Classroom* (Holt, Rinehart & Winston, New York, 1968).
16. E. ZIGLER and L. PHILLIPS, *J. Abnorm. Soc. Psychol.* **63**, 69 (1961). See also R. K. FREUDENBERG and J. P. ROBERTSON, *A.M.A. Arch. Neurol. Psychiatr.* **76**, 14 (1956).
17. W. MISCHEL, *Personality and Assessment* (Wiley, New York, 1968).
18. The most recent and unfortunate instance of this tenet is that of Senator Thomas Eagleton.
19. T. R. SARBIN and J. C. MANCUSO, *J. Clin. Consult. Psychol.* **35**, 159 (1970); T. R. SARBIN, ibid. **31**, 447 (1967); J. C. NUNNALLY, Jr., *Popular Conceptions of Mental Health* (Holt, Rinehart & Winston, New York, 1961).
20. A. H. STANTON and M. S. SCHWARTZ, *The Mental Hospital: A Study of Institutional Participation in Psychiatric Illness and Treatment* (Basic, New York, 1954).
21. D. B. WEXLER and S. E. SCOVILLE, *Ariz. Law Rev.* **13**, 1 (1971).
22. I thank W. MISCHEL, E. ORNE, and M. S. ROSENHAN for comments on an earlier draft of this manuscript.

Section II

Psychopathology

Traditionally, psychopathology has been studied in terms of more or less discrete classes or subdivisions. Long before man had much of an understanding of the causes of behavioral abnormality, he made attempts to classify it. In fact, he often seems to have thought that by classifying abnormality he could understand it better. Certain disorders, like manic-depressive psychosis, were described in the Bible and in the writings of classical Greece. Others, like schizophrenia, were not even beginning to be conceptualized in their present form until the late nineteenth century or even more recently. Despite the many disadvantages and potential pitfalls of the business of creating nosologies, such systems have tended to cut the behavioral pie into certain kinds of slices that then draw specific attention.

This section presents examples of research and theories that have been developed about the various major subdivisions of abnormal behavior. The number of pages devoted to each slice of the abnormal behavioral pie bears little relation to the severity of that problem for society. Instead, it reflects the amount of attention devoted to the problem by professionals. Therefore, while there are far fewer people suffering from psychoses than from personality disorders, much more professional attention has been devoted to psychoses, especially schizophrenia.

3 Psychoneurosis

Neurotic problems became a major concern of the mental health professional only after Freud devoted much time and thought to them. His perceived success in understanding and treating such disorders was a potent impetus to the development of a variety of personality theories. It was also the basis for considerable faith that all behavior could be fathomed eventually. Certainly one of the major legacies of the early work on psychoneurosis was a redefinition of the field of abnormal psychology that broadened it out from the narrow involvement with the psychoses that had characterized it earlier. This expansion also laid the groundwork for a still further enlargement of the mental health worker's area of concern that was to come.

SIGMUND FREUD

My Views on the Part Played by Sexuality in the Aetiology of the Neuroses

One cornerstone of the psychoanalytic theory of psychoneurosis is the basic role seen to be played by infantile sexuality in personality development. In the following paper, which was written in 1905, Freud attempts to explain the basis for his conclusions concerning the key role of sexuality in the life of the very young child and the way in which inadequacies in sexual development lead to neurotic problems. It is a valuable testament to the way his theoretical approach was shaped by his clinical experience.

Reprinted with permission from Chapter XIV in *The Collected Papers of Sigmund Freud*, Vol. I, edited by Ernest Jones, translation under the supervision of Joan Riviere. Published by Basic Books, Inc. by arrangement with The Hogarth Press Ltd. and The Institute of Psycho-Analysis, London.

My theory of the aetiological importance of the sexual factor in the neuroses can best be appreciated, in my opinion, by following the history of its development. For I have no desire whatever to deny that it has gone through a process of evolution and been modified in the course of it. My professional colleagues may find a guarantee in this admission that the theory is nothing other than the product of continuous and ever deeper-going experience. What is born of speculation on the contrary, may easily spring into existence complete, and thereafter remain unchangeable.

Originally my theory related only to the clinical pictures comprised under the term 'neurasthenia,' among which I was particularly struck by two, which occasionally appear as pure types and which I described as 'neurasthenia proper' and 'anxiety neurosis.' It had, to be sure, always been a matter of common knowledge that sexual factors *may* play a part in the causation of these forms of illness; but those factors were not regarded as invariably operative, nor was there any idea of giving them precedence over other aetiological influences. I was surprised to begin with at the frequency of gross disturbances in the *vita sexualis* of nervous patients; the more I set about looking for such disturbances—bearing in mind the fact that everyone hides the truth in matters of sex—and the more skilful I became at pursuing my enquiries in the face of a preliminary denial, the more regularly was I able to discover pathogenic factors in sexual life, till little seemed to stand in the way of my assuming their universal occurrence. It was necessary, however, to presuppose from the start that sexual irregularities occurred with similar frequency in our ordinary society under the pressure of social conditions; and a doubt might remain as to the degree of deviation from normal sexual functioning which should be regarded as pathogenic. I was therefore obliged to attach less importance to the invariable evidence of sexual noxae than to a second discovery which seemed to me less ambiguous. It emerged that the form taken by the illness—neurasthenia or anxiety neurosis—bore a constant relation to the nature of the sexual noxa involved. In typical cases of neurasthenia a history of regular masturbation or persistent emissions was found; in anxiety neurosis factors appeared such as *coitus interruptus*, 'unconsummated excitation,' and other conditions—in all of which there seemed to be the common element of an insufficient discharge of the libido that had been produced. It was only after this discovery, which was easy to make and could be confirmed as often as one liked, that I had the courage to claim a preferential position for sexual influences in the aetiology of the neuroses. Furthermore, in the mixed forms of neurasthenia and anxiety neurosis which are so common it was possible to trace a combination of the aetiologies which I had assumed for the two pure forms. Moreover, this twofold form assumed by the neurosis seemed to tally with the polar (i.e. the masculine and feminine) character of sexuality.

At the time at which I was attributing to sexuality this important part in the production of the *simple* neuroses,[1] I was still faithful to a purely

[1] In my [first] paper on anxiety neurosis (1895*b*).

psychological theory in regard to the *psychoneuroses*—a theory in which the sexual factor was regarded as no more significant than any other emotional source of feeling. On the basis of some observations made by Josef Breuer on a hysterical patient more than ten years earlier, I collaborated with him in a study of the mechanism of the generation of hysterical symptoms, using the method of awakening the patient's memories in a state of hypnosis; and we reached conclusions which enabled us to bridge the gap between Charcot's traumatic hysteria and common non-traumatic hysteria (Breuer and Freud, 1895). We were led to the assumption that hysterical symptoms are the permanent results of psychical traumas, the sum of affect attaching to which has, for particular reasons, been prevented from being worked over consciously and has therefore found an abnormal path into somatic innervation. The terms 'strangulated affect,' 'conversion' and 'abreaction' cover the distinctive features of this hypothesis.

But in view of the close connections between the psychoneuroses and the simple neuroses, which go so far, indeed, that a differential diagnosis is not always easy for inexperienced observers, it could not be long before the knowledge arrived at in the one field was extended to the other. Moreover, apart from this consideration, a deeper investigation of the psychical mechanism of hysterical symptoms led to the same result. For if the psychical traumas from which the hysterical symptoms were derived were pursued further and further by means of the 'cathartic' procedure initiated by Breuer and me, experiences were eventually reached which belonged to the patient's childhood and related to his sexual life. And this was so, even in cases in which the onset of the illness had been brought about by some commonplace emotion of a non-sexual kind. Unless these sexual traumas of childhood were taken into account it was impossible either to elucidate the symptoms (to understand the way in which they were determined) or to prevent their recurrence. In this way the unique significance of sexual experiences in the aetiology of the psychoneuroses seemed to be established beyond a doubt; and this fact remains to this day one of the corner-stones of my theory.

This theory might be expressed by saying that the cause of life-long hysterical neuroses lies in what are in themselves for the most part the trivial sexual experiences of early childhood; and, put in this way, it might no doubt sound strange. But if we take the historical development of the theory into account, and see as its essence the proposition that hysteria is the expression of a particular behaviour of the individual's sexual function and that this behaviour is decisively determined by the first influences and experiences brought to bear in childhood, we shall be a paradox the poorer but the richer by a motive for turning our attention to something of the highest importance (though it has hitherto been grossly neglected)—the after-effects of the impressions of childhood.

I will postpone until later in this paper a more thorough-going discussion of the question whether we are to regard the sexual experiences of childhood as the causes of hysteria (and obsessional neurosis), and I will now return to the form taken by the theory in some of my shorter preliminary publications during the years 1895 and 1896 (Freud, 1896*b* and 1896*c*). By laying stress on the supposed aetiological factors it was possible at that time to draw a contrast between the common neuroses as disorders with a *contemporary* aetiology and psychoneuroses whose aetiology was chiefly to be looked for in the sexual experiences of the remote past. The theory culminated in this thesis: if the *vita sexualis* is normal, there can be no neurosis.

Though even to-day I do not consider these assertions incorrect, it is not to be wondered at that, in the course of ten years of continuous effort at reaching an understanding of these phenomena, I have made a considerable step forward from the views I then held, and now believe that I am in a position, on the basis of deeper experience, to correct the insufficiencies, the displacements and the misunderstandings under which my theory then laboured. At that time my material was still scanty, and it happened by chance to include a disproportionately large number of cases in which sexual seduction by an adult or by older children played the chief part in the history of the patient's childhood. I thus over-estimated the frequency of such events (though in other respects they were not open to doubt). Moreover, I was at that period unable to distinguish with certainty between falsifications made by hysterics in their memories of childhood and traces of real events. Since then I have learned to explain a number of phantasies of seduction as attempts at fending off memories of the subject's *own* sexual activity (infantile masturbation). When this point had been clarified, the 'traumatic' element in the sexual experiences of childhood lost its importance and what was left was the realization that infantile sexual activity (whether spontaneous or provoked) prescribes the direction that will be taken by later sexual life after maturity. The same clarification (which corrected the most important of my early mistakes) also made it necessary to modify my view of the mechanism of hysterical symptoms. They were now no longer to be regarded as direct derivatives of the repressed memories of childhood experiences; but between the symptoms and the childish impressions there were inserted the patient's *phantasies* (or imaginary memories), mostly produced during the years of puberty, which on the one side were built up out of and over the childhood memories and on the other side were transformed directly into the symptoms. It was only after the introduction of this element of hysterical phantasies that the texture of the neurosis and its relation to the patient's life became intelligible; a surprising analogy came to light, too, between these unconscious phantasies of hysterics and the imaginary creations of paranoics which become conscious as delusions.[2]

[2] [This passage was Freud's first explicit published intimation of his change of views on the relative importance of traumatic experiences and unconscious phantasies in childhood, apart from a brief allusion in his *Three Essays* (1905*d*; this volume, p. 190). In fact, however, he had become aware of his error many years earlier, for he revealed it in a letter to Fliess on September 21, 1897 (Freud, 1950*a*, Letter 69). The effects on Freud's own mind of the discovery of his mistake are vividly related by him in the first section of his 'History of the Psycho-Analytic Movement' (1914*d*) and in the third section of his 'Autobiographical Study' (1925*d*).]

After I had made this correction, 'infantile sexual traumas' were in a sense replaced by the 'infantilism of sexuality.' A second modification of the original theory lay not far off. Along with the supposed frequency of seduction in childhood, I ceased also to lay exaggerated stress on the *accidental* influencing of sexuality on to which I had sought to thrust the main responsibility for the causation of the illness, though I had not on that account denied the constitutional and hereditary factors. I had even hoped to solve the problem of choice of neurosis (the decision to which form of psychoneurosis the patient is to fall a victim) by reference to the details of the sexual experiences of childhood. I believed at that time—though with reservations—that a passive attitude in these scenes produced a predisposition to hysteria and, on the other hand, an active one a predisposition to obsessional neurosis. Later on I was obliged to abandon this view entirely, even though some facts demand that in some way or other the supposed correlation between passivity and hysteria and between activity and obsessional neurosis shall be maintained.[3] Accidental influences derived from experience having thus receded into the background, the factors of constitution and heredity necessarily gained the upper hand once more; but there was this difference between my views and those prevailing in other quarters, that on my theory the 'sexual constitution' took the place of a 'general neuropathic disposition.' In my recently published *Three Essays on the Theory of Sexuality* (1905d [this volume p. 125]) I have tried to give a picture of the variegated nature of this sexual constitution as well as of the composite character of the sexual instinct in general and its derivation from contributory sources from different parts of the organism.

As a further corollary to my modified view of 'sexual traumas in childhood,' my theory now developed further in a direction which had already been indicated in my publications between 1894 and 1896. At that time, and even before sexuality had been given its rightful place as an aetiological factor, I had maintained that no experience could have a pathogenic effect unless it appeared intolerable to the subject's ego and gave rise to efforts at defence (Freud, 1894*a*). It was to this defence that I traced back the split in the psyche (or, as we said in those days, in consciousness) which occurs in hysteria. If the defence was successful, the intolerable experience with its affective consequences was expelled from consciousness and from the ego's memory. In certain circumstances, however, what had been expelled pursued its activities in what was now an unconscious state, and found its way back into consciousness by means of symptoms and the affects attaching to them, so that the illness corresponded to a failure in defence. This view had the merit of entering into the interplay of the psychical forces and of thus bringing

[3] [This particular solution of the problem of 'choice of neurosis' is most clearly expressed in Freud's second paper on the 'Neuropsychoses of Defence' (1896*b*) and his French paper of the same date (1896*a*). His interest in the general question of choice of neurosis goes back at least to the beginning of the same year (Draft K in Freud, 1950*a*) and he used the term itself in a letter to Fliess of May 30, 1896 (Letter 46). He was to return to the subject a few years later in special reference to obsessional neurosis (1913*i*), and indeed the problem never ceased to occupy his mind.]

the mental processes in hysteria nearer to normal ones, instead of characterizing the neurosis as nothing more than a mysterious disorder insusceptible to further analysis.

Further information now became available relating to people who had remained normal; and this led to the unexpected finding that the sexual history of *their* childhood did not necessarily differ in essentials from that of neurotics, and, in particular, that the part played by seduction was the same in both cases. As a consequence, accidental influences receded still further into the background as compared with 'repression' (as I now began to say instead of 'defence').[4] Thus it was no longer a question of what sexual experiences a particular individual had had in his childhood, but rather of his reaction to those experiences—of whether he had reacted to them by 'repression' or not. It could be shown how in the course of development a spontaneous infantile sexual activity was often broken off by an act of repression. Thus a mature neurotic individual was invariably pursued by a certain amount of 'sexual repression' from his childhood; this found expression when he was faced by the demands of real life, and the psychoanalyses of hysterics showed that they fell ill as a result of the conflict between their libido and their sexual repression and that their symptoms were in the nature of compromises between the two mental currents.

I could not further elucidate this part of my theory without a detailed discussion of my views on repression. It will be enough here to refer to my *Three Essays* (1905*d*), in which I have attempted to throw some light—if only a feeble one—on the somatic processes in which the essential nature of sexuality is to be looked for. I have there shown that the constitutional sexual disposition of children is incomparably more variegated than might have been expected, that it deserves to be described as 'polymorphously perverse' and that what is spoken of as the normal behaviour of the sexual function emerges from this disposition after certain of its components have been repressed. By pointing out the infantile elements in sexuality I was able to establish a simple correlation between health, perversion and neurosis. I showed that *normality* is a result of the repression of certain component instincts and constituents of the infantile disposition and of the subordination of the remaining constituents under the primacy of the genital zones in the service of the reproductive function. I showed that *perversions* correspond to disturbances of this coalescence owing to the overpowering and compulsive development of certain of the component instincts, while *neuroses* can be traced back to an excessive repression of the libidinal trends. Since almost all the perverse instincts of the infantile disposition can be recognized as the forces concerned in the formation of symptoms in

[4] [Actually the term '*Verdrängung*' ('repression') had made its first published appearance as early as in the Breuer and Freud 'Preliminary Communication' (1893). Many years later, in *Inhibitions, Symptoms and Anxiety* (1926*d*; see particularly Section X *c*), Freud once more returned to the term '*Abwehr*' ('defence') as denoting a comprehensive concept, of which 'repression' represented only a single form.]

neuroses, though in a state of repression, I was able to describe neurosis as being the 'negative' of perversion.

I think it is worth emphasizing the fact that, whatever modifications my views on the aetiology of the psychoneuroses have passed through, there are two positions which I have never repudiated or abandoned—the importance of sexuality and of infantilism. Apart from this, accidental influences have been replaced by constitutional factors and 'defence' in the purely psychological sense has been replaced by organic 'sexual repression.' The question may, however, be raised of where convincing evidence is to be found in favour of the alleged aetiological importance of sexual factors in the psychoneuroses, in view of the fact that the onset of these illnesses may be observed in response to the most commonplace emotions or even to somatic precipitating causes, and since I have had to abandon a specific aetiology depending on the particular form of the childhood experiences concerned. To such a question I would reply that the psycho-analytic examination of neurotics is the source from which this disputed conviction of mine is derived. If we make use of that irreplaceable method of research, we discover that *the patient's symptoms constitute his sexual activity* (whether wholly or in part), which arises from the sources of the normal or perverse component instincts of sexuality. Not only is a large part of the symptomatology of hysteria derived directly from expressions of sexual excitement, not only do a number of erotogenic zones attain the significance of genitals during neuroses owing to an intensification of infantile characteristics, but the most complicated symptoms are themselves revealed as representing, by means of 'conversion,' phantasies which have a sexual situation as their subject-matter. Anyone who knows how to interpret the language of hysteria will recognize that the neurosis is concerned only with the patient's repressed sexuality. The sexual function must, however, be understood in its true extent, as it is laid down by disposition in infancy. Wherever some commonplace emotion must be included among the determinants of the onset of the illness, analysis invariably shows that it is the sexual component of the traumatic experience—a component that is never lacking—which has produced the pathogenic result.

We have been led on imperceptibly from the question of the causation of the psychoneuroses to the problem of their essential nature. If we are prepared to take into account what has been learnt from psycho-analysis, we can only say that the essence of these illnesses lies in disturbances of the sexual processes, the processes which determine in the organism the formation and utilization of sexual libido. It is scarcely possible to avoid picturing the processes as being in the last resort of a chemical nature; so that in what are termed the 'actual' neuroses[5] we may recognize the *somatic* effects of disturbances of the sexual metabolism, and in the psychoneuroses the *psychical* effects of those disturbances as well. The similarity of the neuroses to the phenomena of intoxication and abstinence after the use of certain

[5] [I.e. those with a contemporary aetiology (neurasthenia and anxiety neurosis).]

alkaloids, as well as to Graves' disease and Addison's disease, is forced upon our notice clinically. And just as these last two illnesses should no longer be described as 'nervous diseases,' so also the 'neuroses' proper, in spite of their name, may soon have to be excluded from that category as well.[6]

Accordingly, the aetiology of the neuroses comprises everything which can act in a detrimental manner upon the processes serving the sexual function. In the forefront, then, are to be ranked the noxae which affect the sexual function itself—in so far as these are regarded as injurious by the sexual constitution, varying as it does with different degrees of culture and education. In the next place comes every other kind of noxa and trauma which, by causing general damage to the organism, may lead secondarily to injury to its sexual processes. It should not, however, be forgotten that the aetiological problem in the case of the neuroses is at least as complicated as the causative factors of any other illness. A single pathogenic influence is scarcely ever sufficient; in the large majority of cases a *number* of aetiological factors are required, which support one another and must therefore not be regarded as being in mutual opposition. For this reason a state of neurotic illness cannot be sharply differentiated from health. The onset of the illness is the product of a summation and the necessary total of aetiological determinants can be completed from any direction. To look for the aetiology of the neuroses exclusively in heredity or in the constitution would be just as one-sided as to attribute that aetiology solely to the accidental influences brought to bear upon sexuality in the course of the subject's life—whereas better insight shows that the essence of these illnesses lies solely in a disturbance of the organism's sexual processes.

Vienna, June 1905

[6] [Cf. *Three Essays*, this volume p. 216 and footnote.]

JOSEPH WOLPE

Experimental Neuroses as Learned Behavior

Joseph Wolpe has risen in prominence in recent years as founder of one branch within a psychotherapeutic movement called behavior therapy. This approach emphasizes the understanding of the development and treatment of neurotic problems on the basis of learning principles uncovered in the psychology laboratory,

Abridged from the *British Journal of Psychology*, **43** (1952), 243–268 with the permission of the Cambridge University Press and Dr. Wolpe.

often through work with animals. This paper includes Wolpe's analysis of the experiments of others, which have produced "neurotic-like" behavior in animals, as well as a report of his own work with such phenomena. This paper is significant because it presents a view of how neuroses develop that is quite different from the psychoanalytic position that preceded it and commanded a considerable following. Furthermore, it proposes a therapeutic approach that has come to attract considerable attention from researchers and therapists alike in recent years.

The editing done on this paper to conserve space eliminated part of Wolpe's comprehensive and detailed review of studies done in the area of experimental neurosis and his criticisms of previous theories developed to explain such phenomena. The reader who is interested in these details should consult the article in the original.

I. Introduction

In a recent issue of this *Journal* Russell (39) presented a very lucid review of experiments in which neuroses have been artificially produced, and of the theories that have been put forward in explanation. He did not pronounce on the relative merits of the theories, as he felt that further experimental and logical studies were prerequisite. In the present paper a new analysis is made of previously reported experimental neuroses; and then some new experiments are described which, it is believed, clarify our understanding of the mechanisms by which these conditions are produced. The study as a whole supports the conclusion that experimental neuroses constitute a variety of learned behaviour.

Definition

An animal is said to have an experimental neurosis if it displays unadaptive responses that are characterized by anxiety, that are persistent, and that have been produced experimentally by behavioral means (as opposed to direct assault on the nervous system by chemical or physical agencies such as poisonings or extirpations).

An *adaptive response* is defined by Warren (41) as "any response which is appropriate to the situation, i.e. which favours the organism's life processes." This implies that it is a response that has the *effect* of leading directly or indirectly to the reduction of the organism's needs or to the prevention of pain or fatigue. An *unadaptive response*, on the other hand, does not lead to either.

II. Analysis of Previous Experimental Findings

Russell (39), like previous reviewers (5, 22), seems to have been too ready to accept without question the interpretations the various experimenters have given of their own work. It will be seen in the paragraphs that follow that these interpretations often ignore important factors in the experiments, and that if these factors are consistently taken into account all the neuroses so far recorded can be understood as being the outcome of one or other (perhaps sometimes both) of two basic situations—the exposure of the organism to ambivalent stimuli or its exposure to noxious stimuli, in either case under conditions of confinement. It will be argued that these two kinds of situation have an effect in common upon which the development of the neuroses depends.

In the account that follows the neuroses are grouped according to the basic situation which seems to have determined their production, and it will be seen repeatedly how experimental procedures may differ widely in other respects and yet provide the same kind of basic situation.

(*i*) *Neuroses produced by situations of ambivalent stimulation*

An *ambivalent stimulus situation* is a situation to which opposing responses tend to be elicited simultaneously in more or less equal measure. The range of meaning is narrower than would be implied by "conflict situation," for not in every conflict are the opposing response tendencies equal. Examination of the literature reveals that three varieties of situations involving ambivalent stimulation have been effective in producing experimental neuroses. These will be considered under their headings below.

(*a*) *Neuroses produced by difficult discriminations.* Although the expression "difficult discrimination" carries an unwanted suggestion of conscious weighing-up, it is a conveniently brief term of reference for the ambivalent stimulus situation that occurs under the following circumstances: a positive and a negative response having respectively been conditioned to two stimuli at different points on a continuum, the animal is confronted with a stimulus at an intermediate point on the continuum such that the opposing responses are evoked in more or less equal strength.

Pavlov's experiment on neurosis-production based on difficult discrimination was the first to be reported (36, pp. 290–1). The projection of a luminous circle on to a screen in front of a dog was repeatedly followed by feeding. When the alimentary response to the circle was well established, an ellipse with semi-axes in the ratio of 2 : 1 began to be projected among presentations of the circle, and was never accompanied by feeding.

> A complete and constant differentiation was obtained comparatively quickly. The shape of the ellipse was now approximated by stages to that of the circle (ratios of semi-axes of 3 : 2, 4 : 3 and so on) and the development of differentiation continued . . . with some fluctuation, progressing at first more and more quickly, and

> then again slower, until an ellipse with ratio of semi-axes 9 : 8 was reached. In this case, although a considerable degree of discrimination did develop, it was far from being complete. After three weeks of work upon this differentiation not only did the discrimination fail to improve, but it became considerably worse, and finally disappeared altogether. At the same time the whole behaviour of the animal underwent an abrupt change. The hitherto quiet dog began to squeal in its stand, kept wriggling about, tore off with its teeth the apparatus for mechanical stimulation of the skin, and bit through the tubes connecting the animal's room with the observer, a behaviour which never happened before. On being taken into thc experimental room the dog now barked violently.

Because of its close resemblance to the circle the 9 : 8 ellipse presumably generated at least as great a positive ailmentary response tendency due to primary stimulus generalization (18, p. 184) from the circle as negative alimentary response tendency due to generalization from previous ellipses. Since primary stimulus generalization depends on the common neurones activated by similar stimuli (47), if the 9 : 8 ellipse activated a preponderating number of neurones in common with the circle, the negative response tendency to the ellipse could never become completely dominant, however often it were presented to the animal without reinforcement. Consequently, this ellipse would always evoke ambivalent response tendencies.

Karn (21) has described the production of a neurosis in a cat by a method that is of special interest in that a difficult discrimination of *intraorganismal cues* was involved. The animal was trained in a maze that was in effect a T-maze, with the left turn followed by two further left turns, and the right turn by two further right turns, all segments being the same length as the stem of the T. The only place where food was ever given was at the end of the final segment. The animal was required to learn at the choice point the double alternation—right, right, left, left. After 230 trials of the sequence it attained an average of 90% correct in the last 30 trials. During the 232nd trial, at its second arrival at the choice point, the animal hesitated much longer than usual, and then raced to the right end point. During the remainder of the trial it moved slowly, whimpering. From this time onwards the cat resisted being put into the maze, and mewed loudly and micturated at the choice point, especially at the second of the two occasions for a right turn. At later trials the signs of disturbance seemed to get worse, and accuracy of performance became progressively poorer. (In a later article, Karn (22) states that he and E. R. Malamud have produced a neurosis in a dog by the above technique, and that Keller has done likewise with a rat.)

It is reasonable to interpret the results as follows. Each time the cat arrived at the choice point the external cues were the same, and these were equally conditioned to a turn in either direction. In the case of a first arrival at the choice point the distinctive cue of a completely empty stomach must have become strongly conditioned to right-turning. Difficulty would occur at the second arrival, for the internal cues conditioned to right-turning would be the proprioceptive cues from the right-turning movements of one run, plus cues consequent on having eaten once; while conditioned to left-turning would be the proprioceptive cues from the right-turning movements of two runs plus the internal cues consequent on having eaten twice. It is easy to believe that the difference between these two combinations of internal stimuli is minimal, so that at each second (and third) arrival at the choice point the right- and left-turning tendencies would be almost equal, constituting an ambivalent stimulus situation.

(*b*) *Neuroses produced by increasing the delay before reinforcement of a delayed conditional response.* In Pavlov's laboratory (36, pp. 293–4), a dog with a predominant tendency of excitation had become conditioned to make the alimentary response to any of six stimuli. Food was presented when a stimulus had been acting for 5 sec. The duration of action of the conditioned stimulus before presentation of food was now prolonged by 5 sec. daily. All six stimuli were treated in this manner concurrently. When the delay reached 2 min., "the animal began to enter into a state of general excitation, and with a further prolongation of the delay to 3 min. the animal became quite crazy, increasingly and violently moving all parts of its body, howling, barking and squealing intolerably. All this was accompanied by an unceasing flow of saliva. . . ."

This neurosis is regarded as produced by ambivalent stimulation because of the following considerations. Pavlov (36, p. 92) found that when a delayed conditioned reflex has been established, salivation is delayed until some time after the commencement of the conditioned stimulus. Presumably, then, certain durations of the conditioned stimulus have become conditioned to an inhibition of the alimentary response, and other, longer durations to an excitation of that response. If the delay until presentation of food is now increased in stages, at each stage a duration of the stimulus which had previously stimulated the response would begin to be conditioned to an inhibition thereof. Whenever the positive and negative tendencies were more or less equal the stimulus would be an ambivalent one according to the definition given above.

(*c*) *Neuroses produced by rapid alternation of stimuli eliciting opposing responses.* In the two types of ambivalent stimulus situation just described the ambivalent effects are produced in the last resort by a single stimulus. The situation would be quite similar if the two opposing responses were elicited each by its own stimulus, provided that the stimuli followed each other rather closely. In one of Pavlov's dogs, among other positive and negative alimentary conditioned reflexes, conditioning was established positively to a tactile stimulation of 24 per minute and negatively to 12 per minute. One day the positive rate was made to follow the negative without any interval. For the first few days after this it was found that all positive conditioned reflexes had disappeared. This was followed by a period in which there were changing relations between the magnitudes of response to the various stimuli. The disturbances are said to have lasted $5\frac{1}{2}$ weeks, but neither in Anrep's translation (36, pp. 301–2) nor in Gantt's (37, pp. 343–4) are any other changes in behavior described.

(ii) *Neuroses produced by noxious stimuli*

A noxious stimulus is one that causes tissue disturbance of a kind that leads or tends to lead to withdrawal behaviour. In man it is correlated with the experience of pain or discomfort.

In certain experiments in which noxious stimuli have been used to produce neuroses a "clash" between excitation and inhibition has been involved in one way or another. In other experiments, feeding reactions have been interfered with by the presentation of the noxious stimulus. Because in both categories conflict is in some sense present it has been regarded as the centre point of the aetiology in both. Nevertheless, these neuroses are grouped here among those due to noxious stimuli and not to ambivalent stimulation; the first category for reasons given below in the course of an examination of the experiments, the second for the following reasons. First, as was shown above, to result in a neurosis, conflicting tendencies must be of approximately the same strength at the same time, whereas when the reaction to a noxious stimulus has interfered with feeding it has been overwhelmingly stronger than the feeding tendency. Secondly, in experiments to be described below, the writer has found that noxious stimuli, alone and without the aid of any conflict, can be an entirely adequate cause of neurotic reactions. If anything, a more severe neurosis tends to be produced by shock alone than by shock associated with feeding.

In the following account of the various procedures that have been employed more specific comments will be made. To unify the commentary the procedures are grouped according to what the experimenter has believed to be the crux of his method.

(*a*) *Noxious stimuli in experiments involving 'clash' between excitation and inhibition.* The most extensive series of experiments coming under this heading has been reported from the Cornell Behaviour Farm by Liddell & Bayne (25), Anderson & Liddell (1), Anderson & Parmenter (2), and Liddell (24). Sheep, goats, dogs and pigs were used. It will be noticed that some of the experiments parallel those of Pavlov, mentioned above, among the ambivalent stimulation neuroses, but the 'unconditioned response' is a shock-avoidance reaction in place of the alimentary reaction. The basic procedure is described as follows by Anderson & Liddell (1):

> The sheep to be conditioned was led to the laboratory. It ascended a platform and stood on a table where it might eat from a basket of oats. Its freedom of movement was restricted by loops passing under the legs and attached to a beam overhead. With the incentive of food at the beginning and end of the experiment, the sheep within a few days would run on leash to the laboratory from the barn, mount the table and remain quietly for as long as two hours. A leather bracelet wrapped with brass wires was attached to the shaved skin of the upper part of the foreleg. . . . A brief tetanizing shock, not

> painful to the experimenter's touch . . . evoked a brisk flexion of the sheep's foreleg, after which the animal became quiet. . . . If the shock was regularly preceded by some neutral stimulus such as the ticking of a metronome, soon the ticking of the metronome would elicit movement of the leg in anticipation of the shock. . . . The signal that a shock was coming was invariably followed by the shock. The animal quieted down within a few seconds after the shock had been administered.

(*b*) *Noxious stimuli interrupting conditioned feeding responses.* Dimmick, Ludlow & Whiteman (8) were the first to produce animal neuroses by a method that falls under this heading, although they attributed their results to difficult discrimination—mistakenly, as will be shown. Using an experimental cage 36 × 28 × 16 in. they trained cats to raise the lid of a food-box in respose to a lamp switched on simultaneously with the ringing of a bell. When 100% correct responses had been acquired the cat would be shocked through a grid on the floor of the cage if he opened the food-box at any time except while the conditioned stimuli lasted or 6 sec. thereafter. (This shocking, of course, constituted an interruption of the feeding response conditioned, incidentally, to such stimuli as the sight of the food-box.) A varying number of sessions after this was begun, it was found that the cat would stretch towards the food-box at the conditioned stimuli but not touch it. When this happened the animal would be shocked at the end of the "correct" period for opening the food-box. The effect of this was to produce progressively more negative behaviour towards the experimental situation, and such symptoms as yowling, crouching, and clawing at the sides of the cage developed as responses to the conditioned signals. Also, the cats became less friendly in their living quarters.

(*c*) *Noxious stimuli used alone.* The only previous report of neurosis production conforming to this heading appears to be that of Watson & Rayner (42). They found that a usually phlegmatic 11-month-old infant called Albert would react fearfully to the sound of an iron bar loudly struck behind his head. They contrived to strike the bar just as the child's hand touched a white rat. This was done 7 times and then repeated after a week. It was subsequently found that the child reacted with fear to the white rat, and also to a rabbit, a beaver fur, and a dog. A month later these fear reactions could still elicited. After this the child was lost sight of.

III. Present Experiments in Neurosis Production

These experiments were performed between June 1947 and July 1948 in the Department of Pharmacology of the University of the Witwatersrand. The present account is an abbreviated version of a more detailed one written in 1948 (43).

(*i*) *Subjects and apparatus*

The subjects were twelve domestic cats ranging in age from about 6 months to 3 years. They were housed in large, airy cages built into a brick cage-house on the roof of the department. When experimentation began an animal would have been in these quarters for at least 4 weeks. Experiments were always done between 11 a.m. and 1 p.m., when the animals had not eaten for 19–21 hr., except, occasionally, when prolonged observations were necessary.

The experimental centre was a laboratory on the floor below the cage house. Animals were carried to and from the laboratory in 'carrier cages' of which the dimensions were 9 × 9 × 16 in.

The experimental cage (40 × 20 × 20 in.) was practically identical with that of Masserman, except that the long sides and roof were made of stout $\frac{3}{4}$ in. wire-netting in the place of glass. A metal funnel delivered pellets of minced beef into the food-box as required. The conditioned signals used were auditory—a buzzer, and a whirring sound made by the armature of an automobile hooter (inaccurately referred to as a 'hoot'). The grid on the floor of the cage could be charged by depressing a telegraph key in the secondary circuit of an induction coil continuously vibrating 25 ft. away. The current delivered, being of high voltage but low amperage, was very uncomfortable to the human hand but not productive of tissue damage.

In the course of the experiments it became evident that the experimental laboratory, and, indeed, the experimenter himself, could well be regarded as part of the apparatus. For convenience the experimental laboratory was called room A. Experiments were also conducted in three other rooms which were labelled respectively B, C and D. These rooms, in the order stated, seemed, to the human eye and ear, to have decreasing degrees of resemblance to room A. Rooms A and B were both situated about 30 ft. above ground-level overlooking eastwards a fairly busy street, but room A was the brighter of the two, as it also had windows on its north side. Both rooms contained very dark laboratory furniture, the greater quantity being in room A. Room C faced south, was about half the size of A or B, and contained laboratory furniture lighter in colour and less in quantity than that in B. It was out of earshot of the street. Room D was situated on the roof of the Medical School, and was extremely bright with white-washed walls and large windows north and west. Besides a concrete trough and odd packages it contained only a light-coloured kitchen sink in one corner.

(*ii*) *Procedure*

Experimentation was commenced only after an animal's original reactions had been recorded to the experimental cage, to the auditory signals and various other sounds, and to one or more of the rooms B, C and D. In all cases these reactions were found to be inconsequential.

Six experimental animals were subjected to the main experimental procedure (schedule I) and six to a control procedure (schedule II). In brief, it may be said that schedule II corresponds to the method for producing neuroses described by Masserman (29), and schedule I differs from it in omitting what Masserman would regard as an essential step—the conditioning of a feeding response.

Schedule I. Not more than 2 days after the control observations detailed above, the cat was reintroduced into the experimental cage and given five to ten grid-shocks, each immediately preceded by a "hoot" lasting 2 to 3 sec. The grid shocks were separated by irregular intervals ranging from 15 sec. to 2 min. With the exception of cat 8 who received five shocks in all, these animals were subjected to a second series of shocks 1 to 3 days later.

Schedule II. The first part of this schedule consisted of conditioning animals to perform food-approach responses to the buzzer. There were two variations differing from each other in a minor respect. Four of the six animals were trained to raise the lid of the food-box to the stimulus, the other two to orientate themselves to the *open* food-box. When either response had been strongly reinforced over eight to sixteen experimental sessions each consisting of about twenty reinforcements, each animal would be subjected to shocks from the floor of the cage, as follows. The buzzer had just sounded, the cat had made its learned response, the pellet had fallen into the food-box, and now the animal was moving forward to seize it. Before the pellet could be reached a grid-shock was passed into the cat which immediately recoiled, howling. Shocking under these conditions was repeated until the cat ceased to make its previous conditioned response to the buzzer. Two or three shocks were usually sufficient to accomplish this, but one cat required nine shocks distributed over three separate sessions.

(*iii*) *Immediate effects of the shock*

The immediate responses to shock followed the same pattern in all cats, whether they had previously acquired a feeding response in the experimental situation or not. This pattern was made up of various combinations of the following symptoms—rushing hither and thither, getting up on the hind-legs, clawing at the floor, roof and sides of the experimental cage, crouching, trembling, howling, spitting; mydriasis, rapid respiration, pilo-erection, and, in some cases, urination or defecation.

(*iv*) *Lasting effects of the shock*

(*a*) *Effects noted in the experimental cage.* When tested at subsequent sessions, *all* animals, irrespective of the schedule employed, displayed neurotic symptoms in the sense of the definition given at the beginning of this paper. The effects of the two schedules were broadly the same, but a few differences will be mentioned below. Three manifestations were constant and common to all animals: (1) resistance to being put into the experimental cage; (2) signs of anxiety when inside the cage (muscular tension and mydriasis were invariable); (3) *refusal to eat meat pellets anywhere in the cage even after 1, 2 or 3 day's starvation.*

Quantitative change in general activity was almost invariable. An increase or decrease was usually constant for an individual animal. Increased activity took the forms of restless roving, clawing at the wire-netting, butting the roof with the head, and ceaseless vocalizing. Decreased activity varied between tense infrequent movements in the standing posture and very intense immobile crouching.

Symptoms that were observed intermittently in all animals were hypersensitivity to "indifferent" stimuli, pilo-erection, howling, crouching, and rapid respiration.

Certain cats displayed special symptoms in addition to those that were common to all. The respiratory rate of cat 9 always rose from about 30 to about 60 as soon as he was put into the cage. Cat 15, who had micturated while being shocked, invariably micturated a few seconds after being placed in the cage. Cat 6 manifested almost continuous trembling. Cat 8 developed a symptom that it seems permissible to call hysterical. He jerked his shoulders strongly every few seconds in the experimental cage, and also in his living cage *if the experimenter entered it.* This jerking suggested an abortive jumping movement, and may well have had its origin in the fact that on the first occasion on which this animal was shocked he jumped through a hatch in the roof of the cage that had been left open inadvertently. It is worth noting that all but the first-mentioned of these four cats have been through schedule I.

Whatever symptoms an animal showed in the experimental cage were invariably *intensified by presentation of the auditory stimulus* that had been contiguous with the occurrence of the shock.

(*b*) *Generalization of neurotic responses outside experimental cage.* All cats showed some symptoms outside the experimental cage of the same kind as inside it. In two schedule I animals and four schedule II animals these effects were limited to slight tenseness and fluctuating mydriasis in the experimental room, together with inhibition of feeding responses anywhere in the room at the sound of the buzzer or "hooter" as the case might be. However, in the remaining six cats (four of schedule I, and two of schedule II) such symptoms were very marked, and were observed also outside the confines of the experimental laboratory. That is to say, they were observed in one or more of the rooms B, C and D. One animal also refused meat pellets in the passage in front of the living cages. Any animal that showed symptoms of tension in room D showed them more strongly in room C, and still more in room B. A cat free of symptoms in room B would also be free in rooms C and D. Thus it would appear that the anxiety-producing effect of these various rooms was a function of their resemblance to room A as judged in a rough way by the human eye and ear. More exactly, the magnitude of the anxiety response in room C, for instance, seems to have depended upon the number of stimuli common to rooms A and C. As will be seen below, the successful use of these rooms to build up a conditioned inhibition of the anxiety responses provides strong support for this supposition.

(*c*) *Neurotic responses to the experimenter.* Three schedule I animals developed phobic reactions towards the experimenter which were manifested even in the living cages. The jerking shoulders of cat 8 when the experimenter entered his cage have already been mentioned. Two others would crouch with pupils widely dilated as soon as they saw even his entry into the cage-house. Such effects were never noted in schedule II animals.

(*d*) *A note on some differences between the effects of the two schedules.* The general similarity between the effects of the two schedules has been mentioned. However, it is only to be expected that the preliminary conditioning of feeding reactions in schedule II animals would result in some differences. The fact that only schedule I animals became phobic towards the experimenter was noted in the last paragraph. The explanation seems to be that for schedule II cats "approach" attitudes towards the experimenter had at first been built up as a result of his previous association with feeding responses; and at the time of shocking, the experimenter was relatively remote as a stimulus since the animal was usually almost continuously oriented towards the food-box. Schedule II animals were alone found to show phobic responses to meat pellets dropped in front of them wherever they might be—starting with pupils widely dilated. This is easily understood, as these animals were responding strongly to the sight and smell of these pellets when they were shocked.

IV. Curative Measures Involving Reciprocal Inhibition

The fact that the neurotic reactions of the cats were associated with inhibition of feeding suggested that under different conditions feeding might inhibit the neurotic reactions: in other words, that the two reactions might be reciprocally inhibitory.

In order actively to inhibit the anxiety reactions the feeding would have to occur in the presence of anxiety-producing stimuli. Either, then, some factor that would favour feeding had to be added to the stimulus situation in the experimental cage, or else feeding had to be attempted somewhere *outside* the experimental cage where anxiety-producing stimuli would be less numerous and less potent. Both principles were used, as described below.

(*i*) *The addition to the experimental environment of a factor favouring feeding*

(*a*) *The human hand as a stimulus of feeding.* Since in their living cages the cats were accustomed to have food cast to them by the human hand, it was expected that the hand had become conditioned to evoke approach responses to food. Consequently, the experiment was tried of placing an animal in the experimental cage and moving towards its snout pellets of meat on the flat end of a 4 in. rod held in the experimenter's hand, in the hope that the presence of the hand would overcome the inhibition to eating. This procedure was applied to nine animals (six schedule I, and three schedule II), and after some persistence four of them (three schedule I, and one schedule II) were induced to eat. These animals at first approached a pellet hesitantly, sometimes refusing it. But after several had been eaten, they ate fairly freely from the rod, and soon after would also now and then eat a pellet on the floor of the cage or in the food-box. In the case of cat 3, the only one of these four cats that had been through schedule II (in which shock interrupted a movement towards the food-box), eating out of the food-box did not occur until he had eaten more than fifty pellets on the floor of the cage in the course of several sessions. As the number of pellets eaten in the situation increased, each of these animals ate more freely, moved about the cage with greater freedom, and showed decreasing anxiety symptoms. By the time cat 10 had eaten about fifty pellets and cat 11 about eighty they were jumping spontaneously out of the carrier into the experimental cage; and inside the cage were showing no sign of anxiety whatever. Cat 8, who, it will be remembered, had the 'hysterical' jerking movement of the shoulders, lost all traces of his symptoms only after he had eaten 216 pellets in the experimental cage in the course of eleven sessions.

(*b*) *Masserman's "forced solution."* The three schedule II cats on which the human-hand technique was not tried were each subjected to procedures based on the "forced solution" described by Masserman (29, p. 75), with like results. The essence of this method is that a hungry neurotic cat in the experimental cage is gradually pushed by means of a movable barrier towards the open food-box which contains appetizing food. This accentuates the manifestations of anxiety, but after a while the animal snatches at the food in one or more hurried gulps. Repeating the procedure over several days has the effect of diminishing and then eliminating the neurotic reactions.

(*ii*) *Feeding in the presence of relatively weak anxiety responses*

It has already been stated that the inhibition of eating, together with the rest of the neurotic picture, occurred not only in the experimental cage but also anywhere in the experimental room and in other rooms resembling this room in various ways—an effect presumably due to primary stimulus generalization (18, p. 184; 47). The slighter the resemblance of a given room to the experimental room the less marked were the anxiety reactions. In the case of the five cats who had remained unaffected by the delivery of food in the experimental cage by the human hand, it was decided to try to obtain feeding responses in the rooms where the anxiety reactions were less marked. It was thought that somewhere in this "hierarchy" of rooms there would be found for each animal a place where the anxiety responses were mild enough to permit eating at least at times. Starting in the experimental room (room A), each cat was patiently plied with meat pellets on the floor. If it did not eat after about 30 min. the experiment was repeated on the following day in the next room lower in the "hierarchy." One cat ate initially in room A, one in room B, one in room C, and one in room D. The fifth animal could not be persuaded to eat even in room D, but did so eventually in the passage that separated room D from the living cages. Once an animal had eaten in a given place it was given about twenty pellets there, always responding to their presentation with increasing rapidity, and with decreasing signs of anxiety. The next day it was tested in the room next in order of resemblance to room A. (From time to time control tests of response in the experimental cage were also made.) By this method of gradual ascent all the animals were eventually enabled to eat in room A. Then, within the room, gradual approach was made to the experimental cage in similar fashion, the animal being fed on the floor increasingly close to the experimental table, then on the table next to the cage, on the roof of the cage, and at last inside the cage. It was found that when feeding became possible in the cage anxiety reactions were much more rapidly eliminated there when the pellets were tossed at widely distributed points than if they were confined to the food-box. Apparently, scattered placing of the pellets resulted in reciprocal inhibition of the anxiety responses to stimuli from all parts of the experimental situation, and this made possible the development of conditioned inhibition of the responses to all parts (according to the mechanism discussed below), so that after 50–100 pellets had been eaten in the cage, manifestations of anxiety ceased to be observed.

(*iii*) *The elimination of neurotic responses to the conditioned auditory stimuli*

The fact that an animal, after subjection to the procedures just described, would behave without anxiety in the experimental cage can be attributed to the elimination of the neurotic responses that had previously been conditioned to the various visual (and olfactory) cues in the vicinity of the cage. But if the *auditory* stimulus that had preceded the shocks was now presented the animals again manifested a high degree of anxiety. The effect was such that the animal could be inhibited by the auditory stimulus from completing any movement towards a pellet of meat in the experimental cage, and, in most cases, at various points in the experimental room as well. The problem was to present the auditory stimulus in such a way that the anxiety reactions would be weak and there would be no inhibition of eating. There were two possible solutions to this: (1) diminishing the strength of the stimulus either by reducing its physical intensity or by increasing the distance between the animal and the stimulus; or (2) making use of the stimulus trace and the fact that the effects of a brief sensory stimulus on the nervous system gradually decline in intensity with passage of time (1). The first solution was applied to two animals and the second to seven.

(*a*) *Feeding in conjunction with the auditory stimulus at reduced strength.* Both cats upon whom this procedure was used had been through schedule I. The minimum distance at which cat 11 would eat with the conditioned auditory stimulus ("hooter") sounding continuously was found by trial and error to be 40 ft. Here, though continuously tense and mydriatic, the animal ate eight pellets, but would not eat at a point 10 ft. nearer. The next day, after two pellets at 40 ft., he ate ten at 30 ft., at first only when dropped a few inches away from him, but afterwards even at distances of 3 or 4 ft. Pellets were then dropped increasingly near the "hooter," and by the time eight more had been given he had eaten two only 17 ft. away. After eating each pellet he would run back to the 30 ft. point, or even beyond it. Day by day, the distance at which the animal would eat was reduced. When he had had a total of 160 pellets at progressively decreasing distances he was at last able to eat inside the experimental cage during the sounding of the "hooter," although manifesting considerable anxiety. At the end of his fourth session spent in eating in the cage, by which time he had eaten a total of eighty-seven pellets there, the note was made, "There is now absolutely no sign of avoidance reaction or anxiety to the auditory stimulus."

Cat 8, whose anxiety responses to the auditory stimulus were much milder than those of cat 11 at the commencement of this procedure ate as little as 20 ft. away from the "hooter" in the beginning, and required only thirty-three pellets at decreasing distances to enable him to eat in the presence of the sound in the experimental cage. He lost all tenseness there after forty-five pellets given over four sessions.

(*b*) *Feeding in the presence of the trace of the conditioned auditory stimulus.* Four of the cats treated in this way had been through schedule I and the other three through schedule II. The animal was placed inside the experimental cage, and though showing no sign of disturbance was given one or two meat pellets on the floor of the cage. Then, after an interval of about a minute, the auditory stimulus was sounded for about one-fifth of a second, and *immediately afterwards* a pellet was dropped in front of the animal, who had in the meantime become tense and hunched-up, with pilo-erection and mydriasis. After a variable interval, usually about 30 sec., the animal would have lost most of its tenseness and would move forward cautiously to the pellet and eat it. Not less than 1 min. later, the auditory stimulus would again be presented, making the cat tense, and be followed by a meat pellet, but this time the animal would eat after a shorter interval. This procedure was repeated 10 to 20 times during a session, and the interval before the eating of the pellet would gradually diminish until the animal ate without delay. In illustration of the above, the intervals recorded (in seconds) for one cat during the first session of this kind were: 40, 15, 20, 7, 5, 6, 6, 6, 4, 8, 8, 11, 4, 6, 4, 4, 5, 3, and 4. At the next session the invervals were 3, 3, 2, 3, 2 and 2 sec. for the first six presentations of stimulus, and thereafter she consistently responded practically at once.

The next step was *to increase the duration of the auditory stimulus.* First, every fourth or fifth stimulus was given a duration of about a second; and then, gradually, depending on the responses of the animal, the duration was increased. Eventually, the animal would show no vestige of anxiety even to a stimulus of 30 sec. duration, and would make alert food-seeking movements as soon as she heard the auditory stimulus.

(*c*) *Demonstration that the neurotic reactions were not merely overshadowed.* Whichever of the above two procedures had been employed, the question remained whether the neurotic reactions had really been eliminated or had merely been overshadowed by a stronger reaction of feeding beneath which they lay dormant. The decisive experiment was *to extinguish the food-seeking response to the auditory stimulus* and then observe whether or not the neurotic reactions were reinstated. Each of the animals was given thirty irregularly massed extinction trials on each of three successive days. Long before the end of the third day's session they all showed almost complete indifference to the auditory stimulus. Immediately after the conclusion of the third extinction session the following test was made. A pellet was dropped on the floor of the experimental cage about 2 ft. away from the animal, and as he began to approach it the auditory signal was sounded continuously, to see if extinction had reinstated the inhibitory effect on eating that had originally been noted. *In no instance was there observed any semblance of the restoration of an anxiety response or any suggestion of an inhibition of eating.* Moreover, observation for many weeks afterwards never revealed recurrence of anxiety responses in any animal.

V. Interpretations of the Present Results

(*i*) *Conformity of the behaviour changes to definition of experimental neurosis*

According to the definition given at the beginning of this paper an experimental neurosis has to satisfy criteria of anxiety, unadaptiveness and persistence. The prominence of anxiety is sufficiently obvious from the account of the experiments and need not be discussed further.

Unadaptiveness was shown in two ways—the inhibition of feeding responses in a hungry animal in a situation in which feeding would not again be followed by shock (and in the case of schedule I animals had never been followed by shock); and the mere fact that the anxious responses were causing fatigue without in any way favouring the organism's life processes (i.e. were without reward).

The criterion of persistence was satisfied by: (1) maintenance of tenseness and other manifestations at an undiminishing level throughout a long session; (2) recurrence of manifestations at unabated strength session after session; and (3) re-evocation of manifestations after long periods free from experimentation, for example, in all of three cats rested for 6 months.

The following extract from the protocols of cat 7 (schedule I) illustrates the unremittingness of the neurotic tension and shows how complete the inhibition of feeding could be.

> On September 1, 1947, seven days after she had been shocked, cat 7 was taken when hungry to the experimental laboratory. She resisted being put into the experimental cage. Inside the cage, she crouched with pupils widely dilated. She was kept there for 2 hours, during which her pupils remained dilated, although their size fluctuated a good deal, reaching a maximum at any sharp sound or sudden movement. At times

> she became very restless, mewed plaintively, and clawed at the sides of the cage. She showed no response at all to meat pellets put in front of her nose on an ebony rod, and left untouched a pellet which lay on the floor of the cage during the whole of her two hours' confinement.

(ii) *Why the behaviour changes are regarded as learned*

In order to decide whether or not the neurotic behaviour was learned it is necessary first to define what is to be understood by the term *learning*. Learning may be said to have occurred if a response has been evoked in temporal contiguity with a given sensory stimulus, and it is subsequently found that the stimulus can evoke the response although it could not have done so before. If the stimulus could have evoked the response before but subsequently evokes it more strongly, then, too, learning may be said to have occurred.

In the case of our experimental cats there was no qualitative difference between the immediate responses to the shock and the later responses to the experimental environment. In other words, the responses produced by the shock in the originally "neutral" experimental environment were subsequently found to be producible by the experimental environment itself. This clearly implies the occurrence of learning as defined above. It was particularly well shown in the development of the "special" symptoms noted earlier. For example, the cat that displayed the jerking shoulders was the one that had once jumped out of the cage when shocked, and the one that regularly micturated in the experimental cage and micturated when shocked.

Furthermore, it will be seen below that these experiments embody other features that make the results easily explicable in terms of modern knowledge of the learning process.

(iii) *The present results in the light of modern learning theory*

(*a*) *Preliminary remarks on modern learning theory*. By modern learning theory is meant the recently developed body of psychological theory associated largely with the name of C. L. Hull (18). Involving a rigorous scientific discipline and placing much emphasis on quantification, this body of theory has gone far towards raising the methodological level of psychology to that of the older sciences. To-day it increasingly dominates the literature of American experimental and theoretical psychology.

A few of the basic notions of modern learning theory must be briefly mentioned. They derive essentially from Hull's classic work (18), but are modified in certain respects out of consideration of recent neurophysiological knowledge (44, 45, 47, 48, 49).

In 1938, Culler (7) showed in dogs that when a semitendinosus response was established to a tone, stimulation of a point found by trial and error on the exposed cortex also evoked the response, and ceased to do so if the response to the tone was extinguished. This finding strongly supports the supposition that learning is subserved by the development of conductivity between neurones in anatomical apposition. Numerous experiments have demonstrated that in a given learning situation there is a direct quantitative relationship between the amount of learning that occurs and the magnitude of the associated drive reduction. It has been argued elsewhere (45) that if learning has a neural basis, then it is through reduction of a feature common to all drives—*central neural excitation*—that drive reduction subserves learning. The strength of central neural excitation can be appraised indirectly by knowledge of stimulus strength or of response strength. (In the case of human subjects, some indication of strength of drive can, of course, be obtained from reports of experience.)

The process of *elimination* of learned reactions is conceived to involve the weakening of neural connexions previously formed during learning. The process occurs in either of two ways—extinction or reciprocal inhibition, and in both of them drive reduction plays as important a part as in learning. In the case of *extinction* the drive concerned is the fatigue-associated state of disequilibrium having its origin in the effector organs subserving the response—the Mowrer-Miller hypothesis (18, p. 277; 32, 35). *Reciprocal inhibition* implies that in the presence of stimuli that would lead to the given response, another, incompatible and stronger response is enabled to occur, and the given response is inhibited (49). In such cases, an obvious drive reduction is always provided by the reciprocal inhibition of the excitation that would have led to the given response; and if the response that was dominant is rewarded its drive is also reduced.

(*b*) *The learning process in the present experiments.* Reasons were given above for deciding that the neurotic reactions of our cats were learned. The high intensity of the reactions after very few shocks can be accounted for on the basis that a very powerful drive reduction occurred *at the cessation of each shock.* The responses occurring at the time of the cessation became strongly connected thereby to stimuli from the experimental environment. These responses comprised musculoskeletal movements tending away from the situation and autonomic responses evidenced, for example, by muscular tenseness, mydriasis, and pilo-erection. The whole picture was one of "anxiety."

After the first shocking, stimuli from the experimental environment were already able to elicit some measure of anxiety responses, and these, of course, had an anxiety-drive state as an antecedent. In other words, the environmental stimuli had become able to arouse a secondary (i.e. learned) drive state. Reduction of this secondary drive by the removal of the animal from the experimental environment would further reinforce the anxiety responses as responses to the stimuli of that environment. O. H. Mowrer (33, 34) was the first to recognize the role of anxiety reduction as a reinforcing agent. Other workers who have demonstrated this are Farber (13), May (30), and Miller (31).

(*c*) *The factor of confinement.* Anderson & Liddell (1) have pointed out that all animal neuroses have been produced in conditions of confined space. Cook's experiments (6), employing different degrees of space constriction with other factors constant, indicate that it is a potent factor in neurosis production. There are at least three ways in which confinement could exert its influence.

First, the prevention of an effective escape response allows the cumulative action on the animal of stimuli that have become conditioned to anxiety, so that there is a rising magnitude of potentially reducible anxiety drive. Secondly, the drive reductions occur in the presence of a limited number of stimuli, and the anxiety responses can be conditioned to these in greater strength than would be the case if the environment were a changing one. Thirdly, it seems likely that autonomic responses are stronger when freed from the reciprocally inhibiting effects of musculo-skeletal responses (51).

(*d*) *The reason for persistence of the neurotic responses* (*resistance to extinction*). As stated under (*a*), learned responses that are unrewarded (and so unadaptive) ordinarily undergo extinction by a mechanism that is associated with fatigue. Since fatigue occurs whether there is reward or not, there is *always* a fatigue-associated drive state that tends towards a weakening of the connexion between the response and the stimulus that led to it. But it is only when there is no significant reward that the connexion is *actually* weakened (18, p. 298). When reward counteracts this tendency towards weakening it does so through reducing the central drive state due to, say, hunger.

Now, the neurotic responses are unrewarded (unadaptive). Yet they necessarily have a central state of drive as an antecedent. This drive is automatically reduced by the retreat of the organism from the anxiety-producing stimulus, or by any other means that removes the organism from the action of this stimulus. Any responses that may be occurring at such a time will be reinforced, and their fatigue-associated tendency to be extinguished will be counteracted. Farber (13) has presented a clear demonstration in rats of the manner in which anxiety drive reduction interferes with extinction.

Frequently repeated or continuous consequents of the anxiety drive (of which the autonomic responses are an example) are much more likely to coincide in time with drive reductions than are responses that occur only occasionally. That is why, in our experiments, the autonomic responses, whose evocation was continuous, were always persistent, whereas such intermittent responses as clawing the sides of the cage were soon extinguished. It is important to note that these autonomic responses were reinforced even though they did not themselves bring about removal from the shock.

(*e*) *The mechanism of cure.* The effectiveness of the procedures that overcame the neurotic responses can be accounted for as follows: in every instance feeding was made possible in the presence of stimuli conditioned to anxiety responses which, under other circumstances, inhibited feeding. When stimuli to incompatible responses are present simultaneously the occurrence of the response that is dominant in the circumstances involves the reciprocal inhibition of the other. As the number of feedings increased, the anxiety responses gradually became weaker, so that to stimuli to which there was initially a response of the anxiety pattern there was finally a feeding response with inhibition of anxiety. This "permanent" change implies a new positive conditioning *pari passu* with a conditioning of inhibition, and this could have been subserved by at least two drive reductions—hunger drive reduction, and reduction by the reciprocal inhibition itself of the drive antecedent to the anxiety responses. That the conditioned inhibition was due to a *neural change* and was not merely a correlate of the occurrence of the alternative response seems a clear inference from the fact that eventual extinction of the alternative response did not result in reinstatement of the original one. This mechanism has been more fully discussed elsewhere (49).

At this point it is necessary to comment on Masserman's interpretation of the cures obtained by the "forced solution." He states (29, p. 203) that with the cat maximally hungry and the food very attractive, at a certain proximity to the food, the food-approach drive reached such an intensity as to break through the animal's inhibitions; and 'once the motivational impasse was disrupted, the feeding behaviour soon became more natural . . . and the other neurotic manifestations rapidly diminished in intensity.' Now, it can scarcely be doubted that the creation of a very intense drive to feed makes it possible to overcome the inhibitory effects of the anxiety state at a given moment. But it is still necessary to explain how the feeding results in a "permanent" decrease in anxiety. It is by no means self-evident that the momentary overcoming of an inhibition implies the breaking of a *habit* of inhibition, as Masserman seems to think.

VIII. Clinical Implications

Since 1947 the writer has studied a large number of human cases of neurosis with a view to determining to what extent their causation parallels that of the experimental neuroses. The findings of these investigations can only be summarily mentioned here.

From the outset, the fact that in human case-histories, too, conflict or trauma or both are invariably found seemed to support the idea of a common basis; and the experience of the past 4 years has encouraged belief in the hypothesis that experimental and clinical neuroses are parallel phenomena. Some of the similarities, discussed at some length in a dissertation (43), have been briefly reported (46).

The human subject is not often forced to undergo his conflicts or his traumata in physically confined space. He is usually kept in the anxiety-producing situation by the force of habits previously learned. For instance, a woman entangled in a humiliating marriage may be unable to get out of it because her earlier training has given a horror to the idea of divorce. Besides confining her within the marriage, this feeling of horror, being in conflict with escape tendencies, makes possible the development of a high level of emotional tension (anxiety). This tension becomes increasingly conditioned to contiguous stimuli through the drive reductions that follow every partial escape from the causative situation.

In therapy, the writer has concentrated on seeking means of obtaining reciprocal inhibition of anxiety responses, after the pattern that was so successful in animals. In the great majority of cases reciprocal inhibition of anxiety has in fact been procurable, either in the interview situation or the life situation, always with results that are beneficial, sometimes in a most dramatic way. The methods used and their effects are discussed in detail elsewhere (50). In an earlier communication (46) reasons were given for supposing that the similar amounts of success obtained by therapies differing widely in character are largely due to something common to all interview situations—reciprocal inhibition of anxiety responses by more powerful antagonistic emotional responses evoked in the patient by the therapist and by the interview situation in general.

References

1. ANDERSON, O. D., & LIDDELL, H. S. (1935). Observations on experimental neurosis in sheep. *Arch. Neurol. Psychiat.* XXXIV, 330–54.
2. ANDERSON, O. D., & PARMENTER, R. (1941). A long term study of the experimental neurosis in the sheep and dog. *Psychosom. Med. Monogr.* II, nos. 3 and 4.
3. BABKIN, B. P. (1938). Experimental neuroses in animals and their treatment with bromides. *Edinb. Med. J.* XLV, 605–19.
4. BAJANDUROW, B. (1932). Zur Psychologie des Sehenanalysators bei Vogeln. Z. *vergl. Physiol.* XVIII, 288–306. Quoted by Cook (5).
5. COOK, S. W. (1939). A survey of methods used to produce 'experimental neurosis.' *Amer. J. Psychiat.* XCV, 1259–76.
6. COOK, S. W. (1939). The production of 'experimental neurosis' in the white rat. *Psychosom. Med.* I, 293–308.
7. CULLER, E. (1938). Observations on direct cortical stimulation in the dog. *Psychol. Bull.* XXXV, 687–8.
8. DIMMICK, F. L., LUDLOW, N., & WHITEMAN, A. (1939). A study of 'experimental neurosis' in cats. *J. Comp. Psychol.* XXVIII, 39–43.
9. DWORKIN, S. (1939). Conditioning neuroses in dog and cat. *Psychosom. Med.* I, 388–96.
10. DWORKIN, S., BAXT, J. O., & DWORKIN, E. (1942). Behavioural disturbances of vomiting and micturition in conditioned cats. *Psychosom. Med.* IV, 75–81.
11. DWORKIN, S., RAGINSKY, B. B., & BOURNE, W. (1937). Action of anaesthetics and sedatives upon the inhibited nervous system. *Curr. Res. Anaesth.* XVI, 238–40.
12. ESTES, W. K. (1944). An experimental study of punishment. *Psychol. Monogr.* LVII, no. 263.
13. FARBER, I. E. (1948). Response fixation under anxiety and non-anxiety conditions. *J. Exp. Psychol.* XXXVIII, 111–31.
14. FENICHEL, O. (1945). *The Psychoanalytic Theory of Neurosis.* New York: Norton.
15. FINGER, F. W. (1945). Abnormal animal behaviour and conflict. *Psychol. Rev.* LII, 230–40.
16. GANTT, W. H. (1944). Experimental basis for neurotic behaviour. *Psychosom. Med. Monogr.* III, nos. 3 and 4.
17. HEBB, D. O. (1947). Spontaneous neurosis in chimpanzees: theoretical relations with clinical and experimental phenomena. *Psychosom. Med.* IX, 3–16.
18. HULL, C. L. (1943). *Principles of Behaviour*, New York: Appleton.
19. ISCHLONDSKY, N. E. (1944). Quoted by Gantt (16), pp. 180–1.
20. JACOBSEN, C. F., WOLFE, J. B., & JACKSON, T. A. (1935). An experimental analysis of the functions of frontal association areas in primates. *J. Nerv. Ment. Dis.* LXXXII, 1–14.
21. KARN, H. W. (1938). A case of experimentally induced neurosis in the cat. *J. Exp. Psychol.* XXII, 589–92.
22. KARN, H. W. (1940). The experimental study of neurotic behaviour in infrahuman animals. *J. Gen. Psychol.* XXII, 431–6.
23. KRASNOGORSKI, N. I. (1925). The conditioned reflexes and children's neurosis. *Amer. J. Dis. Child.* XXX, 754–68.

24. LIDDELL, H. S. (1944). Conditioned reflex method and experimental neurosis. In Hunt, J. McV., *Personality and the Behaviour Disorders*. New York: Ronald Press.
25. LIDDELL, H. S., & BAYNE, T. L. (1927). The development of 'experimental neurasthenia' in sheep during the formation of difficult conditioned reflexes. *Amer. J. Physiol.* LXXXI, 494.
26. MAIER, N. R. F. (1949). *Frustration: The Study of Behaviour Without a Goal.* New York: McGraw-Hill.
27. MAIER, N. R. F., & GLASER, N. M. (1942). Studies of abnormal behaviour in the rat. IX. Factors which influence the occurrence of seizures during auditory stimulation. *J. Comp. Psychol.* XXXIV, 11–21.
28. MAIER, N. R. F., & LONGHURST, J. V. (1947). Studies of abnormal behaviour in the rat. XXI. Conflict and audiogenic seizures. *J. Comp. Psychol.* XL, 397–412.
29. MASSERMAN, J. H. (1943). *Behaviour and Neurosis.* Chicago: University of Chicago Press.
30. MAY, M. A. (1948). Experimentally acquired drives. *J. Exp. Psychol.* XXXVIII, 66–77.
31. MILLER, N. E. (1948). Studies of fear as an acquirable drive. I. Fear as motivation and fear-reduction as reinforcement in the learning of new responses. *J. Exp. Psychol.* XXXVIII, 89–101.
32. MILLER, N. E. & DOLLARD, J. (1941). *Social Learning and Imitation.* New Haven: Yale University Press.
33. MOWRER, O. H. (1939). A stimulus-response analysis of anxiety and its role as a reinforcing agent. *Psychol. Rev.* XLVI, 553–65.
34. MOWRER, O. H. (1940). Anxiety-reduction and learning. *J. Exp. Psychol.* XXVII, 497–516.
35. MOWRER, O. H., & JONES, H. M. (1943). Extinction and behaviour variability as a function of effortfulness of task. *J. Exp. Psychol.* XXXIII, 369–86.
36. PAVLOV, I. P. (1927). *Conditioned Reflexes.* Transl. G. V. Anrep. London: Oxford University Press.
37. PAVLOV, I. P. (1928). *Lectures on Conditioned Reflexes.* Transl. W. H. Gantt. New York: Liveright.
38. PETROVA, M. K. (1935). New data concerning the mechanisms of the action of bromides on the higher nervous activity. Moscow. Quoted by Babkin (3).
39. RUSSELL, R. W. (1950). The comparative study of 'conflict' and 'experimental neurosis.' *Brit. J. Psychol.* XLI, 95–108.
40. THORNDIKE, E. L. (1932). Reward and punishment in animal learning. *Comp. Psychol. Monogr.* VIII, no. 39.
41. WARREN, H. C. (1935). *Dictionary of Psychology.* London: Allen and Unwin.
42. WATSON, J. B., & RAYNER, R. (1920). Conditioned emotional reactions. *J. Exp. Psychol.* III, 1–14.
43. WOLPE, J. (1948). An approach to the problem of neurosis based on the conditioned response. M.D. Thesis, University of the Witwatersrand.
44. WOLPE, J. (1949). An interpretation of the effects of combination of stimuli (patterns) based on current neurophysiology. *Psychol. Rev.* LVI, 277–83.
45. WOLPE, J. (1950). Need-reduction, drive-reduction, and reinforcement: a neurophysiological view. *Psychol. Rev.* LVII, 19–26.
46. WOLPE, J. (1950). The genesis of neurosis: an objective account. *S. Afr. Med. J.* XXIV, 613–16.
47. WOLPE, J. (1952). Primary stimulus generalisation: a neurophysiological view. *Psychol. Rev.* LIX, 8–11.
48. WOLPE, J. (1952). The neurophysiology of learning and delayed reward learning. *Psychol. Rev.* LIX, 192–9.
49. WOLPE, J. (1952). The formation of negative habits: a neurophysiological view. *Psychol. Rev.* LIX, 290–9.
50. WOLPE, J. (1952). Objective psychotherapy of the neuroses. *S. Afr. Med. J.* (In the press.)
51. WOLPE, J. (1952). Learning theory and 'abnormal fixations.' To be published.

BERNARD J. SOMERS

Reevaluation Therapy: Theoretical Framework[1]

Cathartic approaches to treatment of behavior disorders have risen in popularity in recent years. Many group movements as well as individual therapeutic approaches, such as Gestalt Therapy, Reichian analysis, and the dramatic "Primal Scream" therapy originated by Janov, heavily stress the release of primitive feelings presumably inhibited and stored over many years as a consequence of life's frustrations.

The following paper by Somers details the theoretical underpinning of a cathartic approach originated by Harvey Jackins, as well as the therapeutic procedures that follow from this theory. Presumably, the theory can be used to account for psychotic as well as neurotic behavior. However, Jackins' clinical work, and that of most therapists stressing catharsis has been done primarily with neurotics and personality disorders.

In the editing of the article, material comparing Jackins' approach to other therapeutic approaches has been omitted. The reader interested in this aspect of the presentation is invited to consult the original source.

Introduction

This article presents the theoretical framework for the practice of Reevaluation Therapy and describes similarities with the concepts and methods of other orientations in counseling and psychotherapy. An earlier paper (Somers, 1971) described a special modality within Reevaluation Therapy known as the *cocounseling workshop* in which group members are trained to exchange effective help in therapeutic partnerships. A future paper will present empirical findings regarding the outcome of cocounseling workshops. The

[1] The author is thankful to Harvey Jackins, Jerry Saltzman, and Leonora Somers for their attentive reading of an earlier draft of this paper.

Abridged from *Journal of Humanistic Psychology*, **12** (1972), 42–56, with the permission of the Association for Humanistic Psychology and Dr. Somers.

article by Scheff (1972) presents a discussion of Reevaluation Therapy viewed as a peer self-help movement and considers its social implications.

Recent Developments in the Therapy Field

In the past decade we have observed an accelerated interest in a philosophically based as well as scientifically rooted approach to psychotherapy—the former known as the humanists and the latter as the behaviorists in counseling and psychotherapy.

The humanistic group favors a holistic and value-based orientation in the helping relationship (Bugental, 1967). A democratization of this relationship is sought by some (Steinzor, 1969). Authenticity of presence for both helper and helped is often endorsed. The human being is regarded as a full organism, not an empty vessel into which experience is poured and shaped by contingency alone. Their focus is also upon the positive, creative, loving and cooperative forces in each of us. Workers such as Rogers (1957), May (1969), Bugental (1965), Otto (1969), Maslow (1967), and Shostrom (1967), and the Gestalt therapists and the developers of growth centers are examples of persons working within the broad humanistic framework. Within this humanistic cluster there are frameworks which fail to be explicit enough to generate testable hypotheses. And often there is a failure to specify therapeutic procedures necessary to implement the humanistic values so eloquently articulated. In some instances, the detailed specification of procedures is applicable only to a narrow clinical or nonclinical population.

Behavior therapy has become an active force in the therapy field, in training and practice as well as research. It has a creditable list of accomplishments in the modification of a variety of disturbed and fixated behaviors (Yates, 1970). Behavior therapists also have raised fundamental questions about the claims, theories and methods of traditional, dynamically oriented therapies as well as the newer therapies in our field (Ullman & Krasner, 1969). Their procedures are rather clearly specified and replicable. The value-orientation is usually implicit rather than explicit in the work of the behaviorist. Underlying assumptions about the positive forces in each of us are typically unexamined yet pervade the work of behavior therapists. The major emphasis in the behavioristic therapeutic procedure is in the creation of contingencies which reinforce certain responses and extinguish others. The inner, recovery capacitites of the patient are not designated. Facilitating conditions which will activate and release these positive forces within the individual are also not fully specified.

A theoretical framework is needed which assumes and specifies the positive, creative, actualizing forces in all of us, and indicates the nature of those internal and external conditions which stifle and limit these positive forces. Maslow's theoretical system lies in this direction, yet it is not linked in a specific manner with a therapeutic system of concepts and procedures. From a set of hypotheses describing what happens to impede the basic, growth-producing forces in all of us, we can specify the conditions and procedures which will activate those forces seemingly absent or partially obscured in people.

Reevaluation Therapy[2]

Man's core being

Reevaluation Therapy proceeds with the working hypothesis that all humans possess a *core being* comprising qualities of lovingness, zest, intelligence, cooperativeness, curiosity and communicativeness. Specifically, the perspective holds that our basic tendency as humans is to: love ourselves and one another; act rationally; enjoy what we do; cooperate with one another; explore and discover more about each other, our planet and the cosmos, past, present and future; communicate well with one another. These assumptions are more specific than those of the humanistic group (Cantril, 1965). They permeate the consciousness and the activities of the reevaluation therapist because of his own experience in contacting his core self through the continuing process of Reevaluation Therapy.

Many therapists of different persuasions work with at least some of these assumptions about man's core being. For example, Rogers (1957) has specified certain conditions that facilitate movement in psychotherapy (i.e., therapist's transparency or congruency, empathy, and unconditional positive regard). The helper's experiencing of his own core being is the more critical condition that is generating Rogers' necessary and sufficient conditions for movement in psychotherapy. The helper who has made firm and full contact with his own core being freely gives attention to the patient and believes in the patient's underlying core being. Too often the helper maintains an aware intellectual belief in the growth potential of his patient at the sacrifice of his own emotional well-being. His theoretical system and/or his own therapeutic experiences have not sufficiently confirmed a belief in man's core being.

Distress and Discharge

If all human beings possess this core being, then the obvious questions are: Whatever happened to us? What went wrong? How is it that our core being is so often fully or partially obscured?

As every young child moves through his or her world with natural curiosity, zest and interest, there occur various contingencies which *distress* him or her: indifference, frightening events, scoldings, frustrating obstacles and disappointments, punishment, physical hurts, and ridicule. The events are

[2] Much of what follows is based on the work of Harvey Jackins who, over a twenty-year period, has developed the principles and practice of Reevaluation Therapy and the modality of cocounseling (Jackins, 1964, 1965).

experienced in the form of noxious emotions such as fear, pain, anger, grief, disappointment, sadness, humiliation, embarrassment, shame, etc. If the distressed child is not exposed to interference by others, he or she will discharge the distress thoroughly in the presence of an attentive, noncritical, supportive person. The *discharge process* has its external manifestations in: crying, shaking, trembling, shivering, laughing, raging, screaming, violet movements, blushing, perspiring, yawning, stretching, and eager and reluctant non-repetitive talking. The unsocialized child discharges spontaneously. As socialization takes place, the young child is conditioned to limit or extinguish discharge entirely. Males in our culture are exposed to greater taboos about discharge than are females. Zaslow and Breger (1969) call this distress-discharge cycle the "stress-relaxation" cycle. They point out the importance of the parenting one helping the stressed child to remain in physical contact with the adult so that the stress reaction can be "worked through," that is, the child can return to his normal state of relaxation and spontaneity. They emphasize the working through of rage—yet note the acceptance of their patient's crying and laughter. In our theoretical framework, other distresses and forms of discharge would be included in Zaslow and Breger's concept of the stress-relaxation cycle.

The child is helped to discharge, as adults are also, by the existence of a proper balance of attention in the distressed person. This balance of attention is between present time (some other person who is warmly attentive and supportive) and the reactive material (the inner, experienced distress). The child who is frightened by the barking dog next door will, upon seeing his mother, begin to shake, more likely to cry and talk about the event. When he stops crying and the mother maintains her warm, noninterfering attention, the child will resume crying, talking, trembling and follow a sequence of various types of discharge. When there is an absence of an attentive person for the child, some discharge may occur, although there may be none, and the child may be overwhelmed with his distress. The continuing free attention of a supportive adult will help the child drain off *all* of his hurt, fear, anger, disappointment, embarrassment, etc., by discharge. Typically, adults, including us therapists, are not concious of the need for *full* discharge in the distressed child as well as adult.

When the conditions of safety and noninterference with the distressed person are met, discharge tends to proceed in a sequence from "heavy" forms of discharge to "light" forms: crying and sobbing; shaking and trembling; laughter and cold perspiration; shouting, violent movement and warm perspiration; reluctant talking, animated talking and laughter, to happy relaxation and the turning of attention away from the distress. Adults discharging on old, stored-up distresses seem to follow the sequence once they reach the crying form of discharge.

Discharge, then, is a natural recovery process easily available to all human beings in infancy and early childhood. It is still potentially available, though inhibited to different degrees for adults. Reevaluation Therapy views each person, whether adult or child, as capable of regaining all of his or her discharge capacity. The term "recovery process" indicates that what is recovered, with adequate discharge, is our core being, which was temporarily obscured by the distress.

Misstorage and restimulation

What happens when the discharge does not take place or is interrupted prematurely? The internal distress tends to persist in consciousness. The distressed person receives *all* of the information of the distress incident. Cognitive processes and other aspects of the core being are constricted. The cognitive processes include: free attention (the person's alertness; openness to experience; absence of perceptual set; self-transcending objectivity); reasoning; conceptualizing skills; planning; remembering; and decision-making skills. The brain seems to misstore the information recorded during the event along with the negative emotion itself. This process may be likened to repression. Ego defense mechanisms are active in maintaining repression at the cost of intellectual efficiency. The distressed person is not able to think clearly. The negative emotions interfere with the free attention available to a person when he is not distressed. Rationality, used here to embrace all cognitive processes, is normally available in large amounts to the undistressed person. Rationality is the synthesizing capacity of each of us to provide a specific, appropriate, and unique response to each and every encounter with the human and nonhuman world. Distress prevents this peculiarly human function from operating. Discharge allows rationality to return to function. Accumulated, undischarged distress becomes associated with the repeated constriction and weakening of rationality. As the result of such repetitive constriction and weakening, we can assume that most of us are functioning on a very small percentage of our inherent rational capacity.

If discharge does not take place on the original, primary distress, recurrence of cues similar to the originally distressing one will cause *restimulation.* The originally undischarged distress is again experienced in restimulation. Most, if not all, of the cognitive aspects of the original event are not functional. Restimulation brings forth all of the controlling and coping mechanisms associated with handling the inner distress and the external stimulus evoking the distress (e.g., scolding from foreman arouses hurt and anger, based on undischarged distress from an earlier, familial experience; person withdraws, avoids foreman and others while restimulated, and stops the instigation to discharge; person cannot think of rational ways to deal with the foreman on a direct or indirect basis). Restimulation has some similarity to the transference reaction. It is seen here as some negative emotion, never fully discharged, and accompanying cognitive aspects, which are aroused by an experience in one's present life which is, in some respects, similar to another from the past that was the source of distress.

Reevaluation and responsibility

When old distress is discharged, information and cognitive processes associated with the distressing event return to awareness. With the return to awareness of information and activation of the cognitive processes constricted by the undischarged distress, we can expect: increased rationality; freer attention; insight and behavior change. In sum, *reevaluation* of the distress incident and information contained therein takes place. Insight and behavioral change are based on a fuller appraisal of oneself, and the relationships and events associated with the distressing experience. The "insight work" is in the hands of the patient, taking place spontaneously and correlatively with the flow of discharge as well as afterwards. Reevaluation has some similarity to the psychoanalytic concept of abreaction in which the patient, through free associational activity, experiences the "return of the repressed," the reliving of the experience followed by insight. In abreaction the patient usually discharges. From the perspective of Reevaluation Therapy, abreactions are usually incomplete discharges. Following exhaustive discharge, the patient will recall the distressing events and information in much greater detail. Some therapists knowingly work to help their patients repeat their abreactions again and again until the discharge is complete.

As reevaluation takes place with greater frequency due to frequent discharge on different distresses, the person experiences a greater sense of control over himself and his environment. Rationality, comprising all cognitive or ego functions, is heightened. One's core being becomes more operative, exerting greater dominance over feeling and behavior. Such a state of existential affairs is synonymous with owning responsibility for oneself, freedom to experience a rich variety of alternatives and make the most rational choice among them. With more discharge, and therefore more reevaluation, there is an increase in the individual's hopefulness for himself and others, and a forgiving attitude towards those persons who have distressed him in the present as well as the past. The increase in rationality makes it possible to create the most effective solution for those conditions and people in one's life that continue to oppress and distress.

Chronic and intermittent patterns

As restimulation occurs in much of one's waking existence, distresses accumulate to a great depth in all people. Restimulation involves re-experiencing of such feelings as hurt, anger, pain, fear, humiliation and disappointment without discharge, along with the addition of newly received information to the rigid pattern. As the distresses are restimulated and reexperienced sufficiently, certain patterns of thought, word, posture and action become chronic. Additional ways of communicating the distress are added. Attempts to cope with the distressing feelings and situations are made and are also added to the total reaction. The person in his chronic pattern has diminished rationality and loss of free attention and judgment. Reasoning, conceptualizing and information retrieval skills are lessened. In addition to the primary distress reexperienced under restimulation, the chronic pattern tends to create additional (secondary) distress. Secondary distresses are evoked by the reactions of others who are alienated, frightened, frustrated and/or hurt by the chronic pattern of the person. Each adult has chronic patterns—behaviors that are present during a large part of one's waking existence.

In summary, a chronic pattern is the fusion of: restimulation of old distress: repeated reenactment in some form of the original distress experience, modified and added to by later restimulating experiences; acquired mechanisms of control over the instigation to discharge; coping mechanisms that reduce the negative affect chronically restimulated; acquired behavior that seeks to terminate or avoid the distressing cues and restimulation; secondary distresses stimulated by feedback from others distressed by the person's chronic pattern. Several examples of chonic patterns will illustrate the components just described.

Complaining depressive—Chronic restimulation: Both external and internal cues continuously present themselves, and restimulate old disappointments, losses, hurts, sadness, perhaps anger and fear, while cognitive aspects of the old experiences remain in the background. Control over discharge: Subvocal statements such as "I mustn't cry," "Only babies cry," "I shouldn't scream." Coping mechanisms that reduce the negative affect: Anger, blaming, and self-doubting may control distressing cues; the person refuses to accept flattery, or avoids an encounter where success or acceptance is possible but not certain. Anticipatory behavior: The person looks sad much of the time and talks of anticipated failure. Secondary distress: Others are irritated and feel rebuffed by the complainer's preoccupation with criticism and lack of attention to the listener as a person—the listener rejects or avoids the complaining depressive.

Paranoid behavior—Chronic restimulation: Cues which are internal, but more likely perceived as external, present themselves continuously, restimulating primary distresses of hurt, fear and humiliation in which the persons who originally caused the distress typically denied their culpability. Control over discharge: The instigation to discharge is often obscured, with feelings of humiliation and attendant rage controlled by dramatized attribution and blame. Coping mechanisms that reduce the negative affect: Rumination and referential thinking. Behavior that seeks to terminate or avoid the distressing cues: Withdrawal, attack. Anticipatory behavior: The anxious suspicious look communicating an expectation of harm, criticism, etc. Secondary distress: Evoked when others retaliate with hostility and avoidance on being accused of doing or conspiring to do harm.

In addition to chronic patterns, there are *intermittent* or *episodic patterns* which express the individual's characteristic style of responding to a restimulating event that does not occur on a frequency basis. (Example: In the face of meeting people for the first time, an individual may be very fearful, appear glassy-eyed, stutter, and generally seem to be decompensating.) All of the components of the chronic pattern referred to previously would apply in the case of an intermittent pattern.

The therapeutic relationship

One of the tasks of Reevaluation Therapy is to facilitate the reinstatement of the natural recovery process of discharge. As mentioned earlier, this discharge process takes place under conditions of balanced attention on the part of the distressed person. The balance is between the reactive material (the distress) and the present time (the therapist and the reassuring environment). There is some elasticity in the amount of attention that can be given to one aspect at the expense of the other. And there are limits to the imbalance that can be tolerated while still permitting discharge to take place. For example, the patient can be so attentive to the therapist that he cannot attend to his own distresses, thus preventing discharge. On the other hand, the patient can be so involved with his reactive material that he is overwhelmed by negative affect, does not discharge and may, in fact, experience some distressing physical symptoms such as headaches and nausea. In addition to the proper balance of attention that facilitates discharge, such conditions as experiencing trust and the therapist's expectation of the patient's imminent discharge should also be included.

Even where the proper balance of attention has been struck between subjectively felt distress and the warm, attentive listener, discharge may still not take place. *Control mechanisms* are operating which prevent discharge. These mechanisms are part of the distress recording itself. They include external, visible actions as well as internal, sometimes subliminal ones. They are usually added to the recording in a social context and follow operant principles. From our earliest years we are admonished to stop crying, screaming, shaking, raging, etc. The cultural conditioning is pervasive and nearly consistent. Ritualistic phases are used when we are distressed and on the verge of discharge: "Don't get excited"; "Crying is for babies"; "Act strong"; "Don't cry"; "That doesn't hurt"; "Don't make a scene." Physical posturing and facial expressions may be learned as controls over discharge. Rapid or slowed speech when distressed, changing the subject, elaborate detailing of the distressing event, etc., all may be devices for repressing discharge. Therapists are very familiar with many of the ways in which patterns manipulate humans to avoid some emotional experience. The therapist's task is to find an appropriate interruption of the control pattern.

The therapist's tasks go beyond facilitating the proper balance of attention and the interruption of the control pattern's inhibition of discharge. Chronic patterns require *interruption* as well. For example, for the "complaining depressive," the therapist warmly and consistently invites and insists that the patient talk positively about himself and others. The therapist validates the patient by telling him of the traits, talents and other aspects of the person which are attractive, positive, etc. He may invite the patient to say things, act in expressive styles (e.g., smile and brag about himself), etc. that directly contradict the chronic pattern. Discharge usually follows as temporary resistance to the invitation from the therapist is overcome.

A basic principle in dealing with a chronic pattern is rather akin to those articulated by therapists such as Greenwald (1969) and others. The therapist does not "speak" with or to the chronic repetition of some invalidating attitude towards self and others. He interrupts by communicating with the patient's core being and about the distresses the patient has experienced. (Example: Paranoid person in acute persecutory state reports incident which "proves" they are after him; therapist says, "It's scary, huh?" and "I know you can handle it." Patient explodes in anger and therapist facilitates discharge. The hurt and fear in the distress pattern then become more accessible for discharge.)

Through our developing years we are conditioned to the view that heavy discharge, especially crying and trembling, are "wrong," painful, and even a sign of decompensation. Sobbing and trembling only lead to decompensation when they are aborted and the distress continues to mount in the person, leading to self-defeating control and coping mechanisms. The acquired social meaning of crying can be so embarrasing, humiliating, "unmasculine," etc. that the crying may be perceived as painful. The therapist helps the patient unlock himself from this cultural encapsulation since he has unlocked himself from the same cultural taboo about discharge.

Validation and *self-appreciation* are fundamental aspects of the therapeutic relationship. Validation comprises the therapist's consistent appreciation of the core being of the patient, all of the latent and manifest talents of the patient, and a believable sense of hopefulness for the person communicated quite overtly and frequently. Self-appreciation is suggested to the patient and expected of him or her. In self-appreciation, the patient is asked to do what the therapist has done in validating him. The particular content of self-appreciation is the choice of the patient, of course, but deepened and persisted in through the encouragement of the therapist. In both validation and self-appreciation, what follows is: The contradiction and destimulation of chronic patterns of criticism of self and others; the un-numbering and reexperiencing of some old distress; and discharge in the patient and possibly in the therapist as well.

The reevaluation therapist has discharged on many of his own distresses and continues to do so. Discharge frees his attention for listening to and observing his patient just as it frees his patient's own attention for more rational considerations in daily life. The therapist's rationality can operate through warm, attentive listening, to assess when the patient is distressed, near or far from discharge, overwhelmed by distress, controlling the discharge, in a chronic or intermittent pattern, etc.

The therapist has a deeply held conviction about the loving, zestful, intelligent, curious, cooperative and communicative nature of people. Consistently, he adheres to this positive framework about his patient. If he finds himself departing from this framework, he works on his own restimulations and discharges. He listens and views his patient in a realistic manner, always aware that the patient's hostility, withdrawal, and other negative aspects are part of undischarged distress and chronic patterns. All of the therapist's techniques are implemented in the context of his perspective of man's core being. Because he has interrupted many of his own critical patterns, he is able to maintain a steadfast position as he warmly interrupts and contradicts all of his patient's critical patterns, which may include pessimism, cynicism, complaining, fault-finding, blaming of self and others. Inevitably, the therapist finds himself contradicting a very pervasive characteristic of North-American culture: relating to others through criticism, competitiveness and self-criticism (Somers, 1970). As he maintains this contradicting approach, he finds that it elicits discharge in his client and sometimes in himself.

Since the therapist has experienced the cocounseling group, one in which he and a peer take turns working with each other toward discharge, he is free to discharge with his patient when he feels distressed and it seems appropriate (i.e., does not interrupt his patient). If he finds that his discharging constricts his own free attention for his patient, or hinders the patient's discharge, he waits until he can discharge under more appropriate conditions which do not require that he have free attention for a patient. Therapists work in a very restimulative environment and need ample opportunities for discharge. Naturally, the therapist cannot rely upon discharging only with patients.

The therapist's own attitude toward discharge is rather different from that of the culture and his patient senses this very quickly. Distressed people have a desire to be rid of their distresses and will often seek out a listener for that purpose. The listener's active presence, through free attention and the expectant attitude, has a salutary effect upon the distressed patient in facilitating discharge. The therapist, paying attention to the distress/discharge sequence, is able to redirect the patient over and over again to the phrase, the look, the expression that brought the discharge on its heels. Some Gestalt therapists, and Janov (1970) in his primal theory, have made this discovery. In the case of the Gestalt school, the patient is directed to attend to his awareness. If he discharges this is accepted. But Gestalt theory leaves the direction to the patient. Often the patient's control mechanisms or chronic patterns takes over, thus preventing the exhaustive discharge that is necessary. Janov limits his conception of discharge to the "primal" which is discharge of a limited although important variety, and which is focused largely on a particular period of childhood. His conception of the types of discharge is much too narrow, excluding laughter and not mentioning yawning, stretching, etc.

The reevaluation therapist does not usually lead or interview his client. The client's phenomenal world often provides the lead—he brings up his own material. The therapist is active in interrupting control and chronic patterns and directing and redirecting the client to the material that produces discharge. He is also active with the deeply distressed person in directing him to neutral or positive material that will help develop more free attention. The therapist does not interpret to the client, offer insight or direct the patient to this kind of work. As mentioned earlier, the patient is fully capable, after sufficient discharge, of reevaluation—recall of information, new awareness of self and others, planning, and decision-making activity.

Reevaluation Therapy proceeds in stages where necessary. Individual one-way therapy, where required to help the patient achieve more free attention, may precede participation in a cocounseling workshop. In the workshop members choose partners, known as cocounselors, and are trained in the group in the theory and techniques which they will use with each other to exchange effective help in sessions outside of the workshop meetings.

References

BUGENTAL, J. (1965). *The Search for Authenticity.* New York: Holt, Rinehart and Winston, Inc.

BUGENTAL, J. (ed). (1967). *Challenges of Humanistic Psychology.* New York: McGraw-Hill.

CANTRIL, H. (1965). *The Pattern of Human Concerns.* New Brunswick, N. J.: Rutgers University Press.

GREENWALD, H. (1969). Play and self-development. In H. A. Otto & J. Mann (eds.), *Ways of Growth.* New York: Viking Press.

JACKINS, H. (1964). *The Human Side of Human Beings.* Seattle: Rational Island Publishers. (P.O. Box 2081, Main Office Station, Seattle 98111).

JACKINS, H. (1965). *Basic Postulates of Reevaluation Counseling.* Seattle: Rational Island Publishers.

JANOV, A. (1970). *The Primal Scream.* New York: Putnam.

MASLOW, A. (1967). Self-actualization and beyond. In J. F. T. Bugental (ed.), *Challenges of Humanistic Psychology.* New York: McGraw-Hill.

MAY, R. (1969). *Love and Will.* New York: W. W. Norton.

OTTO, H., & MANN, J. (eds.). (1969). *Ways of Growth.* New York: Viking Press.

ROGERS, C. (1957). The necessary and sufficient conditions of therapeutic personality change. *Journal of Consulting Psychology*, **21**, 95–103.

SCHEFF, T. (1972). Reevaluation counseling: social implications. *Journal of Humanistic Psychology*, **12** (1).

SHOSTROM, E. (1967). *Man, the Manipulator: The Inner Journey from Manipulation to Actualization.* Nashville, Tenn.: Abingdon.

SOMERS, B. (1970). Social factors limiting intimacy in psychotherapy. *Voices: The Art and Science of Psychotherapy*, **6** (2).

SOMERS, B. (1971). The cocounseling workshop: training people to exchange effective help. Mimeographed ms., Department of Psychology, California State College, Los Angeles, California 90032.

STEINZOR, B. (1969). *The Healing Partnership: The Patient as Colleague in Psychotherapy.* New York: Harper and Row.

ULLMANN, L., & KRASNER, L. (1969). *A Psychological Approach to Abnormal Behavior.* Englewood Cliffs, N.J.: Prentice-Hall.

YATES, A. (1970). *Behavior Therapy*, New York: John Wiley.

ZASLOW, R., & BREGER, L. (1969). A theory and treatment of autism. In L. Breger (ed.), *Clinical-cognitive Psychology.* Englewood Cliffs, N.J.: Prentice-Hall.

BERNARD T. ENGEL, DAVID SHAPIRO, HERBERT BENSON, HENRY SLUCKI, GEORGE B. WHATMORE, ALAN H. HARRIS, and LOUIS VACHON

The Use of Biofeedback Training in Enabling Patients to Control Autonomic Functions

Recent research in psychosomatic disorder has moved from an attempt to find relationships between physiological syndromes and general personality characteristics to an effort to relate rather specific behaviors to specific physiological reactions. Associated with this recent approach is the discovery that many physiological functions thought not to be under voluntary control actually can, under the proper circumstances, be controlled. The following summary of the program of research by Dr. Bernard T. Engel and his colleagues describes recent research on the use of biofeedback to enable patients to control autonomic functions. The application of these techniques to the treatment of specific psychosomatic disorders is also discussed. One of the most exciting aspects of this work is that it promises to bypass the symptomatic treatment of these disorders through the use of drugs. Instead, it offers behavioral techniques for controlling the physiological functions that set in motion processes leading to tissue changes.

In abridging this paper, the editors have omitted major sections describing research relating autonomic processes to such specific disorders as asthma, cardiac arrhythmia, hypertension, and so on. Readers interested in this material should consult the original source.

In the future specialists treating patients with a variety of psychosomatic diseases may have the option of using training instead of relying exclusively on drug therapies. Psychologists, working with physicians, particularly in the realm of cardiovascular illness, have shown that there are behavioral aspects to the etiology of illness, and similarly, behavior can be reshaped to modulate the symptoms. A new concept of the autonomic nervous system is emerging

---

Abridged from J. Segal (ed.), *Mental Health Progress Reports*, **5** (1971), 349–375, with the permission of B. T. Engel.

in Western medicine, for it is clear that both animals and man can exert fine control over aspects of organic function that had been thought to be involuntary. In some instances the investigators have been using instruments that would sense, amplify, and feed back to the subject an inner change such as blood pressure, or stomach acidity that he might not ordinarily be aware of, thus allowing him to recognize these physiological functions and to gain control over them. This technique has been known as biofeedback. Other researchers have not fed back the internal signal in a manner the subject could recognize, but instead have rewarded him for producing a certain kind of change, in the traditional manner of operant conditioning. The distinction between biofeedback and operant conditioning depends upon whether or not an individual is rewarded for the correct response. Sometimes, however, the distinction is obscure, for a person with hypertension often will be rewarded merely by seeing that he has moved his blood pressure down. The important point is that the instruments that feed back internal changes to a person allow him to "see" his own physiological responses and then to control functions that formerly lay outside his awareness. In general, experimenters using animals employ operant conditioning, while many of the human experiments rely on feedback, thus the term biofeedback has become popular.

Psychosomatic Illness and Response Specificity

Among many people with the symptoms of hypertension, ulcers, or other psychosomatic illness, it is almost a commonplace that stress can activate symptoms. Articulate patients, for example, have described feeling restrained rage as "a knot in the stomach," or "bursting in the head." Over the last two decades quite a number of psychiatrists, psychologists, and clinicians in other specialities have conjectured that for various reasons individuals may react to stress in specific physiological ways. One person might brace himself, habitually, by tensing the muscles of his back and neck, while another might respond with the rapid breathing and cardiac changes that would be appropriate if he were preparing to fight. These changes throughout the nervous system, endocrine system, and musculature galvanize a person to meet a physical threat, but in the context of a purely intellectual challenge, such physiological changes might become a damaging habit.

In the early 1960's, Dr. Bernard T. Engel and his colleagues began to study healthy young people and patients with psychosomatic diseases to see whether they showed very specific tendencies when they responded to stressful or neutral events. Pulse rate, blood pressure, respiration, and skin temperature and resistance were measured in healthy young nurses under a number of conditions—while solving arithmetic problems very quickly, or immersing a foot in ice water, or being subjected to a loud automobile horn. The kinds of responses depended in part on the stimulus. However, each individual seemed to have his own manner of reacting physiologically to stressful stimuli. These individual propensities were not very clear in the healthy volunteers;

however, patients with essential hypertension showed a marked tendency to respond with changes in systolic blood pressure.

A second study was designed to compare patients with hypertension and patients with rheumatoid arthritis. In this study, the stimuli were relatively mild, statements that demanded a free association response. Test phrases, such as "I am constantly pressured," were recited to the patients. The patients did not reveal many differences in their reactions to the test phrases, but they did respond differently to the entire experimental situation, in which they were wired with sensors and given relaxation periods. These periods were exceedingly revealing. During the rests, the arthritic patients never adapted by relaxing the muscle groups spanning joints that had been giving them pain, and the hypertensive patients did not lower their blood pressure.

There is a voluminous literature on the subject of response specificity, but none of it gives data clear enough to predict which psychosomatic ills a particular person will develop, since genetic differences and the myriad of influences in an individual's lifetime make the etiology very complex. In some subtle fashion, however, it appears possible that a person's habitual responses to stress may ultimately lead to symptoms, or may influence the course of the disease whatever the cause.

Disponesis

Dr. George B. Whatmore and his colleagues in Seattle, Washington, have been using instrumental feedback to "retrain" many patients with symptoms such as headaches, backaches, depression, extrasystoles, and exhaustion. Dr. Whatmore has postulated that these people have come to react to environmental events, bodily sensations, thoughts, and emotions with specific but undetected covert expenditures of energy. This covert energy expenditure is not a vague entity. It consists of measurable action-potentials in the neuromuscular system with consequent covert muscular contraction and biochemical change. This "dysponesis" appears to have pronounced effects upon the autonomic nervous system and endocrine system. Bracing—holding the skeletal musculature partially contracted and thus the body rigid and on guard—can enhance a person's arousal and intensify a sense of fear and anxiety. It can also disturb the function of smooth muscle, thus disturbing digestion and can lead to ulcers, colitis, and other conditions. Since patients who are making such characteristic efforts do so unknowingly, it takes considerable training for them to recognize what they are doing. By amplifying, processing, and displaying in audiovisual forms the covert tensing and relaxing of various muscles, Dr. Whatmore has enabled patients to identify and control their covert efforts. Gradually they are trained to continue their control during conversations on stressful subjects. The patient is then encouraged to practice this control in daily life. It may require two years of training; however, follow-up studies have demonstrated that patients have overcome symptoms of backache, headache, or depression so severe that they formerly required hospital care. Dr. Whatmore's careful and cautious clinical work over nearly two decades suggests that neurophysiologic retraining may reach some of the origins of symptoms, returning to the individual some responsibility and also ability to protect his own health. One might say that this returning of responsibility to the patient is now becoming a philosophical trend in medicine.

Feedback for Sensing Internal Changes

Many researchers are reaching toward a similar mode of therapy. Perhaps, ideally, we should begin to use all available techniques so that youngsters and young adults might learn to "tune in" to their inner sensations discovering how they respond to unpleasant events and how to control their responses. It is easy to show a child how to throw a ball, by demonstrating, and moving his arm. Ultimately, with feedback from his own action, the child's practice will make him accomplished. It is, however, difficult to tell a child how to control his bladder, or his intestines, or any internal processes. Most of us are relatively insensitive to small events in that interior hinterland of our bodies, and while we will put ointment on a burn, we may tolerate a developing duodenal ulcer for months without seeing a doctor.

Dr. Henry Slucki, a psychologist at the University of Southern California Medical School, has indicated that it may be a lack of interoceptive discrimination training that permits us to go through life so bluntly insensitive to events within our skins. Even animals in the laboratory take longer to learn a response that is attached to an internal stimulus than to respond to a light, or sound, external to the body.

If serious illness is to be prevented, individuals must begin to apprehend incipient symptoms at the earliest possible time. Today, most people go to the doctor too late, after they feel pain, or have seen a serious disruption in their own behavior, an inability to concentrate, or great fatigue. Because our culture encourages a kind of puritan fortitude, children, who often do anticipate their illnesses by responding to the gentle prodding within, are taught to ignore such feeling and may be accused of malingering because they do not yet have a fever. Could early diagnosis and preventive medicine be enhanced by reversing this attitude and training people to monitor events in their bodies?

A coworker of Dr. Slucki, Gyorgi Adams, found that when volunteers swallowed inflatable balloons, their brain waves, by desynchronizing, registered the fact that the balloon in the stomach had been inflated even when the individual did not report "feeling" anything. Moreover, volunteers quickly adjusted, or became habituated to the balloons, although they appear to learn spatial discrimination when there were two balloons. The inflation of a second balloon also showed up in desychronized brain waves, even though the individuals were not consciously aware of it and could not verbalize what was happening internally. In order to find out whether interoceptive training (training in internal sensitivity) would be possible without contamination from the effects of verbal suggestion or the emotional complexities of human beings, Dr. Slucki began working with animals.

In an initial study with Drs. Gyorgi Adam and Robert W. Portive, five macaque monkeys were implanted with an inflatable loop in the small intestine and with electrodes at sites in the brain. These animals quickly learned to press a lever rapidly for a sugar pellet. Much like the human volunteers, they seemed to go on pressing unperturbably even when the balloon was inflated, as though they didn't feel it. Occasionally one of them would look around. Generally, they seemed not to show any sign of noticing the internal stimulation, although their EEGs became desynchronized each time the balloon was slightly inflated. Thus, in some fashion, the cortex was receiving the internal news, although the animal acted unaware of stimulation. Then the monkeys were rewarded only for bar pressing when the balloon was inflated. As if they had learned to "feel" they quickly became adept at pressing the moment the balloon inflated. In a subsequent study, a similar procedure was performed using the colon, and the monkeys showed the same ability to respond to a formerly overlooked internal stimulus. Learning, indeed, did seem to increase their sensitivity. After they had learned to "feel" and respond to the sizeable inflation of a balloon, they became sensitive to a very tiny balloon inflation that they could not "sense" at first. Internal conditioning seems to proceed very much like any external training, in which an individual first learns to respond to gross properties, and later to more refined and delicate qualities. In psychology this is known as stimulus discrimination.

In a similar study with female monkeys, water at body temperature was infused through a catheter into the bladder, thus increasing pressure on the bladder, and the animals were conditioned to press a lever at each increase in bladder pressure. In this way the animals became aware when the bladder volume became high and they relaxed their bladder in order to reduce pressure. These studies might enable adults to make toilet training easier for children by giving them more explicit verbal instructions, relating pressure and urination. Sensitivity to pressure, to tension and relaxation throughout the intestinal system might indeed enable people to anticipate, perhaps even prevent themselves from incurring such symptoms as spastic colon, or colitis. This kind of training is being used to enable both discrimination of internal events and control over many autonomic functions.

In quite a few laboratories, other researchers are using instrumental conditioning to find out to what extent that various functions of the body may be controlled by training. At Duke University, for instance, in Durham, North Carolina, Drs. Ben Feather and Malcolm Robinson have shown that animals can learn to control the output of bile in the spleen. Dr. Louis Vachon and his associates at Boston University have begun investigation to determine whether biofeedback training might elicit some voluntary control over the regulation of respiratory resistance which is the key symptom in asthma.

References

BENSON, H., HERD, J. A., MORSE, W. H., & KELLEHER, R. T. (1969). Behavioral induction of arterial hypertension and its reversal. *Amer. J. Physiol.*, **217**, 30–34.

BENSON, H., SHAPIRO, D., TURSKY, B., & SCHWARTZ, G. E. (1971). A behavioral approach to clinical hypertension. For presentation to the American Society for Clinical Investigation. Atlantic City, May.

BRADY, J. V., FINDLEY, J. D., & HARRIS, A. H. (1971). Experimental psychopathology of emotion. In H. Kimmel (ed.), *Experimental Psychopathology*, in press. New York: Academic Press.

ENGEL, BERNARD T. (1960). Stimulus-response and individual-response specificity. *AMA Archives of General Psychiatry*, March, 305–313.

ENGEL, B. T., & BICKFORD, A. F. (1961). Response specificity. *Archives of General Psychiatry*, November, **5**, 478–489.

ENGEL, B. T., & GOTTLIEB, S. H. (1970). Differential operant conditioning of heart rate in the restrained monkey. *Journal of Comparative Physiological Psychology*, **73** (2), 217–225.

ENGEL, B. T., & HANSEN, S. P. (1966). Operant conditioning of heart rate slowing. *Psychophysiology*, **3** (2), 176–187.

ENGEL, B. T., & CHISM,R. A. (1967). Operant conditioning of heart rate speeding. *Psychophysiology*, **2** (4), 418–426.

ENGEL, B. T., & CHISM, R. A. (1967). Effect of increases and decreases in breathing rate on heart rate and finger pulse volume. *Psychophysiology*, **4** (1), 83–89.

ENGEL, B. T., & MOOSE, R. H. (1967). The generality of specificity. *Archives of General Psychiatry*, May, **16**, 574–581.

GUTMANN, M. C., & BENSON, H. Interaction of environmental factors and systemic arterial blood pressure. Submitted for publication, 1971.

LEVINE, H. I., ENGEL, B. T., & PEARSON, J. A. (1968). Differential operant conditioning of heart rate. *Psychosomatic Medicine*, **30** (6), 837–844.

MOOS, R. H., & ENGEL, B. T. (1963). Psychophysiological reactions in hypertensive and arthritic patients. *Psychosomatic Medicine*, 227–241.

SCHWARTZ, G. E., SHAPIRO, D., & TURSKY, B. (1971). Learned control of cardiovascular integration in man through operant conditioning. *Psychosomatic Medicine*, **33**, 57–62.

SCHWARTZ, G. E. (1970). Operant conditioning of human cardiovascular integration and differentiation. Presented to the Society for Psychophysiological Research. New Orleans, November.

SHAPIRO, D., CRIDER, A. B., & TURSKY, B. (1964). Differentiation of an automatic response through operant reinforcement. *Psychon. Sci.*, **1**, 147–148.

SHAPIRO, D., TURSKY, B., GERSHON, B., & STERN, M. (1963). Effects of feedback and reinforcement on the control of human systolic blood pressure. *Science*, 588–590.

SHAPIRO, D., TURSKY, B., & SCHWARTZ, G. E. (1970). Control of blood pressure in man by operant conditioning. *Circul. Res.*, 26–27: Suppl. 24–41.

SHAPIRO, D., TURSKY, B., & SCHWARTZ, G. E. (1970). Differentiation of heart rate and systolic blood pressure in man by operant conditioning. *Psychosomatic Medicine*, **32**, 417–423.

SHAPIRO, D., SCHWARTZ, G. E., & TURSKY, B. (1970). Control of diastolic blood pressure in man by feedback and reinforcement. Presented to the Society for Psychophysiological Research, New Orleans, November.

SLUCKI, H., MCCOY, F. B., & PORTER, R. W. Interoceptive S^d of the large intestine established by mechanical stimulation. *Psychological Reports*, **24**, 35–42.

SLUCKI, H., ADAM, G., & PORTER, R. W. (1965). Operant discrimination of an interoceptive stimulus in rhesus monkeys. *Journal of the Experimental Analysis of Behavior*, **8**, 405–414.

TURSKY, B., SHAPIRO, D., & SCHWARTZ, G. E. An automated constant cuff-pressure system for measuring average systolic and diastolic blood pressure in man. Submitted for publication in 1971.

WEISS, T., & ENGEL, B. T. Operant conditioning of heart rate in patients with premature ventricular contractions. *Psychosomatic Medicine*, in press, 1971.

WHATMORE, G. B., & KOHLI, D. R. (1968). Dysponesis: a neurophysiologic factor in functional disorders. *Behavioral Science*, March, **12** (2), 102–124.

4 The Psychoses

Psychosis is the most severe mental illness and, as a result, very often requires hospitalization for the protection of both the psychotic individual and others around him. Because psychosis is very severe, lay people find it difficult to think of disorders subsumed in this category as understandable entities and often dismiss it as "crazy" and beyond comprehension. Most psychologically oriented theorists prefer to think that psychotic behavior and thought represent an attempt to express something meaningful, albeit in a difficult and idiosyncratic manner.

OTTO ALLEN WILL, Jr.

Human Relatedness and the Schizophrenic Reaction

The author of the paper to follow, Dr. O. A. Will, has had a long and distinguished career as a psychotherapist working primarily with schizophrenic patients. In this paper he provides interesting case material concerning his therapeutic relationship with two schizophrenic patients, as well as some generalizations concerning the psychogenic basis of schizophrenia to which he was led as a result of these relationships.

The editors have omitted a discussion of physical death and its relationship to a sense of unrelatedness, as well as a discussion of therapeutic technique with schizophrenics. The reader interested in these materials should consult the original paper.

Reprinted from *Psychiatry*, **22** (1959), 205–223, by special permission of The William Alanson White Psychiatric Foundation Inc., and Dr. Will.

Some time past I was called upon to serve as physician to a young woman who had passed many years as a patient in a series of psychiatric hospitals. She spent the greater portion of her time in a closed room barren of furniture and decoration; she tore to pieces clothing and other objects, barricaded her door against visitors, and ran from them when she could. For many years she had not eaten freely, saying that her food was poisoned, and struggling against the efforts made to feed her. She was known by various names descriptive of fragments of her behavior, and the person which she had been was concealed behind a façade of stereotypes. Referred to as "assaultive," "negativistic," "hostile," a "feeding difficulty," as "the one who runs away," and so on, she was seen more as a problem than a person.

The information about Catherine, as I shall call her, was slight, recent accounts adding little to those of earlier periods. She was said to have been an amiable, good, and intelligent child who had displayed no gross difficulties in her course of development, having been more than adequate as athlete, student, and participant in social affairs. It was evident, however, that some matters troublesome to her had not been communicated clearly to her associates; in her late teens she became markedly preoccupied, showed a distaste for the company of others, and attempted to kill herself, revealing to no one her thoughts about her indisposition. Her apparent depression was then obscured by symptoms suggestive of a physical disorder; she suffered from constipation, loss of appetite, and a persistent decline in weight.

The diagnosis of a pituitary disease was made, but medications effected no cure, and she was finally hospitalized as a "mental" patient—emaciated, increasingly withdrawn, and hostile. She was moved from one institution to another, received the currently popular treatments with insulin and electricity without noticeable benefit, worsened, and was thought by some to show evidence of a "deterioration" of the brain.

Catherine cried out that she hated all things medical, and made every effort to run away from the hospital. She had little to do with her ward associates, rarely called anyone by name, and revealed nothing of her past life to others, acting as if she guarded a terrible secret. She denied that she had difficulties other than those associated with being incarcerated against her will, and resisted all approaches made to her. At times she experienced panic, acting as if she had been caught up in a horrible nightmare, assaulting those near her, and attempting to hurt or destroy herself.

Here were displayed anxiety, fear, loneliness, and the corroding effects of social isolation. But anyone who sought to help her was, without exception, driven away by her contempt or anger, or by their fear of her aloneness, seeking to account for this retreat and despair by saying that Catherine was afflicted with a strange "organic" illness, was "hopeless," "unable to love," or lacking in certain "essential human qualities." Thought of as less than human, she was referred to as "empty" and "hollow," as if she were a nonliving object.

Catherine showed no enthusiasm concerning my visits. Although I came regularly, she did not acknowledge my name or our appointments, denied that I was a physician, and turned her back on me. As I persisted she grew more tense, ran from me or attacked me, screamed that I was injuring her by my presence, was mute for long periods, and noticeably grew worse. I continued my visits, but my enthusiasm as a therapist declined on occasion. My varied approaches were seemingly ineffective, my theories were often without apparent relevance to the patient's behavior, and I frequently felt angry, discouraged, humiliated, and inept.

During the long silences—extending over many of our meetings—I would at first think of Catherine's difficulties and possible explanations for them; then I would consider our reactions together, puzzling about the reasons for our behavior; but shortly my thoughts would turn more to myself, to my own hopes and apprehensions; and in time I seemed to be abandoning all but a few repetitive and unprofitable ideas, which evidenced no clear connection to a past or future, and had their existence in an unchanging and seemingly unalterable present. Catherine was then not clear in my thinking, and I was engrossed with such generalizations as the "meaninglessness" of the situation to me and my "inadequacies" as a therapist, with anger at the institution and feelings of "despair."

What was at that time obscure later became more evident. Although I was in the room with Catherine, I was drawing back from her, it having soon become laborious for me to think of her for any length of time. Thoughts of her were replaced by abstractions, which in turn gave way to recurrent banalities and vaguely directed emotions. That which I called despair reflected difficulties in the organization and use of previous and current experience in the exercise of foresight; that is, 'hope'—which includes expectation—does not flourish when anxiety so disturbs comprehension of past and present that the concept of an evolving 'future' cannot be grasped.

Although I came to see Catherine with the purpose of helping improve her living, her responses often led me to feel ineffective and brutal. As I entered her room one day, she turned on me, saying: "I don't want to see you. You are cruel and punishing. You hurt people. You come here so you can laugh at me; you never listen to me. You are bitter and see only the dark side of things. You are unkind and you ought to be killed." I felt attacked unjustly, but as I listened I understood a little better how isolated, embittered, and pessimistic this woman was.

In this situation of anxiety and guarding, Catherine and I often held stereotyped and rigid views of each other. To me she was becoming just a patient with a diagnosis, and to her I was as follows: "You are a nothing," she said, "You are pompous, and cruel, and think you know it all, and you just want to tell people how to live as you think they ought to live. All doctors look, and act, and think alike; they aren't persons—they're just robots."

During one of the periods of silence Catherine and I, each unknown to the other, wrote about our views of what was taking place. On one occasion she wrote as follows:

> They just want to hurt you in this place and I am going mad. . . . You, doctor, are a piece of stone. . . . Your heart is ice. I shall die. . . . I shall sit and weave my fantasies into the wall. I shall never get well. . . . I feel crushed so that nothing is left. . . . I want to grow younger and younger until I don't exist any more. . . . Leave me alone; you are only a machine with all the feelings left out.

At approximately the same time I wrote:

> This woman seems brittle, cold, and hollow. With her I usually feel ignored and frozen out; I feel crushed, discouraged, and useless. I think that my personality has defects which disqualify me for this work.

Despite our silences and our withdrawals it was apparent that to some extent Catherine's experiences were being made clearer to me. It was not easy to put these matters into words, and in some instances I was reluctant to hear what she had to say, finding the message disturbing to me, and attempting to 'explain' my discomfort by saying that my personality was unsuited to the task.

There was a period during which I felt unusually alone, isolated from my colleagues, and unable to tell them much of my work with Catherine. To one of them I said: "I might as well not be here. It's like being in a cemetery; there isn't any life." Here is an excerpt from Catherine's writing at that time, read by me some months later:

> People are too terrible to live with. They have killed and the unremovable blood lies on their conscience. . . . Sorrow comes by day, and at night comes the evil. . . . I think that I am mad, because no living human being understands what I say. I feel in pieces and confused. At times I fall into the dark, going down with nothing to stop me—and then there are the voices, and I feel that I go away for a long time. I don't know who I am. I think I have been dead for many years, but didn't know it. Maybe that's why you say I can't go home; because I am dead. Death is lonely, and I am a stranger to all of you and to me. I can't make a move; someone else will have to take the first step.

But my first steps often seemed to be misdirected or ill-timed. One day as I sat in silence Catherine suddenly turned and struck me. I held her arms and she wept, saying: "I haven't been able to hear you. You've been staying behind that wall of glass. It had to get broken somehow."

Thereafter Catherine and I spoke more freely with each other, and our isolation tentatively receded. During the several years of our meeting together she had said that she did not dream. Now she told me of a dream: "It was all very clear. I was almost afraid to look. I was afraid that it might go away, or that something would happen to it. But it was all right. It was just a picture. There was an ocean, and a white sand beach; and at the edge of the sand were some trees." I asked if there were any people in the dream. "Oh, no. Not even I. There was no one. Nothing moved—no wind—the sea was quiet; but the sun was shining. . . . But I wasn't afraid. It all seemed natural enough."

Of a later dream Catherine said: "It was like the first dream. There was the water, the beach, and the trees. But there was some surf, and I felt good. . . . And there was something else—a bird flew across the sky."

Catherine's behavior was called schizophrenic, and the events described above are not uncommon in the experience of such patients. There are certain aspects of the account which I wish to emphasize:

The patient's isolation. She was isolated, and had become involved in a situation promoting the development and maintenance of stereotyped thinking and behavior. She had great needs, but seemed to be unaware of them or denied their existence, and those who attempted to help often misinterpreted her requirements, or did not respond in ways acceptable to her. She often spoke of being free and independent, and of being separate from all people, as if her memories of relatedness were intolerable, and any hopes of comfortable closeness with another had been abandoned.

Her difficulty in communicating in words. Catherine's difficulties in adolescence had been obscured by her social success; at that time no one thought of her as ill. She made a suicidal attempt, became depressed, developed signs of an "organic" illness, and was finally called "mentally" disordered. It was as if her case could not be stated in words, her entire organism being involved in a responsiveness that included communicative as well as defensive and survival values. Thus the nonverbal aspects of our association were of great significance.

My reflections of my patient's feelings. There were times when my own[1] sentiments—anxiety, loneliness, depression, anger, uncertainty about myself and my function—were reflections of my patient's feelings, and these shared experiences were the rudimentary beginnings of our using a more highly symbolic form of communication.

Our growing mutuality. Our contacts were marked by recurrent approaches and retreats, without, however, a complete abandonment of a growing mutuality. Despite mutual rebuff and withdrawal I felt increasingly bound to Catherine, and she said: "You are a fool for getting caught up in this—this nothingness, this evil." Evil or otherwise, there were ties which were strengthened.

The concept of relatedness. My earlier thoughts were concerned with such concepts as "her" ability to relate to me, or mine to her. As we went on, I thought of *our* relatedness, the mutuality of the therapeutic field becoming more apparent to me.

As Catherine and I continued our meetings, her anxiety subsided somewhat and her behavior became less disturbed. At this point some of her family members wished to terminate her treatment, saying that not enough was being

[1] "My own" is an inappropriate locution, as it seems to imply the operation of ideas apart from the interpersonal field.

accomplished; this was at the very time when there first appeared some evidence of useful change in the patient. There was no openly expressed serious complaint about the therapy, and the relatives had always spoken of their grave concern with the young woman's betterment, although they had often remarked that she was probably something to which they referred as "beyond recovery." I talked with the parents, finding them to be evasive, uneasy, and seemingly under some unclear but powerful pressure to "change things." I reminded Catherine's mother of her frequently expressed wish that her daughter get "well," and again asked what that term meant to her. The reply was: "I want it to be like it used to be when we all seemed all right together. She's getting different now—she doesn't seem to be a part of us any more."

I had witnessed such events before. Why should those who wished for the betterment of the patient frequently appear uncertain, anxious, and unsympathetic at the very point of his improvement and growing independence?

In thinking about this question I recalled John, a young man who improved from a schizophrenic reaction during the course of therapy with me. There was a point at which he became fearful and hesitant and wished to terminate our meetings, finally saying that he might kill me. I eventually learned from him that as our association developed he was at times afraid that I could not tolerate either his closeness to me or his independence. He stated matters this way:

> I felt that there was a destructiveness in me that would involve you and kill you. I tried to tell you, but you didn't seem to hear. I'd get to feeling all right, but then we'd seem to be getting tied together so that neither one of us could be separate—or free—something like that. It was like we'd be lost, or eaten up, if we got close. So I wanted you to go away. If you stayed on and were destroyed, I'd lose you. But if you went away—I'd have you in my memory. . . . Then I got to feeling that something would happen to you if I went out on my own. It's crazy—but it's like you couldn't stand to let me get well—or go away.

In discussing John's experience, we discovered that his feelings about me resembled those he held for his mother. She had often spoken with enthusiasm about her pleasure in thinking of him as becoming more independent, but she also suggested that she could not live adequately without him, and that she might die or succumb to depression should he leave her. So it was that John grew anxious in his work with me. He needed me, but he expected that I, for my own necessities, would attempt to control him and resist his achievement of maturity and separation. We talked about all of this, and kept on with the work. John's mother seemingly accepted the changes in her son, but thereafter grew more aloof and developed a malignancy of which she died. Referring to this, John said: "When you spoke of my getting well I felt as if you were telling me to be a murderer—that somehow you, or me, or someone—like my mother—was going to get killed. That sounds crazy, but I felt that way."

This may indeed sound crazy. I am not talking about simple cause and effect, and I do not know why John's mother sickened as she did. I do suggest that the family is a social field in which the patient plays an important functional role, subtle accommodations being made by other members to the development of his disordered ways of living, and a definite importance being attached to their perpetuation.[2] The patient, including what one may think of as his "sickness," is not only an expression of the family culture, but also an integral factor in the maintenance of its uncertain equilibrium. Changes in the patient, for example, threaten that stability, and necessitate reciprocal adjustments on the part of others, who are required to alter their behavior in some way, becoming more expressive, more participant, or more withdrawn. If the more independent, self-sufficient actions of the patient cannot be met by similar action on the part of others, those others may respond with the display of what are called "emotional" and "physical" disorders. To avoid such alterations, often felt to be disruptive and threatening, attempts may be made to reinclude the patient unchanged in the family field, the move being rationalized in terms of his being "hopeless" or requiring some other form of treatment.

In brief, the schizophrenic reaction reflects the family social system, and changes in the one require accompanying changes in the other. In such systems growth, which involves greater self-identification and accommodation to new experience, may be looked upon as productive of destruction and loss, and may lead to powerful—and seemingly hostile or meaningless—efforts to retain the status quo. One may look upon such phenomena as

[2] See, for example, the following incomplete list of articles concerned with family relationships. Studies of the patient's family increasingly emphasize the function of that organization as a social unit, the structure of which is mirrored in (and requires) the behavior of the patient, and reflects the larger culture of which it is a part (see Caudill). The problem is considered in various ways, as follows: (1) the teaching to the children of distorted and personal family concepts of the culture (Lidz and others); (2) the involvement of various members in the anxiety of any one member (Limentani); (3) disturbances in communication systems within the family (Bateson and others); (4) the family system as a trap from which the patient cannot extricate himself without significant alteration in the system (Wynne and others).

The list is as follows: Nathan W. Ackerman, "Toward an Integrative Therapy of the Family," *Amer. J. Psychiatry* (1958) 114 : 727–733; Gregory Bateson, Don D. Jackson, Jay Haley, and John Weakland, "Towards a Theory of Schizophrenia," *Behavioral Science* (1956) 1 : 251–264; William A. Caudill, *Effects of Social and Cultural Systems in Reaction to Stress*; New York, Social Science Research Council, Pamphlet 14, 1958; Donald L. Gerard and Joseph Siegel, "The Family Background of Schizophrenia," *Psychiatric Quart.* (1950) 24 : 47–73; Melvin L. Kohn and John A. Clausen, "Parental Authority Behavior and Schizophrenia," *Amer. J. Orthopsychiatry* (1956) 26 : 297–313; Theodore Lidz, "Schizophrenia and the Family," *Psychiatry* (1958) 21 : 21–27; Theodore Lidz, Alice Cornelison, Dorothy Terry, and Stephen Fleck, "Intrafamilial Environment of the Schizophrenic Patient: VI. The Transmission of Irrationality," *AMA Arch. Neurol. and Psychiat.* (1958) 79 : 305–316; Davide Limentani, "Symbiotic Identification in Schizophrenia," *Psychiatry* (1956) 19 : 231–236; Benjamin B. Wolman, "Explorations in Latent Schizophrenia," *Amer. J. Psychotherapy* (1957) 11 : 560–588; Lyman C. Wynne, Irving M. Ryckoff, Juliana Day, and Stanley I. Hirsch, "Pseudo-Mutuality in the Family Relations of Schizophrenics," *Psychiatry* (1958) 21 : 205–220.

evidence of interrelatedness of the participants in a social field in which the pattern or mode of interaction must be comprehended in order to clarify the transactions involving any two members.[3] The parent who responds anxiously to his child's growth is not necessarily resisting change for evil motives; he may not recognize the need for alteration in himself, or he may think of himself as incapable of such development. In this last instance his child's increasing separateness may be experienced as a threat—of loss of the child, or as destruction of the parent who continues to need the child to maintain his own sense of integrity. As the interrelatedness of behavior is recognized, provision may be made for the mutuality of change, and growth will be equated with life rather than with death.

I have reported that Catherine was thought to have a pituitary disorder—sometimes called *Simmond's Cachexia*[4]—prior to the onset of that behavior described as schizophrenic. In the course of treatment there came to be no further evidence of such a state, and she was eventually no longer looked upon as "physically" or "mentally" ill.

I thought of other patients who had shown marked disturbances of organ systems prior to the establishing of the diagnosis of schizophrenia. Charles was eighteen years old when he developed a colitis; a year later he was obviously schizophrenic, but the colitis persisted during the first three years of psychotherapy, and then disappeared. James was thought to be suffering from multiple sclerosis before the appearance of schizophrenic behavior, and neurological signs were evident at times during the earlier period of his psychotherapy, although the original diagnosis was not confirmed.

I then thought of Steven, a college student who consulted me many years ago with a complaint of pain in the groin, and the fear that he might have a rupture. I examined him, assured him that there was no evidence of hernia, and was surprised to find that he was not relieved at this intelligence. We talked further and I discovered that he had engaged recently in a sexual venture. He feared that he might have contracted a venereal infection, and hoped that in the course of my examination for hernia I might comment on the absence—hopefully not the presence—of such a disease. When I did not mention his genitals he was troubled, but was at first unable to question me because of being ashamed. But this was not all; he was concerned with the feeling that he had committed the unpardonable sin in having a sexual affair, and he was hesitant to speak of this, not wishing to appear insane. I asked him what he meant by the sin, and he said: "I felt as if I had done something very terrible, and that I'd be punished. That's crazy—but I felt as if I would lose my mind. How could I talk of that?"

[3] In this sense the schizophrenic reaction is not considered to be a reflection of an earlier (or persistent) interaction between 'schizophrenogenic' mother and child, or 'inadequate' father and child. The object of study becomes the character of the social field, reflecting the participation of significant members in it.

[4] Simmond's disease: Cachexia hypophysea (pituitary cachexia).

"What do you mean by '*that*'?" I asked.

He gave me a plain answer: "I just wouldn't *be* any more. There would be no one."

Steven was describing his experience of severe anxiety, but he was also telling of his great difficulty in relating to another human. The physical symptom, pain in the groin, enabled him to see a physician, and because I had time and was somehow not too harsh with him, he learned more of himself, speaking finally not so much of sexual matters, but of his great need for and fear of any relationship, and his shame at being so alone.

Each of my patients displayed behavior which at times involved various organ systems and frequently required the expert consultation of the internist and other specialists. Often these physical symptoms were more pronounced when verbal communication was failing and social withdrawal increasing—as in the earlier stages of onset, prior to the appearance of clearly evident psychosis, and at intervals during the course of psychotherapy. In this sense the bodily disturbances had a quality of communication. They could not be translated directly into speech (so far as I am concerned), but they were suggestive of the patient's struggle with his need to express himself without terrible risk to his self-esteem; his contacts with others were fragile and failing, his words were not adequate for the maintenance of both security and communication, and his entire organism responded strongly to the threat of an increasing unrelatedness.

I shall now say something of the course of human development, as a preliminary to discussing how the schizophrenic way of life has its beginning. The human animal moves from one developmental era to another in gaining the experiences through which he can become more fully human. In each era readied behavioral potential must be met by the social situation appropriate to its expression in order for proper growth to occur. Defects in development resulting from inadequate meeting of ability and opportunity in one era may not be fully corrected in later periods, the resulting deficiencies in learning, dissociation of aspects of experience, and deformities of behavior being, in some instances, so prominent and troublesome that the personalities concerned are referred to as examples of mental illness.

The human infant—if he is fortunate—has much bodily contact with a mother who is happy in her love for him and somewhat pleased with herself as a person. In such an accepting situation he begins to differentiate himself from others without undue anxiety, and accepts with increasing pleasure and responsiveness the tenderness available to him. The child, increasing his linguistic skill, learns more of his particular cultural prescriptions, advances in his ability to distinguish between those matters labeled by his group as "reality" or "fantasy," and discovers others outside his home. The juvenile improves his social skills, learns something of group activities involving competition and cooperation, hopefully corrects certain gross distortions learned in the home, discovers the often destructive short cuts available through the use of stereotypes, and makes increasing use of foresight. The preadolescent refines his abilities for group participation and discovers the wonder of love and communication as he finds a friend. There follows the patterning of sexual behavior and the achieving of a greater coincidence of lustful and loving interests.

In all of these steps the human has become more involved with his fellows. So that he may feel secure—tolerably free of anxiety—he requires the approval of his kind. His need for tenderness has developed into a need for intimacy, for collaboration with others, for the giving, as well as the receiving, of affection. He has gained what he has of his humanity from others, and his fate is inextricably and finally bound to theirs. Being attached to others, he will know loss and loneliness, but these he can endure if he does not deny his relatedness.

The schizophrenic reaction may be looked upon as the expression of complicated patterns of behavior adopted by the organism in an effort to deal with a gross inadequacy in relating to other humans, the appearance of the clinical syndrome being a late expression of the accumulating disasters of many years. The behavior exhibited is a reflection of response to stress; is evidence of a disorder of personality structure—that is, the organization of the interrelatedness of person and environment; has a communicative aspect; and enables the person to preserve some sense of security and comfort.

It is my impression that the schizophrenic way of life has its beginnings in infancy, that period during which the young human is remarkably dependent upon those who care for him, is vulnerable to their anxiety, and is subject to their teaching. It is then that the fundamental pattern of relationship is formed. That pattern may be marked by anxiety, fear, and insecurity, with accompanying attempts at correction—refinements of human behavior which are referred to as sublimation, repression, substitution, obsessionalism, projection, and so on—or by relative comfort and acceptance of human associations.

By *stress* I refer to the following elements which, if uncorrected by later experience, may contribute to the deviation of personality which may eventuate in a schizophrenic response:

First, severe and recurrent anxiety in the mothering person, complicating the infant's attainment of a clear concept of himself or others.[5]

[5] See, for example, the following: Sylvia Brody, *Patterns of Mothering: Maternal Influence During Infancy*; New York, International Univ. Press, 1956; William Goldfarb, "Emotional and Intellectual Consequences of Psychologic Deprivation in Infancy: A Revaluation," pp. 105–119; in *Psychopathology of Childhood*, edited by Paul H. Hoch and Joseph Zubin; New York, Grune and Stratton, 1955; Lawson G. Lowrey, "Personality Distortion and Early Institutional Care," *Amer. J. Orthopsychiatry* (1935) 10 : 576–585; Margaret Schoenberger Mahler, "On Child Psychosis and Schizophrenia: Autistic and Symbiotic Infantile Psychoses," pp. 286–305; in *The Psychoanalytic Study of the Child*, Vol. 7; New York, International Univ. Press, 1952; M. F. A. Montagu, "Constitutional and Prenatal Factors in Infant and Child Health," pp. 148–210; in *The Healthy Personality*, edited by M. J. E. Senn; New York, Josiah Macy, Jr. Foundation, 1950; M. A. Ribble, "Disorganizing Factors of Infant Personality," *Amer. J. Psychiatry* (1941) 98 : 459–463; L. W. Sontag, "Differences in Modifiability of Fetal Behavior and Physiology," *Psychosomatic Med.* (1944) 6 : 151–154; René A. Spitz, "Anxiety in Infancy: A Study of Its Manifestations in the First Year of Life," *Internat. J. Psycho.-Anal.* (1950) 31 : 138–143.

Second, a multiplicity of conflicting, incomplete, and obscure messages from those who care for the infant, before he has attained much skill in the use of language. The discrepancies between action and speech lead to uncertainty about his position in relation to others and to persisting unclarity as to the significance of what is said and done.

Third, repeated threats to the continuance of the relationship of the infant with those who care for him. The result may be the dissociation of aspects of behavior which seem to jeopardize the relationship essential for survival; and the keeping of such matters out of awareness will interfere with further learning and contribute to later perceptual distortions.

Fourth, a warped and peculiarly personal view of the culture, taught to the child by members of his family through the necessities of their own anxieties.

Fifth, the development of a fear of people, interfering with learning, the verification of ideas with others, and the correction of early misapprehensions of the culture.

The human has certain *goals* toward which he tends, among which are:

First, the continuance of his growth toward a greater realization of potential.

Second, the attainment of learning which will increase the comprehension of experience and the capacity to cope with it.

Third, the maintenance of the relatedness required for survival.

Fourth, the preservation of some feeling of security and freedom from anxiety.

Fifth, the awareness of some dependable concept of himself in relation to his family, his culture, and his universe; that is, the establishing of some sense of permanency and predictability regarding the social field in which he exists.

In order to attain anything resembling such goals, the person who has experienced the stress suggested above must keep dissociated important aspects of interpersonal experience, which requires that he move with great caution among people who may threaten to increase his anxiety and disturb his precarious security, and that he distort his perception of events in the service of his prestige needs. With increasing involvement in the complexities of living and a greater need for self-identification, the defensive operations may no longer suffice to maintain anxiety at a tolerable level, and behavior characteristic of the onset of schizophrenia may appear.

There comes a time—usually in adolescence in this culture—at which one must declare himself; he must identify himself as a person apart from his family, establish intimacy with a friend or face loneliness, pattern his sexual behavior, and consider such matters as further formal education, marriage, work, and life in a community. All of these activities require increased self-identification, the ability to relate, and the revelation of self to others. The move toward intimacy involves increasing anxiety; the failure to make the move brings loneliness and the threat of unrelatedness. The extreme of either course is panic and the feeling of impending, if not actual, dissolution and death. Many of the phenomena observable during the development of disorder reflect efforts to escape the intolerables of anxiety[6] and aloneness.

From the point of view presented here schizophrenia is not looked upon as a disease, but as a reaction to, and an expression of, the social scenes in which an organism with certain biological endowments—usually adequate, so far as I know, to the task of becoming fully human—has its being.[7]

The schizophrenic person has become involved in a relatedness which has been complicated by his fear that he cannot measure up to expectations of him, by the anxiety associated with people, by deficiencies of learning, and by the warped views held by those who participate with him in the disorder. Such a person is not unrelated; he values relatedness and is so fearful of losing that which he has that he may fail to improve his state, the anxiety of human contact being equated with the loss of all contact.

The human who develops his ability to experience some degree of intimacy with another is subject to loneliness, a tension so strong that on occasion one may endure anxiety to escape it. Loneliness, which is a refinement of intimacy in human relationship, is marked by a quality of hopefulness, in that there is the possibility of its relief through action. Unrelatedness does not have this quality, but implies the loss of human contacts without discernible ways for regaining them. The failure to develop the needed relatedness in infancy leads to the marasmic death. The loss of relatedness later in life leads to panic, to a sense of the loss of self, and, in some instances, to death.

[6] By the word *anxiety* I refer to an interpersonal phenomenon in which one is related to another in such fashion that his feeling of security and personal worth seems subject to that one's approval. This anxiety is man-made, having its origin and continuance in the relationships between humans. Although this unpleasant sentiment, which is so destructive to human intimacy, reflects the anticipation (and experience) of disapproval, it is, I think, more basically associated with the apprehension that separation and unrelatedness will follow upon rejection. By anxiety I do not refer to any more basic discomfort supposedly associated with growth, new experience, or death. I think that anxiety is manmade, and that processes of growth, including death, are not 'naturally' accompanied by any anxiety other than that reflecting human experience.

I make these rather limited remarks in order to emphasize my concern with what I think of as the necessity for man to direct his attention to the part which he plays in the reduction and destruction of himself. Should man 'explain' or seek to 'justify' his destructiveness as being evidence of his 'fate,' or his 'nature,' or the unfathomable 'wisdom' of unidentified forces, he might overlook his proper responsibilities and seal his own fate; that is, he might begin to accept the symbolic structure of his culture as somehow an unmodifiable reality, and die a victim of the symbolization of his personal inadequacy. The therapist, without abandoning wonderment for his universe and recognition of his own limitations, and without espousing a biological reductionism, is well advised to seek for anxiety in the interpersonal field, avoiding any tendency to ascribe interhuman discomfort to the extrahuman. (Of interest in regard to the concept of anxiety is the following: Hubert Benoît, *The Supreme Doctrine, Psychological Studies in Zen Thought*, New York, The Viking Press, 1959; Chapter 5.)

[7] I do not speak of 'disease of the ego,' not being content with a dividing of the personality into parts, and being impressed by the totality of the organism's response to situations of stress.

ALAN F. FONTANA

Familial Etiology of Schizophrenia: Is a Scientific Methodology Possible?[1]

Many who regard schizophrenia as a disorder having primarily psychogenic causes have looked for those causes within the dynamics of the family producing a schizophrenic member. While intra-familial relationships would seem to be the simplest and most sensible area in which to attempt to understand the psychological forces that provoke a schizophrenic reaction, unfortunately, conducting research in this area is extraordinarily difficult methodologically. The paper by Fontana, which follows, reviews a number of studies of familial factors in the etiology of schizophrenia and evaluates the methodology used in such studies. In addition to serving as a significant reference for those who would do research in this area, Fontana's paper also describes many of the interesting findings emanating from familial studies that have been done in the recent past.

The 3 major research approaches toward identifying familial etiological factors in schizophrenia are examined from a methodological viewpoint. Both the clinical observational and retrospective recall methods are judged to be inadequate. The 3rd approach, direct observation and recording of family interactions, is concluded to be free of intrinsically disqualifying inadequacies, given the limiting assumption that the variables under investigation are etiological in nature. Although the limitations of this assumption can only be overcome by a longitudinal approach, family interaction studies are considered to be an indispensable, practical precondition to the formulation of longitudinal studies. Results from a subset of methodologically adequate studies are examined and conclusions drawn. Several cautions and recommendations for future research are offered.

[1] The preparation of this paper was supported by Research Grant MH 08050 from the National Institute of Mental Health, United States Public Health Service. The author wishes to thank Edward B. Klein and Carmi Schooler for their critical reading of the manuscript.

Reprinted from *Psychological Bulletin*, **66** (1966), 214–227, with the permission of the American Psychological Association and A. F. Fontana.

The functional role of the family in the development of schizophrenia[2] has been the subject of intensive investigation. Researchers have reported that several personality characteristics differentiate between parents of schizophrenics and nonschizophrenics, and that several aspects of family interaction patterns differ in the families of schizophrenics and nonschizophrenics. However, reviewers (Frank, 1965; Meissner, 1964; Rabkin, 1965; Sanua, 1961) have not shared the optimism and conclusions of the majority of researchers. The recent review by Frank (1965) states that in the last 40 years of research, *no* factors have been found which either differentiate between the families of psychopathological and normal members, or among families of pathological members who are classified according to different diagnostic categories. That author's pessimism extends to the more general issue concerning the applicability of the scientific method to the study of human behavior:

> Apparently, the factors which play a part in the development of behavior in humans are so complex that it would appear that they almost defy being investigated scientifically and defy one's attempt to draw meaningful generalizations from the exploration which has already been done [p. 201].

Frank is quite correct in raising the issue of methodology. It is a truism that any body of scientific facts must rest upon a scientifically sound methodology. The conclusions from any study not so based cannot be considered scientific, no matter how scholarly they may be. Some of the previous reviewers have paid insufficient attention to the methodology of individual studies. Rather, their approach has been to tabulate positive and negative results without evaluating the methodological adequacy of individual studies. This approach may have obscured some consistent empirical trends which can be found in well-designed studies.

The purpose of this paper is to examine the scientific status of the three major research approaches, first methodologically and then in terms of empirical results. The sources of data for the approaches to be considered are: (*a*) clinical observations and psychiatric impressions of family members in treatment, (*b*) retrospective accounts of child-rearing practices, and attitudes obtained from family members' responses to interviews and questionnaires, and (*c*) current patterns of interaction among family members directly recorded and systematically coded by the investigator. Rabkin (1965) and Sanua (1961) have presented excellent critiques of much of the work in this area, particularly those

[2] It is assumed that the term "schizophrenia" applies to a subset of behaviors or processes which differentiates persons so labeled from others. The reliability of psychiatric diagnosis has been a topic much discussed and argued. It is clear from the extant literature that schizophrenia, as a major category, is the most reliable of the diagnoses. The possibility exists, however, that psychiatric and psychological professionals are inconsistently "over-inclusive" or "underinclusive" in applying schizophrenia as a concept, and for this reason "schizophrenics" may be just as different from each other as they are from others. The crucial question is, of course, "What is schizophrenia?" In attempting to answer this, there seems to be little choice but to study people *called* schizophrenic.

studies classified under the first two headings above. Their papers provide extensive coverage of inadequacies, such as the lack of control groups and nonspecification of subjects' demographic characteristics, which are not essential to the viability of the methodology itself. The present analysis will focus on issues concerning the scientific appropriateness of the methodology per se.

Clinical Observational Studies

The major limitation inherent in the methodology of clinical observational studies is that the theoretical biases of the therapists tend to become inextricably interwoven with the recording and obtaining of data. Since there is no mechanical recording of the data, the therapist becomes the recording instrument. The therapist typically makes notes after the therapy session has been completed. Thus not only are his perceptions of the moment colored by his biases, but his recollections are subject to primacy-recency effects. Acquisition of the data is also likely to be affected by the therapist's preconceptions. Verbal conditioning studies have demonstrated that people's verbal productions can be shaped to a marked degree by the listener's expressions of interest. Therapists are likely to be unaware that they are selectively reinforcing certain aspects of their patients' behavior.

There is some evidence that many of the theoretical concepts that serve as a framework for therapists' descriptions of the familial characteristics of schizophrenics are not accurate (Jackson, Block, Block, & Patterson, 1958). Jackson et al. asked 20 well-known psychiatrists, who had had considerable experience with schizophrenics and their families, to perform two *Q* sorts on 108 statements according to their conceptions of the schizophrenic's mother and father. Factor analysis produced three factors for each parent. The six factors were considered to represent the conceptions of mothers and fathers of schizophrenics most widely held in the field of psychiatry. The conceptions were correlated with descriptions of the parents of 20 autistic and 20 neurotic children which had been made by *Q* sorts of the same 108 items. None of the conceptions showed even a trend toward differentiating the two groups of parents. The results of the Jackson et al. study provide an empirical example and documentation of the inadequacies of this method. Whereas the clinical observational method is valuable as a source of provocative hypotheses and potentially fruitful insights, intrinsic difficulties make it unsuitable as a firm basis for a scientific methodology.

Retrospective Studies

The validity of interviews and questionnaires for ascertaining the actual parental child-rearing practices and attitudes during the subject's childhood rests upon several assumptions: (*a*) that people conceptualize their lives in terms of the language used by the investigator so that their understanding of the questions is similar to that of the investigator; (*b*) that people can accurately recall events and feelings of many years past with minimal forgetting; (*c*) that people will report unpleasant events without selective forgetting, defensive distortion, and justification of actions by inaccurate elaboration; and (*d*) that people will report past events unaffected by social desirability or other response sets. Fortunately, there is a substantial amount of empirical data available for evaluating the tenability of these assumptions. McGraw and Molloy (1941) interviewed mothers twice concerning their retrospective accounts of the developmental history of their children. The first time, they conducted the interviews in the usual manner of an intake interviewer. One month later they interviewed the mothers again with more detailed and specific questioning, including pictorial representations of many of the developmental skills involved in the questions. The accuracy of the reports, when compared to staff examination of the children during their development, increased markedly from first to second interview for many questions, particularly for those accompanied by pictorial representations. These results demonstrate the considerable lack of commonality of meaning between investigator and subject when questions are phrased in their typical, unelaborated form. Moreover, questions dealing with feelings and attitudes are not amenable to the pictorial specificity possible in other areas.

The ability of people to recall past events and feelings reliably has been investigated in wider, longitudinal research projects. Haggard, Brekstad, and Skard (1960), Robbins (1963), and Yarrow, Campbell, and Burton (1964) have compared retrospective parental reports to historical parental reports, and Jayaswal and Stott (1955), McGraw and Molloy (1941), Pyles, Stolz, and Macfarlane (1935), and Yarrow et al. (1964) have compared parental recollections to observational material obtained by a research staff during the children's development. All these studies found considerable unreliability in retrospective reports, as well as large intrasubject variability in accuracy across items.

Content of the material to be recalled has an important effect on accuracy of recall. Questions asking for recall of quantitative information and concrete events are answered more reliably than inquiries about attitudes and feelings (Haggard et al., 1960; Yarrow et al., 1964). Haggard et al. (1960) have reported, further, that the greater the initial anxiety associated with an attitude, the less accurately the attitude is recalled. In fact, recall of attitudes originally associated with great anxiety is almost completely unreliable. Kohn and Carroll (1960) found that the picture of past events varied considerably depending upon the member of the family doing the reporting. Heilbrun (1960) found no difference between the way the mothers of schizophrenic and of normal daughters described their child-rearing attitudes, but did find that schizophrenic daughters described their mothers as more pathological in their attitudes than did normal daughters. On the other hand, Jayaswal and Stott (1955) reported that young adults and their parents showed high agreement in their descriptions of the young adults as children. However, neither set of descriptions bore much relation to teachers' descriptions of the young adults obtained when they were children.

Many empirical studies have shown that social desirability and other response sets affect subjects' responses to questionnaire items. There are some data to indicate that responses to questions in an interview are subject to similar biases. McGraw and Molloy (1941) and Pyles et al. (1935) have shown that maternal inaccuracies in recall tended to be made in the direction of precocity in their children, that is, mothers tended to under-estimate the age at which their children acquired developmental skills and the time taken to acquire the skills. Robbins (1963) has reported a variation on this finding. Inaccuracies tended to reflect the recommendations of a noted contemporary child-rearing expert.

The results of studies evaluating the reliability of retrospective reports make the assumptions underlying the method untenable. Kasanin, Knight, and Sage (1934), Rabkin (1965), and Sanua (1961) have pointed out additional weaknesses in this method. Two are peculiar to the use of interview material from case history folders. These records vary widely in their completeness, with the result that many are rejected because of missing data. Overprotective mothers give more information about their children's background, so that a selective bias influences the characteristics of the records accepted. Offspring of such mothers are very likely over-represented in samples drawn on the basis of completeness. Another bias derives from the manner in which the case histories are obtained. The intake interviewer asks questions and records the data according to his theoretical biases. This same limitation was discussed in connection with the clinical observational method. There is one reservation peculiar to questionnaire data. A high and consistent relationship between current attitudes and current behavior has not yet been empirically demonstrated. It would seem to be an almost insurmountable task to demonstrate a high and consistent relationship between past attitudes and past behavior. For all the above reasons, the retrospective report method is judged to be an inadequate foundation for a body of scientific facts.

Family Interaction Studies

A criticism that has been applied to each of the preceding methods of investigation is that, in many cases, the data are not recorded and coded objectively and systematically. Haley (1964) and Rabkin (1965) have extended this criticism to family interaction studies, pointing out that high interjudge reliabilities may occur as a result of two or more judges coding within the framework of the same theoretical biases. Thus, one could not be sure that the data were free of inferences from the observer. Haley has suggested and used automatic recording and tabulating of interactional indices by electronic instruments (Haley, 1962, 1964). This insures highly reliable coding, but is purchased at a high price. In one study, Haley (1964) used a machine to tabulate automatically the number of times one person followed another in conversation. However, it is impossible to tell from the data whether the second person interrupted, asked a question, answered a question, disagreed, agreed, said something irrelevant, or was even talking to the first person. The meaningfulness of the data is questionable when they are stripped of such categories. It should be possible, however, to make increased use of instrumentation without sacrificing most of the content of the interaction. Even at best, instrumentation would not solve the problem completely, since the investigator must still program his instruments to code selected aspects of the interaction. A balance must be reached between unchecked observer contamination and such rigid control of possible contamination that essential aspects of the phenomenon under investigation are obscured. At the present time, establishment of high interjudge reliabilities seems to be a workable solution to the dilemma.

Family interaction studies that seek to discover factors which are etiologically relevant to the development of schizophrenia necessarily assume that the causal factors lie in the characteristics of the family interaction pattern. Many people have made the opposite assumption that it is the schizophrenia of the child which has caused the family to develop certain interactional characteristics. Thus, if family interaction studies could demonstrate differences between familes of schizophrenics and nonschizophrenics, the question would still be moot as to the locus of cause and effect. At the present time, one assumption is as valid as the other. The assumption that the family interaction patterns are the causal factors in the development of schizophrenia is important for present purposes because it implies several other assumptions concerning methodology. The first is that the interaction patterns in the experimental setting are the usual family patterns and the subjects' usual behavior is not altered by the knowledge that they are being studied by professional experts. This assumption is particularly dubious for those studies in which a hospitalized schizophrenic group is compared to a nonhospitalized control group. The two groups of families undoubtedly have different perceptions of the meaning of the experimenter's request for participation. For the families of schizophrenics, participation is probably perceived as a way of helping their children; while for the families of nonhospitalized controls, it may well be seen as a test of their psychological health or normality. Each family's perception of its role in the research program would probably affect its mode of interaction. For example, Cheek (1964a) has found that mothers of normals were significantly more ego defensive than mothers of schizophrenics. A similar trend was also obtained for fathers (Cheek, 1965). The problem of differential defensiveness can be largely circumvented by utilizing families of other institutionalized and stigmatized groups as controls so that all are recruited on the same basis and are likely to share the meaning of the request for participation. People could still be expected to react to being studied, but the groups would not be differentially affected. The possibility (and probability) that people's behavior will be affected by the knowledge that they are being observed is present in all areas of psychology.

A second assumption, related to the first, is that current interaction patterns are unchanged from their characteristics before the child became a patient. This means that the way family members interact is unaffected by the hospitalization, and consequent change in status. It is particularly unlikely that this assumption would be valid for chronic patients. If a person has been hospitalized for a long time or for a large number of times, the family is likely to incorporate his status as a mental patient into its image of him. Likewise, the person could be expected to modify his self-concept to include the attributes of the chronic mental patient. Institutionalization effects can be lessened by using only families of acute patients, for whom hospitalization would more likely be perceived as transitory. An even more desirable group would be families of persons on outpatient or trial visit status.

A third assumption is that current interaction patterns are essentially unchanged from their characteristics at the time the child was becoming schizophrenic. In order for this assumption to be valid, there must have been no essential change over time due to aging of the parents and maturation of the child. The crucial aspect of this position revolves around the word "essential." The extent to which basic personality and interactional characteristics are modifiable beyond the first few years of life is still an issue of considerable dispute.

A fourth assumption is also made that the task around which the interaction is organized does not alter the pattern in some unique way so that it is specific to that task and a circumscribed group of similar tasks. Rather, it is assumed that the families react to the experimental task as they characteristically react to most tasks.

A fifth assumption is that family interaction patterns are the same when some members are absent as they are when all members are present. This assumption appears of dubious validity, but whether different groups of families are affected differentially by missing members is unknown. Siblings of the patients or control subjects could be included in the interactions in order to investigate this possibility.

Consideration of these five assumptions highlights the tentativeness of etiological conclusions that might be drawn from family interaction studies. Nevertheless, the study of family interaction holds promise for providing valuable guidelines for the design and hypothetical formulations of longitudinal studies, from which appropriate cause and effect statements can be made. If the inconclusiveness of the etiological assumption is granted and accepted, then there are no apparent, intrinsic methodological inadequacies to the study of family interaction which would disqualify it as a scientific endeavor. The possible limitations of method arising from the etiological assumption can be largely circumvented or minimized by careful attention to specific controls. With this in mind, let us proceed to an examination of family interaction studies, first from a methodological viewpoint and then from the perspective of empirical results from the better designed studies.

Difficulties of Interpretation and Evaluation

Studies employing the direct recording and systematic coding of actual family interactions have been few in number and recent in origin. This reviewer is aware of only 20 reports subsequent to the year 1950 which fall into this category, with the earliest published in 1958. The paucity of such studies is primarily due to two factors: (*a*) the recent interest in the study of interpersonal relations, and (*b*) the difficulty in conducting such studies. In view of the latter factor, it is unfortunate that the results of the labor and effort invested in the majority of studies have been negated by insufficient attention to essential controls. On the basis of considerations arising from the etiological assumption and from data demonstrating the possible confounding effects of certain variables, nine criteria were selected for evaluating the methodological adequacy of studies in this area. This reviewer's judgments of the methodological status of family interaction studies are summarized in Table 1. It is apparent from the table that there is great variability among the studies, and that much desired information is unavailable from the published reports. It is important that control and experimental groups be comparable on as many demographic variables as possible, but particularly on ages of parents and children, sex and birth order of the children, family size, and social class of the family.

Different rates of interaction and patterns of participation could be expected between parents and offspring, depending on the ages of both. All parents might plausibly be expected to be more indulgent of a small child than of a young or middle-aged adult. Similarly, adult patients and control subjects could be expected to relate somewhat differently to their parents if the latter were middle-aged than if they were close to retirement age.

The importance of keeping the sexes separate in the data analysis has been demonstrated in a number of studies. Cheek (1964b) found that schizophrenic women were more active in family interactions than were normal women, and schizophrenic men were less active than normal men. In addition, women were higher than men in acknowledgements, tension release, giving opinions, and asking for opinions. Ferreira (1963) reported a difference in frequency of coalitions with each parent in normal families, depending on the sex of the child. Same-sex coalitions were more frequent than opposite-sex coalitions. This same relationship was found in a subsequent study (Ferreira & Winter, 1965) in terms of the initial private agreement between parents and children, and observed to increase with increasing age of the children. Again, this relationship only occurred in normal families. Baxter, Arthur, Flood, and Hedgepeth (1962) found that families of male and female schizophrenics differed in amount of conflict, depending on whether conflict was coded from the extent of initial, private agreement among members or from disagreements arising during family interaction. Also, families of male patients tended to have more mother-

TABLE 1 *Methodological summary of family interaction studies*

Author	Demographic comparability of control and schizophrenic groups	Sex of subjects[a]	Hospital status of schizophrenic group	Subdivision of schizophrenic group	Control group	"Blind" coding of data	Reliability of coding	Members in interaction[h]	Task characteristics
Baxter et al. (1962)	No control group	m & f	Acute	Poor premorbid[d]	—	Ns	Good	F,M,C	Joint interview
Baxter & Arthur (1964)	No control group	m	Acute	Poor & good premorbid	—	Ns	Good	F,M	Joint interview
Behrens & Goldfarb (1958)	Questionable	m & f	Ns	—[e]	Maladjusted persons	No	Fair	F(u)	Home interactions
Caputo (1963)	Good	m	Chronic	—	Normals[g]	Ns	Vs	F,M	RDT[j]
Cheek (1964a)	Fair	m & f[b]	Convalescent	—	Normals	Ns	Vs	F,M,C	RDT
Cheek (1964b)	Fair	m & f[b]	Convalescent	—	Normals	Ns	Vs	F,M,C	RDT
Cheek (1965)	Fair	m & f[b]	Convalescent	—	Normals	Ns	Vs	F,M,C	RDT
Farina (1960)	Fair	m	Acute	Poor & good premorbid	Tubercular patients[g]	Ns	High	F,M	RDT
Farina & Dunham (1963)	No control group	m	Acute	Poor & good premorbid	—	Ns	High	F,M,C	RDT
Ferreira (1963)	Questionable	m & f	Ns	—	Normals, maladjusted persons	Ns	Ns	F,M,C	RDT
Ferreira & Winter (1965)	Good	m & f	Ns	—	Normals, delinquents, maladjusted persons	Ns	Ns	F,M,C	RDT
Fisher et al. (1959)	Good	m	Ns	—	Neurotics,[g] normals,[g] normals	Yes	High	F,M	Family discussion, TAT story construction
Haley (1962)	Fair	m & f	Ns	—	Normals	Mt	High	F,M,C	Game
Haley (1964)	Questionable	m & f	Ns	—[e]	Normals	Mt	High	F,M,C	RDT, TAT story construction
Lennard et al. (1965)	Fair	m	Ns	—[e]	Normals	Ns	Ns	F,M,C	Family discussion
Lerner (1965)	Good	m	Ns[c]	High & low genetic level[f]	Normals[g]	Ns	High	F,M	RDT
McCord et al. (1962)	Good	m	Prehospitalization	—[e]	Maladjusted persons	Yes	Good	F,M,C	Home interactions
Meyers & Goldfarb (1961)	Fair	m & f	Ns	Organic & nonorganic	Normals	No	Ns	F(u)	Home interactions
Morris & Wynne (1965)	Questionable	m & f	Ns	—	Neurotics[g]	Yes	Un-obtained	F,M[i]	Joint therapy
Stabenau et al. (1965)	Good	m & f	Ns	—	Delinquents, normals	Ns	Ns	F,M,C,S	RDT

Note.—Ns = not stated, Vs = vaguely stated, Mt = machine tabulated.
[a] m = male, f = female.
[b] Analyzed separately.
[c] Schizophrenic and control groups were equated on length of current hospitalization.
[d] Premorbidity rated according to the Phillips' (1953) scale.
[e] Included unspecified psychotics.
[f] According to Becker's (1956) system of Rorschach analysis.
[g] Hospitalized.
[h] F = father, M = mother, C = child, S = sib, F(u) = family (unspecified).
[i] Patient present but not a verbal contributor.
[j] Modification of the Revealed Difference Technique, after Strodtbeck (1951).

father conflict, while mother-patient conflict tended to be greater in the families of female patients. Investigators in most studies using the families of both male and female subjects have not equated their experimental and control groups for the number of each sex, while, at the same time, they have summed their interaction indices across sex. It is impossible to tell how much confounding this procedure may have introduced into the data analysis.

A control related to sex effects, which no study has considered, concerns the possible effects of birth order on interaction behavior. Schooler has used birth order as an independent variable in several studies of schizophrenia. He found that female schizophrenics disproportionately come from the last half of the birth order regardless of social class, while lastborn male schizophrenics disproportionately come from middle-class families and firstborns from lower-class families (Schooler, 1961, 1964). In two other studies, female schizophrenics born in the first half of the birth order were found to be more sociable than those born in the last half (Schooler & Scarr, 1962), and firstborn male schizophrenics were observed to perform better than middle borns who in turn performed better than lastborn patients on a task where their performance was seen as helpful to another person (Schooler & Long, 1963). These findings parallel those of Schachter (1959), obtained with normal women.

Closely allied with birth order is the issue of family size. It seems reasonable to expect that parents might have more contact with each of their children, the fewer of them there are. Also, the number of children in the family might reflect differences in parental attitudes and behavior toward their offspring.

Schooler (1964) and Cheek (1964b) have identified an important qualification which must be applied to all studies using hospitalized persons as subjects. It is most appropriate to generalize only to hospitalized schizophrenics and not to all schizophrenics. Schooler noted that latter-born female schizophrenics manifested more noticeable symptomatology, such as hallucinations and suicidal tendencies, than did their counterparts born in the first half of the birth order. He has suggested that the florid character of their symptoms might lead to latter borns being hospitalized more readily, therefore being disproportionately represented in hospitals. In a similar vein, Cheek has suggested that overactive females and underactive males manifest interaction patterns deviant from societal norms, which may result in their being hospitalized more readily than those whose activity patterns are congruent with socially normative behavior. If many symptom characteristics turn out to be epiphenomena of a more basic, common schizophrenic process, the search for schizophrenic-specific factors will be somewhat confounded by society's attitudes toward different symptoms.

Social class embodies many attitude, value, knowledge, and social skill differences between people and, for this reason, is an extremely important variable to keep comparable among groups. Baxter and Arthur (1964) have provided striking evidence of how social class can interact with an independent variable to confound the results of the unwary investigator. These authors found that social class interacted with the premorbid adjustment of their male schizophrenic patients, so that middle-class parents of patients who had made a relatively adequate premorbid adjustment showed more conflict in interaction than did middle-class parents of patients who had made an inadequate premorbid adjustment, with the reverse results obtaining for lower-class groups of parents. All differences disappeared when the data were analyzed by social class or premorbidity alone. These results also argue for a subdivision of the schizophrenic sample according to some criteria such as good-poor premorbid adjustment or the process-reactive distinction. Both of these subdivisions have been empirically demonstrated to have prognostic validity (Becker, 1959; Phillips, 1953), to reduce the heterogeneity of schizophrenic performance (Garmezy & Rodnick, 1959; Herron, 1962), and to be highly interrelated (Solomon & Zlotowski, 1964). Thus, either subdivision makes an empirically meaningful distinction within schizophrenia, and holds promise of indicating a fruitful theoretical distinction as well.

Religion and ethnicity are two interrelated variables which have rarely been controlled. Sanua (1961) has argued that reports of contradictory results in the literature might be reconciled by closer consideration of differences in the subjects' religion and ethnicity. In an exploratory study, he (Sanua, 1963) found that parental characteristics differed widely according to the religion and social class of the families. These data are only suggestive however, since some essential methodological controls were not employed. A well-controlled study in this area has been reported by McClelland, de Charms, and Rindlisbacher (1955). These investigators questioned Protestant, Jewish, Irish-Catholic, and Italian-Catholic parents about their expectations concerning their children's mastery of several independence skills. In addition to main effects for sex of parent, level of parental education, and religion, they found a complex triple interaction of these variables with the expected age of mastery. There also tended to be a difference within religion between the expectations of Irish and Italian parents. The available evidence is sufficiently strong to warrant attention to the religious and ethnic composition of the subject sample. Certainly, it would be hazardous to ignore sizable religious and ethnic differences between experimental and control groups by assuming on an a priori basis that such differences are irrelevant to the style of family interaction.

A minority of studies specify the characteristics of their hospitalized samples in terms of the acuteness-chronicity dimension. In view of one of the assumptions of the method and the unknown effects of institutionalization on relatives and patients, it would seem to be a highly relevant variable.

Most studies have utilized some mechanical means of recording data, yet some have relied on an interviewer to manually record the interaction as it occurs or even after it has occurred. Most reports do not state whether the data were coded in a "blind" fashion or not, that is, with the coder unable to identify the group membership of the families. In many cases, the reliability of the coding procedure is not stated or is so vaguely stated as to be of unknown value.

Difficulties of Comparison

Aside from differing degrees of methodological adequacy among studies, there are two factors which complicate direct comparison of results. One is the differing group membership comprising the "family." In some cases only parental interaction has been measured, while in other cases, interaction has included the contributions from the parents and the patient or control child, and in one case assessment was made of the interaction among parents, patient or control child, and another child of the family. It is difficult to assess the possible differential effects of group size, role diversity, and other factors which accompany variation in the number of members in interaction.

A second factor is the difference in task characteristics utilized in the studies. The majority have used modifications of the revealed difference technique (RDT) initially developed by Strodtbeck (1951). The RDT essentially consists of having each member of the family privately state his solutions to a number of problem situations. Then the experimenter asks the family to discuss each problem and to arrive at a group solution. The family discussion is recorded and coded for interaction indices such as agreement, yielding, interruption, and compromise. In studies employing the RDT, however, the range of problem situations extends from highly loaded interpersonal situations involving parent-child conflict to rather trivial, neutral situations. The focus of attention on the structure of family interaction has led to a neglect of the content, around which the interaction is organized, as a factor worthy of systematic study itself. It is not readily apparent that family reactions to situations involving parent-child conflict are structurally indistinguishable from reactions to differences among members concerning trivial preferences, such as choice of colors for an automobile or choice of food from a restaurant menu.

Instead of the RDT, other investigators have used joint interviews, family discussions, joint construction of TAT stories, home interactions, game playing, and joint therapy sessions. Haley (1964), using both the RDT and the construction of stories in the TAT, found that each task yielded somewhat different results, though each individually was inferior to the two combined in differentiating families of normals from those of psychiatric subjects. One must conclude that task characteristics do affect results, but that the extent of influence is currently undetermined.

Empirical Results

The methodology of most family interaction studies leaves much to be desired. Several controls which are either essential or desirable have been suggested. The five most essential controls have been selected as the bases for determining the subset of studies with sufficiently sound methodology to permit comparison of results and evaluation of conclusions. Four studies have (*a*) utilized only schizophrenics in an experimental group, (*b*) analyzed the data separately by sex, (*c*) made some statement indicating attention to reliability of coding, (*d*) specified adequate comparability of control and experimental groups on demographic variables, and (*e*) included at least one hospitalized control group (Caputo, 1963; Farina, 1960; Fisher, Boyd, Walker, & Sheer, 1959; Lerner, 1965). The Baxter and Arthur (1964) and Farina and Dunham (1963) studies did not include control groups, but are reviewed here because they were designed to test specific points concerning premorbidity differences in Farina's (1960) study. In addition, Cheek's (1964a, 1964b, 1965) reports of her study will be reviewed. Since neither the experimental nor the control group was hospitalized at the time of data collection, the extent to which this difference may have affected her data in comparison to the data of the other studies is unknown.

One of the most widespread and persistent notions concerning schizophrenic etiology is that of the "schizophrenogenic" mother (Fromm-Reichmann, 1948). According to this notion, the family pattern of a strong, dominant mother and a weak, passive father deprives the son of an adequate model of identification. The son reacts to the stresses of this culturally atypical pattern by becoming schizophrenic. As a result of the popularity of this notion, the most frequently coded aspects of family interaction have been maternal and paternal dominance. Fisher et al. (1959) have reported that mothers of normals talked more than did mothers of neurotics or schizophrenics.[3] The latter two groups did not differ. There were no differences among the fathers of the three groups in amount of talking or initiation of conversation. Caputo (1963) found that the fathers of schizophrenics were generally more dominant than the mothers, with the fathers winning more disagreements than mothers. The parents of normals did not differ in the number of disagreements won. Lerner (1965) obtained no differences for mothers and fathers of normals and of two groups of schizophrenics in yielding to the other's position. Cheek (1964a, 1964b, 1965) found no support for the notion of the domineering "schizophrenogenic" mother. In the families of males, each member of the normal's family interacted in a more dominant way than each corresponding member of the schizophrenic's family. Thus *all* members of the schizophrenic's family were more passive than members of the normal's family when the offspring were males. The reverse tended to be true for fathers and offspring in the families of females: each of these members of the schizophrenic's family acted in a more dominant way than each corresponding member of the normal's family. On the other hand, mothers of both male and female normals were more dominant than mothers of schizophrenics. When pairs of means for indices relating to dominance are compared for mothers and fathers, the largest discrepancies between parents occur most often for the parents of normals. In other words, there tended to be a greater imbalance in dominance between parents in the families of normals than in the

[3] All differences reported in this review have been found to be statistically significant at the .05 level or less, unless they are otherwise stated herein as tending to be the case, as trends, or as not significant.

families of schizophrenics. The most notable exception to this trend was for the index, Total Interaction, for which fathers of both male and female schizophrenics tended to be more active relative to their wives, than fathers of normals. All of these findings are counter to what would be expected according to the schizophrenogenic mother notion.

Rodnick and Garmezy (1957; Garmezy & Rodnick, 1959) have proposed a theory which essentially states that the pattern of the schizophrenogenic mother can be found in the families of patients with a poor premorbid adjustment (Poors), while the reverse pattern can be observed in the families of schizophrenics with a relatively good premorbid adjustment (Goods). The adequacy of premorbid adjustment and degree of pathology are presumed to be causally related to the sex of the dominant parent, with the Poors being "sicker" because of the cultural atypicality of their family pattern. Discrepancy in parental dominance is held to be one of the pathognomonic factors predisposing to schizophrenia. One of the keystone studies testing the theory was conducted by Farina (1960). He found that the parents of Poors and Goods were different on all seven of his dominance indices, with Poors being mother dominated and Goods father dominated. However, enthusiasm for this finding as support for the theory must be tempered by consideration of other aspects of these and subsequent data. The parents of Poors were not different from the normals on any of the dominance indices. Goods differed from normals on four of the seven indices. However, two of the nonsignificant indices involved the extent of yielding of one parent to the other. Thus, although the parental dominance pattern for Poors is quite different from that of Goods, neither is strikingly different from the pattern for normals. It is particularly puzzling that the lesser difference from normals was found where the greater difference could have been expected from the theory, that is, in the families of Poors.

Farina also coded the interactions for conflict. It seems reasonable that initiation of conflict could be another way of viewing dominance. Inspection of the index means for conflict reveals that, in all groups, mothers tended to interrupt more and to disagree and aggress more than did fathers. The parental differences are not significant, but the data indicate that the mothers in all groups initiated conflict at least as much as fathers did. A later study by Farina and Dunham (1963) investigated the interactions of mother, father, and patient for groups of Poors and Goods. Although some differences exist, this study can be considered an approximate replication of the Poor-Good comparisons in Farina's study. In the replication, the parental differences for the means of the dominance indices were not as consistent in direction as in the initial study, nor were any of the differences statistically significant. These studies neither support the proposition that the schizophrenogenic pattern is uniquely characteristic of the families of poor premorbid schizophrenics, nor do they offer strong or consistent support for the proposed interaction between parental dominance pattern and adequacy of the patients' social and sexual premorbid adjustment.

Another popular conception is that the schizophrenic's family, in many cases, is characterized by high levels of parental hostility and conflict (Lidz, Cornelison, Fleck, & Terry, 1957). Fisher et al. (1959) found that the parents of schizophrenics and neurotics disagreed more than the parents of normals when they were discussing their sons. The parents of schizophrenics and neurotics did not differ in amount of disagreement. When parents worked jointly on constructing a TAT story, the parents of schizophrenics were higher in disagreement than parents of neurotics who were higher than parents of normals. Caputo (1963) reported that parents of schizophrenics disagreed more and displayed more hostility toward one another than did parents of normals. In Lerner's (1965) study, parents of normals compromised their differences more than either schizophrenic group did, although there were no significant differences among groups in lack of agreement without distortion. However, when lack of agreement with distortion was coded from the interaction, parents of the low genetic level schizophrenic group scored higher than parents of the high genetic level and normal groups. The theoretical significance of this distinction will be elaborated in the next section dealing with clarity of communication. Farina (1960) coded parental interactions on 10 indices of conflict. Parents of Poors manifested more conflict than parents of normals on seven of the indices, while parents of Goods and normals did not differ on any of the indices. Three indices showed differences within schizophrenia, with parents of Poors consistently higher than parents of Goods. The Farina and Dunham (1963) replication provided some support for the differences within schizophrenia obtained by Farina. It will be recalled that Baxter and Arthur (1964) found an interaction between social class and premorbidity affecting parental conflict scores. They suggested that Farina's Poor-Good differences in conflict may have resulted from the particular social-class characteristics of his groups and may not be attributable to premorbidity alone. In brief, the evidence consistently favors support of the contention that there is more conflict in the families of schizophrenics (particularly in the families of the more pathological patients, poor premorbids, and those with a low genetic level of development) than in the families of normals. Whether there is more conflict in the families of schizophrenics than in those of other psychiatric groups is less clear. Systematic variation of social class in this area is necessary for clarification and generalization of present trends.

A fourth theoretical position which can be evaluated in terms of the present data is that the etiological family factor pathognomonic for schizophrenia is lack of clarity in parental communication patterns. This idea has been most systematically developed by Wynne and Singer (1963a, 1963b). They have proposed that the unique characteristic of schizophrenia is disorder of the thought processes, particularly inability to focus attention on thematic material in a consistent and prolonged manner. The thought disorder is learned by imitation of parental patterns of communication, in which meanings are blurred by subtle shifts in attention to progressively tangential material.

These authors have reported several successful attempts at differentiating the parents of schizophrenics from the parents of other groups on the basis of their projective test protocols (Singer & Wynne, 1963, 1965a, 1965b). Morris and Wynne (1965) have reported similar success using excerpts from joint therapy sessions. It is evident that these authors have engaged in a systematic research approach. However, before their results can be considered to be scientifically demonstrated, their research needs the introduction of some basic methodological controls such as specification of an objective coding system and establishment of acceptable interjudge reliabilities. Fortunately, the studies of Fisher et al. (1959) and Lerner (1965) provide more scientifically established evidence relevant to this theoretical position. Fisher et al. (1959) found that parents of normals were less ambiguous in their communication with each other than were the parents of neurotics and schizophrenics when they were discussing their sons, and were less ambiguous than parents of schizophrenics when jointly constructing a TAT story. It will be recalled that in the Lerner (1965) study there were no differences among parental groups of high and low genetic level schizophrenics and normals in extent of agreement without distortion of communication. When interactions were coded for lack of agreement *with* distortion, parents of the low genetic level group scored higher than parents of the high genetic level and normal groups. The latter two groups did not differ significantly. In addition, parents of the low genetic level group yielded more often than parents of the other two groups by "masking," that is, by claiming that they held a position different from the one which they had previously endorsed privately. These data lend support to Wynne and Singer's position that communication between parents of schizophrenics is less clear and comprehensible than it is between parents of normals.

Conclusions and Recommendations

Studies obtaining data by clinical observation or by retrospective recall are unsuitable bases for a scientific body of etiological facts since the data are confounded by intrinsic methodological inadequacies. Interpretation of data acquired from direct recording and systematic coding of family interactions is subject to the cautions and tentativeness necessitated by the etiological assumption. *If the etiological assumption is granted and if the behavior sample is characteristic of the families' usual behavioral repertoire*, there are no apparent, intrinsic methodological inadequacies which disqualify this approach as unscientific. The greatest value of current studies of family interaction seems to lie in the guidelines the findings might provide for longitudinal research. Truly appropriate etiological conclusions can only be drawn from careful longitudinal studies. This reviewer doubts that sufficient knowledge is currently available to warrant the great expenditure involved in longitudinal research at the present time.

Four general findings are consistently supported by the few methodologically adequate research studies reviewed here: (*a*) there is no evidence for the proposed "schizophrenogenic" pattern of dominant mother–passive father, (*b*) there is little support for the proposed interaction between parental dominance pattern and premorbid adjustment of patients, (*c*) there is more conflict between the parents of schizophrenics (or a schizophrenic subgroup) than between the parents of normals, and (*d*) communication between parents of schizophrenics (or a schizophrenic subgroup) is less clear than it is between the parents of normals. These generalizations apply mainly to hospitalized white males. Future research on family interaction and schizophrenia would seem to require (*a*) use of families of recently institutionalized persons only; (*b*) comparability of control and experimental groups on social class, religion and ethnicity of the family, and sex, birth order, and premorbidity of the patients and control subjects; (*c*) inclusion of other institutionalized and stigmatized groups as controls, for example, nonschizophrenic psychiatric patients, tubercular patients, and prisoners; (*d*) investigation of the interaction of parents of schizophrenics with their nonschizophrenic children as a control condition; and (*e*) objective data recording, "blind" coding, and attainment of high interjudge reliabilities.

Handel (1965) and Haley (1962) have argued that it is premature to attempt to differentiate between the families of normal and pathological subjects or to attempt to differentiate among the families of pathological individuals. In their opinion, before such differentiation is attempted, a typology of families according to dimensions and characteristics peculiar to intimate groups is needed. This reviewer believes that the most fruitful approach would direct attention to the two goals concurrently. Certainly the typology and classification of individuals according to traits and motives, independent of theoretical concerns, has not been very effective in the more traditional realms of psychology. A similar approach to family psychology could not reasonably be expected to have a different history.

References

Baxter, J. C., & Arthur, S. C. (1964). Conflict in families of schizophrenics as a function of premorbid adjustment and social class. *Family Process*, **3**, 273–279.

Baxter, J. C., Arthur, S. C., Flood, C. G., & Hedgepeth, B. (1962). Conflict patterns in the families of schizophrenics. *Journal of Nervous and Mental Disease*, **135**, 419–424.

Becker, W. C. (1956). A genetic approach to the interpretation and evaluation of the process-reactive distinction in schizophrenia. *Journal of Abnormal and Social Psychology*, **53**, 229–236.

Becker, W. C. (1959). The process-reactive distinction: A key to the problem of schizophrenia? *Journal of Nervous and Mental Disease*, **129**, 442–449.

Behrens, M. L., & Goldfarb, W. (1958). A study of patterns of interaction of families of schizophrenic children in residential treatment. *American Journal of Orthopsychiatry*, **28**, 300–312.

Caputo, D. (1963). The parents of the schizophrenic. *Family Process*, **2**, 339–356.

Cheek, F. E. (1964). The "schizophrenogenic mother" in word and deed. *Family Process*, **3**, 155–177. (a)

CHEEK, F. E. (1964). A serendipitous finding: Sex roles and schizophrenia. *Journal of Abnormal and Social Psychology*, **69**, 392–400. (b)

CHEEK, F. E. (1965). The father of the schizophrenic. *Archives of General Psychiatry*, **13**, 336–345.

FARINA, A. (1960). Patterns of role dominance and conflict in parents of schizophrenic patients. *Journal of Abnormal and Social Psychology*, **61**, 31–38.

FARINA, A., & DUNHAM, R. M. (1963). Measurement of family relationships and their effects. *Archives of General Psychiatry*, **9**, 64–73.

FERREIRA, A. J. (1963). Decision-making in normal and pathologic families. *Archives of General Psychiatry*, **8**, 68–73.

FERREIRA, A. J., & WINTER, W. D. (1965). Family interaction and decision making. *Archives of General Psychiatry*, **13**, 214–223.

FISHER, S., BOYD, I., WALKER, D., & SHEER, D. (1959). Parents of schizophrenics, neurotics, and normals. *Archives of General Psychiatry*, **1**, 149–166.

FRANK, G. H. (1965). The role of the family in the development of psychopathology. *Psychological Bulletin*, **64**, 191–205.

FROMM-REICHMANN, F. (1948). Notes on the development of treatment of schizophrenics by psychoanalytic psychotherapy. *Psychiatry*, **11**, 263–273.

GARMEZY, N., & RODNICK, E. H. (1959). Premorbid adjustment and performance in schizophrenia: Implications for interpreting heterogeneity in schizophrenia. *Journal of Nervous and Mental Disease*, **129**, 450–466.

HAGGARD, E. A., BREKSTAD, A., & SKARD, A. (1960). On the reliability of the anamnestic interview. *Journal of Abnormal and Social Psychology*, **61**, 311–318.

HALEY, J. (1962). Family experiments: A new type of experimentation. *Family Process*, **1**, 265–293.

HALEY, J. (1964). Research on family patterns: An instrument measurement. *Family Process*, **3**, 41–65.

HANDEL, G. (1965). Psychological study of whole families. *Psychological Bulletin*, **63**, 19–41.

HEILBRUN, A. B. (1960). Perception of maternal child rearing attitudes in schizophrenia. *Journal of Consulting Psychology*, **24**, 169–173.

HERRON, W. G. (1962). The process-reactive classification of schizophrenia. *Psychological Bulletin*, **59**, 329–343.

JACKSON, D. D., BLOCK, J., & PATTERSON, V. (1958). Psychiatrists' conceptions of the schizophrenogenic parent. *Archives of Neurology and Psychiatry*, **79**, 448–459.

JAYASWAL, S. R., & STOTT, L. H. (1955). Persistence and change in personality from childhood to adulthood. *Merrill-Palmer Quarterly*, **1**, 47–56.

KASANIN, J., KNIGHT, E., & SAGE, P. (1934). The parent-child relationship in schizophrenia. I. Overprotection-rejection. *Journal of Nervous and Mental Disease*, **72**, 249–263.

KOHN, M. L., & CARROLL, E. E. (1960). Social class and the allocation of parental responsibilities. *Sociometry*, **23**, 372–392.

LENNARD, H. L., BEAULIEU, M. R., & EMBRY, N. G. (1965). Interaction in families with a schizophrenic child. *Archives of General Psychiatry*, **12**, 166–183.

LERNER, P. M. (1965). Resolution of intrafamilial role conflict in families of schizophrenic patients. I: Thought disturbance. *Journal of Nervous and Mental Disease*, **141**, 342–351.

LIDZ, T., CORNELISON, A. R., FLECK, S., & TERRY, D. (1957). The intrafamilial environment of schizophrenic patients: II. Marital schism and marital skew. *American Journal of Psychiatry*, **114**, 241–248.

MCCLELLAND, D. C., DE CHARMS, R., & RINDLISBACHER, A. Religious and other sources of parental attitudes toward independence training. In D. C. McClelland (ed.) (1955). *Studies in Motivation*. New York: Appleton-Century-Crofts, pp. 389–397.

MCCORD, W., PORTA, J., & MCCORD, J. (1962). The familial genesis of psychoses. *Psychiatry*, **25**, 60–71.

MCGRAW, M. B., & MOLLOY, L. B. (1941). The pediatric anamnesis: Inaccuracies in eliciting developmental data. *Child Development*, **12**, 255–265.

MEISSNER, W. W. (1964). Thinking about the family-psychiatric aspects. *Family Process*, **3**, 1–40.

MEYERS, D. F., & GOLDFARB, W. (1961). Studies of perplexity in mothers of schizophrenic children. *American Journal of Orthopsychiatry*, **31**, 551–564.

MORRIS, G. O., & WYNNE, L. C. (1965). Schizophrenic offspring and parental styles of communication. *Psychiatry*, **28**, 19–44.

PHILLIPS, L. (1953). Case history data and prognosis in schizophrenia. *Journal of Nervous and Mental Disease*, **117**, 515–525.

PYLES, M. K., STOLZ, H. R., & MACFARLANE, J. W. (1935). The accuracy of mothers' reports on birth and developmental data. *Child Development*, **6**, 165–176.

RABKIN, L. Y. (1965). The patient's family: Research methods. *Family Process*, **4**, 105–132.

ROBBINS, L. C. (1963). The accuracy of parental recall of aspects of child development and of child rearing practices. *Journal of Abnormal and Social Psychology*, **66**, 261–270.

RODNICK, E. H., & GARMEZY, N. An experimental approach to the study of motivation in schizophrenia. In M. R. Jones (ed.) (1957). *Nebraska Symposium on Motivation: 1957*. Lincoln: University of Nebraska Press, pp. 109–184.

SANUA, V. D. (1961). Sociocultural factors in families of schizophrenics. *Psychiatry*, **24**, 246–265.

SANUA, V. D. (1963). The sociocultural aspects of schizophrenia: A comparison of Protestant and Jewish schizophrenics. *International Journal of Social Psychiatry*, **9**, 27–36.

SCHACHTER, S. (1959). *The psychology of affiliation*. Stanford, Calif.: Stanford University Press.

SCHOOLER, C. (1961). Birth order and schizophrenia. *Archives of General Psychiatry*, **4**, 117–123.

SCHOOLER, C. (1964). Birth order and hospitalization for schizophrenia. *Journal of Abnormal and Social Psychology*, **69**, 574–579.

SCHOOLER, C., & LONG, J. (1963). Affiliation among chronic schizophrenics: Factors affecting acceptance of responsibility for the fate of another. *Journal of Nervous and Mental Disease*, **137**, 173–179.

SCHOOLER, C., & SCARR, S. (1962). Affiliation among chronic schizophrenics: Relation to intrapersonal and birth order factors. *Journal of Personality*, **30**, 178–192.

SINGER, M. T., & WYNNE, L. C. (1963). Differentiating characteristics of parents of childhood schizophrenics, childhood neurotics, and young adult schizophrenics. *American Journal of Psychiatry*, **120**, 234–243.

SINGER, M. T., & WYNNE, L. C. (1965). Thought disorder and family relations of schizophrenics. III. Methodology using projective techniques. *Archives of General Psychiatry*, **12**, 187–200. (a)

SINGER, M. T., & WYNNE, L. C. (1965). Thought disorder and family relations of schizophrenics. IV. Results and implications. *Archives of General Psychiatry*, **12**, 201–212. (b)

SOLOMON, L., & ZLOTOWSKI, M. (1964). The relationship between the Elgin and Phillips measures of process-reactive schizophrenia. *Journal of Nervous and Mental Disease*, **138**, 32–37.

STABENAU, J. R., TUPIN, J., WERNER, M., & POLLIN, W. (1965). A comparative study of families of schizophrenics, deliquents, and normals. *Psychiatry*, **28**, 45–59.

STRODTBECK, F. (1951). Husband-wife interaction over revealed differences. *American Sociological Review*, **16**, 468–473.

WYNNE, L. C., & SINGER, M. T. (1963). Thought disorder and family relations of schizophrenics. I. A research strategy. *Archives of General Psychiatry*, **9**, 191–198. (a)

WYNNE, L. C., & SINGER, M. T. (1963). Thought disorder and the family relations of schizophrenics. II. Classification of forms of thinking. *Archives of General Psychiatry*, **9**, 199–206. (b)

YARROW, M. R., CAMPBELL, J. D., & BURTON, R. V. (1964). Reliability of maternal retrospection: A preliminary report. *Family Process*, **3**, 207–218.

MARGARET THALER SINGER and LYMAN C. WYNNE

Differentiating Characteristics of Parents of Childhood Schizophrenics, Childhood Neurotics, and Young Adult Schizophrenics

In recent years, researchers interested in schizophrenia have turned to a study of family interaction patterns in the hope that the illness can be understood as a product of such factors. In this very exciting research study by Singer and Wynne, efforts were made to distinguish among a large group of parents having either childhood schizophrenic, childhood neurotic, or young adult schizophrenic children on the basis of the way these parents related to people. The style of relating was inferred from responses on a Thematic Apperception Test. The hypotheses guiding the distinctions made by the authors derived from their observations of the family relations of schizophrenics. The fact that the authors could successfully determine which parents had offspring suffering from each type of disorder is more than a parlor trick. It can be taken as a validation of the parental behavioral styles that seem to be related to the development of such disorders.

During the course of a long-range research program on the family relations of schizophrenics, we have developed criteria by which families with late adolescent and young adult schizophrenic offspring can be differentiated from families whose offspring have other kinds of psychiatric disturbances (1–5). In this paper we shall present data from parents of child psychiatric patients, and compare the findings with those from the parents of patients studied earlier.

Our research has assumed that innate and experimental factors are co-determinants of behavior. Additionally, we have hypothesized that certain parental forms of focusing attention, communicating and interpersonal "relating" are intimately linked to the forms of ego impairment found in

---

Reprinted from the *American Journal of Psychiatry*, **120** (1963), 234–243, with the permission of the American Psychiatric Association and Drs. Singer and Wynne.

offspring. *Form* or style of parental behaving has been emphasized rather than the *content* of thoughts and attitudes.

Schizophrenia does not appear to be a single entity; rather, there are various forms of individual schizophrenic illness. Similarly, there is no single pattern for families of schizophrenics; instead, subgroups of schizophrenics have families which share similar characteristics. Thus, among adult patients, the family patterns of patients with different forms of thought disorder can be blindly distinguished (5). We hypothesized that the family relations of the various kinds of childhood schizophrenics would similarly differ from each other and from the parents of the various kinds of adult schizophrenics.

This paper delineates certain of these differences through the study of projective test data from (a) the parents of 20 autistic, schizophrenic children, (b) 20 neurotic children (10 "acting-out," aggressive children and 10 withdrawn children), and (c) 20 schizophrenics who became overtly ill in late adolescence or young adulthood.[1]

Selection of Subjects. The parents of the two groups of child patients (median age, 8 years) had been selected for another study (6) in the following way:[2] First, the parents of the schizophrenic children were selected. A clinical consensus in the diagnosis of "schizophrenic reaction, childhood type," was used, with cases eliminated having any serious physical illness, demonstrable neurological findings,[3] or recognizable mental deficiency.

Our review of the clinical records following the test analyses indicated that 14 of the "childhood schizophrenic" patients clearly fell into the group originally described by Kanner (7) under the heading of "early infantile autism" and recently reviewed by Rimland (8). The other 6 patients fitted the designation "childhood schizophrenia with autistic traits." Eighteen had clear-cut autistic symptoms well before age 2, and the other 2 clearly had these symptoms soon after their second and third birthdays. At ages 4–7 most of these children were without communicative speech, had almost no contact with people, and showed idiosyncratic repetitive behavior, such as unscrewing screws, twiddling paper, and stacking items. All patients would be in the group described by Mahler (9) as "autistic psychoses" rather than "symbiotic psychoses." The findings reported in this paper should not be assumed to be generally applicable to the families of other varieties of patients.

[1] Similar data from the parents of 20 chronically physically ill children and 20 asthmatic children, along with additional material about various kinds of adult schizophrenics and neurotics, will be reported subsequently.

[2] We wish to express our appreciation to Drs. Jeanne Block and Virginia Patterson, who made available to us a major portion of the tests from the parents of the young children. The schizophrenic children were patients of the Langley Porter Children's Service, San Francisco. Dr. S. A. Szurek, Director, and Dr. A. J. Gianascol gave access to the clinical records on these patients and families after the test analyses were completed. Responsibility for the interpretation of the data rests with the authors. The families of the neurotic and other children were secured from various clinics in the San Francisco area.

[3] Although none of the patients had neurological findings on examination, 7 histories (5 in an early infantile autism group) revealed an unusually difficult pregnancy or delivery; 2 of these, plus one other patient, all in the early infantile autism group, later had a history of seizures.

These families were used as the base for selecting comparison families. The families of the schizophrenic and the neurotic children were individually matched using the method of "precision controls" (10) for the following 5 variables: (a) age of child within 3 years; (b) age of parents in relation to child; (c) number of children in family (the parents of an only child were matched with parents of an only child; where there was more than 1 child, the number was held roughly equivalent); (d) educational and occupational level of parents; (e) participation of at least the mother in a psychotherapeutic relation. Fifteen of the 20 schizophrenic children were also matched with 15 of the neurotic children on the basis of sex. Thirty-three of the child patients were male and 7 were female (S : 6 female, 14 male; N : 1 female, 19 male).

The families of the young adult schizophrenics[4] could not, of course, be matched so well with respect to age. The median age of the young adult patients was 23 years, and 56 years for their parents. The median age of the parents of the child patients was 37 years. In other respects, including size of family, and educational and occupational level, the parents of the young adult patients were comparable. It is important to note that in all the families the parents themselves had raised the children.

Procedures

1. Using general hypotheses drawn from earlier work, the projective test data from the 40 pairs of parents of the childhood schizophrenics (CS) and childhood neurotics (CN) were studied blindly in a preliminary fashion. The Thematic Apperception Test and the Rorschach were the main tests used in this study. Preliminary groupings of the parents into predicted CS and CN groups were rank-ordered by one of us (MTS) in terms of the degree of confidence with which the designations were made. Dr. Virginia Patterson,[4] who held the code of correct classification of these parents, indicated that the first 5 CS and the first 5 CN designations were correct.

2. These 10 sets of tests were then used for developing more specific criteria differentiating the CS and CN parents. In the second phase of the blind differentiations, the remaining 30 sets of tests from the child patients were blindly differentiated, first, into the CS and CN groups.

3. The tests from those parents who were correctly identified as having neurotic children were blindly differentiated with respect to whether their offspring were in the acting-out group or the withdrawn neurotic group.

4. Criteria were specified for the differences in the TAT test behavior of the 4 sets of parents—the parents of the childhood schizophrenics, the

[4] We also wish to express our appreciation to Dr. Theodore Lidz of Yale University, who made available tests from 9 pairs of parents of the young adult schizophrenics. The parents of the other adult schizophrenic patients were tested at the NIMH by Mr. Charles Odell and Mr. George Usdansky. The parents of the adult patients constitute only an early portion of the NIMH data which was specifically comparable to the data from the families of the child patients.

acting-out children, the withdrawn neurotic children, and the young adult schizophrenics.

5. Finally, various special Rorschach ratings were analyzed and compared statistically for the 4 groups of parents: (a) thinking disorder and related schizophrenic features; (b) genetic-level scores; (c) affective symbolism, particularly hostility scores and the presence of a hostile or threatening component to the first Rorschach response of each individual.

Results

1. In the preliminary blind differentiation and rank-ordering of the projective tests from the parents of the child patients, the Rorschach and TAT tests from each marital pair were considered simultaneously as a family unit. Most studies have considered fathers and mothers separately; the present study is concerned with what emerged when both parents' tests were examined in relation to each other and were considered together as compounding, confusing, or correcting the impact of each parent as an individual.

Selecting the 10 sets of tests which could be designated with the greatest confidence as belonging in either the CS or CN groups, resulted in an entirely accurate differentiation. That is, the 5 pairs of parents which were expected to have schizophrenic children were all designated correctly, and the 5 sets of parents which were predicted to have neurotic children were also designated correctly, with no errors. Using Fisher's exact test for categorical data, this differentiation is significant statistically ($p = .005$).[5]

2. In the second phase of the blind differentiations, the remaining 30 sets of tests from the parents of the child patients were differentiated using the more detailed criteria developed on the basis of the 10 most distinctive sets of tests. Twenty-four of the 30 sets of parents were then correctly identified either as parents of autistic schizophrenic or of neurotic children. Twelve of 15 in both the schizophrenic and the neurotic groups were correctly placed, giving a statistically significant level of accuracy ($p < .005$, using Fisher's exact test).

3. The next stage of the blind differentiation combined the 5 sets of parents of the neurotic children who were used in the preliminary development of criteria and the 12 others who were correctly predicted as having neurotic children. The rater did not know which were parents of acting-out or withdrawn children. Thirteen of the 17 sets of parents were blindly labeled correctly; parents of 7 acting-out children out of a total of 9 were correctly designated; and the parents of 6 withdrawn children out of 8 were correctly designated (using Fisher's exact test, $p = .044$).

TAT Criteria for Differentiation. On theoretical grounds we expected that the parents of autistic schizophrenic children would be different from the parents of young adult schizophrenics previously studied. Contrasting core

[5] We wish to express our appreciation to Dr. Donald Morrison, Biometrics Branch, NIMH, for his invaluable assistance in the statistical analysis of the data of this study.

problems exist. The autistic children do not appear to relate to others, or do so in extremely restricted ways; the young adult schizophrenics have thinking and experiencing disorders. If learning, "conditioning" and experiential factors are related to the behavior of autistic children and of adult schizophrenics, then, in far over simplified terms, the role of *relating* is crucial in families with autistic children and the parental contribution to *thinking and attention defects* is central in the families of those who become designated as schizophrenic at a later age. The parents of autistic, childhood schizophrenics, we surmised, have forms of behavior which would rebuff, impair, and interfere with the very beginnings of relationships they might have with the child, and would continue to do so later.

In the earlier studies of the families of adult schizophrenics who had grown up in intact families, we had been impressed by a family subculture in which the parent-child relationships are not by any means prevented from developing nor are they totally shattered. Rather, the focusing of attention and the achievement of subjectively meaningful experience are impaired, blurred, and fragmented but with enduring parent-child relatedness.[6] The *content* of what these parents say is not so critical as the level at which focal attention[7] is impaired. Criteria which have been helpful in identifying the parents of the young adult schizophrenics include such maneuvers as amorphously and implicitly shifting the area to which attention is given, vaguely shifting the context of reference, externalizing the sources of attention, scattering and fragmenting attention over such a large series of items that meaningfulness cannot be integrated, *etc.* (5).

The further study of the CS and CN criterion groups highlighted two major distinguishing qualities in the TAT behavior of the parents of these autistic children: *disaffiliation* and *dissatisfaction* as characteristic and pervasive expectancies about the way any interaction is going to turn out.[8]

A. Parents of autistic childhood schizophrenics

DISAFFILIATION. Persons are seen moving away from each other, moving out of relationships, and avoiding closeness. Interactions appear inherently unpleasant and failing to satisfy. Relationships are viewed with cynicism, distrust and pessimism. At best there is something uncomfortable about interacting with others.

At least four pathways to disaffiliation are discernible. In each pair of

[6] Earlier communications from the larger NIMH research group have used such terms as pseudomutuality and pseudohostility to characterize the essence of the oddly held-together relationships of these families (1, 3).

[7] The term focal attention is used here as described by Schachtel (11): acts of attention appear directional, specific, aim at mental grasp via a sustained approach and with renewed approaches to the object or thought, and flexibly exclude extraneous stimuli (p. 253).

[8] A partial replication based upon these criteria and utilizing the TAT parental tests alone was carried out by another rater (LCW). Nine out of 10 cases of the child patients (5 autistic and 5 neurotic withdrawn) were correctly differentiated in this replication.

the CS parents, both have some of the following qualities, which appear *either* within the TAT stories, or in the manner of telling the story and interacting with the examiner.

1. *Cynical outlook.* Approximately 70% of the CS parents were in this group. They expect the worst possible motivation in people. They sound embittered, disenchanted, and describe warmth, closeness and tender motivations with contempt, skepticism, or scorn. Often their criticism conveys an active, destructive quality, with a sadistic finality about people leaving one another.

In their TAT stories these CS parents were vindictive toward persons for trying to establish and maintain relationships. They doubt the worthwhileness of relating and interacting; people disaffiliate into empty lives. Some indicate "things are not as they seem," not true or real. Some parents of CN children and parents of young adult schizophrenics are pessimistic but imply one keeps on trying to establish relationships, and to trust people.

Certain CS parents covertly imply that nothing endures, and therefore one should not affiliate or attach oneself to people or objects.

2. *Passivity and apathy about interacting.* Others convey resignation, withdrawal, disinterest and avoidance when characterizing interactions between persons. They imply, "Why bother interacting. It's useless and going to turn out poorly anyhow." They create an air of passive pessimism.

3. *Superficiality.* Certain parents treat potentially moving, touching scenes with great superficiality. They seem unable to sense the persons in the cards might be involved in touching, feelingful experiences. They treat everything in a superficial "surfacey" way. Nothing has depth or poignancy and only the most blatant, overt, concrete actions are noted. When they try to describe close, tender and warm human transactions, their stories become parodies and travesties. Sometimes there is a seeming mockery present.

Facetiousness appears particularly in the tests of parents who might be classed as either cynical or superficial. Both imply there is a lack of genuineness about tender, positive scenes and they facetiously flaunt and degrade tenderness, closeness and positive emotions and interactions. They doubt their genuineness, imply they denote weakness, are maudlin and to be scorned.

4. *Obsessive, intellectualized distance.* Some parents convey a sense of disaffiliation via detachment and intellectualized distance. This has to be differentiated from certain CN parents who are obsessive and intellectualizing but who seem to bury themselves in busily trying to figure out what is going on in a transaction, but become obsessively involved and participating in the test task, rather than dismissing it.

DISSATISFACTION. Overlapping with disaffiliation is dissatisfaction, a quality which is pervasive, but difficult to characterize briefly because it hinges upon reading and analyzing whole tales or the over-all test protocol. Disaffiliation can be described via actions and expectancies. Dissatisfaction is seen in TAT characters having lives that are non-rewarding. Their efforts, work, and patterns of life are chronically dissatisfying.

Praise, recognition, and admiration are almost absent from the CS parent tales.[9] Often when they see a person striving, they impute selfish motives, and predict that he will be punished or will collapse. For example, one card shows a man climbing a rope. The CS parents deride his physique and his mentality, impute self-centered motives, and usually have him fall or injure himself for showing off, trying to be strong, etc.

In one way or another most of the stories of these parents are negatively toned. Certain CS parents create a relatively positive story, but append side comments, bored yawns, and add denouements which ruin the impact of any pleasant content by a final coup de grâce which belies sincerity or belief in the content of the story.

When parents with these intense, disaffiliating, distancing, unempathic tendencies have an infant with a low innate capacity to elicit appropriate responsiveness, transactional failures crippling to ego development will necessarily begin at birth. Parents who are psychologically able to stand apart from others, including their infant, will be relatively objective, clear and definite in their thinking, and in their capacity to differentiate self and other, and in their capacity to direct their activities, including telling TAT stories, with relative coherence, unity, and point. Diversions do occur, but these parents manage to convey that they have maintained or can return to an over-all point. They seem to "remember" where they came from and where they are going with their stories. Thus, they do not ordinarily shown significant attention defects.

B. Parents of young adult schizophrenics

In contrast, the TATs of these parents of the young adult schizophrenics are marked by a failure to develop and hold a set, to focus and sustain attention. Their stories neither unfold with coherence nor with a clear sense of point and meaningfulness, nor conclude with closure.

The persons in these stories are not depicted as disaffiliated and detached but as interacting in frustrated or pointless ways. Sometimes the persons are together in parallel, each doing something but failing to interact productively. Others have people in the tales intruding into other persons, trying to control and manipulate them, usually to no avail. They convey feelings of aloneness, frustration, and meaninglessness about transactions even though the persons are together.

> 1. *Fragmentation.* Tangential ideas, side themes, and distracting comments are prominent. Their tales are replete with fragments of alternative meanings and alternative feelings, usually none of which are selected and completed. Often when the examiner asks for further steps or details, as well as when the teller recalls the instructions, there is a "jump" or almost non-sequitur appending of the next part. The teller seems to fail to realize he needs to move the listener with him to

[9] Boatman and Szurek (12), summarizing clinical impressions from more than 200 childhood schizophrenics and their parents, including those whose tests are used here, noted (p. 415), "Exchange of tender words, admiration and approbation is also scanty."

a conclusion or next step. Frequently words and phrases are omitted. This is especially apparent in verbatim, tape-recorded tests. Non-sequiturs and misperceptions seem to occur because intrusive, secondary associations get into these parents' main stream of attention.

2. *Perseveration.* Concomitant with the fragmented quality of these attention-meaning defects, mild to open perseverative tendencies may be present. These parents' attention does not focus flexibly. Occasionally there is a failure to "clear" either a detail or a global essence from a previously attended idea; this influences subsequent perceptions and associations unduly.

3. *Pointlessness.* There is a feeling upon reading most of the stories that a point really never was developed. Even if apparent closure is achieved, the reader is left with a sense of pointlessness. Various wordy trappings often conceal that the production is merely a card description or "filler material."

4. *Indefinite referents.* A subgroup of these parents gives stories which seem relatively concise and with closure, but inspection reveals a great non-specificity about the referents of experience.

C. Parents of acting-out children

The TAT stories of the parents of the aggressive, acting-out children are distinctive from either of the schizophrenic groups. There is an absence of thought disorders, rambling communication, fragmented attention, low mood tones, anergy, and pessimism. They are not concerned about doing well. They fail to strive, in contrast to the parents of the CS who show contempt for others' striving. Some fail to sense tacit implications of social behavior. The following qualities do stand out:

1. *Facetiousness.* They directly or indirectly taunt about authority. They are facetious toward rules and amenities, while the autistic children's parents are facetious toward feelings, especially positive and tender ones.

2. *High activity.* They sound like active, energetic persons and have strong empathies with persons seen. In comparison with the parents of CS children and young adult schizophrenics, they are more likely to stimulate action in others.

3. *Clear communication.* Percepts are relatively clear, ideas conventional, language orderly and concise. Almost none have genuinely obsessive tests. They have a lack of concern about doing well. They fail to strive, in contrast to the parents of the CS who show contempt for others' striving. Some fail to sense tacit implications of social behavior.

4. *Relatively "normal" tests.* In general their tests are those of active, somewhat hostile persons. Yet their hostile tales do not convey the sadism implied in the records of certain parents of CS children. Additionally, a sparseness of conflictual content conveys an aura of "normalcy" even though raters can detect propensities for disturbed moods and impulses.

D. Parents of withdrawn neurotic children

1. *Lower mood.* In contrast to the tests from the parents of acting-out children, these tests contain lower mood tones, less open energy, and less acting-out potentials.

2. *Coherence.* In contrast to TATs from parents of young adult schizophrenics, these parents do not have gross attention difficulties, nor do they feel resigned or deeply pessimistic. A few low-mood tone parents are moderately fragmentary, and their tests may seem "schizoid." However, they have people relating and staying together in spite of adversities. Some may talk in generalities and abstractions (masculinity versus femininity, viewing the sky equals thinking of the future, *etc.*), but do it within a framework of relating, striving, and attempts at coherence and cohesiveness.

3. *Affiliation and satisfaction.* In contrast to tests from parents of autistic children, these tests express a belief in the "basic goodness of men and life in general" even though mood tones may be low. There is a minimum of disaffiliation. When someone gets rejected, these parents have identified with the rejectee and not the rejector (as with autistic parents) and imply they would want to go back into the relationship and are sad over its loss. People may feel anxious, inadequate, or ambivalent, but they strive to maintain relationships. They recognize it is best to comply, even though they may not want to. Inner drives may tempt one to do evil, but these should be overcome. Control is often an issue—one person over another, nature over man, *etc.* Control can be seen as intrusive, but it keeps children and others close. Satisfactions, accomplishments and pleasure from work can come to people.

Table 1 contrasts the TAT characteristics of the four groups of parents. These are expressed in terms of TAT features of prototypic parents. The underlined items are considered particularly distinctive qualities.

Rorschach measures

A. Thinking disorders. These formulations have generated further specific hypotheses which we have tested with measures from the Rorschach protocols of these four parent groups. In work with the families of young adult schizophrenics, we have been impressed with striking links between the underlying form of thinking of parents and their offspring. We attempted to evaluate this question from Rorschach data through criteria developed by M. T. Singer, using cues from Benjamin (13) and Rapaport (14). We compared the frequency and kinds of thinking disorder and related schizophrenic features in the various groups of parents studied. Hypothetically, in terms of the considerations discussed from the TAT data, the parents of the acting-out children, would be most free of thinking disorders amongst these four parent groups. The next clearest thinking group would be the parents of the autistic schizophrenic children and the most disturbed in thinking processes would be the parents of the young adult schizophrenics. Considering that the withdrawn children were perhaps a somewhat heterogeneous nosologic group, we expected that the parents of these patients would be intermediate in frequency and severity of thinking disorders.

As Table 2 indicates, the predicted ranking of Rorschach-rated thought

TABLE 1 *Summary of TAT features of parents*

Parents of autistic children	Parents of withdrawn children
*1. Feel dissatisfied, bitter, critical.	1. Feel sad, with low mood.
2. Disaffiliate via many modes.	2. Seek to stay in relationships, despite the mood tone.
3. Tell coherent tales with a point and unity.	3. Have a point and unity to stories.
4. Have clear percepts; depict people, events, feelings, consequences clearly compared to parents of adult schizophrenics.	4. Have relatively clear, specified percepts; may, however, dwell obsessively on details or on abstract qualities; appear introspective.
Parents of adult schizophrenics	**Parents of acting-out children**
1. Feel unhappy, hopeless, resigned.	1. Have various moods, including orneriness, rebelliousness, sadness; are active, energetic.
2. Have frustrating interaction, experienced as pointless.	2. Have people relate and interact to an ordinary level—not an outstanding feature.
3. Convey over-all sense of directionlessness; tell stories in which closure not achieved, without unity.	3. Tell unified stories; do not strive to do outstandingly well on tests.
4. Have people, events, feelings, consequences remain global, abstract, overly general; attention appears fragmented or amorphous.	4. Have well defined, clear percepts; do not appear genuinely introspective.

*1. Mood.
2. Relationship Style.
3. Capacity for Over-all Point and Coherence.
4. Clarity of Percept and Thought.

TABLE 2 *Schizophrenic features, especially thought disorder, in Rorschachs of parents*

	Percent of parents with schizophrenic Rorschach features			
Parental pairs	**Parents of young adult schizophrenics (20 pairs)**	**Parents of withdrawn children (10 pairs)**	**Parents of autistic schizophrenic children (20 pairs)**	**Parents of acting-out children (10 pairs)**
Neither parent	0%	20%	50%	90%
One parent	5	20	30	10
Both parents	95	60	20	0
Individual Parent Totals	38/40 (95%)	14/20 (70%)	14/40 (35%)	1/20 (5%)

disorder and schizophrenic features in the four groups of parents was confirmed. Ratings by independent psychologists[10] using Singer's criteria, achieved perfect agreement on the tests from the parents of the adult patients and the neurotic children with some disagreement among raters on 6 of the 40 parents of the autistic children. These 6 cases were resolved by consensus. Nearly all of the parents of the young adult schizophrenics had evidence of thought disorder in their Rorschach records, while almost none of the parents of the acting-out children had such features, with the other two groups intermediate in the predicted direction. These groups were significantly different ($p = .001$) (chi square test of homogeneity).

These differences were still more sharply apparent in terms of the severity of disorder. Briefly, the forms of thinking seen in the Rorschachs of the parents of the adult schizophrenics reflected relatively severe forms of rambling, loose, paralogical thought disorders, with marked attention problems and peculiar content, sufficiently prominent so that the raters had easily noted these features. The CS parents showed a fairly large number of mild features, but rarely loose, scattered, or fragmented forms of thinking. The features found in their records included: pseudoprofundity, forms of concreteness, original but rather odd contents, and repetitious returns to particular themes. They cut off secondary confabulatory associations and focused attention in a relatively constricted, orderly fashion without rambling or loose associations.

B. Genetic-level Rorschach scores. Another way of scoring Rorschach data which is relevant to our conceptualizations is in terms of degree of psychological differentiation, the "genetic" level of perceptual development, as suggested by Heinz Werner's theory (15). Using Becker's method for Rorschach Genetic-level scoring (16), the parents of the four groups, treated as pairs, differentiate in a multi-variate analysis of variance at the 0.01 level of confidence (See Table 3).

The higher the genetic-level score is, the more mature the perceptual quality of the over-all responses. The parents of the young adult schizophrenics who are prone to blur and fragment attention, give responses of a significantly less differentiated and less integrated quality than found in the other parents. They are not, however, a homogeneous group. We have noted elsewhere the importance of distinguishing the parents of schizophrenics who are especially amorphous and undifferentiated in their thinking from those who are relatively better differentiated but still fragmented and unintegrated (5).

The acting-out children, where one expects little ego impairment of this basic labeling of "reality," had parents who tended to give the most articulated and integrated percepts. The parents of the autistic schizophrenic children show a higher level of psychological differentiation than the parents of either the withdrawn neurotic or the young adult schizophrenic groups.

[10] We wish to thank Dr. Jerome Fisher and Mr. Frank Gorman of the Langley Porter Neuropsychiatric Institute and Dr. George DeVos of the University of California for their test evaluations.

TABLE 3 *Genetic-level Rorschach scores*

Group	Mothers		Fathers	
	Mean	SD	Mean	SD
Acting-out children (N = 20)	3.70	0.369	3.71	0.302
Schizophrenic young children (N = 40)	3.45	0.319	3.59	0.373
Withdrawn children (N = 20)	3.29	0.291	3.06	0.508
Schizophrenic young adults (N = 40)	3.11	0.553	3.08	0.512

This finding appears to be consistent with the Rorschach ratings of thought disorder in that the frequency of thought disorder in the various parent groups increased in the same order: acting-out children, autistic children, withdrawn neurotic children, and young adult schizophrenics.

C. HOSTILE AFFECT. We have described our impression that the parents of the autistic schizophrenic children tend to disrupt actively and hostilely the very beginnings of transactions and relationships. It appears possible to be openly disaffiliating only if relatively clear capacity for self-other differentiation has been achieved. Among the group of parents of autistic children, those who seem most explicitly and, often, brutally disaffiliating have relatively clear, genetically "mature" perceptions and little indication of schizophrenic Rorschach features.

The parents of the young adult schizophrenics are rarely so openly and directly disaffiliative as the parents of most of the autistic children. They may be hostile, but are more prone to stay in a transaction, even if only as inert spectators. Although not all parents of the autistic children use a hostile path to disaffiliation, the impression of a greater frequency of this trend in these parents seemed worth while checking out statistically.

Over-all hostile affect: As a partial measure of this tendency, each parent's Rorschach responses were scored for affective symbolism (17). Each response was scored either neutral, hostile, anxious, body preoccupation, dependency, positive, or miscellaneous affect.[11] We reasoned that the CS parents would show the highest hostility scores, with the parents of the acting-out children next, but the parents of the young adult schizophrenics and the withdrawn children were expected to be lower. For the mothers, this hypothesis (child schizophrenic and acting-out parent groups > adult schizophrenic and neurotic withdrawn) was confirmed at the 0.01 level of confidence;

[11] Dr. Joseph C. Speisman, NIMH, independently scored the records for genetic-level and affective symbolism, achieving 89% agreement with the previous scores. We appreciate his assistance.

for the fathers, at the 0.05 level of confidence. Within the schizophrenic groups alone, the parents of the child patients also had significantly higher hostility scores than the parents of the adult schizophrenics.

Initial hostile responses: It also seemed reasonable to hypothesize that the CS parents, if they characteristically disrupted transactions from their beginnings, would introduce hostile or threatening content very early in associations. A tally of the affective symbolism assigned each parent's very first Rorschach response revealed that 40% of the parents of the child schizophrenics (8 mothers and 8 fathers), but only 15% in each of the other three groups (4 mothers and 2 fathers of young adult schizophrenics, and 1 mother and 2 fathers each of the acting-out and withdrawn groups) had a hostile or threatening component to their first response. (Comparing parents of adult and child schizophrenics, chi square, 5.08, p. $<$ .025.) A larger portion of the parents of child schizophrenics had this initial tendency to think of a hostile or threatening association. This quick arousal of hostile or threatening content, associated with a general presence of greater hostility content among the CS parents, is suggestive that not only the presence of hostile associations, but where they enter in the transaction seems relevant.

Summary

Research at the NIMH on the families of schizophrenics is broadened in this study to include the parents of child psychiatric patients. Previous studies in this program (5) have demonstrated that the families of young adult schizophrenics can be blindly differentiated from the families of young adult neurotics when criteria are used which emphasize form or style of thinking and focusing attention. In the present study we show that relationship disorders, rather than the thinking disorders which are so prominent in the families of the adult schizophrenics, are especially pertinent to the differentiation of families of autistic schizophrenic children from families of neurotic children.

The criteria for predicting autistic illness in an offspring from parental data were derived from the psychodynamic hypothesis that primary disruption and impairment in the child's relationship to parental figures is crucial in early autistic disorders. We have assumed that an infant's congenital incapacity can contribute to such relationship failure. Nevertheless, in this series of families it has been possible to distinguish blindly those parents who have autistic children from the manner in which they appear to rebuff, impair, and interfere with the very beginning of any tender or nurturant relationship, as judged from projective test protocols.

The parents of 20 autistic children were blindly differentiated at a statistically significant level of accuracy from sociologically matched parents of 20 neurotic children. The parents of the neurotic children, half withdrawn and half aggressive, acting-out, were in turn successfully differentiated into these two groups on the basis of the parental projective tests.

This research suggests the importance of considering mental disorders, including schizophrenia, both in childhood and later, as heterogeneous, and studying the links between definable varieties of individual mental disorder and definable varieties of family patterns.

Criteria applicable to TAT data for distinguishing the parents of the three varieties of child patients and the parents of young adult schizophrenics were described. The disaffiliative tendencies of the parents of the autistic young children were especially significant, while the parents of patients whose schizophrenia did not become overt until late adolescence or young adulthood appeared to let relationships develop but distorted and impaired the focusing of attention and the acquisition of clear meanings. The parents of the acting-out children in this series were active and energetic in their relationships, though often with various disturbed moods and impulses, and were relatively well-defined and clear in their percepts. Parents of a group of withdrawn neurotic children showed especially sadness, together with serious strivings to maintain relationships. The behavior of the offspring in all of these families appeared "logical" and developmentally meaningful in the sense that the forms of behavior seen in the patient-offspring would fit in with major formal transactional patterns seen in the parents.

The formulations made in this paper are applicable, we wish to stress, only to those varieties of patients and families which we have thus far studied; we do not regard these findings as applicable, for example, to the families of childhood schizophrenics who have gross neurological impairment (18).

These formulations generated additional hypotheses which were tested through blind ratings of Rorschach data from these parents. It was found that the frequency of thinking disorders, genetic-level of psychological differentiation, and frequency of expressions of over-all and initial hostile affect found in the four groups of parents were in predicted directions.

The data presented here support a developmental theory of familial contributions to ego impairment which is being evolved in the family studies at the NIMH. The present data especially emphasize parental *styles* of thinking and relating as a crucial co-determinant—other experiential and innate factors are also co-determinants—of enduring patterns of behavior in offspring.

References

1. WYNNE, L. C., et al. (1958). *Psychiatry*, **21**, 205.
2. RYCKOFF, I. M., DAY, J., & WYNNE, L. C. (1959). *A.M.A. Arch. Psychiat.*, **1**, 93.
3. WYNNE, L. C. (1961). The study of intrafamilial alignments and splits in exploratory family therapy. In Ackerman, N. W., et al (eds.), *Exploring the Base for Family Therapy*. New York: Fam. Service Asso.
4. SCHAFFER, L., et al. (1962). *Psychiatry*, **25**, 32.
5. WYNNE, L. C., & SINGER, M. T. (1963). Thought disorder and the family relations of schizophrenics: I, II, III, and IV. *Arch. Gen. Psychiat.*, **9**, 191–206; **12**, 187–212.
6. BLOCK, J., et al. (1958). *Psychiatry*, **21**, 387.
7. KANNER, L. (1949). *Am. J. Orthopsychiat.*, **19**, 416.

8. Rimland, B. (1963). *Early Infantile Autism: Review, Theory and Implications.* New York: Appleton-Century-Crofts.
9. Mahler, M. S. (1952). *Psychoanal. Study Child*, **7**, 286.
10. Some observations on controls in psychiatric research. Group advance. *Psychiat. Report*, 42, 1959.
11. Schachtel, E. G. (1959). *Metamorphosis.* New York: Basic Books.
12. Boatman, M. J., & Szurek, S. A. (1960). A clinical study of childhood schizophrenia. In Jackson, D. D. (ed.), *The Etiology of Schizophrenia.* New York: Basic Books.
13. Benjamin, J. (1950–1954). Personal communication.
14. Rapaport, D. (1946). *Diagnostic Psychological Testing*, Vol. II. Chicago: Year Book Publishers.
15. Werner, H. (1961). *Comparative Psychology of Mental Development.* New York: Science Editions.
16. Becker, W. C. (1956). *J. Abnorm. Soc. Psychol.*, **53**, 29.
17. DeVos, G. A. (1952). *J. Proj. Techniques*, **16**, 133.
18. Meyer, D., & Goldfarb, W. (1962). *Am. J. Psychiat.*, **118**, 902.

DAVID ROSENTHAL, PAUL H. WENDER, SEYMOUR S. KETY, FINI SCHULSINGER, JOSEPH WELNER, and LISE ØSTERGAARD

Schizophrenics' Offspring Reared in Adoptive Homes

Although many have attempted to understand schizophrenia as a disorder resulting almost exclusively from a reaction to psychological forces, an equally enthusiastic group of researchers have seen schizophrenia as deriving primarily from genetic or constitutional predisposition. Supporters of this viewpoint have tended to do large-scale surveys which generally demonstrate that schizophrenia occurs far more frequently among the children of schizophrenics than among the children of normal parents. However, since the children of schizophrenic parents are not invariably schizophrenic, it may be argued that schizophrenia is not caused by a dominant gene. Furthermore, those emphasizing the importance of psychological forces in the etiology of schizophrenia can explain its higher incidence among the offspring of schizophrenic parents on the grounds that schizophrenic parents are more likely to provide a stressful psychological setting in which one is likely to grow up disturbed.

Reprinted from D. Rosenthal and S. S. Kety (eds.), *The Transmission of Schizophrenia.* Oxford, England: Pergamon Press, 1968, pp. 377–391, with the permission of Pergamon Press and Dr. Rosenthal.

As a compromise between the strict genetic or constitutional viewpoint and the strict psychogenic position, the diathesis-stress hypothesis has been advanced. This hypothesis states that a predisposition for developing schizophrenic behavior is inherited and that such development can take place only within a particularly stressful psychological environment. Thus, those born without the predisposition will never become schizophrenic despite exposure early in life to a very stressful environment. Those born with the predisposition who are fortunate to grow up in an environment that is relatively nonstressful, will also avoid developing schizophrenia. Only those having the genetic predisposition and the misfortune to grow up in a particularly adverse psychological environment can be expected to succumb to the disorder.

Until very recently no studies had been done to test the diathesis-stress hypothesis. In recent years Heston did one such study involving children whose mothers were schizophrenic but who were adopted very early in life into families where there was no schizophrenia. A similar study is the one that follows by Rosenthal and several colleagues, carried out in Denmark where it was possible to follow a large group of adoptees whose mothers were schizophrenic and who grew up in homes where there was no schizophrenia. In addition, Rosenthal was able to identify a group of adoptees whose parents were not schizophrenic but who grew up in homes where the adoptive mother became schizophrenic. The unique opportunity for locating such subject samples has resulted in a particularly fascinating and significant study on the etiology of schizophrenia.

This is the first of a projected series of reports on what Dr. Kety, Dr. Wender and I call the Adoptees Study.[1] The one that Dr. Kety presented we call the

[1] The American authors originally formulated the principal strategy of this study together. Our Danish collaborators include: Dr. Fini Schulsinger, who did much to implement the strategy of the study, to enlist the cooperation of Danish authorities, to provide the facilities for the examinations, to supervise the on-the-scene administrative aspects of the study, and who did the psychiatric interviews when Dr. Welner was ill; Dr. Joseph Welner, who performed the psychiatric examinations and evaluations of subjects, and who supervised the day to day administration of the study's research aspects; and Prof. Lise Østergaard, who helped to choose some of the tests used and who selected and supervised the project psychologists. Other participating professional personnel include: Psychiatrists who prepared the R-forms and assisted in the diagnoses of the parents: Dr. Hans Søvsø, Dr. Harriet Thieme, Dr. P. Freitag, Dr. Kirsten Bjerke, Dr. B. Jacobsen; Psychologists: Mr. Vestberg Rasmussen, Mrs. Kirsten Boman, Mr. Rasmus Jordan, Mrs. Ulla Praetorius and Mrs. Brita Jørgensen; Social workers: Mrs. Birgit Jacobsen and Mrs. Skat Andersen. Secretaries and clerks: Lene Monrad Hansen, Agnathe Beck, Ida Bech and Kitty Scharf. Dr. Sarnoff A. Mednick suggested that we carry out our studies in Denmark and use the facilities of the Psychological Institute, of which he is Director. Mr. John L. Van Dyke, Bethesda, assisted in the analysis of the data and in the selection of Control subjects.

Extended Family Study and the one that Dr. Wender presented we call the Adoptive Parents Study. The names may help to distinguish the studies in future discussions of them.

This is a preliminary as well as a first report, since we are still very much in the midst of our extensive research activities. We will be finding and examining subjects for at least another year. In June 1967 we began the third year of this project.

The reader will observe a strong resemblance, as well as important differences in conception and method, between the Adoptees Study and the study reported by Heston. We want to point out that our study was conceived and planned years before we learned of Heston's remarkable feat, and it was well under way for some time before Heston's report appeared.

Although all our studies attempt to assess the relative contributions of heredity and environment to schizophrenia, the major focus of the Adoptees Study is somewhat different. Here we are trying to obtain evidence that a diathesis-stress theory of schizophrenia is correct. What we would like to do is to detect and describe some behavioral and psychological aspects of that inherited diathesis. Paul Meehl would call it the "schizotype," which is a perfectly good name for it.

Another way to get at this assumed diathesis is to examine the non-schizophrenic twin in discordant monozygotic pairs. Several investigators are taking a closer look at such twins and, hopefully, the various studies will support and complement one another. In twins, one has the task of evaluating the effects, both prenatal and experimental, of the twinship *per se*. We do not run into such problems in the Adoptees Study.

A research design such as Mednick and Schulsinger's hinges on the deliberate selection of what they correctly call high-risk subjects. These are children born of schizophrenic mothers. Most of them were reared in the parental home, or in various institutions or foster-homes. From the usual environmentalist point of view as well as the genetic, these are indeed high-risk subjects. Therefore, behavioral differences between them and a control group could reflect both genetic and environmental effects. For this reason their subjects are less useful in the search for the schizotype, but are very well suited to their main purpose, viz. the delineation of behavioral precursors of schizophrenia.

Selection of Subjects

We begin with a pool of subjects who were given up for nonfamilial adoption at an early age. These are the same adoptees that were found, identified and coded by number in the Extended Family Study reported by Dr. Kety. There were slightly less than 5500 such children in the years 1924 to 1947. The number-coding that identified each adoptee was done sequentially on special forms, which we call A-forms. The A could stand for

Adoptee. On each A-form was listed the names of, and other identifying information about, the biological and adoptive parents.

It is the approximately 11,000 biological parents who now become our focus of attention. Unfortunately, in about 25% of the cases, the biological father was not known. This leaves us with about 10,000 known biological parents. We want to find out who among them was schizophrenic.

To begin this search, clerks compare the parents' names and birth dates listed on the A-forms with the names in the Psychiatric Register of the Institute of Human Genetics. The same search is made at the Bispebjerg Hospital, which does not report to the Human Genetics Institute. A large number of biological mothers must first be screened in the Folke-register in order to learn all their changes of names. When a parent's name is found in the Register, the information in his file is copied. We then request his case record from every psychiatric hospital or other facility that he attended.

Psychiatrists read through the case records and dictate a summary of the case in English, emphasizing the main areas stipulated on another prepared form, which we call the R-form. The R could stand for the parent's case Record. The R-forms are number-coded sequentially, and the A-form number of the corresponding adopted child is recorded on each. The psychiatrist preparing the R-form reports the parent's name(s), birthdate and sex; all institutional admissions, including the dates, length of stay, and discharge diagnoses; behavior leading to admission; major features of life history; major features of the premorbid personality; known precipitating factors; major features of the illness noted at the first admission; additional major symptoms noted in the subsequent course of the illness; and clinical course and outcome. The psychiatrist then makes his own final diagnosis and another according to a code which was worked out primarily by Dr. Wender, with some minor assists from Dr. Kety, Dr. Schulsinger and myself. This is the same code described by Dr. Kety in his report on the Extended Family Study.

The R-forms are then sent to Bethesda as soon as they are completed and typed. Initially, Dr. Kety, Dr. Wender and I reviewed each R-form independently and made our separate coded diagnoses. Subsequently, since Dr. Kety left for a year in Paris, Dr. Wender and I have been making the diagnoses without him. In each case where we have a full consensus that the parent is in the schizophrenic range (coded B_1, B_2 or B_3), the child he or she gave up for adoption is selected as an Index Case.

Now, the A-form number of the Index child is copied from the R-form. We then enter a file where we keep all the A-forms, which are arranged in number sequence. We find the A-form and record from it the adoptee's name, sex, birthdate, age of transfer to his adoptive parents, age at formal adoption, and the adoptive parent's occupation, income and "fortune", as it is called in Denmark. Beginning at the place in the file occupied by this A-form, we search systematically forward and backward in the file until we find at least four other adoptees who are of the same sex as the Index Case, and who have approximately the same age, age of transfer, age at adoption, socio-economic status of their adoptive or rearing parents, and who do *not* have a parent with an R-form or known psychiatric diagnosis. These data for the four or more subjects are recorded on another form. I and one other person, Dr. Wender or a psychologically trained research assistant, independently rank the four or more subjects according to how closely each resembles the Index Case in these several respects weighed together. The subject with the highest summed rank is selected as the Control. If he refuses to or cannot participate in the study, the subject with the next highest rank is substituted as the Control, and so on down the list.

The mingled A-form numbers of both Index and Control subjects are then sent to Copenhagen. Of course, we send only the numbers. We do not say which numbers represent Index Cases or which represent Controls. We say only that these are new subjects. The examining staff never knows if the subject before them is an Index Case or not. Even the psychiatrist who obtains a history from the subject cannot know, since the adoptee himself does not know about his biological parents,[2] and the psychiatrist does not actively seek this information, though he is permitted to pursue the matter if the adoptee himself volunteers to talk about it. To date, the examining psychiatrist has not known whether any subject was an Index Case or not. The psychologists do not even have the possibility of finding out. It is especially this aspect of the study which makes it so esthetically appealing, as well as scientifically sound.

The social worker who receives the A-form numbers first sends a specially prepared form letter to the prospective subjects and then contacts them by telephone to try to arrange an examination date or to make an appointment for a personal visit to discuss the matter further. The subjects are told that a scientific study is being conducted on the relation between environment and health, that all strata of the population are included, and that such studies require that all subjects selected participate since the results might otherwise be invalidated. The social worker uses all her skills to persuade the subjects to come to Copenhagen's Kommunehospitalet to participate in the study. An examination lasts 2 days. The subject is offered compensatory pay for salary he may be missing, or for the cost of a baby sitter. His transportation is paid, as are his hotel bills if he must stay at an hotel. If he wishes to have another person accompany him, that person's transportation is paid as well. In addition, each subject is given a modest sum of money as a bonus or added incentive.

Selection of Examination Procedures

Let us assume now that the subject has agreed to come. We have 2 precious days in which to examine this scientifically precious person. What should we do in this time?

[2] One subject said that her adoptive father had told her that he was also her biological father. We rechecked the records. They gave different names for adoptive and biological fathers.

If one has a specific theory in mind, the question is easily answered. Mednick, for example, could tailor his procedures so that each one would bear on one or more aspects of his neatly formulated theory. We, on the other hand, were more or less committed to a broad conceptual framework which, in *The Genain Quadruplets* (Rosenthal, 1963), I called diathesis-stress theory. This is less a theory than a designation for a class of theories. It says nothing specific about either the nature of the diathesis or of the stress.

We are making a series of assumptions. The first was that heredity was an important contributor to schizophrenia. The second was that this inherited factor manifested itself in the behavior or personality of persons who were not frankly schizophrenic. The third was that these manifestations could be detected by tests or in one or two interviews. The fourth was that we would know which questions to ask or which tests to use to detect these manifestations.

Lacking a clearcut theory, we had recourse to three broad strategies to guide our decisions about what or what not to do. The first was that differences found between schizophrenics and normal controls on various psychological or behavioral tests might reflect inherited differences, and that we should therefore use these tests in hopes of finding similar differences, but perhaps of lesser degree, between our two groups of subjects. This strategy is a shaky one since the differences found in the schizophrenia studies may simply reflect the clinical condition itself, the consequences of being ill rather than the causes. Nevertheless, when a simple task such as reaction time discriminates schizophrenics and normals so well, and when one considers that reaction time may indeed reflect hereditary influences, one feels almost compelled to include such a procedure. Actually, a few of our tests are based on this strategy, including reaction time.

The second strategy seemed more promising. It was based on the idea that we should find the same kinds of traits and aberrations in our Index group as in the premorbid personality of known schizophrenics. Of course, those who become schizophrenic must be different in some way from those who do not, and since we could expect only a few of our subjects to become schizophrenic, we might be focusing on the wrong traits. Moreover, the literature on the premorbid personality of schizophrenics was hardly exciting. It was based on retrospection, or on past clinical records prepared in service settings for reasons not necessarily coinciding with ours.[3] Formulations thus derived emphasized traits like shyness, timidity, passivity, sex difficulties, introversion, and others. We would, of course, look for such traits, but we hoped for a more fine-grained description of the inherited diathesis than that. We included a self-assessment procedure whose items were based on such literature and on our own clinical observations or impressions as well.

A third strategy was simply to emulate success. Mednick, for example, was able to discriminate his Index and Control groups using autonomic indices

[3] The Judge Baker Guidance Center reports (Fleming, 1967; Waring and Ricks, 1965) had not appeared or were not known to us when we began this study.

in a conditioning procedure. However, the possibility existed that environmental factors were contributing significantly to this discrimination. Would it occur as well when rearing factors were more balanced between the two groups? It was a question worth asking in our study. Moreover, to the extent that heredity plays a role at all in Mednick's theory, it implies that it is the propensity for high anxiety levels that is inherited in, and is critical for, the development of schizophrenia. An alternative hypothesis would be that the critical inherited factor is cognitive rather than affective, if one can make this conceptual distinction at the inherited level. Nevertheless, we included a conditioning procedure similar to Mednick's but with a few tactical modifications, and we added an habituation and "demandingness" procedure used successfully at the NIMH to discriminate schizophrenic and control groups (Zahn et al., in press).

In emulating success, we attended especially to the work of Wynne and Singer. They were able to discriminate relatives of schizophrenic and neurotic subjects with respect to cognitive, attentional and transactional factors elicited by projective tests. The possibility existed that it was exactly such moderately deviant behaviors that were inherited. We invited Dr. Singer to Denmark where she spent 2 weeks lecturing to our psychologists (and others) and consulting intensively with Dr. Lise Østergaard, who is the senior psychologist in the Adoptees Study and who is a leading authority on cognitive disturbances in border-line schizophrenics. Dr. Østergaard has since worked out a system for evaluating cognitive and projective test performance, combining in it features of both her own and Dr. Singer's approach to such test evaluation. Consequently, we included several such tests in our battery.

In addition, we were not above playing hunches, and a few tests were included on that basis. It would take much too long to describe all the tests and procedures selected; and of course there were many others that we would like to have included, but could not.

Dr. Joseph Welner and I hammered out together the nature and orientation of the psychiatric interview he would employ. The interview is taped. The subject is encouraged to speak freely, and to set his own pace and direction. However, there are 26 categories of information that the interview is supposed to cover, and if the subject does not lead into them himself, Dr. Welner at opportune moments guides the interview towards those categories still not covered. The interviews have lasted from 3 to 5 hours. Afterward, Dr. Welner dictates a psychiatric summary in which he not only formulates his characterization and diagnosis of the subject, but also describes the information elicited for each category separately. In this way, we can compare our Index and Control subjects category by category.

Before we began the actual examination of our own subjects, we ran several known border-line schizophrenics through the entire 2-day examination on a dry run basis. This was done to synchronize all procedures, to trim the timing so that we could stay within our limited schedule, and to help each examiner develop familiarity and skill with the procedures he would use.

The Sample

The diagnoses and sex of the sick parents of our Index Cases are shown in Table 1.

You will be surprised to learn that a number of Index Cases had parents who carried a diagnosis of verified or possible manic-depressive psychosis. We did not want to bring up this point when we were describing our method of case finding, which was already complicated enough. These cases were included for two reasons. The first was one of expediency. There were periods when we simply did not havc enough schizophrenic parents processed and the staff in Copenhagen had no subjects to examine. The second and more important reason derived from this question: What if we should find differences between our Index and Control groups; how could we know that these differences were specific to a schizophrenic genotype? Might they not represent the severity dimension of a general factor of mental illness? If we had a comparison pathology group, we might be able to learn something about the specificity problem. As a bonus, we might also learn something about the possible genetic relationship between schizophrenia and manic-depressive psychosis, and about the nature of the assumed inherited diathesis for manic-depressive psychosis.

In 56 cases, the parent was clearly schizophrenic by our criteria, although in 10 of these we differed as to the subcategory of schizophrenia in which he

TABLE 1 *Consensus diagnoses and sex of the sick parents*

Diagnosis*	N	Sex ♂	Sex ♀
B_1	36	8	28
B_2	7	2	5
B_3	3	1	2
B_1/B_3	2	2	0
B_1/B_2	6	2	4
B_2/B_3	2	0	2
D	1	1	0
B_1/D_1	1	0	1
B/M	1	0	1
D/M	1	1	0
M?	1	1	0
M	8	5	3
Total	69	23	46

* B_1 = chronic schizophrenia. B_2 = acute schizophrenic reaction. B_3 = border-line or pseudoneurotic schizophrenic. D = doubtful schizophrenia. M = manic-depressive psychosis.

belonged. In 2 cases we could not decide between schizophrenia or doubtful schizophrenia and manic-depressive psychosis.

Among the 56 schizophrenic cases, the ratio of mothers to fathers is about $2\frac{1}{2}$ to 1. There is a slight excess above expectancy of mothers over fathers, and it could result from the fact that about 25% of all biological fathers were not known. In the main, this distribution speaks well for the representativeness of the sample. Among the manic-depressive parents, there are actually more fathers than mothers, but the numbers are small. They do suggest, however, that this is indeed a different diagnostic group.

Among the Index adoptees, we find 31 males and 38 females. The difference from expectancy is small, but the possibility exists that there may have been a slight preference for adopting girls in past years.

It may be important to know whether the sick parent was psychotic before the adoptee was born, or if the illness had its onset after the birth and transfer of the child. Some data relevant to this point are shown in Fig. 1. in which the date of the parent's first admission for psychosis has been subtracted from the birthdate of the child. If the parent's admission occurred first, the difference is negative.

Of the 69 parent-child pairs, in only 11 instances (16%) had the parent been admitted before the child's birth, and of the 11, only 5 were mothers. In this respect, then, our sample differs strikingly from Heston's, since all his schizophrenic mothers were actively psychotic and hospitalized when his Index children were born. Is it possible that the active pyschosis, with concomitant hospitalization and treatment, provided gestational conditions detrimental to the subsequent mental health of the offspring, apart from genetic factors? It is at least a point worth keeping in mind. Although 84% of our parents were

Fig. 1. *Years between birth of child and first admission for psychosis of the sick patient.*

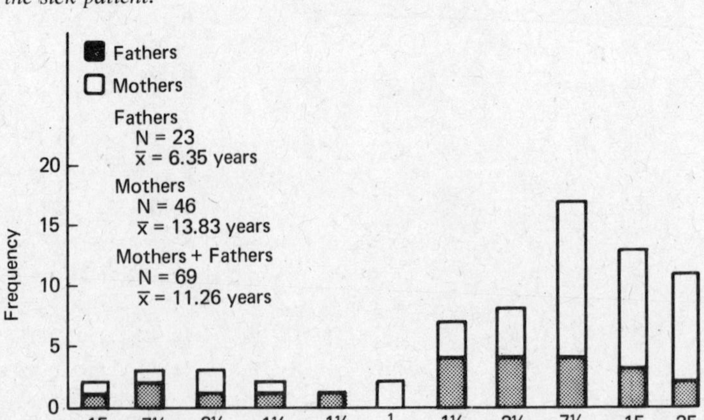

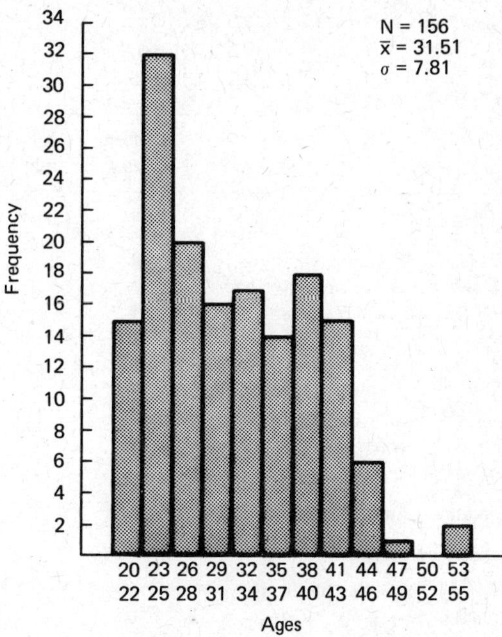

Fig. 2. *Age of index and control subjects.*

not hospitalized until after the child's birth, it is of course still possible that a number of them may have been ambulatory psychotics for years before their first admission. We will look at such temporal relationships carefully in the future and check on their possible bearing on mental illness in our adoptees.

The age distribution of our Index Cases is shown in Fig. 2. The sample is still a young one. The mean age is 31·51 years, the standard deviation 7·81 years.

Findings and Discussion

Now let us show you some of the salient features characterizing our Index and Control groups (see Table 2).

As of the day we began to prepare this paper, 28 April 1967, we had sent the A-form numbers of 155 adoptees to Copenhagen to be subjects in this study. The reason we have more Controls than Index Cases is that when a selected Control cannot or will not participate, we send another Control to replace him. When an Index Case refuses to participate, no replacement is possible.

We had reason to expect that most refusals would occur among the Index group. In fact, the refusals are evenly distributed among the two groups. The possibility exists, however, that those who refuse are a particularly pathological

TABLE 2 *Some demographic characteristics of the adoptees sample*

	Index cases	**Control subjects**
Number sent	69	86
Refused to participate	14	15
Number of refusals who have had contact with a psychiatric facility	1	3
Died	2	4
Congenital idiot	1	0
Living in Norway or Sweden	2	1
Migrated elsewhere	1	5
Could not locate	0	2
Hospitalized for schizophrenia	1	0
Incarcerated for crimes	0	1
Other psychiatric hospitalization	2	1
Suicidal attempts	0	2
Examined	39	47

group whom it would be important for us to examine. We will obtain as much data as possible from other sources about these people to check this possibility. However, since in the Extended Family Study the name of every adoptee was searched in the Psychiatric Register and in the files of the 12 major mental hospitals in Denmark, we are reasonably certain that only four of the persons who refused had ever been seen at a psychiatric facility. Three of these were Control subjects, and none was in the schizophrenic spectrum.

The possibility remains, too, that the reasons underlying the refusals differ between the two groups. We examined the first 25 refusals to check this possibility, but could see no obvious pattern differentiating the two groups. Perhaps the Controls on the whole were less ambivalent in their refusals. One Control thought she was selected because she was living with a man to whom she was not married, and she was opposed to speaking of personal matters. One Index Case said he had simulated disease in military service and was fearful of being found out. One Control was a 41-year-old woman who still lived with her mother and kept an unlisted telephone number. One 37-year-old Index male lived with his parents, and his mother said he would refuse. He had been admitted to the Kommunehospitalet at age 11 because of behavior problems in school. Now he is a travel guide. The total group of refusals included about twice as many women as men. The Index refusals included proportionately more people in their young twenties. It is difficult to say what these figures mean. We will continue to try to persuade these people to come for examination, but will in any case learn as much as possible about them.

Not as many Index children died as Control children. The figures, however, throw no light on the question of possible increased mortality among the offspring of schizophrenic parents. Not only are the figures small, but it is usually *infant* mortality that is at issue, and it is clear that most of such cases, if they did indeed exist, would have died before they could have been adopted. The one congenital CNS syndrome that occurs in the sample is in fact an Index Case.

One might have expected the Index subjects to be more migrant, but the opposite seems to be the case. We do not know to where one of the Index Cases migrated. The 5 subjects who definitely left Scandinavia were all Controls. They migrated to England, France, Spain, Switzerland and Singapore. Maybe Index Cases are less bold and adventurous. Of the 2 Controls who could not be located, 1 disappeared from view during the war.

Among the entire sample of 155 subjects, only 1 had ever been hospitalized for schizophrenia. This is a low rate, of course, and is consistent with the rate for the general Danish population. The 1 hospitalized schizophrenic was an Index Case. We should expect a greater number of such cases, based on Heston's findings. Our sample is about 5 years younger than Heston's but that is probably not an important factor. We will soon show you why our data are in good agreement with his in regard to schizophrenic psychopathology.

Where our data *dis*agree with his is in the area of criminality and psychopathy, which occurred with high frequency in his non-schizophrenic Index Cases. In our sample, the only instance of criminality occurs in a Control subject who served 6 years at the Horsens psychopathic hospital for 4 petty crimes that he committed as a young man. He was the only subject in our sample diagnosed as a frank psychopath. We should pay close attention to this difference between Heston's study and ours because it suggests that whether an individual with the assumed diathesis that we are talking about becomes psychopathically antisocial or not is determined in overriding fashion by environmental factors. And it suggests that such factors are much more prevalent in the United States than in Denmark. It is also possible that prenatal factors among Heston's hospitalized mothers may have somehow contributed to psychopathy in their children.

There is one other point in Table 2 that warrants comment. Two of our examined Index Cases who were not schizophrenic had been admitted at some time in their lives to a psychiatric hospital. In each case, the issue was relatively minor and transient, involving affective or depressive reactions to unhappy personal affairs, and very brief hospital stays. These are counter-balanced by one similar episode and two suicidal attempts among the Control subjects, who also had what could be described as affective reactions. Thus, there are no appreciable differences between the groups in these respects.

Now, let us return to the question of schizophrenic psychopathology. Dr. Welner made a carefully formulated diagnostic evaluation of each case examined. Both he and Dr. Schulsinger, who pinch-hit for him when Dr. Welner was ill, have an appreciation of the nuances of diagnosis which is too often discounted in the United States. In addition, both have had training and supervision in psycho-analysis, and both have been psycho-analyzed. Thus, they are attuned to both the symptomatic and dynamic factors in each case they examine. We would like to present their detailed diagnostic formulations regarding every case in the study, but that would take much too long. If we did, the reader would have a better appreciation of the richness of the material and of the wide variety of symptoms and personalities represented in both groups of subjects. Some time in the future, Dr. Welner will present much of this material himself. For now, however, we will present only those thumbnail diagnostic formulations which we may consider to be in the realm of schizoid–schizophrenic psychopathology (Table 3).

First, note that 3 subjects are diagnosed as schizophrenic, and all 3 are Index Cases. Seven cases are called clear border-line schizophrenics. Six of the seven are Index Cases. There are 13 Index Cases in the schizophrenic spectrum as compared to 7 Control subjects. Note, too, that among the Controls the diagnoses tend to be more qualified, as though the examiner sees the psychopathology as not quite so severe. For example, 1 case is said to be "near border-line", but not quite. Another is "probable" borderline, but not surely. The 2 schizoid subjects are said to be "moderately" or "not too vulnerably" schizoid. And the subject in the paranoid spectrum is called "subparanoid". The two qualifications in the Index group include 1 case called "border-line schizophrenia or pervert", a matter of some indecision regarding the differential diagnosis although the emphasis was on border-line

TABLE 3 *Diagnoses in the schizophrenia spectrum (by Dr. Joseph Welner)*

Parent D_x	**Index** (N = 39)	**Control** (N = 47)
B_1/D_1	Schizophrenia, hospitalized	Border-line Sz
B_1	Schizophrenia, never hospitalized	Pre-Sz character, near border-line
B_1/B_2	Schizophrenia, never hospitalized	*Schizoid or premorbid Sz personality
B_1	Border-line Sz	Probable border-line paranoid
B_1	Border-line Sz	*Moderately schizoid
B_1	Border-line Sz	Not too vulnerable schizoid
B_2	Border-line Sz	Subparanoid personality
B_1	Border-line Sz or pervert	
M	Border-line pseudoneurotic Sz	
B_1	Schizoid, paranoid border-line	
M?	Schizoid	
B_1/B_3	*Vague schizoid tendencies	
B_3	Paranoid character	

* These diagnoses were made by Dr. Fini Schulsinger.

schizophrenia, and the second case was said to have "tendencies" that are vague and schizoid. Since the 13 Index Cases were so diagnosed from among 39 Index Cases examined, one-third fall in the schizoid-schizophrenic spectrum. This is a high proportion indeed. Since the 7 Controls were so diagnosed from among 47 subjects, or about 1 in 7, the rate is more than two times as great for the Index group. Moreover, the more severe disorders cluster primarily among the Index subjects.

It is worth pointing out that if such findings were reported in the usual study, where the diagnostician knows which subjects are Index Cases and which are Controls, they would be mighty suspect indeed. Here there is no question of the diagnostician being influenced by such information.

Does the particular form of the diagnosis in the parent make any difference with respect to the frequency of schizophrenic spectrum diagnoses in the children?

We can read the answer to this question in Table 4. The frequency among the B_1 offspring, where we are dealing with hard-core schizophrenia, seems to be no higher than for the less severe types of schizophrenia. Moreover, the rate for the offspring of manic-depressives seems to be in the same range. Among the other three offspring of manic-depressives, one was called repressive, with alcohol bouts and a bad memory, a second was said to be slightly overreactive but functioning well, and the third had some mild neurotic features but was also functioning well. Such data suggest that the inherited core diathesis is the same for both schizophrenia and manic-depressive psychosis, but that manic-depressives may have other modifying genes or life experiences which direct the clinical manifestations of the diathesis in a different way.

It is important, too, to note that the rate of schizophrenic spectrum diagnoses among the Controls is 15%, a figure which is not negligible and

TABLE 4 *The percent of schizophrenia spectrum diagnoses in the offspring according to the subcategory diagnosis of the parent*

Parental diagnosis	Number of cases examined	Number in the schizophrenia spectrum	Percent in the schizophrenia spectrum
B_1	24	7	29
B_2	5	1	20
B_3	2	1	50
B/	3	2	67
M or M?	5	2	40
None	47	7	15
	—	—	—
Total	86	20	23

which is actually half the rate found in the offspring of B_1 parents, although the disturbances among the latter tended to be more severe. It is possible that a number of the biological parents of Controls might have been called psychiatrically ill if they had been personally examined in the same way as the Adoptees. Since many of these parents are now old or dead, it is questionable whether there would be any appreciable value in trying to bring them in for such examination. All we know is that they probably have never had contact with a psychiatric facility.

There are two other questions we must ask ourselves. One concerns the events in the life of the Adoptees that occurred between birth and transfer to the adoptive family. The Index and Control adoptees are matched for age of transfer, but perhaps that is not enough. We are now in process of collecting as much information as possible about birth, time spent with biological parents or in institutions, and some other data relevant to this question. We should eventually be in a position to determine whether the length of time spent with a psychotic or pre-psychotic parent during this earliest phase of life is related to degree or type of psychopathology.

The other question concerns the possibility that the rearing of the Index Cases differed from that of the Controls. Possibly, for some reason not clear, those people who adopted children of schizophrenics may have themselves been more psychopathological or more psychonoxious to the child. We have left this factor uncontrolled and assumed randomness across both groups in reard to it. However, we will in the near future control the factor of psychopathology in the rearing parents and evaluate its contribution to possible psychopathology in their adopted children.

One inference ought to be drawn from these data: that is, if we are going to learn anything more about the genetics of schizophrenic disorders, we can no longer rely on statistics based only on hospitalized cases. Had we done so in this study, we would have concluded that heredity did not contribute significantly to schizophrenia, or that, if it did, the gene was probably recessive. Moreover, such data imply what many of us have long recognized, that the dichotomy of schizophrenia *vs.* non-schizophrenia is artificial and masks an underlying continuity of severity of pathology in this spectrum of disorders. Although such continuity of symptomatology suggests a polygenic theory with respect to the probably inherited diathesis, we should have a better appreciation of the contribution of environmental agents of various kinds before we accept this theory unqualifiedly.

It is probably not necessary, but let us remind you that the figures presented today are not final. We are still collecting subjects. The patterns we have seen so far could change. In a year or two we will be able to present the final figures, with somewhat larger N's and a more complete assessment of the material.

We would have liked to present many results from our testing program. Unfortunately, we are able to present only fragments of findings from two of our procedures. These are really self-assessments rather than tests. One involves a widely used and studied set of such assessments, the MMPI. The other involves a set of items that we thought might have particular relevance to the assumed diathesis. We call them the Self-rating Scales.

There are 52 such scales. Each has 7 points. The midpoint is assigned a score of 4 and represents an evaluation of self as average with respect to that item. Scores 5, 6 and 7 represent the more-than-average direction, scores 3, 2 and 1 the below-average direction.

We had misgivings about self-assessments, for many reasons, but we thought that the self-concept might be a readily visible reflection of the inherited diathesis, and a harbinger as well of a trend toward clinical schizophrenia. The confronting problems were again methodological. Could subjects see themselves as they really were, i.e. could they represent their true self-concept accurately? And if they could, would they? We could do nothing about the first question, except to hope that the self-assessments would not be too distorted. To maximize cooperativeness and candor, the Self-rating Scales were administered during the first morning of the 2-day examination. The subject was told to answer all items as best he could and that later that afternoon a psychiatrist would discuss his ratings with him. In fact, the psychiatrist did so, as part of his interview. Whether the anticipation of an inquiry about their ratings loosened subjects' defenses in this respect, we cannot say. In any case, the statistically significant results are shown in Table 5.

One item is significant at the 0·01 level, two at the 0·025 level, and three at the 0·05 level. Three items go in the predicted direction, and their t values are printed in italic figures; three go in the reverse direction. Such findings could be due to chance. Nevertheless, we ought not dismiss them out of hand. They may be meaningful. We do not want to spend too much time with possible explanations of these findings. The N's are about half of what we expect the final N's to be, and the significant items could change. There are no

TABLE 5 *Comparison of index and control subjects on self-rating scales*

Item	Group means		Difference	t
	Index (N = 30)	Control (N = 29)		
Shy	3·53	4·24	−0·71	2·342
Close friends	4·50	3·90	0·60	2·376
Feel things are unreal	4·00	3·24	0·76	*2·721*
Feel I'm not master of my own fate	3·83	3·24	0·59	*2·029*
A good talker	4·70	4·07	0·63	2·184
Sense of humor	4·33	4·79	−0·46	*2·239*

At $p = 0{\cdot}05$, $t = 2{\cdot}000$, two-tailed.
At $p = 0{\cdot}025$, $t = 2{\cdot}299$, two-tailed.
At $p = 0{\cdot}01$, $t = 2{\cdot}660$, two-tailed.

extreme scores here; all mean values hover around average, ranging from over 3 to less than 5. The mean differences are not large. The three predicted items indicate that the Index Subjects have more feelings of unreality, feel that they are less in control of their own destiny, and have less of a sense of humor. The fact that they say they are less shy, have more close friends and are better conversationalists than the Controls suggests that they may have a distorted self-image or are over-defensive with respect to such traits. It is difficult to explain such self-assessments, and we leave the matter open for now.

How does the MMPI discriminate the two groups? The answer is found in Table 6.

We see that the groups are very similar with respect to their K, F and L scale scores, which are all acceptable. With respect to the 8 pathology scales, not one reaches a statistically significant difference, but the Index group is higher on 7 of them, the Controls scoring slightly higher on Depression. The difference between the groups on the Schizophrenia scale is in the predicted direction, but it is not large and not significant statistically. The Index group scores highest on Hysteria and Hypochondriasis, not Schizophrenia, and scores slightly *lower* than Controls on Social Introversion. The latter finding is again contrary to expectation.

Again, we do not want to dwell on these findings. Here, the N is small and will increase considerably. We may see many changes. The time to discuss theoretical implications will be when all the data are in and analyzed in

TABLE 6 *Comparison of 24 pairs of matched index and control subjects on MMPI scales*

Scale	**Mean T score**		**Difference**	***t***
	Index	**Control**		
K	57·96	57·38	0·58	0·092
F	56·83	55·67	1·16	0·158
L	59·38	59·13	0·25	0·183
HS	63·67	59·21	4·46	1·451
D	61·13	61·92	−0·79	0·071
Hy	65·67	60·96	4·71	1·451
PD	55·83	54·17	1·66	0·656
PA	57·00	53·75	3·25	0·605
PT	54·04	53·63	0·41	0·265
SC	61·33	57·29	4·04	0·913
MA	55·83	54·71	1·12	0·477
SI	51·75	52·93	−1·17	1·085
ES	53·92	55·38	−1·46	0·697

At $p = 0{\cdot}05$, $t = 2{\cdot}07$, two-tailed.
At $p = 0{\cdot}05$, $t = 1{\cdot}71$, one-tailed.

more ways, and in more sophisticated ways, than we were able to marshal for this presentation.

What we have done primarily is to sketch the research design we have used to get some leverage on the possible contribution of heredity to schizophrenia and the nature of that contribution. We have presented some preliminary findings so that readers can obtain some idea of the potential usefulness of such a design. At this point, the story we hope to tell has only begun to unfold. We look forward to learning the full story with all the anticipation that we hope any interested professional audience will feel when it learns about such a study.

References

FLEMING, P. (1967). Emotional antecedents of schizophrenia: inner experiences of children and adolescents who were later hospitalized for schizophrenia, Lecture at NIMH, 19 May.

ROSENTHAL, D. (ed.), et al. (1963). Theoretical overview. In *The Genain Quadruplets.* New York: Basic Books.

WARING, M. and RICKS, D. (1965). Family patterns of children who became adult schizophrenics, *J. Nerv. Ment. Dis.*, **140**, 351–64.

ZAHN, T. P., ROSENTHAL, D. and LAWLOR, W. G. (1968). Electrodermal and heart rate orienting reactions in chronic schizophrenia, *J. Psychiat. Res.*, **6**, 117–134.

NORMAN GARMEZY

Vulnerability Research and the Issue of Primary Prevention

In the paper that follows, Garmezy reviews a number of studies in schizophrenia that focus on individuals identified as high risks for becoming schizophrenic. The various factors accounting for their vulnerability to such serious mental disorder are surveyed, and the implications of such work for eventually developing programs to prevent the occurrence of schizophrenia are discussed. This paper is particularly timely in that it combines the approach to understanding the etiology of schizophrenia, as exemplified by the preceding paper on adoptees, as well as the strong preventive orientation that characterizes the significant segment of the field of abnormal psychology that is concerned with the community approach.

Reprinted from the *American Journal of Orthopsychiatry*, **41** (1971), 101–116, with the permission of the American Orthopsychiatric Association, Inc. and Dr. Garmezy.

For psychiatry, primary prevention is aimed at "modifying the environment and strengthening individual capacities to cope with situations" in order to reduce "the incidence of new cases of mental disorder and disability in a population" (15). Such a goal is a laudatory one for any discipline. To a nation beset with problems, citing mental illness statistics to log still another crisis of our times seems almost gratuitous. But a crisis exists and the number of our emotionally wounded suggests the magnitude of this problem: 19 million citizens suffering from diverse forms of mental or emotional illness that require professional intervention; a rising tide of criminality, delinquency, suicide, drug addiction, alcoholism and assault; a half-million severely mentally ill children joined by four million more whose emotional difficulties can only foster a pattern of social and economic incompetence that will fetter them in adulthood. One can cite endless statistics of despair such as these to justify the need for knowledge that will provide the basis for programs of primary, secondary and tertiary prevention.

Unfortunately, empirical data that would buttress such programs are in small supply. We lack fundamental knowledge for determining and, in many instances, identifying early in development those among our citizens who will, in time, constitute the most vulnerable members of our population. Who will fall to the ravaging effects of mental disorder or who will, despite stress and adversity, remain inviolate to psychopathology remains a problem of mystery and challenge. One can, of course, cite numerous case histories to substantiate many factors that may contribute to breakdown; but a simple declaration of physical, psychosocial or sociocultural resources cannot explain divergent paths to adaptation or to deviance.

High Risk Research

The complexity of this problem is evident in the literature of high-risk studies. We can begin with a question. What are the consequences in adulthood for children born to schizophrenic mothers (or fathers, since the data tend to be comparable)? Mednick and Schulsinger (23) suggest that by the end of the risk period of age 45, perhaps 12%–14% of a sample of such children will themselves have suffered some form of schizophrenic disorder, while an additional 35% or so will likely manifest some alternate form of deviant, atypical behavior. On the other hand, expressed, too, in terms of overt behavior, some 50% can be expected to be functioning adequately and to be symptom-free. And of this latter group a small subset (and this is extrapolated from the work of Heston (14) and Karlsson (16)) may even reveal elements of creative expressiveness in their makeup. This last point deserves elaboration, for it reveals the variability in outcomes so characteristic of psychiatric study.

In his follow-up study of infants born to schizophrenic women and placed away from their mothers shortly after birth, Heston (14), in collaboration with Denney, has reported an interesting finding within this Experimental (risk) group:

> One further result deserves special emphasis. The 21 Experimental subjects who exhibited no significant psychosocial impairment were not only successful adults but in comparison to the Control group were more spontaneous when interviewed and had more colorful life histories. They held the more creative jobs: musician, teacher, home-designer; and followed the more imaginative hobbies: oil painting, music, antique aircraft. It must be emphasized that the finding of what may be especially adaptive personality traits among persons in the Experimental groups was noticed only in retrospect as the material compiled on each person was being reviewed. Such traits were not systematically investigated: Most psychiatric studies focus on pathology, not on the delineation of degrees of normal psychological health and this study was not an exception. Also it is uncertain what influence the known greater variability in intelligence among the relatives of schizophrenics might have had. We wish to report a strong *impression* (authors' italics) that within the Experimental group there was much more variability of personality and behavior but more evidence is required before this can be regarded as confirmed. (p. 371)

Karlsson (16), referring to his genetic study of schizophrenia in Iceland, also alludes to individuals who are "genetic carriers . . . with thought disorders" and who

> seem not infrequently to be persons of unusual ability, such as leaders in society or creative persons with performance records suggestive of a superior capacity for associative thinking (p. 61).

And elsewhere he asks:

> Could it be that some highly creative individuals are nonpenetrant schizophrenics and that society is thus dependent in terms of social and scientific progress on persons with a schizophrenic constitution? This suggestion is compatible with the observation that on certain psychologic tests the same type of response is seen with highly creative persons and schizophrenic patients . . . It is impressive that lists of the most creative contributors to the various fields of art and science are generally found to include individuals who developed psychotic disorders. This is true in the fields of philosophy, mathematics, physics, music, prose literature, poetry, sculpture, painting, etc. (p. 65).

Recently, McNeil (20), using the Adoption Registry for the Copenhagen metropolitan area in Denmark, reported preliminary evidence related to mental illness in adoptees working in creative (e.g. performing and graphic arts, literary) occupations as contrasted with noncreative ones (bookkeeper, bank clerk, factory foreman, etc.). Histories of mental disorder in the adoptees, their biological and adoptive parents and siblings were subsequently checked through the Danish national psychiatric register. Despite the small number of cases, creative ability level was found to be related to mental illness rates among the adoptees and their biological relatives but not to the rates for the adoptive relatives.

These citations are not offered as determinate evidence for a correlation between genius and madness or creativity and emotional disorder. That elusive relationship will demand a more stringent, empirical test. What is suggested, however, is that even in the presence of a markedly deleterious family environment—which some consider to be the most central psychosocial factor determining dysfunction (15)—the outcomes for children born into such families are not invariant. Of course, one can suggest in rebuttal that the presence of a psychotic mother does not *per se* guarantee a deleterious environment; but certainly even the most conservative of clinicians would be loath to point to such a maternal state as a source of strength for the child.

Poverty and the Etiology of Mental Disorder

Perhaps attention to another area of concern in matters of primary prevention may provide additional support for the point I seek to make. With regard to the different social structures that characterize communities and subcultures, Kaplan and Grunebaum (15) have written:

> If a person happens to be born into an advantaged group in a stable society, his social roles and their expected changes over a lifetime will tend to provide him with adequate opportunities for healthy personality development. If, on the other hand, he belongs to a disadvantaged minority, suffers from economic deprivation, . . . he may find his progress blocked and he may be deprived of opportunity and challenge. This may have an adverse effect on his mental health. (p. 333)

These authors are appropriately cautious in expressing this hypothesis. But other professionals have not adopted a comparable restraint in considering the role of slums and poverty as potential etiologic agents for mental disorder. The view that slums induce mental disorder is, as I have noted elsewhere (10), rooted in American social science. It is the product of a long-term concern for the social welfare of disadvantaged citizens as well as a derivative of a political ideology that sees environmental influences as the most powerful forces shaping behavior.

But the hypothesized powerful negative effect of slum life on personal adaptation remains an assumption and not a given. Slums, like other environments, seem to produce individuals who vary markedly in their ability to cope. It is demeaning to suggest that for those reared in our festering slums the prognosis for successful adaptation is inevitably bleak. Such a position ignores the history of an urbanized nation that has been built by a succession of ethnic groups each of which, in turn, has cast off disadvantaged economic status and pestilent neighborhoods without assuming the burdens of psychopathology.

A more sophisticated sociological view of the socially integrative power of a highly disadvantaged environment is found in Suttles' (36) fascinating volume, *The Social Order of the Slum*, in which he details three years of participant observation in one of Chicago's more malignant neighborhoods. Dunham's (5) summary of his epidemiological study of schizophrenia in two subcommunities of Detroit is also congruent with the shift away from viewing a disordered ecology *per se* as an etiologic agent in mental disorder. Dunham challenges and then rejects the prior interpretation of the classical investigation that he conducted in conjunction with Faris (8) of the differential rates of prevalence of mental disorder in Chicago and its environs. Earlier he had assigned conditions of social isolation, culture conflict, social deprivation and stress to the high prevalence rates of psychopathology found in the central city. Dunham now focuses on the "extreme competitiveness" of an open class society and "the personality characteristics of the pre-schizophrenic" that constrict his quest for education and employment.

We can further examine this issue of variation of outcomes in disadvantaged social settings by turning to the significant study by Robins (29) detailed in her superb volume, *Deviant Children Grown Up*. Robins sought to follow up, some 30 years later, a group of children who had been diagnosed and treated in a small child guidance clinic in St. Louis. For controls she selected children from the same lower social class milieu who met the following criteria: they had never been seen in a psychiatric clinic; they had never repeated a full year of elementary school; and they had not left school for reasons of expulsion or transfer to a correctional institution.

Although the slum environment in which the experimental and control children had been reared was extremely similar in terms of the degree of manifest physical deprivation, the controls, when examined in adulthood, were found to be "extraordinarily well adjusted." Some 60% had moved to the suburbs, possessed good jobs, had a high rate of home ownership, a relatively low divorce rate, and an absence of incarcerations, indigence or mental disorder. In Norman Podhoretz' words, they were "making it." Within the clinic group, too, outcomes were found to be variable; antisocial children more typically revealed maladaptive adult behavior, while the prognosis for neurotic problem cases proved to be relatively favorable.

Retrospection, Continuity, and Prediction

What, then, shall we say about primary prevention when the major variables of family and social structure produce such highly diverse outcomes? It would seem more appropriate if we did not presume to use the word "prevention." for it holds greater promise than our mental health disciplines can fulfill. It also suggests a historical basis for our assumption that we know the variables that produce disorder and can stay their action. What is the source of this complacent belief that the factors for programming primary prevention efforts are known to us?

I believe we in psychiatry have become ensnared by restrictions in our traditional method of gathering information. The focus of past efforts at understanding patients has been the case study. As with many medical specialities, the method has served its discipline well (24). For psychiatry, it has been the instrument for bringing order to a bewildering array of symptoms and psychopathologies; it has provided a basis for the taxonomy of psychiatric disorders, and has stimulated insights into developmental events that may help produce a vulnerability to mental illness (33). The case method has led to many studies of prognosis that provide evidence for a continuity of pathological development extending from premorbid adjustment through morbid symptom formation to postmorbid outcome. Furthermore, the case history has generated hypotheses for experimental studies of a psychological, biological and genetic cast.

Given these many virtues, it is difficult to be disparaging of the case history method. And yet we must, for it has served to disfigure our formulations of personality development. Studies of normal families (22, 27, 39) have revealed the unreliability of the case history, with its exclusive reliance on retrospective reconstruction of an earlier time period. These investigations conducted with normal mothers of primary school age (and younger) children provide evidence that not only do mothers suffer deficits in recalling events in the early years of their children's lives but that the deficiency is particularly acute in those very spheres of behavior, such as emotions and affectively-tinged attitudes (13), that are presumed to be potentially significant for the formation of maladjustment in children. The central issue, then, is this: *If normal* mothers engaged in the act of recall of *normal* events related to the growth and development of their own *normal* children are found to have defective memory for such events, then with what confidence can we view the reliability of recall provided by disordered mothers of disordered children? Yet this has not deterred us from creating a substantial edifice for a science of psychopathology (with its attendant view of prevention) using as the structure's foundation data gathered by just such unreliable retrospective procedures.

Why should such retrospective elaborations provide us with this unwarranted degree of comfort regarding the antecedents of behavior disorder? Looking backward, the behavioral scientist can always find support for his belief in the developmental continuities he believes to be evident in personality formation. The scientist is not alone in his belief system. I recently presented 185 competent undergraduates enrolled in an Abnormal Psychology course at a distinguished university with this hypothetical situation:

> Imagine [I told them] that I am capable of dropping a potion into your drink which will, in the brief passage of time, induce a marked psychosis (surely not an outlandish fantasy in these days). You, however, have neither memory nor awareness of this intervening event. Within a day your worried parents take you to a psychiatric center where you and they are interviewed at intake by a social worker followed in turn by a psychiatrist. You are asked to detail the background of your life. Consider this situation tonight and at the next class session let me know whether or not a rational reconstruction of your psychotic state could be inferred from your previous life experiences.

All but two students in this class of 185 indicated that they believed their "fantasy" psychoses would be justified by a recital of events in their lives, despite the evident competencies most of them possessed.

Looking backward from an end point of a developmental sequence, we can construct justification for an outcome marked by either competence or incompetence. Provide us with a slum child who is forging a pattern of strength and we will cast about for environmental surrogates who *must* have served as inoculators against despair, for events that *must* have encouraged hope rather than hopelessness, for inner resources that *must* have proclaimed vitality rather than helplessness. However, were we to convert this same slum child into someone prone to violence or aberration, our focus would be turned with equal efficiency and perhaps even greater facility to alternate figures and facets that would buttress our perception of deviance. Thus do we become victimized by our self-fulfilling clinical prophecies, ignoring the insightful observation of Freud, for whom the case history was the royal road into theory.

In his *Psychogenesis of a Case of Homosexuality in a Woman*, Freud (9) wrote:

> So long as we trace the development from its final outcome backwards, the chain of events appears continuous, and we feel we have gained an insight which is completely satisfactory or even exhaustive. But if we proceed the reverse way, if we start from the premises inferred from the analysis and try to follow these up to the final result, then we no longer get the impression of an inevitable sequence of events which could not have been otherwise determined. We notice at once that there might have been another result, and that we might have been just as well able to understand and explain the latter. The synthesis is thus not so satisfactory as the analysis; in other words, from a knowledge of the premises we could not have foretold the nature of the result.
>
> It is very easy to account for this disturbing state of affairs. Even supposing that we have a complete knowledge of the aetiological factors that decide a given result, nevertheless what we know about them is only their quality, and not their relative strength. Some of them are suppressed by others because they are too weak, and they therefore do not affect the final result. But we never know beforehand which of the determining factors will prove the weaker or the stronger. We can only say at the end that those which succeeded must have been the stronger. Hence the chain of causation can always be recognized with certainty if we follow the line of analysis, whereas to predict it along the line of synthesis is impossible. (pp. 167–168)

I believe too that we are biased in our interpretation of events by those ardently cathected theories that form the base for programs of primary prevention. Let me illustrate this point with reference to a serious contemporary social problem—the threat of bombings from militants of the radical left and the radical right. In an astute analysis of the problem, Thomas R. Brooks in *The New York Times* (Mar. 15, 1970) searched for the roots of the violence espoused by the Weathermen, the most radical fringe of SDS. Indicating that these persons typically tend to be the educated children of middle-class and often wealthy parents, Brooks inquired:

> What prompts them to live the life of terrorists? Are they sensitive idealists turned off by the wrongs of our society and by the greater violence of the Vietnam war?

He cites, on the one hand, the view of Dr. John Spiegel of the Lemberg Center for the Study of Violence at Brandeis University that the motives underlying the violent behavior can be comprehended within a normal context.

> The young people have had protests and riots and disorders—they've done everything one can do in the way of peaceful and unplanned protest, and not much has changed. To that degree there is an increasing sense of desperation, and a sense of vengefulness.

Yet, as Brooks points out, other militants have not chosen the path of violence. I have an able, young SDS iconoclast in one of my seminars who will bow to no man in his distaste for the Establishment, yet who terms the Weathermen "action freaks." He is prone to define their behavior in the context of pathology, as is Mr. Brooks when he writes:

> Nonetheless, it is difficult to escape the feeling that these youngsters are demented. How else explain the admiration for Sirhan Sirhan, the murderer of Senator Robert F. Kennedy, or for Charles Manson, group leader of a band of alleged murderers. Among these youngsters, there are open jokes about assassinations, and a salivating over violence. Witness Bernadine Dohrn: "Dig it, first they killed those pigs (actress Sharon Tate and her friends), then they ate dinner in the same room with them, then they even shoved a fork into a victim's stomach! Wild!"

This is, perhaps, a dramatic, overblown instance of how different our orientations can be when viewing behavior in terms of the presence or absence of manifest pathological content. If we perceive the Weathermen's behavior as the representation of altruism and humanitarian concern, we are quite unlikely to introduce such acts into our concepts of primary prevention. On the other hand, if we view the same behavior as bordering on madness, then the behavior, the instigator and his background will be factors of concern in action programs. The tale of the Weathermen merely demonstrates our lack of clarity regarding the nature of deviance and normality. But, lacking such clarity, is it not premature for the mental health disciplines to assert a readiness to set forth on programs of primary prevention?

The Place of Action Programs

Those concerned with the overwhelming problem of mental disorder nevertheless have every reason to ask: "All right, then, what do we do—wait until we can collect a core of hard data and in the meantime mount no programs at all? Do we turn away from efforts to prevent the onset of disorder and direct our energies solely to the treatment of deviance when it appears?"

I would suggest two replies to these questions; one is pragmatic, the other strategic. No, we cannot sit still and by so doing add to the nation's festering crisis. We will initiate programs as best we can, hoping that through a juncture of heart and mind we can set up efforts at intervention that will restrict disorder, or at worst will do little to enhance its expression. The view seems an appropriate one since much intervention presumably will center on those programs (37) that good government and a responsible society should maintain anyway: adequate prenatal, postnatal and infant care and nutrition; prevention of birth defect; economic security for citizens to insure family stability; extended support for education, including development of preschool and school programs devoted to the enhancement of social and cognitive competence; a more adequately financed and more sophisticated network of social agencies dedicated to meeting the emotional and economic needs of citizens; a plan for the eradication of slums; the pledge of freedom from contaminants and pollutants, etc. Securing these goals is a worthy direction for any society to take. I would urge, however, that we not oversell our power to reduce the numbers of mentally ill and that we do not proclaim to the nation that we stand on the threshold of a preventive breakthrough in psychiatry. Such a promise, emulating the unfulfilled pledge of the mental health community clinic movement that it can provide the base for secondary and tertiary prevention, could bring us well-deserved condemnation from those who take our pledges and promises seriously. There is only one way to strengthen such a pledge, and that is to develop our knowledge of the phenomenon of deviance and its roots. And yet the entire governmental health apparatus is now being turned rapidly toward the delivery of health care services, while neglecting programs of research that in time might provide wiser methods for intervening in the cycle of pathology than those suggested by traditionalists.

A Strategy for Research

This brings me to my central concern, namely the strategies for research in psychopathology that may ultimately provide us with a more adequate return. Roberts (28) has expressed the problem in this manner:

> The development of programmes for primary prevention will require a clear recognition of the inadequacies as well as the possibilities of our present knowledge. Developments in this area must not be deferred because of the inadequacy of present knowledge, rather efforts must be made to prevent disorders and promote mental health. To the maximum extent possible, these efforts should be accompanied by research programmes which will, at this stage, be as much concerned with the development of methodology for such research as they will be with the monitoring of efforts in the field. (p. 37)

One direction in research now being undertaken by investigators here and abroad centers on studies of *high-risk groups* in what can be called generically *vulnerability research.* Vulnerability research involves the selection of those children in a community who are at high risk for the later onset (typically in late adolescence and adulthood) of severe psychopathology. Selection criteria may be based on genetic loading within the family (as revealed by the psychiatric status of parents or relatives), evidence of excessive family disorganization or the undesirable effects generated by a disordered environment. In essence, the status of a child as "vulnerable" or at "high-risk" (as in the case of a genetic predisposition) typically is derived from the three basic models that characterize our speculations about the etiology of mental disorder: 1) genetic transmission of the predisposition or the diathesis, 2) pathological disorganization within the near environment (the family) or 3) within the molar (sociocultural) environment of the child. We can also identify a fourth model that is coming to prominence, although its applicability to adult psychopathology is not yet clear—one stressing deprivation within the prenatal and neonatal period in which faulty maternal care and inadequate nutrition can serve to render the infant vulnerable to subsequent stressors (25, 35).

Once these children are selected, the study of their adaptation or maladaptation, compared with appropriate control groups, becomes the focus of investigation. To evaluate such adaptation, programs of research have used a long-term longitudinal focus (23), a relatively short-term prospective format (2), or a cross-sectional design (10, 12, 30).

The Study of Vulnerability

Investigators of vulnerability in childhood have been concerned with a number of critical issues: the defining of vulnerable groups and attendant controls; the selection of variables to be studied; and the implications for intervention prior to the onset of disordered behavior in risk cases.

Defining High-Risk Groups and Controls

As I have indicated, the determination of what constitutes a high-risk group is a function of one's etiological model. Thus, in the study of schizophrenia, the dominant models have included emphasis on genogenic, psychogenic and sociogenic factors. Of these three major orientations, selection on the basis of genetic disposition has clearly assumed the ascendant position in vulnerability research. To Mednick and Schulsinger (23) must go the credit for initiating the study of high-risk children in a manner that stresses genetic loading: their method utilizes a schizophrenic-mother group as the cohort while their biological children serve as the probands. The expectation that, by this method of selection, the frequency of anticipated schizophrenic outcomes in such children would approximate 14% clearly indicates its base in psychiatric genetics. Since then other projects have followed similar selection procedures, including those of Anthony (2), Beisser (3), Rolf (30), and Garmezy (10). More recently Dr. Erlenmeyer-Kimling (7) has suggested that true high-risk would be more likely to be observed in offspring of marriages in which both parents are schizophrenic, since the prediction of ultimate schizophrenia for such a sample of children would range approximately between 40%–50% (31). Initial efforts by Erlenmeyer-Kimling to locate such children in New York State have convinced her of the viability of selecting for risk in this fashion, despite the manifold methodological difficulties that are involved.

The psychogenic orientation to schizophrenia finds its expression in the study of disordered families and disturbed modes of family interaction. To approach the study of vulnerability in this manner requires the identification of such families either through the medium of survey research, the selection of parents who are themselves being seen for treatment or diagnosis, or by centering on already disturbed children who are known to some clinical resource. The latter method makes two assumptions: that such severely disturbed children typically reflect a disordered or disorganized family; that such children, in time, also contribute heavily to the pool of adult behavior pathology.

An example of subject selection based on a criterion of disturbed children within disordered families can be seen in the research program currently being conducted at UCLA by Rodnick, Goldstein and Judd (12). This group is studying, through departmental clinic intake, groups of children whose differing behavioral modes (withdrawn, social isolation, acting out, passive aggression) may have certain components in common with the coping patterns of the schizophrenic patient. It is the expectation of these investigators that specific family patterns may relate to the form of symptom expression in the offspring, and, in time, may be shown to bear a patterning similar to that observed in families with a schizophrenic offspring. As a strategy for obtaining a high-risk sample, their method appears to have some solid virtues, for the subjects in the UCLA project have already slipped into schizophrenia at a rate not appreciably different from the rates observed by Mednick and Schulsinger in their Denmark project, in which selection is based on mothers' schizophrenia status. Wynne (40) and Singer (34), having in common an orientation to disorder espoused by the UCLA investigators, have recently suggested that a program of risk research be initiated with groups selected on the basis of deviant modes of parental communication, on the assumption that the preschizophrenic will more often be found among offspring within such family constellations. Thus one can start from a base of disordered families or disordered offspring with the common thread to be found in the importance assigned to faulty parent-child and parent-parent relationships. The search for disturbance is given a locus in the investigation of communication networks, role structure and transactional patterns within the family—an orientation far more sophisticated than that of the earlier studies that examined child-rearing patterns against such simplistic attributes as parental "dominance," "over-protection," "rejection," etc.

A third source of vulnerability to schizophrenia is to be found in studies of the sociology of mental disorder and the inverse relationship that has been consistently found to exist between prevalence rates for schizophrenia and social status (19). Whether one believes that such a correlation reflects the role of diathesis or stressor, the evidence of studies cast in a sociological context remains a challenge for high-risk researchers and a guide to the importance of social class variables in the design of their studies.

Controls

An examination of risk studies now underway reveals considerable diversity in the choice of controls. Many factors contribute to the heterogeneity that is evident in subject selection: theoretical views regarding etiology, availability of various subject pools, beliefs about demographic variables that may contribute to later psychopathology, etc.

Most ongoing risk programs employ normal control subjects; the UCLA project does not, however, since it perceives controls to be present in the several constituent adolescent experimental groups that differ largely in the mode of sympton expression. Several projects have used other psychopathological groups as controls, although the reasons for the choice of the specific forms of disorder selected are not always evident.

In the first study of our own Minnesota high-risk project, Dr. Jon Rolf (30), now at the University of Vermont, measured the social and academic competence of a variety of high-risk, vulnerable and control groups. Rolf's cohorts included not only children born to schizophrenic mothers but those born to neurotic depressive mothers as well. Use of a third group of acting-out character disordered mothers was contemplated and then postponed when the logistical demands of Rolf's design became apparent.

The rationale behind the selection of these groups was not happenstance. Data drawn from a number of recent genetic studies of schizophrenia (14, 17) have suggested that there exists a *spectrum of schizophrenia* in which pathologic outcomes appear to cohere around schizophrenia, sociopathic personality and impulse disorders; tending to fall outside the spectrum are the depressions and anxiety neurosis. These data are congruent with symptom linkages suggested by Zigler and Phillips (41) and by Phillips (26). On these grounds the selection of groups of mothers whose disorders may be schizophrenia-linked together with representation of other non-linked psychopathologies (e.g. depression) would appear to be warranted in high-risk research. Such a method of selection would provide for manifest disturbance in mothers who varied in the adequacy of their premorbid and postmorbid adaptation.

Since the basis for selecting these cohorts does bear a strong genetic emphasis, efforts must also be made to tap groups that would reflect psychogenic speculations about schizophrenic outcomes. Here Rolf chose to focus on two types of disordered children who had already come to psychiatric attention. One group, termed *externalizers* (1, 38), had been referred to clinics for destructive, acting-out behavior in the community; the second group comprised an internalizer set of children whose symptomatology included fearfulness, excessive inhibition, phobic and avoidance behaviors. Since there is strong evidence that antisocial behavior frequently eventuates in malignant outcomes including sociopathy and schizophrenia (18, 29), whereas neurotic behaviors of children do not, the stage was set for the inclusion of these two groups in Rolf's study. This decision was given more meaning as a possible road into psychogenic hypothesizing by the empirical evidence of characteristically marked disorganization in the families of externalizing children—a situation that does not obtain to the same degree with children prone to internalizing symptomatology (1, 38).

An indirect test of the sociogenic hypothesis (although not a very adequate one) was attempted by Rolf, who chose a matched (for age, academic and intellectual ability, intactness of the family and occupation of the breadwinning parent) and a random control child within the same classroom in which each target child was finally located. Thus, for each child in the four vulnerable groups (schizophrenic and depressive mothers; externalizing and internalizing children), there were two controls who shared a comparable neighborhood setting with the child who was at high risk. Since many of these triads came from the more depressed and often less stable areas of the city, while others were drawn from stable, middle-class neighborhoods, it is possible to relate degrees of effectance in these children to area of residence.

Of course, a more adequate test of a sociogenic hypothesis will have to involve, among other things, an extended knowledge of community disorganization including incidence and prevalence rates for mental disorder, incarcerations, indigence, quality of adaptation of families selected randomly from high as well as low prevalence areas, a more extended study of the adjustment of children born within such families, etc. Nevertheless, Rolf's design suggests the complexity of a model necessary for testing the multiple hypotheses that have been posited regarding the etiology of schizophrenia. Certainly, it seems likely at this point that the decision as to what kinds of groups to evaluate in vulnerability research will prove to be far more complex than is evident in most projects now underway.

The Choice of Variables

What aspects of behavior may be most fruitfully studied in the high-risk child? Typically what one observes in reviewing risk research is that the researcher's decision may be based on a variety of considerations. Choices may be theoretically-based, as in the case of Mednick and Schulsinger's (23) Denmark project. Several of the most central dependent variables of this program involve measures of autonomic responsivity, latency of arousal and decay of the autonomic response, generalization and habituation. The source for such measures is to be found in Mednick's theory of the etiology of schizophrenia, in which he has placed great emphasis on these factors: 1) a biological predisposition for rapid arousal; 2) an attendant pattern of excessive generalization induced by the heightened anxiety state; 3) the reinforcement of deviant thought as an escape from anxiety arousal. But one need not be bound by the constraints of theory. The significance of variables to be studied may arise serendipitously, as can be perceived in Mednick's (21) current preoccupation with prenatal and perinatal complications. Such complications appear to be present in the pregnancy and birth histories of those high-risk adolescents who are now beginning to show signs of significant mental aberration but are absent in comparison with high-risk healthy and normal control subjects.

Unfortunately, theoretical models for the origins of schizophrenia tend not to be circumscribed constructions. Thus, the choice of variables is a complex task for those who bear allegiance to the rather vague doctrine of diathesis-stress theory, since one can not specify either the nature of the predisposition or the stress. As subscribers to such a view, David Rosenthal (32) and his colleagues have faced this difficulty in trying to determine what factors to study in Danish adoptees who have been born to schizophrenic parents but reared in adoptive homes. Their selection of tasks to use in a two-day study of these adoptees, in which time considerations precluded their doing many things they had wished to do, was made on three bases: 1) tasks and procedures that had been shown consistently to distinguish schizophrenics from others; 2) assessment procedures to provide measures of more fundamental trait dispositions; and 3) the choice of other methods that had proved to be successful discriminators for other investigators.

My own view is this: I believe it best that we turn away from a premature fixation on global theorizing about the etiology of schizophrenia and engage in the search for relevant behavioral parameters that can differentiate high-risk-maladaptive from high-risk-adaptive children as well as risk from non-risk subjects. Until we have such a strong empirical predictive base, a long-term longitudinal project seems inadvisable. The ideal design compromise could well entail replicated cross-sectional studies employing Bell's (4) convergence technique with short-term follow-up of different groups of children ranging in age from infancy to late adolescence. Unfortunately, the pattern of subject attrition we have observed within our own project may render such an idealized design difficult to achieve. Furthermore, the competencies of individual investigators will preclude attention to all age segments of the developmental sequence.

As for specific areas of investigation, perhaps some of the parameters we now deem most significant for programs of primary intervention could be tested within high-risk and vulnerability programs: studies of pregnancy and birth difficulties, investigations of stress and frustration tolerance, interaction studies of disordered parents and children, exploration of patterns of attachment and of socialization and dyssocialization, laboratory studies of social competence, peer acceptance, and of cognitive, motivational and perceptual adequacy. More specific studies of processes we know to be deficient in the disordered adult psychotic patient would also be warranted, such as measuring of attention and set, particular forms of cognitive styles (e.g. scanning), associative thought processes, psychophysiological responsivity in relation to arousal and feedback mechanisms, etc.

Goldstein (11) has suggested that a focus on *behavioral continuities* (as exemplified by stimulus processing, deviant thinking, social isolation and withdrawal) be joined with investigations of *developmental continuities* initiated by those socio-environmental conditions that may shape pathology (family structure, family communication, child rearing practices, etc.). Certainly at this point diversity appears to characterize the focus of high-risk projects, but Erlenmeyer-Kimling's (7) suggestion that an effort be made to standardize some measures across studies of comparable high-risk *S*s seems worth implementing.

The Issue of Intervention

Finally, what can be said about the issue of intervention? A conservative viewpoint would hold that intervention, in the absence of knowledge about the process of pathological development, would be premature. And yet the ethical demands placed upon those who study high-risk children can be a powerful force that compels one to look, perhaps with hesitancy, upon the necessity of intervening irrespective of one's confidence in the tools that are available for efforts at prevention and containment. The needs may well be pressing. E. James Anthony (2), who has underway a major program of risk research at Washington University in St. Louis, testing the biological children of schizophrenic mothers or fathers, has found such striking instances of early pathology that he has established a special clinic in which these children can be treated.

We shall undoubtedly be called upon to intervene, but hopefully we can do so in a manner that will free us from the formalisms of contemporary therapeutics. By so doing, we may be able to learn more about these vulnerable children in a therapeutic framework that provides a rich source for observations about their adaptation.

In an earlier article (10), I noted that:

> At the turn of the century, Binet moved into the Paris school system to identify and to cope with those children who appeared unable to profit from instruction. Today there are a larger number of children in our schools whose emotional burdens prevent them from profiting from the one major institution of society that can liberate them from incompetence. Identifying and intervening in such situations requires the collaboration of researchers and practitioners in schools, communities, and clinics. Cognitive compensatory educational efforts for the disadvantaged low-risk child deserve to be matched with compensatory stress training efforts with the disadvantaged high-risk child. (p. 234)

Perhaps in setting forth such compensatory programs we can adopt paradigms and models that in other contexts have been used to induce behavior change: the model of immunization against efforts at attitude change or models designed to foster such changes; the model of learned helplessness suggested by Seligman, Maier, Mowrer, Masserman and others; and the model of behavior change through the use of operant techniques. The questions for study are these: Can we adapt such methods for use with our high-risk children? Can we use our schools and clinics as centers for training these children in more adaptive techniques for coping? Can we use participation in successful play to increase the flexibility of the response repertoires of these children? Can we stimulate adaptive behavior by introducing into such training centers healthy children who can serve as models for the vulnerable child?

Perhaps the mediators of such change should be drawn not from the ranks of middle-class therapists and teachers but rather from mothers who, by attitude, value, and act, have proved capable of producing healthy children. Perhaps, too, we can select mothers drawn from inner-city families who have ably defended their children from the disorganizing consequences of high-risk environments. Such mothers, in many instances, may well be the major factor in the predisposition of their children toward health. Perhaps they can also be agents for helping other less fortunate children.

Invulnerability

In the study of high-risk and vulnerable children, we have come across another group of children whose prognosis could be viewed as unfavorable on the basis of familial or ecological factors but who upset our prediction tables and in childhood bear the visible indices that are hallmarks of competence: good peer relations, academic achievement, commitment to education and to purposive life goals, early and successful work histories. We have seen such children in our inner-city schools. Mary Engel (6) has described them in her study, "Children Who Work." To these children I have assigned the term "invulnerables." School principals not only believe they can identify such children but they resonate to the hopefulness suggested by the concept of an "invulnerable" child. They can produce instances from within their own school settings of children whose intellectual and social skills are not destroyed by the misfortunes they encounter in home and street.

Thus vulnerability research is also concerned with the children of the inner-city, their predisposition to competence (or, in less fortunate circumstances, incompetence) and the various factors within the disadvantaged group that lead some toward disorder while others are seemingly immunized against disorganization. These are the "vulnerables" and the "invulnerables" of a society. "Vulnerables" have long been the province of our mental health disciplines; but prolonged neglect of the "invulnerable" child—the healthy child in an unhealthy setting—has provided us with a false sense of security in erecting prevention models that are founded more on values than on facts.

With our nation torn by strife between races and between social classes, these "invulnerable" children remain the "keepers of the dream." Were we to study the forces that move such children to survival and to adaptation, the long-range benefits to our society might be far more significant than our many efforts to construct models of primary prevention designed to curtail the incidence of vulnerability.

References

1. ACHENBACH, T. M. (1966). The classification of children's psychiatric symptoms: a factor analytic study. *Psychol. Monogr.*, **80**, 37 pp.
2. ANTHONY, E. J. (1968). The developmental precursors of adult schizophrenia. In *The Transmission of Schizophrenia*, D. Rosenthal and S. S. Kety (eds.). Pergamon Press, Oxford.
3. BEISSER, A. R., GLASSER, N., & GRANT, MARSHA (1967). Psychosocial adjustment in children of schizophrenic mothers. *J. Nerv. Ment. Dis.*, **145**, 429–440.
4. BELL, R. Q. (1953). Convergence: an accelerated longitudinal approach. *Child Development*, **24**, 145–152.
5. DUNHAM, H. W. (1965). *Community and Schizophrenia.* Wayne State U. Press, Detroit.
6. ENGEL, MARY (1967). Children who work. *Arch. Gen. Psychiat.*, **17**, 291–297.
7. ERLENMEYER-KIMLING, L. (1968). Studies of the children of schizophrenic parents: pointers for the analysis of gene-environment interaction. Paper presented at the 124th annual meeting of the American Psychiatric Association, Boston.
8. FARIS, R. & DUNHAM, H. W. (1939). *Mental Disorders in Urban Areas.* University of Chicago Press, Chicago.
9. FREUD, S. (1955). The psychogenesis of a case of homosexuality in a woman. In *The Standard Edition of the Complete Psychological Works of Sigmund Freud.* **18**, 146–172. The Hogarth Press and The Institute of Psycho-Analysis, London.
10. GARMEZY, N. (1970). Vulnerable children: implications derived from studies of an internalizing-externalizing symptom dimension. In *Psychopathology of Adolescence*, J. Zubin and A. M. Freedman (eds.). Grune & Stratton, New York.
11. GOLDSTEIN, M. (1969). Studies of high risk children: What to measure? Position Statement. Workshop on Methodological Issues on Research With Groups at High Risk for the Development of Schizophrenia. Center for Studies of Schizophrenia, National Institute of Mental Health, Bethesda, Md.
12. GOLDSTEIN, M. J., et al. (1968). A method for studying social influence and coping patterns within families of disturbed adolescents. *J. Nerv. Ment. Dis.*, **147**, 233–251.
13. HAGGARD, E. A., BREKSTAD, A., & SKÅRD, A. (1960). On the reliability of the anamnestic interview. *J. Abnorm. Soc. Psychol.*, **61**, 311–318.
14. HESTON, L. & DENNY, D. (1968). Interactions between early life experience and biological factors in schizophrenia. In *The Transmission of Schizophrenia*, D. Rosenthal and S. S. Kety (eds.). Pergamon Press, Oxford.
15. KAPLAN, G. & GRUNEBAUM, H. (1967). Perspectives on primary prevention. *Arch. Gen. Psychiat.*, **17**, 331–346.
16. KARLSSON, JON L. (1966). *The Biologic Basis for Schizophrenia.* Charles C. Thomas, Springfield, Ill.
17. KETY, S. S., et al. (1968). The types and prevalence of mental illness in the biological and adoptive families of adopted schizophrenics. In *The Transmission of Schizophrenia*, D. Rosenthal and S. S. Kety (eds.). Pergamon Press, Oxford.
18. KOHLBERG, L., LACROSSE, JEAN, & RICKS, D. (In Press). The predictability of adult mental health from childhood behavior. In *Handbook of Childhood Psychopathology*, B. B. Wolman (ed.). McGraw-Hill, New York.
19. KOHN, M. L. (1968). Social class and schizophrenia: a critical review. In *The Transmission of Schizophrenia*, D. Rosenthal and S. S. Kety (eds.). Pergamon Press, Oxford.
20. MCNEIL, T. F. (1969). The relationship between creative ability and recorded mental illness. Paper presented at Southeastern Psychological Association.
21. MEDNICK, S. A. (1970). Breakdown in individuals at high risk for schizophrenia: possible predispositional perinatal factors. *Ment. Hyg.*, **54**, 50–63.
22. MEDNICK, S. A. & SHAFFER, J. (1964). Mothers' retrospective reports in child rearing research. *Amer. J. Orthopsychiat.*, **33**, 457–461.
23. MEDNICK, S. A. & SCHULSINGER, F. (1968). Some premorbid characteristics related to breakdown in children with schizophrenic mothers. In *The Transmission of Schizophrenia*, D. Rosenthal and S. S. Kety (eds.). Pergamon Press, Oxford.

24. Novey, S. (1968). *The Second Look*. The Johns Hopkins Press, Baltimore.

25. Pasamanick, B. & Knobloch, H. (1961). Epidemiologic studies on the complications of pregnancy and the birth process. In *Prevention of Mental Disorders in Children*, G. Kaplan (ed.). Basic Books, New York.

26. Phillips, L. (1968). *Human Adaptation and Its Failures*. Academic Press, New York.

27. Robbins, L. C. (1963). The accuracy of parental recall of aspects of child development and of child rearing practices. *J. Abnorm. Soc. Psychol.*, **66**, 261–270.

28. Roberts, C. A. (1968). *Primary Prevention of Psychiatric Disorders*. F. C. R. Chalke and J. J. Day (eds.). U. of Toronto Press, Toronto.

29. Robins, Lee N. (1966). *Deviant Children Grown Up*. Williams and Wilkins, Baltimore.

30. Rolf, J. E. (1969). The academic and social competence of school children vulnerable to behavior pathology. Unpublished Ph.D. Dissertation. University of Minnesota, Minneapolis.

31. Rosenthal, D. (In Press). *The Genetics of Psychopathology*. McGraw-Hill, New York.

32. Rosenthal, D., et al. (1968). Schizophrenics' offspring reared in adoptive homes. In *The Transmission of Schizophrenia*, D. Rosenthal and S. S. Kety (eds.). Pergamon Press, Oxford.

33. Rosenthal, D. (1963). *The Genain Quadruplets*. Basic Books, New York.

34. Singer, Margaret T. (1969). Measuring verbal behavior in groups at high risk for schizophrenia: reasoning, roles and scoring rationale. Workshop Position Statement: Workshop on Methodological Issues on Research with Groups at High Risk for the Development of Schizophrenia. Center for Studies of Schizophrenia. National Institute of Mental Health, Bethesda, Md.

35. Stabenau, J. R. & Pollin, W. (1967). Early characteristics of monozygotic twins discordant for schizophrenia. *Arch. Gen. Psychiat.*, **17**, 723–734.

36. Suttles, G. D. (1968). *The Social Order of the Slum*. University of Chicago Press, Chicago.

37. Visotsky, H. M. (1967). Primary prevention. In *Comprehensive Textbook of Psychiatry*, A. M. Freedman and H. I. Kaplan (eds.). Williams and Wilkins, Baltimore.

38. Weintraub, S. A. (1968). Cognitive and behavioral impulsivity in internalizing, externalizing and normal children. Unpublished Ph.D. Dissertation. U. of Minnesota, Minneapolis.

39. Wenar, C. (1961). The reliability of mothers' histories. *Child Development*, **32**, 491–500.

40. Wynne, L. C. (1969). Strategies for sampling groups at high risk for the development of schizophrenia. Workshop Position Statement. Workshop on Methodological Issues on Research with Groups at High Risk for the Development of Schizophrenia. Center for Studies of Schizophrenia. National Institute of Mental Health, Bethesda, Md.

41. Zigler, E. & Phillips, L. (1960). Social effectiveness and symptomatic behaviors. *J. Abnorm. Soc. Psychol.*, **2**, 231–238.

A. T. BECK

Psychological and Psychodynamic Studies (On Depression)

Although depression affects a much larger percentage of the general population than does schizophrenia, it has not received nearly as much attention from researchers and theoreticians. One of the best books in recent years to survey the clinical and research literature on this significant disorder was written by Dr. A. T. Beck. The following selection, a chapter from his book, surveys the psychological and psychodynamic studies done to understand the etiology of depression and is an excellent summary of that work.

Psychomotor Performance

Most clinical descriptions of depression have emphasized psychomotor retardation and have assumed that the patients' complaints of being slowed down in their thinking are an indication of inhibition of thought processes. Objective evidence to substantiate the proposition of an inhibition of psychomotor functions, however, has been lacking.

Rapaport (1945), comparing a depressed group with a schizophrenic group, reported a significant lowering of digit-symbol scores within the depressed group. He concluded that performance on this test is sensitive to the retardation assumed to be associated with depression. A further analysis of Rapaport's data, however, indicated that his depressed group was significantly older than his schizophrenic group and that the difference in age might account for the inferior performances by the depressed patients. To clarify the relationship between depression and performance on tests such as the Digit-Symbol test, we conducted a study with statistical controls for age and intelligence (Beck, Feshbach, and Legg, 1962). The Digit-Symbol test and the vocabulary test were administered to a sample of 178 psychiatric patients. The results indicated that the digit-symbol scores decreased in a stepwise fashion with increasing age, and increased in the same fashion with increasing vocabulary scores. When the variables of age and intelligence were controlled, it was found that there was no relationship between digit-

---

Chapter 10 reprinted from A. T. Beck, *Depression*. Philadelphia: University of Pennsylvania Press, 1972, pp. 154–165, with the permission of the University of Pennsylvania Press, Dr. Beck, and Granada Publishing Limited.

symbol scores and depression. The depressed patients performed as well as did the nondepressed patients.

Granick (1963) performed a comparative analysis of the performances on the Wechsler Adult Intelligence Scale Information and Similarities tests and on the Thorndike-Gallup Vocabulary test of 50 psychotic depressives and 50 normals matched for age, sex, race, education, religion, and nativity. The investigator failed to find any significant difference in performance between the psychotically depressed group and the normal group.

Friedman (1964) administered 33 cognitive, perceptual, and psychomotor tests to 55 depressives and 65 normals matched for age, sex education, vocabulary score, and nativity. In all, 82 test scores were derived from the various tests administered. The depressives ranked lower than did the normal group in only 4 per cent of the test scores, a finding that could be due to chance. The author concluded that actual ability and performance during severe depression is not consistent with the depressed patient's unrealistically low image of himself.

In one of our studies (Loeb et al., 1966), 20 depressed and 20 matched nondepressed male patients were given two card sorting tasks. Although the depressed patients tended to underestimate their performance, their actual performance was as good as that of the nondepressed patients.

Another study that indicates that depressed patients do not have significant impairment of psychomotor ability was conducted by Shapiro et al. (1958). They found that depressed patients following recovery (produced by ECT) did not show any significant change in their performance on a battery of psychomotor tests when compared to a control group.

Tucker and Spielberg (1958) compared the Bender-Gestalt scores of 17 depressed outpatients with those of 19 nondepressed psychiatric outpatients. In general, the various Bender-Gestalt scores did not discriminate between the two groups. Of 20 items, only two, tremor and design distortion, were significant at the 5 per cent level in discriminating between the depressed and the nondepressed group. No test items were significantly different at the 1 per cent level. The finding of only two discriminating items out of 20 could be due to chance. Comparisons were also made of average initial reaction and average response time to each test card. Contrary to expectations, the depressed patients showed a *faster* mean reaction time than the nondepressed group. This finding was short of statistical significance.

In summary, although the depressed patients tend to complain of cognitive inefficiencies, they perform as well in test situations as do nondepressed patients.

Conceptual Performance

Payne and Hirst (1957) investigated conceptual thinking in depressed patients. In a previous study, Payne had found that schizophrenic patients showed a tendency toward "overinclusion" when administered the Epstein Overinclusion test; this finding was consonant with Norman Cameron's formulation that the schizophrenic is unable to preserve his conceptual boundaries so that irrelevant ideas become incorporated into his concepts, making his thinking more abstract and less lucid.

The authors administered the Epstein Overinclusion test to 11 depressed patients and 14 normal controls matched for age, sex, and vocabulary level. Their findings indicated that depressives show a significantly greater tendency towards overinclusion than the normals. They found, in fact, that depressed patients seem to be more extreme with respect to overinclusion of thinking than are schizophrenics. This is inconsistent with Cameron's theory, since he regarded this type of thought disorder as specific to schizophrenics. The authors suggest that the overinclusion tendency may be related to psychosis generally, rather than to any specific psychosis such as schizophrenia or depression.

Perceptual Threshold

Hemphill, Hall, and Crookes (1952) attempted to measure the pain and fatigue tolerance of depressed patients as compared with other psychiatric patients. The depressed patients showed a significantly higher threshold for both pain and fatigue than the other groups. It should be noted, however, that the mean age of the depressed patients was substantially higher than that of the other groups, which could account for the differences in thresholds for perception of fatigue and pain. It is also worth noting that the depressed patients were more persevering in a fatiguing task than were the nondepressed patients. Wadsworth, Wells, and Scott (1962) found no difference in fatigability or work performance between a group of depressives and a group of schizophrenics.

In an attempt to relate perceptual regulation to mental disorders, Dixon and Lear (1962) measured the visual threshold for one eye while presenting neutral and emotive material below the awareness threshold to the other eye. The five depressive patients showed a consistent raising of threshold ("perceptual defense") as compared to the six schizophrenics who showed a lowering of threshold ("perceptual vigilance"). Caution is necessary in interpreting these results because of the small samples and because all the patients were on drug therapy.

Distortion of Time Judgment

Many writers have described a distortion of the time sense in affective disorders. The existential writers in particular have commented on the relevance of time distortion to the existential experience of the patient (Chapter 16). Although it seems fairly well established from the clinical description that depressed patients feel that time is passing more slowly than normal, there is no objective evidence that actual judgment of time is impaired.

Mezey and Cohen (1961) investigated the subjective experience of time and the judgment of time of 21 depressed patients. The study included introspective statements about time experience as well as objective tests involving projection-reprojection and verbal estimation of time intervals ranging from one second to 30 minutes. The authors found that about three-fourths of the patients felt that time was passing more slowly than normal; this feeling tended to disappear on recovery. The objective tests, on the other hand, indicated that the verbal estimation of time under experimental conditions was as accurate during the depressed phase as during the recovery phase.

Distortion of Spatial Judgment

A number of articles have suggested that psychiatric patients experience some changes in spatial perception. Neurotics and schizophrenic patients have been reported to have distortions in the perceived distance between themselves and others. Other phenomena reported to occur in psychiatric patients have been the assignment of different qualities to the right and left aspects of space, and fading of the third-dimensional aspect of objects (Fisher, 1964). There is also some experimental evidence that the individual's mood state influences his spatial perception. Distortion in locating the nearness or distance of objects has been reported to be related to personal insecurity.

Depression has been shown to be related to up-down perception in several studies. Rosenblatt (1956) found that in contrast to manic patients, depressed patients have a tendency to focus on the downward rather than the upward aspect of a spatial situation. Wapner, Werner, and Krus (1957), in a parallel study of college students, related the experience of academic failure to a consequent downward effect on the subjective judgment of eye level ("apparent horizon"). Fisher (1964) tested the specific hypothesis that the degree of downward bias of perception is positively related to the level of sadness or depression. Fifty-two subjects were evaluated. The measure of sad affect was made in terms of the number of sad terms used in describing a series of faces. Upward vs. downward directionality of perception was estimated by means of the autokinetic phenomenon and by judgments requiring the adjustment of a luminous rod to the horizontal. The results supported the proposition that subjects with a sad affect showed a downward bias in perception, whereas subjects with a neutral affect showed an upward bias.

Factor Analytic Studies

Hamilton (1960a) administered a 17-item rating scale to 49 depressed male patients. The product-moment correlations were computed for the 17 variables and the correlation matrix was factored and then transformed to orthogonal simple structure. Four factors were extracted. The first factor was defined by suicidal thoughts, loss of libido, retardation, depressed mood, and loss of insight. The second factor consisted of gastrointestinal complaints, sleep difficulty, loss of interest, body preoccupation, and loss of weight. The third factor consisted of anxiety items. The fourth factor was equivocal.

Grinker et al. (1961) conducted an extensive study to determine the prominent trait-dimensions of depression. In a pilot study, a group of 21 patients diagnosed as depressed by experienced psychiatrists were studied intensively to define the major trait factors. The raw data from the study were translated into a list of "Feelings and Concerns" and a list of "Current Behaviors." The Feelings and Concerns list dealt with the verbalized experiences of the patient such as envy of others, sense of failure, and fear of death or dying. The Current Behavior list dealt with the visible actions of the patient or with traits that require only a low level of inference on the part of the rater. The reliability of the Feelings and Concerns list was high. Factor analysis of the data uncovered three factors. The reliability of ratings on the Current Behavior list was too low to justify factor analysis.

In the large scale study, 96 patients diagnosed as depressive by various psychiatrists were investigated. Ten nondepressed patients were used as a control group. Analysis of the data from this study revealed five factors in the Feelings and Concerns list. The factors made sense psychologically and were described as follows: (*1*) depression; (*2*) projective defense; (*3*) restitution; (*4*) free anxiety; and (*5*) attempt to manipulate the environment.

An analysis of the Current Behavior list revealed ten factors. These were characterized roughly as follows: (*1*) isolation, withdrawal, and apathy; (*2*) retardation of thought processes and speech; (*3*) general retardation in behavior and gait; (*4*) angry, provocative behavior; (*5*) somatic complaints; (*6*) organic syndrome; (*7*) agitation, tremulousness, and restlessness; (*8*) rigidity; (*9*) somatic symptoms such as dry skin and hair; and (*10*) ingratiating behavior.

Certain traits that were expected to be important in depression did not appear in any of the factors. These included loss of interest in oral satisfaction, suicidal ideas, fatigue, wishes to cry, loss of esteem by others, relief after hospitalization, and ambivalence towards important personal issues. In the pilot study, an investigation of precipitating factors suggested that there was rarely a single clear-cut precipitating event or experience. Almost invariably, a series of events led up to the clinical illness.

The factors derived from the Feelings and Concerns list did not correlate with the factors for current behavior. The subjective symptom *anxiety*, for instance, did not correlate with the behavioral factor *agitation*. This finding suggests a lack of correspondence between the self-reports of the patients and the clinicians' inferences based on their overt behavior.

This study by Grinker and his associates is an important pioneering effort to demarcate the important dimensions of depression. The absence of an adequate control group, however, raises questions to whether the factors are characteristic of depression, or whether they are applicable to psychiatric patients generally.

A number of studies of psychotics by Overall and his group (1961, 1962, 1964) have attempted to isolate the basic dimensions of psychiatric disorders. Overall and Gorham (1961) studied 120 chronic schizophrenics in an effort to identify the primary dimensions of change in their symptomatology. Six independent processes were identified. These were labelled as mental disorganization, distortion of thought processes, guilt-conversion, retardation, depression in mood, and anxiety. The depression factor was defined by feelings of inadequacy, depression, and suicidal impulses.

Friedman et al. (1963) obtained factors similar to those previously reported by Grinker. One-hundred-seventy psychotic-depressed patients were rated independently by two psychiatrists on a rating scale of symptoms, traits, and themes. Two experienced psychiatric interviewers rated each patient on the 60 item PPH Depression Rating scale.

Five factors were extracted. Factor A contained the items relevant to the affective component of depression; this included loss of self-esteem, guilt feelings, degree of depression, and loss of satisfaction. Factor B was defined by retardation and apathy, loss of energy, withdrawal and isolation. Factor C was characterized by the vegetative signs of depression such as loss of appetite, sleep disturbance, constipation, and work inhibition. Factor D was defined by items relevant to irritability, preoccupation, complaining and agitation. The fifth factor was equivocal.

McNair and Lorr (1964) attempted to determine the basic mood factors in a neurotic population. A mood scale was administered to a series of psychiatric samples. Five moods were identified: tension; anger; depression; vigor; and fatigue. The depression was defined by a series of adjectives such as worthless, helpless, unhappy, discouraged, and blue.

Pichot and Lempérière (1964) factor analyzed the Depression Inventory. (See Chapter 12 for a more complete account of their findings.) The following orthogonal factors were extracted: (*A*) vital depression; (*B*) self-debasement; (*C*) pessimism-suicide; and (*D*) indecision-inhibition.

Critique

Any comparison of the factors obtained by the various investigators cited above is hampered by each investigator's using different measures. It is possible, however, to find certain regularities among the studies. The vegetative signs of depression, for example, appear as a factor in several studies. Another obstacle to interpreting the findings is that most studies did not include nondepressed psychiatric patients. It is, therefore, not possible to ascertain whether the factors are characteristic of depression, of psychiatric disorders in general, or of the general population. There has not been any independent replication of any of the studies so the findings must be regarded as tentative.

Experimental Studies

An intriguing study concerned with the effect of serum from manic-depressed patients on the behavior of dogs has been reported in the Russian literature. Polyakova (1961) reported that the time taken for five dogs to negotiate a labyrinth increased from a mean of 6.37 seconds to 19 seconds when the dogs received serum from depressed patients. The time decreased to a mean of 5.8 when the blood came from patients in the manic phase. The profound implications of this study certainly warrant independent replication.

In the first of several studies in which depressed patients were exposed to varying experimental conditions, we randomly assigned a group of 20 depressed and 22 nondepressed patients to an experimentally induced superior and inferior performance condition (Loeb et al., 1964). Prior to and immediately following the experimental task, the patients rated their own mood. Indices of self-confidence were also obtained. The depressed patients tended to be more affected by task performance than the nondepressed patients when estimating how they would do in a future task. The groups did not differ, however, in performance effect on self-ratings.

In a later study, we measured the effects of success and failure on mood, motivation, and performance (Loeb et al., 1966). Twenty depressed and 20 nondepressed male patients were selected on the basis of their having, respectively, high or low scores on the Depression Inventory *and* high or low ratings of depression made independently during a psychiatric interview. In an experiment designed as part of the psychiatric outpatient evaluation procedure, the depressed patients were significantly more pessimistic about their likelihood of succeeding and tended to underate the quality of their performances, although their actual output was the same as that of nondepressed patients. On a second task the previous experience of success and failure had contrasting effects on the actual performances of the two groups. Success improved the performance of the depressed patients, and failure improved the performance of the nondepressed patients.

Harsch and Zimmer (1965) selected 62 male and 34 female college students on the basis of their performance on the Zimmer Sentence Completion test. Forty-eight students were considered to exhibit a predominantly extrapunitive behavior pattern, and 48 students were considered to exhibit a predominantly intrapunitive behavior pattern. Since the intrapunitive behavior pattern was considered characteristic of depression, this experiment has relevance to the understanding of depression. The experiment endeavored to produce abandonment of the characteristic behavior pattern and adoption of a different behavior pattern. This was attempted by rewarding subjects for statements contrary to the basic behavior pattern or punishing the subjects for statements conforming to the behavior pattern. As a result of the experimental manipulation, both groups showed significant shifts in behavior pattern as measured by the Zimmer test. The experimentally induced changes in a direction opposite from the starting points persisted over an eight-day follow-up period.

Family Background and Personality

Wilson (1951) investigated the role of family pressures in the socialization of manic depressives. On the basis of his review of case records and the intensive study of 12 patients and their families, he concluded that during childhood the manic depressives felt excessive pressure to conform to the attitudes of their parents and had less freedom than did the control group.

In 1954, Cohen et al. reported the results of an intensive psychoanalytic investigation of 12 cases of manic-depressive psychosis. A consistent finding in all 12 patients was that during the patient's childhood his family felt set apart by some factor that singled it out as "different." Among these factors were membership in a minority group, serious economic reversals, or mental illness in the family. In each case, the patient's family felt the social distinction keenly and reacted to it by trying to improve its acceptability in the community. The family placed a high premium on conformity and made a great effort to improve its social status by raising its economic level or by achieving other symbols of prestige. In order to reach his goal, the children were expected to conform to a high standard of behavior, based primarily on the parents' concepts of what the neighbors expected. The patient's role was experienced by him as being in the service of the family's social striving.

The responsibility for winning prestige was generally delegated by the mother to the child who was later to develop a manic-depressive psychosis. The reason a particular child was selected was either because he was exceptional in terms of intelligence or other gifts or because he was the oldest, the youngest, or the only child. The emphasis on achievement and competition usually caused the child to have serious problems with envy.

Gibson (1957) used a more refined technique to test the findings of Cohen's study. He studied a group of 27 manic-depressive patients and 17 schizophrenic patients from St. Elizabeth's Hospital in Washington, D.C., to determine whether Cohen's description of the early life history and family background could differentiate manic-depressive from schizophrenic patients. Hospital records and interviews with the families by specially trained social workers provided the basic data. The data were evaluated according to a questionnaire specifically designed to measure the degree to which a patient's history conformed to the concepts formulated by Cohen and her group. The 12 patients of the original Cohen study were also evaluated according to the questionnaire.

The two manic-depressive groups were differentiated from the schizophrenic groups on three of the five scales of the questionnaire. The manic depressives were statistically different from the schizophrenics in terms of the following characteristics: (*1*) The manic depressive comes from a family in which there is marked striving for prestige and the patient is the instrument of his parents' prestige needs; (*2*) The manic-depressive patient has a background in which there has been intense envy and competitiveness; and (*3*) The parents of the manic-depressive patients show a high degree of concern about social approval.

Certain methodological inadequacies are apparent in this study. Among these are the possibility of contamination in the social workers' evaluations of their data and the lack of control for age.

Becker and his associates, in a series of systematic studies, attempted to test the hypotheses derived from Cohen's study and the systematic investigation by Gibson. According to their reformulations of Cohen's findings, persons who develop manic-depressive reaction in adulthood have experienced excessive parental expectations for conformity and achievement as children. They react to these demands by adopting the prevailing values of their parents and other authority figures in order to placate them and win approval. The authors attempted to investigate the extent to which chronic dependence on others for guidance and approval is manifested in the opinions and attitudes of the manic-depressive patient. In an initial study, Becker (1960) compared 24 remitted manic depressives with 30 nonpsychiatric controls who were matched for age, education, and literacy level. The manic depressives scored significantly higher than the controls on measures of value achievement, authoritarian trends, and conventional attitudes. The manic depressives did not differ from the non-psychiatric controls in direct self-rating of achievement motivation or on performance output.

In other study, Spielberger, Parker, and Becker (1963) essayed a broader investigation of the formulations derived from the studies of Cohen, Gibson, and Wilson. The subjects of this investigation consisted of 30 remitted manic depressives and 30 nonpsychiatric controls. Four objective psychological scales or tests were administered. These consisted of the California Fascism Scale, the traditional family ideology scale, the value achievement scale, and the need achievement scale. The manic depressives obtained significantly higher scores than the controls on all these experimental measures except need achievement. The authors interpreted their findings as indicating that the adult personality structure of manic depressives is characterized by conventional authoritarian attitudes, traditional opinions, and stereotyped achievement values, but not by internalized achievement motives.

Some doubt of the specificity of these findings is raised by another study by Becker, Speilberger, and Parker (1963). In this study, the scores of manic depressives on various attitude measures were compared with the scores of neurotic depressives, schizophrenics, and normal controls. No significant difference in value achievement or authoritarian attitudes was found between the psychiatric groups, although they differed significantly from the normal controls. The investigators found, however, that age and social class significantly affected the scores; this indicates the need for empirical or statistical control of these variables in personality studies of this kind.

Self-Concept

We developed a self-concept test, consisting of traits and characteristics such as appearance, intelligence, sex appeal, selfishness, and cruelty (Beck and Stein, 1960). Each patient rated himself on each of these traits using a five point scale. He also made ratings of how he felt about having each of these traits (the self-acceptance score). We found a significant correlation (−.66) between self-concept scores and Depression Inventory scores; the correlation between self-acceptance scores and DI scores was also significant (−.42). This study indicated that depressed patients tended to give themselves low ratings on socially desirable traits and high ratings on undesirable traits. We concluded that the self-concept is low in depressed as compared with nondepressed patients.

Laxer (1964) used the semantic differential test to investigate changes in the self-concept of neurotic depressive and other psychiatric patients. The depressives showed a low self-concept on admission to a hospital but moved to a higher concept at the time of discharge. The paranoids, on the other hand, began with a relatively high self-rating and did not change appreciably at the time of discharge.

Summary

There has been a dearth of systematic psychological and psychodynamic studies of depression as compared with the biological studies reviewed in the preceding chapter. In addition to presenting the usual methodological problems such as inadequate attention to diagnosis and the control of extraneous variables such as age, investigations of the psychological and psychodynamic aspects of depression have not been followed by replication studies by other independent investigators. Any conclusions must, therefore, be regarded as tentative.

One interesting group of findings demonstrates that in test situations the depressed patient is able to perform as effectively as matched controls. Experimental studies indicate that the experience of success significantly improves the performance of depressed patients. These findings suggest that the inertia in depression may be related more to factors such as loss of motivation than to physiological inhibition. The studies also indicate that the depressed patients greatly underestimate their capacity and actual performance.

The finding of a high threshold for fatigue also suggests that in actual work situations the depressed patient does not become as fatigued as is generally believed. No objective evidence was obtained to substantiate the notion of a disturbance of judgments of time. Some studies, however, suggest that the depressed patient tends to have a downward bias in spatial perception.

The factor analytic studies have opened a new era for exploration. The differences in clinical and psychometric measures used in the various investigations, however, preclude any definite conclusions about the basic dimensions of depression at this time.

The studies of the personality and of the family backgrounds of depressed patients have not fulfilled early expectations. Efforts to test the hypothesis generated by the clinical studies of M. B. Cohen and her group provided some initial support. Investigations using a tighter design, however, suggest that the obtained differences between depressed and nondepressed patients may be due to extraneous factors such as age, social class, and educational level. Studies of the self-concept indicate that depressed patients rate themselves much lower than nondepressed patients, but return to average ratings upon recovery from the depression.

References

BECK, A. T., FESHBACH, S., & LEGG, D. (1962). The clinical utility of the digit symbol test. *Journal of Consulting Psychology*, **26**, 263–268.

BECK, A. T., & STEIN, D. (1960). *The Self-concept in Depression*. Unpublished study.

BECKER, J. (1960). Achievement-related characteristics of manic-depressives. *Journal of Abnormal and Social Psychology*, **60**, 334–339.

BECKER, J., SPIELBERGER, C. D., & PARKER, J. B. (1963). Value achievement and authoritarian attitudes in psychiatric patients. *Journal of Clinical Psychology*, **19**, 57–61.

COHEN, M. B., BAKER, G., COHEN, R. A., FROMM-REICHMANN, F., & WEIGERT, E. V. (1954). An intensive study of twelve cases of manic-depressive psychosis. *Psychiatry*, **17**, 103–137.

DIXON, N. F., & LEAR, T. E. (1962). Perceptual regulation and mental disorder. *Journal of Mental Science*, **108**, 356–361.

FISHER, S. (1964). Depressive affect and perception of up-down. *Journal of Psychiatric Research*, **2**, 25.

FRIEDMAN, A. S. (1964). Minimal effects of severe depression on cognitive functioning. *Journal of Abnormal and Social Psychology*, **69**, 237–243.

FRIEDMAN, A. S., COWITZ, B., COHEN, H. W., & GRANICK, S. (1963). Syndromes and themes of psychotic depression: A factor analysis. *Archives of General Psychiatry*, **9**, 504–509.

GIBSON, R. W. (1957). *Comparison of The Family Background and Early Life Experiences of the Manic-Depressive and Schizophrenic Patient*. Final report on Office of Naval Research Contract (Nonr-751 (00)). Washington, D.C., Washington School of Psychiatry.

GRANICK, S. (1963). Comparative analysis of psychotic depressives with matched normals on some untimed verbal intelligence tests. *Journal of Consulting Psychology*, **27**, 439–443.

GRINKER, R., MILLER, J., SABSHIN, M., NUNN, R., & NUNNALLY, J. (1961). *The Phenomena of Depressions*. New York: Hoeber.

HAMILTON, M. (1960). A rating scale for depression. *Journal of Neurology, Neurosurgery, and Psychiatry*, **23**, 56–61.

HARSCH, O. H., & ZIMMER, H. (1965). An experimental approximation of thought reform. *Journal of Consulting Psychology*, **29**, 475–479.

HEMPHILL, R. E., HALL, K. R. L., & CROOKES, T. G. (1952). A preliminary report on fatigue and pain tolerance in depressive and psychoneurotic patients. *Journal of Mental Science*, **98**, 433–440.

LAXER, R. M. (1964). Self-concept changes of depressive patients in general hospital treatment. *Journal of Consulting Psychology*, **28**, 214–219.

LOEB, A., BECK, A. T., DIGGORY, J. C., & TUTHILL, R. (1966). The effects of success and failure on mood, motivation, and performance as a function of predetermined level of depression. Unpublished study.

LOEB, A., FESHBACH, S., BECK, A. T., & WOLF, A. (1964). Some effects of reward upon the social perception and motivation of psychiatric patients varying in depression. *Journal of Abnormal and Social Psychology*, **68**, 609–616.

MCNAIR, D. M., & LORR, M. (1964). An analysis of mood in neurotics. *Journal of Abnormal and Social Psychology*, **69**, 620–627.

MEZEY, A. G. & COHEN, S. I. (1961). The effect of depressive illness on time judgment and time experience. *Journal of Neurology, Neurosurgery, and Psychiatry*, **24**, 269–270.

OVERALL, J. E. (1962). Dimensions of manifest depression. *Journal of Psychiatric Research*, **1**, 239–245.

OVERALL, J. E., & GORHAM, D. (1961). Basic dimensions of change in the symptomatology of chronic schizophrenics. *Journal of Abnormal and Social Psychology*, **63**, 597–602.

OVERALL, J. E., HOLLISTER, L. E., MEYER, F., KIMBELL, I. JR., & SHELTON, J. (1961). Imipramine and thioridazine in depressed and schizophrenic patients. *Journal of the American Medical Association*, **189**, 605–608.

PAYNE, R. W., & HIRST, H. L. (1957). Overinclusive thinking in a depressive and a control group. *Journal of Consulting Psychology*, **21**, 186–188.

PICHOT, P., & LEMPÉRIÈRE, T. (1964). Analyse Factorielle d'un questionnaire d'autoévaluation des symptomes dépressifs. *Rev. Psychol. Appl.*, **14**, 15–29.

POLYAKOVA, M. (1961). The effect of blood from manic-depressive psychotics on the higher nervous activity (behavior) of animals. *Zh. Nevropat. I Psikhiat.* (*Moscova*), **61**, 104–108.

RAPAPORT, D. (1945). *Diagnostic Psychological Testing: The Theory, Statistical Evaluation, and Diagnostic Application of a Battery of Tests*, vol. 1. Chicago: Yearbook.

ROSENBLATT, B. P. (1956). The influence of affective states upon body image and upon the perceptual organization of space. Ph. D. Dissertation, Clark University, Worcester, Mass.

SHAPIRO, M. B., CAMPBELL, D., HARRIS, & DEWSBERRY, J. P. (1958). Effects of E.C.T. upon psychomotor speed and the "distraction effect" in depressed psychiatric patients. *Journal of Mental Science*, **104**, 681–695.

SPIELBERGER, C. D., PARKER, J. B., & BECKER, J. (1963). Conformity and achievement in remitted manic-depressive patients. *Journal of Nervous and Mental Diseases*, **137**, 162–172.

TUCKER, J. E., & SPIELBERG, M. J. (1958). Bender-Gestalt Test correlates of emotional depression. *Journal of Consulting Psychology*, **22**, 56.

WADSWORTH, W. V., WELLS, B. W. P., & SCOTT, R. F. (1962). A comparative study of the fatigability of a group of chronic schizophrenics and a group of hospitalized non-psychotic depressives. *Journal of Mental Science*, **108**, 304–308.

WAPNER, S., WERNER, H., & KRUS, D. M. (1957). The effects of success and failure on space localization. *Journal of Personality*, **25**, 752–756.

WILSON, D. C. (1951). Families of manic-depressives. *Diseases of the Nervous System*, **12**, 362–369.

NORMAN CAMERON

The Paranoid Pseudo-Community Revisited

One of the prominent theorists about paranoid disorders in recent years has been Dr. Norman Cameron. His concept of the pseudo-community as a feature of these disorders has been widely known. Here he reformulates that concept and in the process provides a good picture of the development of the paranoid disorder.

A decade of experience with intensive clinical studies of paranoid thinking, in the course of psychoanalyzing psychoneurotics and in the long-term therapy of ambulatory psychotics, has led me to a reworking of the concept of the

---

Reprinted from the *American Journal of Sociology*, **65** (1959), 52–58, by permission of The University of Chicago Press and Dr. Cameron.

pseudo-community as formulated in this *Journal*[1] and further developed elsewhere.[2] The social aspects of the concept require little change. It is in its individual aspects—in a greater concern with the evidence of internal changes and with the signs that forces are operative which are not open to direct observation—that the pseudo-community acquires deeper roots and greater usefulness.

Original presentation. In the normal evolution and preservation of socially organized behavior the most important factor is the developing and maintaining of genuine communication. In each individual, language behavior grows out of preverbal interchange between infant and older person. It evolves in accordance with whatever traditional patterns prevail in the immediate environment, since communication is always, at first, between a child who operates at preverbal levels and older individuals whose language is already a highly organized interactive system. Through sharing continuously in such language and prelanguage interchange, each child develops shared social perspectives and skill in shifting from one perspective to another in time of need.

A highly significant result of this gradual process is that, as time goes on, the child normally acquires an increasingly realistic grasp of how other people feel, what their attitudes, plans, hopes, fears, and intentions are, and in what ways these all relate to his own. Eventually, he is able to take the roles of other people around him in imagination and to view things more or less realistically from their perspectives as well as from his own. In this way he also develops a workable degree of objectivity toward himself, learning to respond to his body, his personality, and his behavior more or less as others do. In the final product, there is considerable difference between the socialization achieved in behavior publicly shared and genuinely communicated and behavior that has remained private and little formulated or expressed in language.

The adult who is especially vulnerable to paranoid developments is one in whom this process of socialization has been seriously defective. His deficient social learning and poorly developed social skills leave him unable to understand adequately the motivations, attitudes, and intentions of others. When he becomes disturbed or confused under stress, he must operate under several grave handicaps imposed by a lifelong inability to communicate freely and effectively, to suspend judgment long enough to share his tentative interpretations with someone else, to imagine realistically the attitudes that others might have toward his situation and himself, and to imagine their roles and thus share their perspectives.

Left to his own unaided devices in a crisis, the paranoid person is able only

[1] Norman Cameron, "The Paranoid Pseudo-Community," *American Journal of Sociology*, XLIX (1943), 32–38. Reprinted in A. M. Rose (ed.), *Mental Health and Mental Disorder: A Sociological Approach* (New York: W. W. Norton & Co., 1955).

[2] Norman Cameron, *The Psychology of Behavior Disorders: A Biosocial Interpretation* (Boston: Houghton Mifflin Co., 1947), and "Perceptual Organization and Behavior Pathology," in R. Blake and G. Ramsey (eds.), *Perception: An Approach to Personality* (New York: Ronald Press Co., 1951); and Norman Cameron and A. Magaret, *Behavior Pathology* (Boston: Houghton Mifflin Co., 1951), chap. xiii, "Pseudo-Community and Delusion."

to seek and find "evidence" that carries him farther in the direction he is already going—toward a more and more delusional interpretation of what seems to be going on around him.[3] This process may culminate in a conviction that he himself is the focus of a community of persons who are united in a conspiracy of some kind against him. It is this supposed functional community of real persons whom the patient can see and hear, and of other persons whom he imagines, that we call the *paranoid pseudo-community.* It has no existence as a social organization and as soon as he attempts to combat it, or to flee, he is likely to come into conflict with his actual social community.

Incompleteness of the descriptive pseudo-community. This, in brief, is the background and structure of the paranoid pseudo-community, as originally described. As it stands, it still seems valid; but it is unnecessarily restricted. In the first place, the account of the delusional development pays scant attention to internal dynamics because of the limits imposed by a behavioristic orientation. Patients, of course, recognize no such limitations. In the course of long-term intensive therapy they can sometimes furnish important information about what is going on within them to a therapist who is ready to receive it. Some of this they describe as it happens, in their own terms, and often in their own idiom. Some of it one can infer from what is said and done, with the help of material communicated in parallel cases. Some of it one must postulate in an effort to make one's observations and direct inferences more intelligible, just as is done in other empirical sciences.

In the original account not enough emphasis was given to the positive achievements of delusion formation. As we shall see, the pseudo-community is the best means a paranoid patient has at the time for bridging the chasm between his inner reality and social reality. Its use for this purpose may lead to a progressive reduction in desocialization and the reappearance of more normal communicative channels.

And, finally, the concept of the pseudo-community needs a background of structural postulates. In order to make sense out of the experiences which people actually have in fantasies, daydreams, and psychoses, one is obliged to go beyond such impermanent concepts as perception, response, and behavior—upon which the writer earlier relied—and to assume probable forces and mechanisms operating within personality systems and interacting subsystems. Here, again, the patient often comes to the rescue with empirical data. And, every now and then, one comes across a patient who describes with naïve simplicity and directness—but consistently over a long period of time—phenomena which seem purely theoretical and highly abstruse, as reported in the literature. Exposed to such material the therapist may still be left with a sense of strangeness; but his previous feeling of their abstruseness and incredulity sooner or later vanishes.

[3] For a detailed discussion of this process of *desocialization* see "Desocialization and Disorganization," in Cameron and Magaret, *op. cit.*, pp. 448–517.

Paranoid loss of social reality. Paranoid delusional development begins with an impairment of social communication. It is preceded by experiences of frustration to which, like many normal persons, the paranoid individual reacts by turning away from his surroundings, and taking refuge in fantasy and daydream. This is the phase of withdrawal and preoccupation which is sometimes obvious even to an untrained observer.

When a paranoid person withdraws like this, he is far more likely than a normal person to lose effective contact with his social environment (i.e., with social reality) and to undergo regression. If this happens, he may abandon social reality for a time completely and become absorbed in primitive regressive thinking and feeling. Occasionally, a patient openly expresses some of his regressive experiences at the time; more often they can be inferred only from what emerges later on.

Precursors of the pseudo-community. I. Beginning restitution. It is a fact, of both clinical observation and subjective report, that paranoid patients, while still withdrawn, preoccupied, and regressed, begin to make attempts to regain their lost relationships with social reality. We may conceptualize these as marking the tapering-off of regression and the beginning of the reintegration of personality. The attempts fail to recover the lost social reality, however, because the patient's internal situation is not what it was before his regression. It is no longer possible for him to regain social reality as, for example, a normal person does when he wakes up in the morning. Instead, as we shall see, paranoid reintegration involves a restitutive process, the construction of a pseudo-reality which culminates in the paranoid pseudo-community.

Paranoid personalities suffer all their lives from defective repressive defenses and a heavy reliance upon the more primitive defenses of denial and projection. If they undergo a psychotic regression, which involves partial ego disintegration, their repressive defenses become still more defective. Primitive fantasies and conflicts now begin to emerge and to threaten ego disruption. The patient is forced to deal with them somehow, if he is to preserve what personality integration he still has and avoid further regression. Since he cannot successfully repress them, he vigorously denies them and projects them. An immediate result of the intense projective defense is that the products of the patient's emerging fantasies and conflicts now appear to him to be coming from outside him. Thus he seems to escape disintegration from within only to be threatened with destruction from without.

Precursors of the pseudo-community. II. Estrangement and diffuse vigilance. In the process of denying and projecting, the paranoid patient makes a start toward regaining contact with his surroundings. But this process neither simplifies nor clarifies the situation for him; and it does not bring about a return to social reality. On the contrary, the surroundings now seem somehow strange and different. Something has unquestionably happened. The patient misidentifies this "something" as basically a change in the makeup of his environment instead of what it actually is, a fundamental change within himself. If he expresses his feelings at this point, he is likely to say that things are going on which he does not understand; and this, of course, is literally true.

It is hardly surprising that the patient, finding himself in a world grown suddenly strange, should become diffusely vigilant. He watches everything uneasily; he listens alertly for clues; he looks everywhere for hidden meanings. Here his lifelong social incompetence makes matters still worse. He lacks even ordinary skill in the common techniques for testing social reality. He is unable to view his threatening situation even temporarily from the perspective of a neutral person. The more anxious and vigilant he grows, the less he can trust anybody, the less he dares to share with anyone his uneasiness and suspicion. He is condemned to pursue a solitary path, beset by primal fears, hates, and temptations which he cannot cope with nor escape.

Precursors of the pseudo-community. III. Increased self-reliance. Strong tendencies toward self-reference are characteristic of paranoid personalities. When a paranoid adult becomes deeply and regressively preoccupied, his habitually egocentric orientation is greatly increased. And when he next resorts to wholesale projection, he in effect converts his environment into an arena for his projected fantasies and conflicts. This destroys whatever neutrality and objectivity the environment may have previously possessed for him. He is now engrossed in scrutinizing his surroundings for signs of the return of what he is denying and projecting. To these he has become selectively sensitive. He is watching out for something that will explain away the strangeness and enable him to escape his frightening sense of isolation.

It is an unfortunate fact that a badly frightened person—even a normal one—is likely to notice things and make interpretations that increase rather than diminish his fear. And this is especially the case if he feels alone, in strange surroundings, and threatened by an unknown danger. Many non-paranoid adults, for example, walking alone through a large cemetery at night, or lost at night in a forest, become extremely alert and feel personally threatened by harmless things wholly unrelated to them. The paranoid adult, who is peopling his surroundings with projected phantoms from his own past, likewise creates a situation in which everything seems somehow dangerously related to him. Since he cannot escape, he tries to understand the situation he has unconsciously created, in the vain hope that he may then be able to cope with it.

Precursors of the pseudo-community. IV. Preliminary hypotheses. Being human, the paranoid patient is driven irresistibly to make hypotheses; but, having partially regressed, and being paranoid as well, he cannot test them. He tends, therefore, to pass from one guess or one suspicion to another like it. Using the materials provided by his environment and by his projected fantasies and conflicts, he constructs a succession of provisional hypotheses, discarding each as it fails to meet the contradictory demands of his internal needs and the environment. This is characteristic also of complex normal problem-solving. It is an expression of what is called the synthetic function of the ego.

Everyone who works with paranoid patients discovers that some kind of delusional reconstruction of reality is essential to their continued existence as persons. Even a temporary and unsatisfactory delusional hypothesis may be at the time a patient's sole means of bridging the gap between himself and his social environment. It gives a distorted picture of the world; but a distorted world is better than no world at all. And this is often a regressed person's only choice. To abandon his projected fears, hates, and temptations might mean to abandon all that he has gained in the reconstruction of reality, to have his world fall apart and fall apart himself. Patients sense this danger, even expressing it in these words, and they rightly refuse to give up their delusional reality. The fear is not unrealistic, for clinically such catastrophes actually occur, ending in personality disintegration.

A great many paranoid persons never go beyond the phase of making and giving up a succession of preliminary delusional hypotheses. Some of them regain a good working relationship with social reality, something approaching or equaling their premorbid status. Some are less successful and remain chronically suspicious, averse, and partially withdrawn but manage even so to go on living otherwise much as they had lived before. They may appear morose, irascible, and bitter; but they do not fix upon definite enemies or take definite hostile action. At most they suffer brief outbursts of protests and complaint without losing their ability to retreat from an angry delusional position. In this paper, however, we are concerned primarily with paranoid patients—by no means incurable—who go on to crystallize a more stable delusional organization.

Final crystallization: the pseudo-community. A great many paranoid persons succeed in crystallizing a stable conceptual organization, the pseudo-community, which gives them a satisfactory cognitive explanation of their strange altered world and a basis for doing something about the situation as they now see it. Their problem is exceedingly complex. It is impossible for them to get rid of the unconscious elements, which they have denied and projected, but which now return apparently from the outside. They cannot abandon or even ignore their environment without facing a frightening regression into an objectless world. Their task is somehow to integrate these internal and external phenomena which appear before them on a single plane into a unified world picture.

The human environment which others share (*social reality*) provides the patient with real persons having social roles and characteristics which he can utilize in making his delusional reconstruction. It also provides real interaction among them, including interaction with the patient himself. Many things actually happen in it, some of them in direct relation to the patient, most of them actually not.

Internal reality provides two sets of functions. One is made up of the previously unconscious impulses, conflicts, and fantasies—now erupted, denied, and projected. This, as noted, introduces imagined motivation, interaction, and intentions into the observed activities of other persons. It gives apparent meaning to happenings which do not have such meaning for the consensus. The other set of functions is included in the concept of ego adaptation. It is the ego synthesis mentioned above, by means of which the demands of internal reality and the structure of social reality are integrated into a meaningful, though delusional, unity.

What the paranoid patient does is as follows: Into the organization of social reality, as he perceives it, he unconsciously projects his own previously unconscious motivation, which he has denied but cannot escape. This process now requires a perceptual and conceptual reorganization of object relations in his surroundings into an apparent community, which he represents to himself as organized wholly with respect to him (delusion of self-reference). And since the patient's erupted, denied, and projected elements are overwhelmingly hostile and destructive, the motivation he ascribes to the real persons he has now organized into his conceptual pseudo-community is bound to be extremely hostile and destructive.

To complete his conceptual organization of a paranoid conspiracy, the patient also introduces imaginary persons. He ascribes to them, as to real persons, imagined functions, roles, and motivations in keeping with his need to unify his restitutional conception and make it stable. He pictures helpers, dupes, stooges, go-betweens, and masterminds, of whose actual existence he becomes certain.

It is characteristic of the pseudo-community that it is made up of both real and imaginary persons, all of whom may have both real and imaginary functions and interrelations.[4] In form it usually corresponds to one or another of the common dangerous, hostile groups in contemporary society, real or fictional—gangs, dope and spy rings, secret police, and groups of political, racial, and religious fanatics. Many paranoid patients succeed in creating a restitutional organization which has well-formulated plans. The chief persecutor is sometimes a relative or acquaintance, or a well-known public figure, while the rest of the imaginary personnel forms a vague, sinister background. Sometimes one finds the reverse—the chief persecutor is unknown, a malevolent "brain" behind everything, while the known dangerous persons play supporting roles in the delusional cast.

The final delusional reconstruction of reality may fall into an integrated conceptual pattern that brings an experience of closure: "I suddenly realized what it was all about!" the patient may exclaim with obvious relief at sudden clarification. The intolerable suspense has ended; the strangeness of what has been "going on" seems to disappear, and confusion is replaced by "understanding," and wavering doubt by certainty. A known danger may be frightening; but at least it is tangible and one can do something about it. In short, the pseudo-community reduces the hopeless complexity and confusion

[4] This is in contrast to the autistic community, which is composed of wholly imaginary persons (see "Autistic Community and Hallucination," in Cameron and Magaret, *op. cit.*, pp. 414–47.

to a clear formula. This formula—"the plot"—the patient can now apply to future events as he experiences them and fit them into the general framework of his reconstruction.

The organization of a conceptual pseudo-community is a final cognitive step in paranoid problem-solving. It re-establishes stable object relations, though on a delusional basis, and thus makes integrated action possible. To summarize what this reconstruction of reality has achieved for its creator:

(*a*) *Reduction in estrangement.* As a direct result of paranoid problem-solving, experienced external reality is distorted so as to bring it into line with the inescapable projected elements. This lessens confusion and detachment and allows the patient to recover some of his lost sense of ego integrity. The world seems dangerous but familiar.

(*b*) *Internal absorption of aggression.* Construction and maintenance of a conceptual pseudo-community absorb aggression internally, in the same sense that organizing a baseball team, a political ward, or a scientific society absorbs aggression. This reduces the threat of ego disintegration which the id eruptions pose.

(*c*) *Basis for action.* Any new cognitive construct can serve as a basis for new action; in this respect the paranoid pseudo-community is no exception. It organizes the drive-directed cognitive processes, leads to meaningful interpretations in a well-defined pseudo-reality structure, and paves the way for overt action with a definite focus. The patient is enabled to go ahead as anyone else might who had powerful urges and felt sure that he was right.

(*d*) *Justification of aggressive action.* Finally, a persecutory pseudo-community justifies attack or flight, either of which involves a direct aggressive discharge in overt action. Fighting or running away is less disintegrative psychologically than prolonged frightened inaction. And under the circumstances, as the patient now conceptualizes them, he need feel neither guilt for attacking nor shame for fleeing.

Paranoid cognition and paranoid action. When a patient succeeds in conceptualizing a pseudo-community, he has taken the final cognitive step in paranoid problem-solving. He now "knows" what his situation is. But he is still faced with his need to do something about it. As a matter of fact, the crystallization of a hostile delusional structure usually increases the urge to take action. A circular process may quickly develop. The imagined threats of the now structured imaginary conspiracy seem to the patient concrete and imminent. They stimulate more and more his anxiety and defensive hostility—and the latter, being as usual projected, further increases the apparent external threat. Often this kind of self-stimulation spirals upward, while more and more "incidents" and people may be drawn into the gathering psychotic storm.

Paranoid action, however inappropriate it may be, still represents the completion of restitutional relationships and the fullest contact with his human environment of which the patient is capable at the time. He switches from his previous passive role of observer and interpreter, with all its indecision and anxiety, to that of an aggressive participant in what he conceives as social reality. For him this is genuine interaction, and he experiences the gratification that comes with certainty and with a massive discharge of pent-up aggressiveness. He may give a preliminary warning to the supposed culprits or make an appeal for intervention to someone in authority before taking direct action himself, which, when it comes, may be in the form of an attack or sudden flight, either of which may be planned and executed with considerable skill.

Making social reality conform to the pseudo-community. Paranoid patients who take aggressive action often achieve a pyrrhic victory. They succeed finally in making social reality act in conformity with the delusional reality which they have created. As long as a patient confines himself to watching, listening, and interpreting, he need not come into open conflict with the social community. But, when he takes overt action appropriate only in his private pseudo-community, a serious social conflict will arise.

Social reality is the living product of genuine sharing, communication, and interaction. Valid social attitudes, interpretations, and action derive continuously from these operations. The restitutional reality in which the patient believes himself to be participating has no counterpart outside of himself: it is illusory. Other persons cannot possibly share his attitudes and interpretations because they do not share his paranoid projections and distortions. Therefore they do not understand action taken in terms of his delusional reconstruction. The patient, for his part, cannot share their attitudes and interpretations because he is driven by regressive needs which find no place in adult social reality.

When an intelligent adult expresses beliefs and makes accusations which seem unintelligible to others, as well as threatening, he may make the people around him exceedingly anxious. This is particularly the case when his words tend to activate their unconscious fantasies and conflicts. And when such a person begins to take aggressive action, which seems unprovoked as well as unintelligible, he inevitably arouses defensive and retaliatory hostility in others. The moment the social community takes action against him, it provides him with the confirmation he has been expecting—that there is a plot against him.

Thus, in the end, the patient manages to provoke action in the social community that conforms to the expectation expressed in his pseudo-community organization. His own internal need to experience hostility from without—as a defense against being overwhelmed by internal aggression—is satisfied when actual persons behave in accordance with his projections. His need for a target against which to discharge hostility is also met. This is his victory and his defeat.

The defeat need not be final. Much will depend, of course, upon the patient's basic personality organization, particularly his emotional flexibility, his potentiality for internal change, and his residual capacity for establishing new ego and superego identifications. The depth and extent of his regression are also important, as are the fixity and the inclusiveness of his delusional structure. Much will also depend upon his potential freedom to communicate, to develop reciprocal role-taking skills with another person, and to include another's alternative perspectives in his own therapeutic orientation.

Therapy. The primary therapeutic consideration, of course, is not the character of the delusional structure but what makes it necessary. A reduction in anxiety is among the first objectives. The source of anxiety lies in the regressive changes and in the threat these have brought of an unconscious breakthrough. But it is also aggravated by anything in the environment which tends to increase the patient's hostility and fear. Once the setting has been made less anxiety-provoking, the most pressing need is for someone in whom the patient can ultimately put his trust—someone not made anxious by the patient's fear and hostility or driven to give reassurances and make demands.

For the paranoid patient who is ready to attempt social communication, an interested but neutral therapist can function as a living bridge between psychotic reality and social reality. Through interacting with such a person, who neither attacks the delusional structure nor beats the drums of logic, a patient may succeed in gaining new points of reference from which to build a new orientation. The therapeutic process now involves another reconstruction of reality, one which undoes the restitutional pseudo-community without destroying the patient's defenses and forcing him to regress further.

As anxiety and the threat of disintegration subside, paranoid certainty becomes less necessary to personality survival. The patient can begin to entertain doubts and consider alternative interpretations. Such changes, of course, must come from within if they are to come at all. If he is able to work through some of the origins and derivatives of his basic problems, the patient may succeed eventually in representing to himself more realistically than ever before how other people feel and think. In this way the conceptual structure of his pseudo-community may be gradually replaced by something approaching the conceptual structure of social reality.

KURT GOLDSTEIN

The Effect of Brain Damage on the Personality

Kurt Goldstein was an eminent clinical neurologist who acquired a great deal of experience with patients suffering brain damage when he served as a German army physician during World War I. As a result of his observations of such patients, he became impressed with the very general disruptive effects brain damage had on personality and behavior, regardless of where it occurred and, within limits, how extensive it was. These common reactions of the brain-injured are described in this paper.

When I was asked to speak before the Psychoanalytic Association about the changes of the personality in brain damage, I was somewhat hesitant because I was not quite sure that I would be able to make myself understood by an audience which thinks mainly in such different categories and speaks in such a different terminology from my own. I finally accepted the invitation, because I thought that members of the Association apparently wanted to hear what I think and because it brought me the opportunity to express an old idea of mine—the idea that it is faulty in principle to try to make a distinction between so-called organic and functional diseases, as far as symptomatology and therapy are concerned (1). In both conditions, one is dealing with abnormal functioning of the same psychophysical apparatus and with the attempts of the organism to come to terms with that. If the disturbances—whether they are due to damage to the brain or to psychological conflicts—do not disappear spontaneously or cannot be eliminated by therapy, the organism has to make a new adjustment to life in spite of them. Our task is to help the patients in this adjustment by physical and psychological means; the procedure and goal of the therapy in both conditions is, in principle, the same.

This was the basic idea which induced a group of neurologists, psychiatrists, and psychotherapists—including myself—many years ago, in 1927, to organize the Internationale Gesellschaft für Psychotherapie in Germany

---

Reprinted from *Psychiatry*, **15** (1952), 245–260, by special permission of The William Alanson White Psychiatric Foundation, Inc.

and to invite all physicians interested in psychotherapy to meet at the First Congress of the Society. Psychotherapists of all different schools responded to our invitation, and the result of the discussions was surprisingly fruitful. At the second meeting in 1927, I spoke about the relation between psychoanalysis and biology (2). During the last twenty years, in which I have occupied myself intensively with psychotherapy, I have become more and more aware of the similarity of the phenomena of organic and psychogenic conditions.

It is not my intention to consider the similarities in this paper. I want to restrict myself to the description of the symptomatology and the interpretation of the behavior changes in patients with damage to the brain cortex, particularly in respect to their personality, and would like to leave it to you to make comparisons.

The symptomatology which these patients present is very complex (3). It is the effect of various factors of which the change of personality is only one. Therefore, when we want to characterize the change of personality, we have to separate it from the symptoms due to other factors: (1) from those which are the effect of *disturbance of inborn or learned patterns* of performances in special performance fields—such as motor and sensory patterns; (2) from those which are the *expression of the so-called catastrophic conditions*; and (3) from those which are the *expression of the protective mechanisms* which originate from the attempt of the organism to avoid catastrophes.

In order to avoid terminological misunderstandings, I want to state what I mean by personality: Personality shows itself in behavior. Personality is the mode of behavior of a person in terms of the capacities of human beings in general and in the specific appearance of these capacities in a particular person. Behavior is always an entity and concerns the whole personality. Only abstractively can we separate behavior into parts—as for instance, bodily processes, concious phenomena, states of feelings, attitudes, and so on (4, pp. 310 ff.).

According to my observation, all the phenomena of behavior become understandable if one assumes that all the behavior of the organism is determined by one trend (5), the *trend to actualize itself*—that is, its nature and all its capacities. This takes place normally in such harmony that the realization of all capacities in the best way possible in the particular environment is permitted. The capacities are experienced by a person as various *needs* which he is driven to fulfill with the cooperation of some parts of the environment and in spite of the hindrance by other parts of it.

Each stimulation brings about some disorder in the organism. But after a certain time—which is determined by the particular performance—the organism comes back, by a process of *equalization*, to its normal condition. This process guarantees the constancy of the organism. A person's specific personality corresponds to this constancy. Because realization has to take place in terms of different needs and different tasks, the behavior of the organism is soon directed more by one than by another need. This does not mean that organismic behavior is determined by separate needs or drives. All such concepts need the assumption of a controlling agency. I have tried to show in my book, *The Organism*, that the different agencies which have been assumed for this purpose have only made for new difficulties in the attempt to understand organismic behavior; they are not necessary if one gives up the concept of separate drives, as my theory of the organism does. All of a person's capacities are always in action in each of his activities. The capacity that is particularly important for the task is in the foreground; the others are in the background. All of these capacities are organized in a way which facilitates the self-realization of the total organism in the particular situation. For each performance there is a definite figure-ground organization of capacities; the change in the behavior of a patient corresponds to the change in the total organism in the form of an alteration of the normal pattern of figure-ground organization (4, p. 109).

Among patients with brain damage we can distinguish between alterations which occur when an area belonging to a special performance field—such as a motor or sensory area—is damaged somewhat isolatedly, and alterations which occur when the personality organization itself is altered. In lesions of these areas—according to a dedifferentiation of the function of the brain cortex (4, p. 131)—qualities and patterns of behavior (both those developing as a result of maturation and those acquired by learning) are disturbed. Indeed, these patterns never occur isolatedly. They are always embedded in that kind of behavior which we call personality. The personality structure is disturbed particularly by lesions of the frontal lobes, the parietal lobes, and the insula Reili; but it is also disturbed by diffuse damage to the cortex—for instance, in paralysis, alchoholism, and trauma, and in metabolic disturbances such as hypoglycemia. The effect of diffuse damage is understandable when we consider that what we call personality structure apparently is not related to a definite locality of the cortex (4, pp. 249 ff.) but to a particular complex function of the brain which is the same for all its parts. This function can be damaged especially by lesions in any of the areas I have mentioned. The damage of the patterns certainly modifies the personality too. Although for full understanding of the personality changes, we should discuss the organization of the patterns and their destruction in damaged patients, that would carry us too far and is not absolutely necessary for our discussion. I shall therefore restrict my presentation to consideration of the symptoms due to damage of the personality structure itself (6).

There would be no better way of getting to the heart of the problem than by demonstrating a patient. Unfortunately I have to substitute for this a description of the behavior of patients with severe damage of the brain cortex. Let us consider a man with an extensive lesion of the frontal lobes (7, 8). His customary way of living does not seem to be very much disturbed. He is a little slow; his face is rather immobile, rather rigid; his attention is directed very strictly to what he is doing at the moment—say, writing a letter, or speaking to someone. Confronted with tasks in various fields, he gives seemingly normal responses under certain conditions; but under other conditions he fails completely in tasks that seem to be very similar to those he has performed quite well.

This change of behavior becomes apparent particularly in the following simple test: We place before him a small wooden stick in a definite position, pointing, for example, diagonally from left to right. He is asked to note the position of the stick carefully. After a half minute's exposure, the stick is removed; then it is handed to the patient, and he is asked to put it back in the position in which it was before. He grasps the stick and tries to replace it, but he fumbles; he is all confusion; he looks at the examiner, shakes his head, tries this way and that, plainly uncertain. The upshot is that he cannot place the stick in the required position. He is likewise unable to imitate other simple figures built of sticks. Next we show the patient a little house made of many sticks—a house with a roof, a door, a window, and a chimney. After we remove it, we ask the patient to reproduce the model. He succeeds very well.

Impairment of Abstract Capacity

If we ask ourselves what is the cause of the difference in his behavior in the two tasks, we can at once exclude defects in the field of perception, action, and memory. For there is no doubt that copying the house with many details demands a much greater capacity in all these faculties, especially in memory, than putting a single stick into a position which the patient has been shown shortly before. A further experiment clarifies the situation. We put before the patient two sticks placed together so as to form an angle with the opening pointing upward (∨). The patient is unable to reproduce this model. Then we confront him with the same angle, the opening downward this time (∧), and now he reproduces the figure very well on the first trial. When we ask the patient how it is that he can reproduce the second figure but not the first one, he says, "This one has nothing to do with the other one." Pointing to the second one, he says, "That is a roof"; pointing to the first, "That is nothing."

These two replies lead us to an understanding of the patient's behavior. His first reply makes it clear that, to him, the two objects with which he has to deal are totally different from one another. The second answer shows that he apprehends the angle with the opening downward as a concrete object out of his own experience, and he constructs a concrete thing with the two sticks. The two sticks that formed an angle with the opening upward apparently did not arouse an impression of a concrete thing. He had to regard the sticks as representations indicating directions in abstract space. Furthermore, he had to keep these directions in mind and rearrange the sticks from memory as representatives of these abstract directions. To solve the problem he must give an account to himself of relations in space and must act on the basis of abstract ideas. Thus we may conclude that the failure of the patient in the first test lies in the fact that he is unable to perform a task which can be executed only by means of a grasp of the abstract. The test in which the opening of the angle is downwards does not demand this, since the patient is able to grasp it as a concrete object and therefore to execute it perfectly. It is for the same reason that he is able to copy the little house, which seems to us to be so much more complicated. From the result of his behavior in this and similar tasks we come to the assumption that these *patients are impaired in their abstract capacity.*

The term "abstract attitude," which I shall use in describing this capacity, will be more comprehensible in the light of the following explanation (9). We can distinguish two different kinds of attitudes, the concrete and the abstract. In the concrete attitude we are given over passively and bound to the immediate experience of unique objects or situations. Our thinking and acting are determined by the immediate claims made by the particular aspect of the object or situation. For instance, we act concretely when we enter a room in darkness and push the button for light. If, however, we reflect that by pushing the button we might awaken someone asleep in the room, and desist from pushing the button, then we are acting abstractively. We transcend the immediately given specific aspect of sense impressions; we detach ourselves from these impressions, consider the situation from a conceptual point of view, and react accordingly. Our actions are determined not so much by the objects before us as by the way we think about them: the individual thing becomes a mere accidental representative of a category to which it belongs.

The impairment of the attitude toward the abstract shows in every performance of the brain-damaged patient who is impaired in this capacity. He always fails when the solution of a task presupposes this attitude; he performs well when the appropriate activity is determined directly by the stimuli and when the task can be fulfilled by concrete behavior. He may have no difficulty in using known objects in a situation that requires them; but he is totally at a loss if he is asked to demonstrate the use of such an object outside the concrete situation, and still more so if he is asked to do it without the real object. A few examples will illustrate this:

The patient is asked to blow away a slip of paper. He does this very well. If the paper is taken away and he is asked to think that there is a slip of paper and to blow it away, he is unable to do so. Here the situation is not realistically complete. In order to perform the task the patient would have to imagine the piece of paper there. He is not capable of this.

The patient is asked to throw a ball into open boxes situated respectively at distances of three, nine, and fifteen feet. He does that correctly. When he is asked how far the several boxes are from him, he is not only unable to answer this question but unable even to say which box is nearest to him and which is farthest.

In the first action, the patient has only to deal with objects in a behavioral fashion. It is unnecessary for him to be conscious of this behavior and of objects in a world separated from himself. In the second, however, he must separate himself from objects in the outer world and give himself an account of his actions and of the space relations in the world facing him. Since he is unable to do this, he fails. We could describe this failure also by saying that the patient is unable to deal with a situation which is only possible.

A simple story is read to a patient. He may repeat some single words, but he does not understand their meaning and is unable to grasp the essential point. Now we read him another story, which would seem to a normal person to be more difficult to understand. This time he understands the meaning very well and recounts the chief points. The first story deals with a simple situation, but a situation which has no connection with the actual situation of the patient. The second story recounts a situation he is familiar with. Hence one could say the patient is able to grasp and handle only something which is related to himself.

Such a patient almost always recognizes pictures of single objects, even if the picture contains many details. In pictures which represent a composition of a number of things and persons, he may pick out some details; but he is unable to understand the picture as a whole and is unable to respond to the whole. The patient's real understanding does not depend on the greater or smaller number of components in a picture but on whether the components, whatever their number, hang together concretely and are familiar to him, or whether an understanding of their connection requires a more abstract synthesis on his part. He may lack understanding of a picture even if there are only a few details. If the picture does not reveal its essence directly, by bringing the patient into the situation which it represents, he is not able to understand it. Thus one may characterize the deficiency as an inability to discover the essence of a situation which is not related to his own personality.

Memory and attention

This change in behavior finds its expression in characteristic changes in memory and attention. Under certain circumstances the faculty for reproduction of facts acquired previously may be about normal. For example, things learned in school may be recalled very well, but only in some situations. The situation must be suited to reawakening old impressions. If the required answer demands an abstract attitude on the part of a patient or if it demands that he give an account of the matter in question, the patient is unable to remember. Therefore he fails in many intelligence tests which may seem very simple for a normal person, and he is amazingly successful in others which appear complicated to us. He is able to learn new facts and to keep them in mind; but he can learn them only in a concrete situation and can reproduce them only in the same situation in which he has learned them. Because the intentional recollection of experiences acquired in infancy requires an abstract attitude toward the situation at that time, the patient is unable to recall infancy experiences in a voluntary way; but we can observe that the after-effect of such experiences sometimes appears passively in his behavior. Such a patient has the greatest difficulty in associating freely; he cannot assume the attitude of mind to make that possible. He is incapable of recollection when he is asked to recall things which have nothing to do with the given situation. The patient must be able to regard the present situation in such a way that facts from the past belong to it. If this is not the case, he is completely unable to recall facts which he has recalled very well in another situation. Repeated observation in many different situations demonstrates clearly that such memory failures are not caused by an impairment of memory content. The patient has the material in his memory, but he is unable to use it freely; he can use it only in connection with a definite concrete situation.

We arrive at the same result in testing attention. At one time the patient appears inattentive and distracted; at another time, he is attentive, even abnormally so. The patient's attention is usually weak in special examinations, particularly at the beginning before he has become aware of the real approach to the whole situation. In such a situation he ordinarily seems much distracted. If he is able to enter into the situation, however, his attention may be satisfactory; sometimes his reactions are even abnormally keen. Under these circumstances he may be totally untouched by other stimuli from the environment to which normal persons will unfailingly react. In some tests he will always seem distracted; for example, in those situations which demand a change of approach (a choice), he always seems distracted because he is incapable of making a choice. Consequently, it is not correct to speak of a change of attention in these patients in terms of plus or minus. The state of the patient's attention is but part of his total behavior and is to be understood only in connection with it.

Emotional responses

The same holds true if we observe the emotions of the patients. Usually they are considered emotionally dull and often they appear so, but it would not be correct to say simply that they are suffering from a diminution of emotions. The same patients can be dull under some conditions and very excited under others. This can be explained when we consider the patient's emotional behavior in relation to his entire behavior in a given situation. When he does not react emotionally in an adequate way, investigation reveals that he has not grasped the situation in such a way that emotion could arise. In fact, we might experience a similar lack of emotion through failing to grasp a situation. The patient may have grasped only one part of the situation—the part which can be grasped concretely—and this part may not give any reason for an emotional reaction. The lack of emotion appears to us inappropriate because we grasp with the abstract attitude the whole situation to which the emotional character is attached. This connection between the emotions and the total behavior becomes understandable when we consider that emotions are not simply related to particular experiences but are, as I have shown on another occasion (10), inherent aspects of behavior—part and parcel of behavior. No behavior is without emotion and what we call lack of emotion is a deviation from normal emotions corresponding to the deviation of behavior in general. From this point of view, one modification of reactions that is of particular interest in respect to the problem of emotions in general, becomes understandable. Often we see that a patient reacts either not at all or in an *abnormally quick manner*. The latter occurs particularly when the patient believes he has the correct answer to a problem. Although this behavior might seem to be the effect of a change in the time factor of his reactivity, it is rather the *effect of an emotional factor*—that is, it is the modification of his emotional feelings because of the impairment of his ability for abstraction—which in turn modifies the time reaction.

Pleasure and joy

These patients are always somewhat in danger of being in a catastrophic condition—which I shall discuss later—as a result of not being able to find the right solution to a problem put before them. They are often afraid that they may not be able to react correctly, and that they will be in a catastrophic condition. Therefore, when they believe they have the right answer, they answer as quickly as possible. Because of impairment of abstraction, they are not able to deliberate; they try to do what they can do as quickly as possible because every retardation increases the tension which they experience when they are not able to answer. The quick response is an effect of their *strong necessity to release tension*; they are forced to release tension because they cannot handle it any other way. They cannot bear anything that presupposes deliberation, considering the future, and so on, all of which are related to abstraction.

This difference in behavior between these patients and more normal people throws light on the nature of the *trend to release tension*. These patients must, so to speak, follow the "pleasure principle." This phenomenon is one *expression of the abnormal concreteness* which is a counterpart to the impairment of abstraction. The *trend to release tension appears to be an expression of pathology*—the effect of a protective mechanism to prevent catastrophic condition. To normal behavior belong deliberation and retardation; but in addition there is the ability to speed up an activity or a part of it to correspond to the requirements of the task, or at least part of the requirements, so that its performance guarantees self-realization. Sometimes the ability to bear tension and even to enjoy it are also a part of this normal behavior. In contrast, the patients that I am talking about are only able to experience the pleasure of release of tension; they never appear to enjoy anything—a fact which is often clearly revealed by the expression on their faces. This becomes understandable if we consider that immediate reality is transcended in any kind of joy and that joy is a capacity we owe to the abstract attitude, especially that part of it concerned with possibility. Thus brain-injured patients who are impaired in this attitude cannot experience joy. Experience with brain-injured patients teaches us that we have to distinguish between *pleasure by release of tension*, and the active *feeling of enjoyment* and freedom so characteristic of joy. Pleasure through release of tension is the agreeable feeling which we experience on returning to a state of equilibrium after it has been disturbed

—the passive feeling of being freed from distress. Pleasure lasts only a short time till a new situation stimulates new activity; we then try to get rid of the tension of the new situation which acts to shorten the span of pleasure. In contrast, we try to extend joy. This explains the different speeds of joy and pleasure. Because of the capacity for joy, we can experience the possibility of the indefinite continuation of a situation. The two emotions of joy and pleasure play essentially different roles in regard to self-realization; they belong to different performances or different parts of a performance; they belong to different moods. Pleasure may be a necessary state of respite. But it is a phenonenon of standstill; it is akin to death. It separates us from the world and the other individuals in it; it is equilibrium, quietness. In joy there is disequilibrium. But it is a productive disequilibrium, leading toward fruitful activity and a particular kind of self-realization. This difference in approach between the normal person and the brain-injured patient is mirrored in the essentially different behavior of the latter and the different world in which he lives. The different significance of the two emotional states in his total behavior is related to their time difference.

Edith Jacobson (11), in the outline of her paper presented to the Psychoanalytic Association, speaks about the speed factor in psychic discharge processes and comes to the conclusion that discharge is not the only process which produces pleasure—that we have to distinguish between different qualities of pleasure in terms of the slow rising and the quick falling of tension. That is very much in accordance with my conclusions derived from experience with brain-injured patients. If one distinguishes two forms of pleasure, one should, for clarity's sake, use different names for them; I think that my use of pleasure and joy fits the two experiences. But I would not like to call them both discharge processes: the one is a discharge process; the other one a very active phenomenon related to the highest form of mental activity—abstraction. From this it becomes clear why they have such an essentially different significance in the totality of performance: the one is an equalization process which prepares the organism for new activity; the other one is an activity of highest value for self-realization. They belong together just as in general equalization process and activity belong together. Therefore they cannot be understood as isolated phenomena.

The phenomenon of witticism

From this viewpoint of the emotions of brain-injured patients, the phenomenon of witticism appears in a new aspect. We can see that even though a patient makes witty remarks, he is not able to grasp the character of situations which produce humor in an average normal individual. Whether or not some situation appears humorous depends upon whether it can be grasped in a concrete way which is suited to producing the emotion of humor. In accordance with the impairment of his ability for abstraction, such a patient perceives many humorous pictures in a realistic way, which does not evoke the expected humor. But of course any of us who might at a given time perceive a humorous picture in a realistic way would respond similarly. On the other hand a patient may make a witty remark in relation to a situation which is not considered humorous by us, because he has experienced the situation in another way. Thus we should not speak of witticism as a special characteristic of these patients. It is but one expression of the change in their personality structure in the same way that their inability to understand jokes under other conditions expresses this change. Indeed, these patients are in general dull because of their limited experience, and their witticisms are superficial and shallow in comparison with those of normal people.

Friendship and love

The drive towards the release of tension, which I have already mentioned, is one of the causes of the strange behavior of these patients in friendship and love situations. They need close relationships to other people and they try to maintain such relationships at all cost; at the same time such relationships are easily terminated suddenly if the bearing of tension is necessary for the maintenance of the relationship.

The following example is illustrative: A patient of mine, Mr. A, was for years a close friend of another patient, Mr. X. One day Mr. X went to a movie with a third man. Mr. X did not take Mr. A along because Mr. A had seen the picture before and did not want to see it a second time. When Mr. X came back, my patient was in a state of great excitement and refused to speak to him. Mr. A could not be quieted by any explanations; he was told that his friend had not meant to offend him, and that the friendship had not changed, but these explanations made no impression. From that time on, Mr. A was the enemy of his old friend, Mr. X. He was only aware that his friend was the companion of another man, and he felt himself slighted. This experience produced a great tension in him. He regarded his friend as the cause of this bad condition and reacted to him in a way that is readily understandable in terms of his inability to bear tension and to put himself in the place of somebody else.

Another patient never seemed to be concerned about his family. He never spoke of his wife or children and was unresponsive when we questioned him about them. When we suggested to him that he should write to his family, he was utterly indifferent. He appeared to lack all feeling in this respect. At times he visited his home in another town, according to an established practice, and stayed there several days. We learned that while he was at home, he conducted himself in the same way that any man would in the bosom of his family. He was kind and affectionate to his wife and children and interested in their affairs insofar as his abilities would permit. Upon his return to the hospital from such a visit, he would smile in an embarrassed way and give evasive answers when he was asked about his family; he seemed utterly estranged from his home situation. Unquestionably the peculiar behavior of this man was not really the effect of deterioration of his character on the emotional and moral side; rather, his behavior was the result of the fact that he could not summon up the home situation when he was not actually there.

Lack of imagination, which is so apparent in this example, makes such patients incapable of experiencing any expectation of the future. This lack is apparent, for instance, in the behavior of a male patient toward a woman whom he later married (12). When he was with the girl, he seemed to behave in a friendly, affectionate way and to be very fond of the girl. But when he was separated from her, he did not care about her at all; he would not seek her out and certainly did not desire to have a love relationship with her. When he was questioned, his answers indicated that he did not even understand what sexual desire meant. But in addition he had forgotten about the girl. When he met her again and she spoke to him, he was able immediately to enter into the previous relation. He was as affectionate as before. When she induced him to go to bed with her and embraced him, he performed an apparently normal act of sexual intercourse with satisfaction for both. She had the feeling that he loved her. She became pregnant, and they were married.

Change in language

Of particular significance in these patients is the change in their language because of their lack of abstract attitude (13, p. 56). Their words lose the character of meaning. Words are not usable in those situations in which they must represent a concept. Therefore the patients are not able to find the proper words in such situations. Thus, for instance, patients are not able to name concrete objects, since as shown by investigation, naming presupposes an abstract attitude and the abstract use of words. These patients have not lost the sound complex; but they cannot use it as a sign for a concept. On other occasions, the sound complex may be uttered; but it is only used at those times as a simple association to a given object, as a property of the object, such as color and form, and not as representative of a concept. If a patient has been particularly gifted in language before his brain is damaged and has retained many such associations or can acquire associations as a substitute for naming something, then he may utter the right word through association, so that an observer is not able to distinguish between his uttering the sound complex and giving a name to something; only through analysis can one make this distinction (13, p. 61). Thus we can easily overlook the patient's defect by arriving at a conclusion only on the basis of this capacity for a positive effect. In the same way we can be deceived by a negative effect which may only be an expression, for instance, of the patient's fear that he will use the wrong word. I have used the term *fallacy of effect* to describe the uncertain and ambiguous character of a conclusion which is based only upon a patient's effective performance. This term applies not only to language but to all performances of the patients. It is the source of one of the most fatal mistakes which can be made in interpretation of phenomena observed in organic patients; incidentally, it is a mistake which can be made also in functional cases.

Frontal lobotomy

In reference to the fallacy of effect, I want to stress how easily one can be deceived about the mental condition of patients who have undergone frontal lobotomy. The results of the usual intelligence test, evaluated statistically, may not reveal any definite deviation from the norm; yet the patient can have an impairment of abstraction that will become obvious through tests which take into consideration the fallacy of effect.[1] My experience with frontal lobotomy patients and my evaluation of the literature on frontal lobotomy leave no doubt in my mind that at least many of these patients show impairment of abstract capacity, although perhaps not to such a degree as do patients with gross damage of the brain. Because of the fallacy of effect, which tends to overlook the defect in abstraction, the reports of the relatives that the lobotomized patient behaves well in everyday life are often evaluated incorrectly by the doctor (14). In the sheltered, simple life that these patients have with their families, the patients are not often confronted with tasks which require abstract reasoning; thus the family is likely to overlook their more subtle deviations from the norm. Sometimes peculiarities of the patient are reported which definitely point to a defect in abstraction, which is more serious than it is often evaluated: for instance, a patient who in general seems to live in a normal way does not have any relationship with even the closest members of his family and manifests no interest in his children; another patient exists in a vacuum so that no friendship is possible with him.

A woman patient after lobotomy still knows how to set a table for guests, and how to act as a perfect hostess. Before lobotomy, she was always a careful housewife, deciding everything down to the last detail; but now she does not care how the house is run, she never enters the kitchen, and the housekeeper does all the managing, even the shopping. She still reads a great number of books, but she does not understand the contents as well as before.

A skilled mechanic, who is still considered an excellent craftsman, is able to work in a routine way; but he has lost the ability to undertake complicated jobs, has stopped studying, and seems to have resigned himself to being a routine worker; apparently all this is an effect of the loss of his capacity for abstraction, which is so necessary for all initiative and for creative endeavor. Thus we see that even when the behavior of the patients appears not to be overtly disturbed, it differs essentially from normal behavior—in the particular way which is characteristic of impairment in abstract attitude. Freeman (15), who was originally so enthusiastically in favor of the operation, has become more cautious about its damage to the higher mental functions. He writes:

> The patients with frontal lobotomy show always some lack of personality depth; impulse, intelligence, temperament are disturbed;

[1] Thirty years ago we constructed special tests when we were faced with the problem of re-educating brain-injured soldiers. (See K. Goldstein and A. Gelb, "Uber Farbennamenamnesie," *Psychol. Forsch.* [1924] 6:127.) These tests, which were introduced in America by Scheerer and myself (reference 9), proved to be particularly useful not only for studying the problem of abstraction in patients, but also for the correct organization of treatment.

> the creative capacity undergoes reduction—the spiritual life in general was affected. They are largely indifferent to the opinions and feelings of others.

He apparently discovered the same personality changes in his patients as those which we have described as characteristic of the behavior of patients with impaired capacity for abstraction. Thus we should be very careful in judging personality change following frontal lobotomy. Although I would not deny the usefulness of the operation in some cases, I would like to say, as I have before, that the possibility of an impairment of abstraction should always be taken into consideration before the operation is undertaken.

I would now like to present a survey of the various situations in which the patient is unable to perform. He fails when he has: (1) to assume a mental set voluntarily or to take initiative (for instance, he may even be able to perform well in giving a series of numbers, once someone else has presented the first number, but he cannot begin the activity); (2) to shift voluntarily from one aspect of a situation to another, making a choice; (3) to account to himself for his actions or to verbalize the account; (4) to keep in mind simultaneously various aspects of a situation or to react to two stimuli which do not belong intrinsically together; (5) to grasp the essence of a given whole, or to break up a given whole into parts, isolating the parts voluntarily and combining them into wholes; (6) to abstract common properties, to plan ahead ideationally, to assume an attitude toward a situation which is only possible, and to think or perform symbolically; (7) to do something which necessitates detaching the ego from the outer world or from inner experiences.

All these and other terms which one may use to describe the behavior of the patients basically mean the same. We speak usually, in brief, of an *impairment of abstract attitude*. I hope that it has become clear that the use of this term does not refer to a theoretical interpretation but to the real behavior of the human being and that it is suitable for describing both normal and pathological personality.

In brief, the patients are changed with respect to the most characteristic properties of the human being. They have lost initiative and the capacity to look forward to something and to make plans and decisions; they lack phantasy and inspiration; their perceptions, thoughts, and ideas are reduced; they have lost the capacity for real contact with others, and they are therefore incapable of real friendship, love, and social relations. One could say they have no real ego and no real world. That they behave in an abnormally concrete way and that they are driven to get rid of tensions are only expressions of the same defect. When such patients are able to complete a task in a concrete way, they may—with regard to the effect of their activity—not appear very abnormal. But closer examination shows that they are abnormally rigid, stereotyped, and compulsive, and abnormally bound to stimuli from without and within.

To avoid any misunderstanding, I would like to stress that the defect in patients with brain damage does not always have to manifest itself in the same way—not even in all frontal lobe lesions. To what degree impairment of abstraction appears depends upon the extensiveness, the intensity, and the nature of the lesion. To evaluate the relationship between a patient's behavior and his defect, we have to consider further that personal experience plays a role in determining whether a patient can solve a problem or not. One patient reacts well—at least at face value—when he is given a task, although another patient has failed the same task; to the first patient the task represents a concrete situation; for the second patient it is an abstract situation. But in both cases, the defect will always be revealed by further examination.

Catastrophic Conditions

Impairment of abstraction is not the only factor which produces deviations in the behavior of patients, as I have stated before. Another very important factor is the occurrence of a catastrophic condition (4, pp. 35 ff). When a patient is not able to fulfill a task set before him, this condition is a frequent occurrence. A patient may look animated, calm, in a good mood, well-poised, collected, and cooperative when he is confronted with tasks he can fulfill; the same patient may appear dazed, become agitated, change color, start to fumble, become unfriendly, evasive, and even aggressive when he is not able to fulfill the task. His overt behavior appears very much the same as a person in a state of anxiety. I have called the state of the patient in the situation of success, *ordered condition*; the state in the situation of failure, *disordered or catastrophic condition.*

In the catastrophic condition the patient not only is incapable of performing a task which exceeds his impaired capacity, but he also fails, for a longer or shorter period, in performances which he is able to carry out in the ordered state. For a varying period of time, the organism's reactions are in great disorder or are impeded altogether. We are able to study this condition particularly well in these patients, since we can produce it experimentally by demanding from the patient something which we know he will not be able to do, because of his defect. Now, as we have said, impairment of abstractions makes it impossible for a patient to account to himself for his acts. He is quite unable to realize his failure and why he fails. Thus we can assume that catastrophic condition is not a reaction of the patient to failure, but rather belongs intrinsically to the situation of the organism in failing. For the normal person, failure in the performance of a nonimportant task would be merely something disagreeable; for the brain-injured person, however, as observation shows, any failure means the impossibility of self-realization and of existence. The occurrence of catastrophic condition is not limited therefore to special tasks; any task can place the patient in this situation, since the patient's self-realization is endangered so easily. Thus the same task produces anxiety at one time, and not at another.

Anxiety

The conditions under which anxiety occurs in brain-injured patients correspond to the conditions for its occurrence in normal people in that what produces anxiety is not the failure itself, but the resultant danger to the person's existence. I would like to add that the danger need not always be real; it is sufficient if the person imagines that the condition is such that he will not be able to realize himself. For instance, a person may be in distress because he is not able to answer questions in an examination. If the outcome of the examination is not particularly important, then the normal person will take it calmly even though he may feel somewhat upset; because it is not a dangerous situation for him, he will face the situation and try to come to terms with it as well as he can by using his wits, and in this way he will bring it to a more or less successful solution. The situation becomes totally different, however, if passing the examination is of great consequence in the person's life; not passing the examination may, for instance, endanger his professional career or the possibility of marrying the person he loves. When self-realization is seriously in danger, catastrophe may occur together with severe anxiety; when this occurs, it is impossible for the person to answer even those questions which, under other circumstances, he could solve without difficulty.

I would like to clarify one point here—namely, that anxiety represents an emotional state which does not refer to any object. Certainly the occurrence of anxiety is connected with an outer or inner event. The organism, shaken by a catastrophic shock, exists in relation to a definitive reality; and the basic phenomenon of anxiety, which is the occurrence of disordered behavior, is understandable only in terms of this relationship to reality. But anxiety does not originate from the experiencing of this relationship. The brain-injured patient could not experience anxiety, if it were necessary for him to experience this relationship to reality. He is certainly not aware of this objective reality; he experiences only the shock, only anxiety. And this, of course holds true for anxiety in general. Observations of many patients confirm the interpretation of anxiety by philosophers, such as Pascal and Kierkegaard, and by psychologists who have dealt with anxiety—namely, that the source of anxiety is the inner experience of not being confronted with anything or of being confronted with nothingness.

In making such a statement, one must distinguish sharply between *anxiety* and *fear*—another emotional state which is very often confused with anxiety (4, p. 293; 16). Superficially, fear may have many of the characteristics of anxiety, but intrinsically it is different. In the state of fear we have an object before us, we can meet that object, we can attempt to remove it, or we can flee from it. We are conscious of ourselves, as well as of the object: we can deliberate as to how we shall behave toward it, and we can look at the cause of the fear, which actually lies before us. Anxiety, on the other hand, gets at us from the back, so to speak. The only thing we can do is to attempt to flee from it, but without knowing what direction to take, since we experience it as coming from no particular place. We are dealing, as I have shown explicitly elsewhere, with qualitative differences, with different attitudes toward the world. Fear is related, in our experience, to an object; anxiety is not—it is only an inner state.

What is characteristic of the object of fear? Is it something inherent in the object itself, at all times? Of course not. At one time an object may arouse only interest, or be met with indifference; but at another time it may evoke the greatest fear. In other words, fear must be the result of a specific relationship between organism and object. What leads to fear is nothing but the experience of the possibility of the onset of anxiety. What we fear is the impending anxiety, which we experience in relation to some objects. Since a person in a state of fear is not yet in a state of anxiety but only envisions it—that is, he only fears that anxiety may befall him—he is not so disturbed in his judgment of the outer world as the person in a state of anxiety. Rather, driven as he is by the tendency to avoid the onset of anxiety, he attempts to establish special contact with the outer world. He tries to recognize the situation as clearly as possible and to react to it in an appropriate manner. Fear is conditioned by, and directed against, very definite aspects of the environment. These have to be recognized and, if possible, removed. Fear sharpens the senses, whereas anxiety renders them unusable. Fear drives to action; anxiety paralyzes.

From these explanations it is obvious that in order to feel anxiety it is not necessary to be able to give oneself an account of one's acts; to feel fear, however, presupposes that capacity. From this it becomes clear that our patients do not behave like people in a state of fear— that is, they do not intentionally try to avoid situations from which anxiety may arise. They cannot do that because of the defect of abstraction. Also from our observation of the patients we can assume that they do not experience fear and that they only have the experience of anxiety.

Anxiety, a catastrophic condition in which self-realization is not possible, may be produced by a variety of events, all of which have in common the following: There is a discrepancy between the individual's capacities and the demands made on him, and this discrepancy makes self-realization impossible. This may be due to external or internal conditions, physical or psychological. It is this discrepancy to which we are referring when we speak of "conflicts." Thus we can observe anxiety in infants, in whom such a discrepancy must occur frequently, particularly since their abstract attitude is not yet developed, or not fully. We also see anxiety in brain-injured people, in whom impairment of abstraction produces the same discrepancy. In normal people, anxiety appears when the demands of the world are too much above the capacity of the individual, when social and economic situations are too stressful, or when religious conflicts arise. Finally we see anxiety in people with neuroses and psychoses which are based on unsolvable and unbearable inner conflicts.

The Protective Mechanisms

The last group of symptoms to be observed in brain-injured patients are the behavior changes which make it possible for the patient to get rid of the catastrophic condition—of anxiety (4, pp. 40 ff.). The observation of this phenomenon in these patients is of special interest since it can teach us how an organism can get rid of anxiety without being aware of its origin and without being able to avoid the anxiety voluntarily. After a certain time these patients show a diminution of disorder and of catastrophic reactions (anxiety) even though the defect caused by the damage to the brain still exists. This, of course, can occur only if the patient is no longer exposed to tasks he cannot cope with. This diminution is achieved by definite changes in the behavior of the patients: They are withdrawn, so that a number of stimuli, including dangerous ones, do not reach them. They usually stay alone; either they do not like company or they want to be only with people whom they know well. They like to be in a familiar room in which everything is organized in a definite way. They show extreme orderliness in every respect; everything has to be done exactly at an appointed time— whether it is breakfast, dinner, or a walk. They show excessive and fanatical orderliness in arranging their belongings; each item of their wardrobe must be in a definite place—that is, in a place where it can be gotton hold of quickly, without the necessity of a choice, which they are unable to make. Although it is a very primitive order indeed, they stick fanatically to it; it is the only way to exist. Any change results in a state of very great excitement. They themselves cannot voluntarily arrange things in a definite way. The orderliness is maintained simply because the patients try to stick to those arrangements which they can handle. This sticking to that which they can cope with is characteristic for their behavior; thus any behavior change can be understood only in terms of this characteristic behavior.

An illustration of this characteristic behavior is the fact that they always try to keep themselves busy with things that they are able to do as a protection against things that they cannot cope with. The activities which engross them need not be of great value in themselves. Their usefulness consists apparently in the fact that they protect the patient. Thus a patient does not like to be interrupted in an activity. For instance, although a patient may behave well in a conversation with someone he knows and likes, he does not like to be suddenly addressed by someone else.

We very often observe that a patient is totally unaware of his defect—such as hemiplegia or hemianopsia—and of the difference between his state prior to the development of the symptoms and his present state. This is strikingly illustrated by the fact that the disturbances of these patients play a very small part in their complaints. We are not dealing simply with a subjective lack of awareness, for the defects are effectively excluded from awareness, one might say. This is shown by the fact that they produce very little disturbance—apparently as the result of compensation. This exclusion from awareness seems to occur particularly when the degree of functional defect in performance is extreme. We can say that defects are shut out from the life of the organism when they would seriously impair any of its essential functions and when a defect can be compensated for by other activities at least to the extent that self-realization is not essentially disturbed.

One can easily get the impression that a patient tries to deny the experience of the functional disturbance because he is afraid that he will get into a catastrophic condition if he becomes aware of his defect. As a matter of fact, a patient may get into a catastrophic condition when we make him aware of his defect, or when the particular situation does not make possible an adequate compensation. Sometimes this happens—and this is especially interesting—when the underlying pathological condition improves and with that the function.

A patient of mine who became totally blind by a suicidal gunshot through the chiasma opticum behaved as if he were not aware of his blindness; the defect was compensated for very well by his use of his other senses, his motor skill, and his knowledge and intelligence. He was usually in a good mood; he never spoke of his defect, and he resisted all attempts to draw his attention to it. After a certain time, the condition improved; but at the same time he realized that he could not recognize objects through his vision. He was shocked and became deeply depressed. When he was asked why he was depressed, he said, "I cannot see." We might assume that in the beginning the patient denied the defect intentionally because he could not bear it. But why then did he not deny it when he began to see? Or we might assume that in the beginning he did not deny his blindness, but that in total blindness an adjustment occurred in terms of a change of behavior for which vision was not necessary; and because of this it was not necessary for him to realize his blindness. The moment he was able to see, he became aware of his defect and was no longer able to eliminate it. The exclusion of the blindness defect from awareness could thus be considered a secondary effect of the adjustment. But in this patient who was mentally undisturbed a more voluntary denial cannot be overlooked. A voluntary denial is not possible in patients with impairment of abstraction as in brain-injured patients. Here the unawareness of the defect can only be a secondary effect—an effect of the same behavior, which we have described before, by which the brain-injured person is protected against catastrophes which may occur because of his defect. As we have said, the patient, driven by the trend to realize himself as well as possible, sticks to what he is able to do; this shows in his whole behavior. From this point of view, the patient's lack of awareness of his defect, as well as his peculiarities in general, becomes understandable. For instance, in these terms, it is understandable why an aphasic patient utters a word which is only on the normal fringe of the word that he needs; for the word that he needs to use is a word that he cannot say at all or can say only in such a way that he could not be understood and would as a result be in distress (13, p. 226). Thus a patient may repeat "church" instead of "God," "father" instead of "mother," and so on; he considers his reaction correct, at least as long as no one makes him aware of the fact that his reaction is wrong. This same kind of reaction occurs in disturbances of recognition, of feelings, and so on.

One is inclined to consider the use of wrong words or disturbances of recognition, actions, and feelings as due to a special pathology; but that is not their origin. Since these disturbances are reactions which represent all that the individual is able to execute, he recognizes them as fulfillment of the task; in this way, these reactions fulfill this need to such a degree that no catastrophe occurs.

Thus the protection appears as a passive effect of an active "correct" procedure and could not be correctly termed denial, which refers to a more intentional activity, "conscious" or "unconscious."

This theory on the origin of the protective behavior in organic patients deserves consideration, particularly because the phenomena observed in organic patients show such a similarity to that observed in neurotics. One could even use psychoanalytic terms for the different forms of behavior in organic patients. For instance, one might use the same terms that Anna Freud (17) uses to characterize various defense mechanisms against anxiety. Both neurotic and organic patients show a definite similarity in behavior structure and in the purpose served by that structure. In organic patients, however, I prefer to speak of protective mechanisms instead of defense mechanisms; the latter refers to a more voluntary act, which organic patients certainly cannot perform, as we have discussed earlier. In neurotics, the development of defense mechanisms generally does not occur so passively through organismic adjustment, as does the development of protective mechanisms in the organic patients; this is in general the distinction between the two. It seems to me that this distinction is not true in the case of neurotic children, however; some of these children seem to develop protective mechanisms in a passive way, similar to organic patients. Such mechanisms can perhaps be found in other neurotics. Thus, in interpreting these mechanisms, one should take into account the possibility of confusing the neurotic patient with the organic patient.

I would like to add a last word with regard to the restrictions of the personality and of the world of these patients which is brought about by this protective behavior. The restrictions are not as disturbing in the brain-injured patients as is the effect of defense mechanisms in neuroses. In a neurotic, defense mechanisms represent a characteristic part of the disturbances he is suffering from; but the organic patient does not become aware of the restriction since his protective mechanisms allow for some ordered form of behavior and for the experience of some kind of self-realization—which is true, of course, only as long as the environment is so organized by the people around him that no tasks arise that he cannot fulfill and as long as the protecting behavior changes are not hindered. This is the only way the brain-damaged person can exist. The patient cannot bear conflict—that is, anxiety, restriction, or suffering. In this respect he differs essentially from the neurotic who is more or less able to bear conflict. This is the main difference which demands a different procedure in treatment; in many respects, however, treatment can be set up in much the same way for both (18). In treating these patients, it is more important to deal with the possible occurrence of catastrophe rather than with the impairment of abstraction, for my observations of a great many patients for over ten years indicate that the impairment of abstraction cannot be alleviated unless the brain damage from which it originated is eliminated. There is no functional restitution of this capacity by compensation through other parts of the brain. Improvement of performances can be achieved only by the building up of substitute performances by the use of the part of concrete behavior which is preserved; but this is only possible by a definite arrangement of the environment.

I am well aware that my description of the personality change in brain damage is somewhat sketchy. The immense material and the problems involved, so manifold and complex, make a more satisfactory presentation in such a brief time impossible. I hope that I have been successful in outlining, to the best of my ability, the essential phenomena and problems of these patients. In addition, I trust that I have shown how much we can learn from these observations for our concept of the structure of the personality, both normal and pathological, and for the treatment of brain-damaged patients and also, I hope, of patients with so-called psychogenic disorders.

References

1. GOLDSTEIN, K. (1924). Ueber die gleichartige functionelle bedingtheit der symptome in organischen und psychischen krankheiten. *Montschr. f. Psychiat. u. Neurol.*, **57**, 191.
2. GOLDSTEIN, K. (1927). Die beziehungen der psychoanalyse zue biologie, in *Verhandlungen d. congresses für psychotherapie in nauheim.* Leipzig: Hirzel.
3. GOLDSTEIN, K. (1942). *Aftereffects of Brain Injuries in War.* New York: Grune & Stratton.
4. GOLDSTEIN, K. (1939). *The Organism: A Holistic Approach to Biology.* New York: American Book Co.
5. GOLDSTEIN, K. (1940). *Human Nature in the Light of Psychopathology.* Cambridge: Harvard Univ. Press, p. 194.
6. GOLDSTEIN, K. (1927). *Handbuch der normalen und pathologischen physiologie.* Berlin: J. S. Springer. Volume 10, pp. 600 ff. and 813.
7. GOLDSTEIN, K. (1936). The significance of the frontal lobes for mental performances. *J. Neurol. & Psychopathol.*, **17**, 27–40.
8. GOLDSTEIN, K. (1936). The modifications of behavior consequent to cerebral lesions. *Psychiat. Quart.*, **10**, 586.
9. GOLDSTEIN, K., & SCHEERER, M. (1941). *Abstract and concrete behavior.* Psychol. Monogr. No. 239.
10. GOLDSTEIN, K. (1951). On emotions: considerations from the organismic point of view. *J. Psychol.*, **31**, 37–49.
11. JACOBSON, EDITH. (1952). The speed pace in psychic discharge processes and its influence on the pleasure-unpleasure qualities of affects. Paper read before the American Psychoanalytic Association, May.
12. GOLDSTEIN, K., & STEINFELD, J. I. (1942). The conditioning of sexual behavior by visual agnosia. *Bull. Forest Sanit.*, **1**, 2, 37–45.
13. GOLDSTEIN, K. (1948). *Language and Language Disturbances.* New York: Grune & Stratton.
14. GOLDSTEIN, K. (1949). Frontal lobotomy and impairment of abstract attitude. *J. Nerv. & Ment. Dis.*, **110**, 93–111.
15. FREEMAN, W., & WATTS, J. (1950). *Psychosurgery*, 2nd ed. Springfield, Ill.: Thomas.
16. GOLDSTEIN, K. (1929). Zum problem der angst. *Allg. ärztl. Ztscher. f. Psychotherap. u. psych. Hygiene*, **2**, 409–437.
17. FREUD, A. (1946). *The Ego and the Mechanisms of Defense.* New York: Internat. Univ. Press.
18. GOLDSTEIN, K. (1949). The idea of disease and therapy. *Rev. Religion*, **14**, 229–240.

5 Personality Disorders

The diagnosis of personality disorder is rapidly becoming the most popular available label in the out-patient situation, and by virtue of this is losing a good deal of meaning. Just as it was once popular to call any behavioral peculiarity "neurotic," more sophisticated individuals now point to these difficulties as personality or character problems. At one time this label was reserved for individuals with behavior problems that led them into difficulties with the law. The diagnostic category that is now used in such a case is sociopathic personality disturbance. Currently, references to personality disorders are more widely used to describe individuals technically diagnosed as personality trait disturbance or personality pattern disturbance. The common feature that cuts across these categories is that the individuals have developed a way of life that creates disharmony in their personal relationships. Instead of placing emphasis on their symptoms or on their subjective discomfort, the focus is on how they get along with others, and in this we usually find some inadequacy, although the patient may not always recognize it as such and often does not recognize his role in disrupting his relationships.

BERNARD C. GLUECK, Jr.

Psychodynamic Patterns in the Sex Offender

Some forms of pathological behavior are particularly abhorrent to society. Sexual offenses are among these. They draw strong, angry reactions from both lay and professional people. As a result, certain stereotypes (generally uncomplimentary and

Abridged from *Psychiatric Quarterly*, **28** (1954), 1–21, with the permission of State Hospitals Press, Utica, N. Y., and Dr. Glueck.

pessimistic) about such offenders tend to be built up; these apply to both their superficial personality and to the prognosis for their future behavior. These stereotypes are often preserved because they help to perpetuate, or do little to contradict, the strong feelings stirred up by such odious actions. Glueck has had the opportunity to observe large numbers of individuals convicted of serious sexual crimes and incarcerated in Sing Sing Prison. In this paper, he presents both the typical stereotype of the sexual psychopath and a discussion of the degree to which the group that he observed conformed or failed to conform to that image.

This paper has been abridged by eliminating some case examples that the author presented. Readers interested in this material should consult the original paper.

Of the many problems that plague our society, that of the sex offender is one of the most disturbing. Society reacts with greater fear, disgust, hysteria and anger to only one other crime, murder. Many explanations can be advanced for this intense emotional reaction, depending upon the particular frame of reference of the individual giving the interpretation. Thus we may have religious, moralistic, philosophical, sociological and psychological explanations, among others. In the course of the last 60 years, largely as a result of the pioneer efforts of Sigmund Freud, and those who followed the trail he blazed, a new approach to the age-old problem of understanding human behavior has been developed, the science of psychodynamics. This is the particular frame of reference for the present remarks.

In the years immediately following World War II, an increasing concern by society about the activities of "sex offenders," spotlighted by a furor in the press over "the depraved machinations of sex fiends," culminated in the establishment in New York State, among others, of a research project under the joint auspices of the commissioners of Correction and Mental Hygiene. Its purpose was to be "the development of information as to the underlying causes of sex crimes and the development of treatment for persons committing such crimes."

The raw material for this research was the group of men incarcerated at Sing Sing Prison, who had been convicted of sex felonies. Included in this group of felonies are: first and second degree rape, first and second degree sodomy, carnal abuse of a child under 10 years, carnal abuse of a minor between 10 and 16—if a second offense, and assault in the second degree with intent to rape, sodomize or carnally abuse. The lesser sexual offenses such as exhibitionism, voyeurism and statutory rape, are not considered felonies, so that men convicted of these offenses are not sentenced to Sing Sing Prison. This selective process has a very important bearing on the statistics gathered by the research group, since only the more serious sex offenses are represented in the men studied. This may account, at least in part, for the marked psychopathology found in the group.

In March 1950, a preliminary report (1) was issued on 102 men who had been studied up to that time. The general conclusions reached included a statement that every man studied suffered from some type of mental or emotional disorder, though not usually so pronounced as to meet the legal definition of mental illness. They were not, in other words, sufficiently psychotic to be certifiable. Additional information on the same men—coming from further psychiatric observation, psychological studies, and the changes in their adjustment to prison, or in a few cases, to parole—as well as information on new cases, confirm the psychopathology present in this group. The major question, at the present writing, is not: Does pathology exist? Instead, we are primarily concerned with an attempt at quantification of the pathology and the development of some kind of adequate diagnostic system which will reflect the psychodynamic aspects of each case, and give a more accurate description of the phenomena observed than the present diagnoses permit. It is unnecessary to stress the benefits from more accurate diagnosis. To mention only two points: There would be improved statistical reporting; and there are possible therapeutic and prognostic implications stemming from a given diagnosis. The last point has an added importance in dealing with psychiatric problems because of the rather divergent attitudes of the extremists who favor either psychotherapy or organic therapy as mutually exclusive techniques, and because of the rather nihilistic attitude of many psychiatrists where the diagnosis of schizophrenia is concerned.

Unquestionably, in the light of present therapeutic results, one tends to be somewhat pessimistic regarding the outcome when a diagnosis of schizophrenia or psychopathic personality is made. There is, however, sufficient evidence available, in the form of well-documented statistics collected over long periods, indicating a basic 30 to 35 per cent remission rate in schizophrenia, regardless of the type of psychosis or kind of treatment. We can, therefore, expect one out of every three schizophrenics to have a remission, even though nothing is done in terms of specific therapy. Furthermore the remission rate can be improved, if only for relatively short periods, by the various therapeutic approaches currently available. The writer is, therefore, of the opinion that the argument against making a diagnosis of schizophrenia, on the grounds of the "death sentence" implications of such a diagnosis, no longer applies, and should not influence decisions about diagnosis. Of even greater importance in forensic psychiatry, is the effect of the diagnosis, when made before trial or sentencing, on the disposition of the particular case.

The present legal interpretations of the terms "sane" and "insane" have been repeatedly challenged by both lawyers and psychiatrists, as being totally inadequate in the light of modern concepts of psychopathology and psychodynamics. The concern of the courts still centers, for the most part, around the need to punish the offender, and the fear that a plea of insanity will protect the "guilty" individual from the just retribution that society demands.

The discovery of extensive pathology in every individual studied by the research group has already been mentioned. All of the men in the first group of 102, covered in the research project's first report were, in spite of clear-cut clinical evidence of psychosis in several cases, and very suspicious symptoms in over half of the group, diagnosed as being without psychosis when examined psychiatrically before trial or sentencing. The same failure to detect overt psychotic symptoms and behavior has been apparent in many of the additional cases studied in the past three years. This has been true in both groups, those entering the prison under the usual short-term definite sentence, and those entering under provisions of the new, indeterminate-sentence law. Failure to establish an accurate diagnosis is especially disturbing in the second group of cases, since one of the provisions of the law is that, "No person convicted of a crime punishable in the discretion of the court with imprisonment for an indeterminate term, having a minimum of one day and a maximum of his natural life, shall be sentenced until a psychiatric examination shall have been made of him and a complete written report thereof shall have been submitted to the court." This examination is made according to certain paragraphs of the code of criminal procedure and involves observation and examination by two qualified psychiatrists.

In spite of these provisions, four men out of 46 who were received at Sing Sing Prison under the new law have been committed to Dannemora State Hospital with overt psychoses. Two of the four were committed within 60 days of reception at Sing Sing, and were held for that interval only to obtain a psychiatric appraisal for the research studies. A fifth individual was suspected of being feebleminded because of his general behavior in the prison community. On psychological testing he was found to have an IQ in the 60's and was committed to the state institution for defective delinquents.

How then can one explain the discrepancies between the pre-trial examination of these men, and the research findings, frequently within one or two weeks? One explanation can be considered and discarded in the same breath; that is the competence of the psychiatrists doing the examinations on these men. They are, for the most part, men of considerable clinical experience, especially in the rapid evaluation of patients hospitalized for psychiatric observation as potential psychotics. In many of the cases studied one finds, in the record, a rather extensive description of symptoms indicative of psychopathological processes, including statements about ideas of reference, persecutory ideas, extreme emotional lability and defective judgement; and yet the diagnosis of a psychotic illness, specifically schizophrenia, is avoided, and the individual is diagnosed as a psychopathic personality, a sexual psychopath, a psychopath with sexual perversions, and so forth. The writer believes that the critical factors influencing the judgement of these psychiatrists are three-fold: first, the patient's antisocial behavior, the fact that he has been indicted for a felony; second, stemming directly from the first, the concern that society, as represented by the prosecution and the court, will complain that the offender is being "protected medically" from receiving proper punishment if a diagnosis of psychosis is made; third, and here one treads on dangerous ground, the psychiatrist's own unconscious reaction to the sexual character of the felony, which may motivate him toward punishment rather than treatment in such a case.

In the writer's opening remarks, he indicated the horror, resentment, anger, fear and demand for retribution that make up society's response to a sexual offense. The reasons for this reaction cannot be gone into in this paper. But the writer does raise the question, on the basis of the psychiatric and psychological appraisals of the sex offenders studied at Sing Sing, of whether punishment is the optimum answer to this problem, or of whether a therapeutically-oriented program would not be preferable. Before arguing the pros and cons of this question, let us consider further the diagnostic problem in these cases.

If these men are psychopathic personalities, sexual or otherwise, they should show specific psychopathological characteristics that are the criteria for diagnosing this condition. In one of the widely-quoted books on the psychopath, Cleckley's *The Mask of Sanity* (2), the characteristics of this type of individual are given as follows, "Superficial charm and good intelligence, absence of delusions and other signs of emotional 'thinking,' absence of 'nervousness' or psychoneurotic manifestations, unreliability, untruthfulness and insincerity, lack of remorse or shame, inadequately motivated antisocial behavior, poor judgment and failure to learn by experience, pathologic egocentricity and incapacity for love, general poverty in major affective reactions, specific loss of insight, unresponsiveness in general interpersonal relations, fantastic and uninviting behavior, with drink and sometimes without, suicide rarely carried out, sex life impersonal, trivial, and poorly integrated, and lastly, failure to follow any life plan." Let us consider these 16 points, one by one, and see whether they fit the data collected from over 200 sex offenders during the course of the project's investigations.

SUPERFICIAL CHARM AND GOOD INTELLIGENCE. The test scores of intelligence in the research project cases range from the middle 60's—four men were transferred to the institution for defective delinquents—to a high of 140, with the mean being slightly over 100. This would indicate that the sex offenders have the same intelligence spread as the general population, and do not fall into a high or low group. They are, however, anything but a charming group, even superficially. Many have definite physical deformities, and they all show marked social awkwardness, stemming from their withdrawn, isolated personality patterns.

ABSENCE OF DELUSIONS AND OTHER SIGNS OF IRRATIONAL THINKING. The men studied do have the ability to cover up ideas and experiences that they have learned are not acceptable when related to their families, friends or others. The distortions in their perception of reality may be very subtle, requiring close contact with the inmate, over a considerable time, to detect. These perceptive disturbances can also be elicited, and this is particularly useful if the subject is trying to cover up, by the use of projective techniques, such as the TAT and the Rorschach examinations. It is the initial perceptive distortions, magnified and further altered by the disturbances of mood and affect, that in many instances lead to the antisocial sexual act; e.g., in the second case, B. relates his discouragement with women, their unreliability, and his lack of satisfaction from contact with them. In the light of his reality situation these would appear to be definite perceptual and reasoning distortions. Cleckley also speaks of the absence of valid depression. About 70 per cent of the cases in this study show mild to severe depression, with some expressing suicidal ideas.

ABSENCE OF "NERVOUSNESS" OR PSYCHONEUROTIC MANIFESTATIONS. The absence of anxiety and tension in the psychopath has been stressed repeatedly. In contrast, the writer has found moderate to severe anxiety in 90 per cent of the project cases, with little or no anxiety appearing only in those individuals with overt psychoses or marked organic cerebral impairment.

UNRELIABILITY. While this is the hallmark of the psychopath, particularly when subjected to the slightest pressure in the form of frustrations of obligations to perform, the opposite is true for the Sing Sing cases. The majority of these men are considered steady, reliable, even compulsive workers, especially in the older age groups, with the exception of their sexual behavior; and, in many of the cases studied, their difficulties with alcohol.

UNTRUTHFULNESS AND INSINCERITY. These qualities are extremely difficult to evaluate in individuals being studied in a prison setting, especially when they feel that their chances for parole may be influenced or determined by the information given to the investigator, a conviction that persists in spite of all reassurances to the contrary. Unquestionably, many of the men studied "put the best foot forward," in that they withold information rather than concoct deliberate falsehoods. There is, however, a sizable group who persistently deny their guilt, in the face of overwhelming evidence in probation records and admissions of guilt at the time of arrest. These are, however, the more seriously-disturbed individuals, largely those with paranoid personality patterns, rather than the typical glib and very plausible psychopath.

LACK OF REMORSE OR SHAME. The amount of depression and guilt, already referred to, in the Sing Sing cases would indicate considerable shame and remorse as a consequence of the antisocial acts. While direct expressions of shame are obtained in less than half the cases studied, indirect evidence, such as the attempt to hide or deny the sex offense from the rest of the prison population, is rather common. This is true even in the group who deny their guilt, since the clinching argument for their innocence is often, "Why I couldn't do such a terrible thing, I'd feel too ashamed."

Inadequately motivated anti-social behavior. While many of the individuals in the Sing Sing group could give no immediate reason for committing their anti-social act or acts, in fact frequently asked for assistance in understanding their aberrant sexual behavior, immediate precipitating factors, such as sexual frustration by their wives, economic reverses, and other threats to status or security were found in about one-third of these men. The absence of such specific events does not, however, imply inadequate motivation. Overwhelmingly influential unconscious motivations can be discovered in these individuals, given an adequate—which does not of necessity mean lengthy—examination. The more bizarre and chaotic the sexual expression becomes, the more severe the degree of schizophrenic involvement, in the writer's experience.

Poor judgment and failure to learn by experience. This is another of the commonly-accepted characteristics of the psychopath, and is one of the factors that makes punishment for his activities so futile. While there are many recidivists in the sex offender group, and while many of them show remarkably poor judgment in the commission of their sexual acts, frequently choosing times and places that appear to invite detection and apprehension, this behavior, as already indicated, does not have the apparent purposelessness of the psychopath, as it is compulsively motivated in most instances. It is likely, however, that the apparent failure to learn by past experience, shown in the repetition of their sexual acts, is the critical factor in determining the diagnosis of "sexual psychopath" made on 95 per cent of the men who have had psychiatric examinations before sentencing to Sing Sing.

Pathologic egocentricity and incapacity for love. Superficial appraisal of the behavior of the "sexual psychopath," with its apparent concentration on the satisfaction of the individual's own sexual needs, to the exclusion of any and all other considerations, would seem to fit the Sing Sing offender into this category very neatly. When one looks beneath this superficial manifestation, however, the anti-social behavior is found to be the resultant of forces, largely unconscious, that have been in conflict for long periods, and that reach external expression—in the majority of the cases—only when the repressive factors are weakened by alcohol, organic brain damage, or the disorganization that accompanies an overt schizophrenic illness. The capacity for object relationships is certainly disturbed in these individuals, largely, one feels, as the result of incapacitating inhibitions and fears over establishing emotional contact and interpersonal give-and-take with others. It is the impression, however, that these disturbances result in a weakened, childish kind of behavior toward libidinal objects, rather than in the absence of capacity for object relationships that is described in the psychopath. Since therapeutic contact is dependent upon the ability to make some kind of object relationship, accurate estimation of this capacity in these individuals has an important bearing on the therapeutic possibilities and therefore on the ultimate prognosis.

General poverty in major affective reactions. In this area, as in the factor just considered, the importance of distinguishing between the "feebleness of affect" of the psychopath, and the affective blunting of the schizophrenic is emphasized by the superficial similarity of behavior in the two groups. This distinction has been attempted in the Sing Sing study by rating each case on "ability for emotional rapport and reactivity." None of the Sing Sing cases has been rated as having a "mature and adequate" ability. Approximately 50 per cent are rated as having ability "present but suppressed," 25 per cent as having "limited" ability, and 25 per cent as having "none or slight." This would indicate a disturbance of affect in all of these cases, the disturbance being both qualitative and quantitative, in contrast to the simple quantitative deficiency in the psychopath. These affective disturbances are interpreted as an indication of the fear experienced by these men when they attempt effective ties with others. As a defense against these fearful situations, they remain emotionally encapsulated, isolated and detached.

Specific loss of insight. Under this heading, Cleckley discusses the psychopath's inability "to see himself as others see him." This is in marked contrast to his perfect orientation, his ability to reason, and his freedom from delusions. The information on this point obtained by the estimates of insight in the Sing Sing prisoners studied, shows normal insight to be lacking. It is found, however, that one-third of the men have partial insight, another 50 per cent have some awareness of their difficulties, while less than 20 per cent are essentially without insight. This last group is comprised of the more overtly psychotic individuals in the series. The majority of the sexual offenders are keenly aware of the attitude of society in general, and prison society in particular, toward their sexual aberration; and they show, as has already been stated, varying degrees of shame and remorse.

Unresponsiveness in general interpersonal relations. The contrast is drawn here between the superficial ease and affability of the psychopath, and his basic lack of response to the usual emotional interplay existing in close interpersonal relationships. The difficulties in interpersonal relations seen in the Sing Sing cases stem, it is felt, from these offenders' marked anxiety and fear of close emotional contact with others, particularly with adults. This is a pervasive difficulty, so that these men show little social ability, and are a significantly isolated and withdrawn group. This isolation continues, even in the prison setting.

Fantastic and uninviting behavior with drink and sometimes without it. The bizarre behavior in all areas of personality-functioning described under this heading in Cleckley's book has rarely been encountered in the Sing Sing cases. Again excluding overtly psychotic individuals, who may exhibit as bizarre behavior as can be imagined, the acting out seen in the majority of the men who were alcoholics tends to be confined to the specific area of their sexual difficulties. In addition, when sober, they are over-controlled, rigid conformists, for the most part.

SUICIDE RARELY CARRIED OUT. In respect to suicide, the psychopath seems to resemble the Sing Sing sex offenders. One encounters mention of suicidal ideas or attempts infrequently, even though depression and guilt are relatively common. Again it is the more disturbed psychotics in the group who have shown the suicidal tendencies found. For example, B. speaks of suicide as an escape from the torment of his immediate situation.

SEX LIFE IMPERSONAL, TRIVIAL, AND POORLY INTEGRATED. This is the third, and perhaps most important area of agreement between the description of the psychopath and the Sing Sing group of sex offenders. In contrast to the generally accepted belief that the sexual offender is a "sex fiend," motivated by an uncontrollable need for sexual gratification, one finds that close to 90 per cent of the men studied show markedly impaired erotic drives. They are satisfying some need other than sexual while performing the aberrant sexual act—such as retaliation or revenge, for the trauma experienced with a hostile, rejecting or castrating mother or wife. There is also a marked lack of integration, extending to chaotic confusion, based primarily on the intense sexual fears generated by their traumatic childhood sexual experiences. A high percentage of such traumatic episodes is found in these men. Analysis of their sexual disturbances reveals a schizophrenic type of disorganization and shallowness, consistent with, and part of, the marked disturbances in interpersonal relationships already described.

FAILURE TO FOLLOW ANY LIFE PLAN. The inconsistency of the psychopath in working toward a definite goal or goals is seldom encountered in this group of offenders. A high percentage are compulsive workers, showing enormous energy and drive in their attempts to gain social and economic status and security. While there may be temporary interruptions because of alcoholism and anti-social sexual activities, they stick closely to patterns of achievement, and have very specific goals and objectives in all areas, including in some instances, fairly realistic sexual goals. Again those in the Sing Sing group who came closest to Cleckley's foregoing description are the more seriously disturbed, disintegrating schizophrenics, who may show very pointless, nomadic and irresponsible lives.

It is found, then, after careful scrutiny of the various characteristics of the psychopath, that the individuals in the present research group, most of them diagnosed as psychopathic personalities, show relatively few of the traits listed by Cleckley as typical of the true psychopath. In fact, in only five of the 16 characteristics given by Cleckley is there even superficial agreement. In four of the five—pathological egocentricity and incapacity for love; general poverty in major affective reactions; unresponsiveness in general interpersonal relations; and sex life impersonal, trivial and poorly integrated—the common psychodynamic denominator is the disturbance of affective capacity which manifests itself in impoverished emotional relationships, and a sharp dampening in external attachments and interests. This autistic withdrawal from interpersonal contacts is one of the earliest, and most significant symptoms of psychological decompensation, an indication of the dangerously narrow margin of competence remaining to the weakened and brittle ego structure of the individual. The fifth factor, poor judgment and failure to learn by experience, is an additional indication of the failure of the ego to perform satisfactorily in all three major areas of its function: the perceptive, integrative, and executive.

That the disintegration or collapse of ego function is not complete, thereby enabling the individual to maintain a façade of normal behavior, does not, in the writer's opinion, vitiate the diagnosis of a schizophrenic illness. The individual is not, to be sure, grossly decompensated, that is, overtly psychotic. But it is precisely because he maintains some semblance of normal behavior that he presents such a problem and threat to the community. The behavior disturbances of the overt psychotic cause him, as a general rule, to be detected rapidly and disposed of properly, in our highly-organized and complex modern society. It is the borderline individual, who can still maintain some semblance of control, but who loses this control episodically, or is about to lose control chronically, who winds up in prison, having had the opportunity to commit one or more antisocial acts, and who is diagnosed as "without psychosis, not mentally defective, psychopathic personality." It is the writer's contention that such a diagnosis does not indicate the true state of affairs, in fact effectively hides the psychodynamic status of the inmate, and causes confusion and apathy regarding treatment and eventual disposition of the inmate.

On the basis of clinical investigations on the Sing Sing sex offenders, corroborated by the findings on psychological examination, the writer would propose that these individuals be diagnosed, for the most part, somewhere along the continuum ranging from schizo-adaptive personality structure (3), through pseudoneurotic schizophrenia (4), pseudopsychopathic schizophrenia (5), and ambulatory schizophrenia to overt, clinically demonstrable schizophrenic psychosis. Without becoming involved in the controversy that is ever present regarding the genetic basis of schizophrenia, the usefulness of the concept of a schizotype—or to use Sandor Rado's term, a schizo-adaptive personality—in dealing with the problems of therapy and prognosis in this group of cases, has become increasingly evident over the past three years. In the field of therapy, for example, while the prognosis in schizophrenia is still not a rosy one, as has been mentioned, therapeutic techniques are available, and do modify the pattern of illness in many patients. On the other hand, there is a universal pessimism, and rightly so, about therapeutic efforts with the psychopath, and this may have an adverse effect upon the treatment of individuals so diagnosed.

In the field of prognosis, which in prison psychiatry includes not only a prediction about the medical future of the inmate patient, but also involves or implies a prediction about his future social behavior, the use of the diagnostic continuum just described, with its implication of movement in either direction, gives a flexibility to statements about therapeutic response that cannot be achieved using terms like "cured" or "improved." Every psychiatrist who has had to decide, or help decide on the ability of a hospitalized patient to adjust to life outside the institution is keenly aware of the difficulties and problems surrounding such decisions. When the "patient" has committed an antisocial act, and may have a history of recidivism, the decision, from the psychiatric standpoint, on his suitability for release, is an even weightier one. The device of attaching a diagnostic label never suffices. The administrative officials in the probation offices, parole boards and courts are increasingly interested in a statement of the psychodynamics of the particular case, reduced of course to understandable lay terminology, and are willing, even eager, to be guided in their decisions by the implications about the future behavior of the individual that are contained in such a statement. In order, therefore, to meet most adequately the dual responsibility which medicine has always accepted—to society on the one hand, and to the individual patient on the other—and which has been intensified in recent years by the willingness of the courts and correctional authorities to accept medical, especially psychiatric, opinion about problems of human misbehavior, we must attempt as accurate a description as possible of the behavior pattern in question. This must be dynamically oriented, if a proper understanding of the motivational context, as well as the actual behavior, is to be achieved. Prediction of future behavior is dependent to a greater extent on a clear understanding of the motivations and goals, both conscious and unconscious, of the individual, than on any other factor.

References

1. Report on Study of 102 Sex Offenders at Sing Sing Prison. Albany. March 1950.
2. CLECKLEY, H. (1950). *The Mask of Sanity*. St. Louis: Mosby.
3. RADO, SANDOR. (1953). Academic Lecture *Am. J. Psychiat.*, **110** : 6, 406, December.
4. HOCH, P., & POLATIN, P. (1949). Pseudoneurotic forms of schizophrenia. *Psychiat. Quart.*, **23**, April.
5. DUNAIF, S., & HOCH, P. (1953). Pseudopsychopathic schizophrenia. Presentation at the meeting of American Psychopathological Association.

DALE C. CAMERON

Facts About Drugs

With the current climate in the United States, the personality disorder that has caused the greatest concern involves the abuse of drugs. Although a drug is any substance which, when taken internally, can modify the structure or functioning of the organism, the term is usually employed within a context that implies that the substance is potentially destructive. There are a great many different types of drugs, and we can expect that they attract different types of users. This article does not deal with the people who use drugs but, rather, with the typical effects that are usually associated with the major drug types. It is important to understand the different effects that drugs have, but it is also important to appreciate that drugs are often unpredictable, with the effect depending upon how much is taken, the context in which it is taken, and the personality and expectations of the user.

The meaning of the word "drug" differs very much depending upon the context in which the word is used. In this article we shall be dealing with drugs in the broadest possible meaning of the word. The WHO Expert Committee on Drug Dependence defined a drug as "any substance that, when taken into the living organism, may modify one or more of its functions."

Drugs of all sorts have long been used and their variety and number keep growing. However, it is primarily those on which a person may become dependent that interest us here. Drug dependence may be described as "a state, psychic and sometimes also physical, resulting from the interaction between a living organism and a drug, characterized by behavioural and other responses that always include a compulsion to take the drug on a continuous or periodic basis in order to experience its psychic effects, and sometimes to avoid the discomfort of its absence. A person may be dependent upon more than one drug."

Since the characteristics of dependence vary with the drug involved, it is important to use the term in specific reference to the type of drug.

Drugs of the *morphine type* (narcotics) are derived, in large part, from opium. Opium is the coagulated juice of the poppy plant *Papaver somniferum L.* which grows well in dry sunny places throughout the world. Opium contains a powerful painkiller and other medically useful drugs can be derived from this

---

Reprinted from *World Health*, **24** (1971), 519–527, with the permission of the World Health Organization and Dr. Cameron.

source. Its principal analgesic action is due to an alkaloid named morphine, after Morpheus, the Greek god of dreams. Morphine can be converted to codeine, a drug with both mild analgesic and cough suppressant actions. Heroin, an opiate readily made from morphine, and opium itself are widely used by narcotic-dependent persons.

A number of non-opiate, synthetic compounds also have narcotic and analgesic properties. Unfortunately, they all share with morphine and opium the capacity to produce dependence of the morphine type.

With narcotics generally, psychic dependence is strong and tends to develop early. The range and paradoxical nature of the effects are astonishing. Narcotics can have both euphoriant and sedative effects, give "relief" from pain and anxiety or "relief" from excessive passivity. Narcotics come as close to being a panacea as any drug yet found by providing different solutions for different people or even for the same person at different points in time. They are used to give "relief," to make someone feel better or just not to feel at all. However, physical dependence also develops early and its intensity roughly parallels the dosage taken. If you were to take ten mg. of morphine every four hours for about two weeks you would develop some physical dependence. Such dependence is an adaptive state of the body which requires *continued* taking of the drug to *prevent* the appearance of an illness or abstinence syndrome that is specific in its signs and symptoms for this group of drugs. Tolerance to narcotics also occurs rapidly, making it necessary to take increasing doses of the drug to achieve the same effect.

The withdrawal or abstinence syndrome, which with morphine or heroin reaches its peak in forty-eight to seventy-two hours after the last dose, is characterized by physical and mental stresses of many sorts ranging from anxiety, restlessness, perspiration, runny nose and eyes, to aches and pains, nausea and vomiting, cramps, weight loss and, in some rare and very extreme cases where no medical care is available, shock and death.

Drugs of the morphine type are most widely used in certain countries of the eastern Mediterranean and in Asia. Until the last ten to fifteen years, opium was generally the drug of choice in most of these areas. At that time, estimates of use ranged up to 6 per cent of the total populations in some countries, but these estimates must be considered as very rough guides. In more recent years, there has apparently been a marked increase in the use of heroin instead of opium, especially by younger persons in these regions, though in some local areas opium remains the drug of choice. Because activities associated with the non-medical use of morphine-type drugs are now illegal in nearly all countries, it is very difficult to obtain good estimates on the prevalence and incidence of such use.

There is believed to be substantial use of opium in the hill areas where Thailand, Burma, Laos and China are in close proximity. Opium and morphine are used in Singapore, while heroin is the drug most taken in Hong Kong and the plains of Thailand. Very rough estimates suggest that users in this general region of the world might be measured in hundreds of thousands.

It has been suggested that there are 120,000 to 180,000 heroin users in the United States of America (1 in 1,140 to 1,700 persons). In the United Kingdom the number of heroin and other opioid users coming to the attention of the Home Office in 1969 was about 2,300, or about 1 person in 24,500. The use of opioids in Europe remains on a small scale despite a recent sharp rise in some countries.

Sedative drugs enjoy a rising popularity as a means of coping with our present hectic way of life. In the past fifty years numerous barbituric acid derivatives have been developed. Some are short and intermediate acting, such as hexobarbital, others are long acting, such as phenobarbital. All are toxic. Those most self-administered by drug users are of the short and immediate acting types, for example, amobarbital, cyclobarbital, hexobarbital, pentobarbital, secobarbital. Certain, but not all, so-called tranquillizers also produce dependence of the barbiturate type. Among those that do are meprobamate, chlordiazepoxide and diazepam. They are used medically to relieve anxiety without producing as much sedation as barbiturates.

With all drugs of this type psychic dependence can be relatively strong. Persons taking these sedatives usually are seeking escape or oblivion, but in some cases sedatives may be taken as part of a drug spree, often in combination with other drugs. The symptoms and signs of chronic intoxication with barbiturates are similar to those seen in alcohol intoxication. Large doses produce lack of motor co-ordination, impairment of mental function and occasionally a toxic psychosis, coma and death. Physical dependence can be strong and usually develops when the daily intake reaches three to four times the usual therapeutic dose.

Tolerance does not develop as rapidly or uniformly as with narcotics. For example, there is little tolerance to the usual minimum lethal dose, so that those who self-administer substantial amounts of barbiturates are often unconsciously skating on the ragged edge of suicide.

The withdrawal syndrome begins twenty-four hours after the last dose and reaches its peak in two to three days. It is characterized by anxiety, tremor, weakness, distortion of visual perception, insomnia, and sometimes grand-mal convulsions and delirium similar to delirium tremens as seen in some cases during withdrawal from alcohol; a major psychotic episode may be provoked.

Alcohol produces psychic dependence of varying degrees from mild (alcohol is missed if not available) to moderate (more than occasional, inappropriate intoxication in a social setting, and often a secret source of supply) to strong (drinking more than is culturally approved, an obsession with the supply of alcohol, and serious interference with personal and social life).

Physical dependence develops slowly and only after fairly heavy consumption. Tolerance develops slowly and is far from complete, especially to doses sufficient to produce coma, and it may diminish to the point of unusual sensitivity in the later stages of alcoholism. Physical dependence and tolerance usually do not develop at social drinking levels.

The withdrawal syndrome is very similar to that of barbiturates and other sedatives. Both types are severe and may result in grand-mal convulsions and/or delirium. It is interesting to note that there is also partial cross-tolerance between alcohol and the barbiturates. That is one reason why barbiturates are relatively effective in controlling the withdrawal syndrome associated with alcohol dependence. These two forms of dependence are essentially a single type.

The moderate use of alcohol in its various beverage forms is not deviant behavior in most countries of the world, although in certain countries in North Africa, the Middle East and the Indian-Pakistani subcontinent such use is considered so; but even in some of them the prevalence seems to be increasing. The immoderate use of alcohol is deviant behavior in essentially all countries. It would appear that, of those who drink at all, a certain percentage do become dependent on alcohol. Estimates made some time between 1945 and 1963 on the rate of alcoholism per 100,000 persons in the population aged 20 or over in selected countries include the following: England and Wales—865 to 1,100; Switzerland—2,100 to 2,700; Chile—3,610 to 4,150; various states of the United States—1,500 to 7,090; and France—5,200 to 7,300 (WHO Expert Committee on Mental Health, 1967). The highest figure is about 8.5 times that of the lowest and illustrates the variability in rates of alcoholism.

However, I want to relate these figures to those given earlier for drugs of the morphine type. In the UK, that figure was 1 in 24,500, as compared with 1 in 99 to 117 for alcoholism. The highest estimated rate of current narcotic use in the world is 1 in 45; the highest alcoholic rate is 1 in 13.7.

Drugs producing dependence of the *amphetamine type* are central nervous system stimulants. Medically, they are effective in treating narcolepsy and certain types of hyperactive behavior in children. However, they are most widely used in medical practice as appetite suppressants. Not all drugs producing dependence of the amphetamine type are amphetamines. Other central nervous system stimulants such as methylphenidate and phenmetrazine are also involved.

This group of drugs produces mood elevation, elation and a sense of heightened awareness. It is these effects that are desired by certain persons and result in their psychic dependence. With large doses, such dependence is often rapid and strong. Tolerance, especially to low doses, is relatively slow to develop and irregular. It may, however, start to develop at usual therapeutic dose levels and can become very marked. When very large amounts are taken, tolerance develops rapidly. Doses several hundred times the therapeutic amount have been taken by highly tolerant persons. There is little, if any, physical dependence and there is thus no abstinence syndrome *per se*, but exhaustion and depression are frequently seen following cessation of intoxication. The visual distortions, hallucinations and sometimes psychotic episodes seen in amphetamine-dependent persons are initiated by intoxication, not withdrawal.

Drugs of the amphetamine type are used in deviant ways in a number of places in the world. One pattern involves the oral self-administration of relatively stable amounts ranging from one or two to several therapeutic doses daily or intermittently. Persons of all ages, especially those of middle age, appear to be concerned. A second pattern involves a rapid escalation over periods of one or two weeks to massive oral and often intravenous doses. Such deviant use is to be found primarily among late adolescents and young adults. One or both of these patterns of use have been identified in Canada, Japan, Sweden, the United Kingdom and the United States of America, among others. Such use in Japan and the United Kingdom has markedly decreased and the trend is said to be downward in Sweden, although deviant use of amphetamine-type drugs is beginning to appear in certain African, European, South American and other countries.

Cocaine, like the amphetamines, is a central nervous system stimulant and produces toxic and euphoriant effects similar to those of drugs producing dependence of the amphetamine type. It is not included among those drugs because, unlike them, it produces no tolerance.

Cocaine is derived from the leaves of the coca plant, which is indigenous to the Andean region of South America. Formerly used in medical practice as a potent local anaesthetic, it has largely been replaced by equally effective anaesthetics without any dependence liability.

Cocaine produces very strong psychic dependence. The drug produces a sense of excitement, heightened and distorted awareness and hallucinations. There is no physical dependence, nor tolerance. However, since the drug is rapidly destroyed in the body, some cocaine-dependent persons take up to ten grams per day during "sprees." There is no withdrawal syndrome *per se*, but there is often marked exhaustion when the intoxication wears off.

The chewing of coca leaves is a very common practice in some localities of the Andean region of South America. Zapata-Ortiz, in 1970, estimated that 6,000,000 persons were regular users in Bolivia and Peru, the principal countries involved. This would mean that 1 in every 2.5 persons of all ages used coca to some extent. Certainly the chewing of coca leaves has a stimulating effect, but the degree of stimulation achieved is simply not to be compared to that resulting from the intravenous use of cocaine.

Many different preparations are derived from the plant *Cannabis sativa L.*, which is ubiquitous in its growth throughout the temperate to tropical zones of the world. These preparations, such as marihuana and hashish, can produce drug dependence of the *cannabis type*. Though still used in some traditional systems of medicine, cannabis has essentially no place in modern medicine.

As with other drugs, the effects of cannabis depend greatly on the amount taken. Cannabis preparations produce effects ranging from anxiety, mood elevation, elation, hilarity, distortions of sensory (particularly visual) perception and loss of inhibitions to delusions, paranoid ideas, depersonalization, agitation, confusion and sedation. These effects lead to a moderate-to-strong psychic dependence on the part of *some* experimenters and are apparently the basis for continued use on the part of heavy users. As with narcotics, the immediate psychic effect produced depends a good deal on the expectations and desires of the user. There is relatively little, if any, tolerance in man, little tendency to increase the dose, little, if any, physical dependence, and hence no regularly reported withdrawal syndrome. Recent reports, however, indicate the need for further studies of tolerance and physical dependence in man.

The use of cannabis in one or another of its several forms—bhang, ganja, charras, marihuana, maconha, kif and hashish, to mention but a few—is particularly widespread in those areas of the world where alcohol is least used. It is also relatively prevalent in some countries where alcohol is widely used. Alcohol is not widely used in India. In certain parts of that country the use of bhang, which is usually taken orally, is neither illegal nor socially unacceptable, while the availability of ganja, a stronger preparation, is controlled and the use of charras is proscribed. Ganja is usually more potent than bhang and marihuana; charras is a resinous material comparable to hashish which is more potent than other commonly used preparations. There is great variation in the potency of cannabis preparations, so that one sample of marihuana may be practically inert while another may be stronger than some samples of ganja or hashish. This, no doubt, accounts for some of the differing views expressed about the "effects of marihuana." The nature of cannabis preparations used varies widely, not only in the Indian-Pakistani subcontinent, but also in certain Middle Eastern, African and South American countries, and their use is gaining popularity in some North and South American and Western European countries.

Drugs of the *hallucinogen type* include lysergide (more popularly known as LSD), mescaline, psilocybin, and dimethyl tryptamine (known as DMT). Lysergide is a synthetic substance; it is readily made from lysergic acid which occurs in ergot, a parasitic fungus that grows on rye and other grains. Psilocybin occurs in certain mushrooms and mescaline in peyote, a form of cactus. Other hallucinogens such as DMT and STP are purely synthetic materials.

Aside from the very local use of hallucinogenic mushrooms and peyote in certain native religious ceremonies, these substances are used largely by those who have more than usual interest in artistic and intellectual pursuits, whether or not they excel in these fields, and by others for "kicks" (changes in sensory perception, development of hallucinations, etc.) and particularly for "expansion of consciousness" and "mystical insight." Such use is to be found primarily in developed countries of the West. Some seek insight into their own emotional problems. Those who *repeatedly* use these drugs in an attempt to achieve the described experience may be said to have psychic dependence. There is no physical dependence. However, tolerance develops rapidly and can be marked. There is cross-tolerance among at least the first four hallucinogens named. The sensations described, as well as the panic reactions and frank psychoses not infrequently produced, are manifestations of intoxication and not of withdrawal.

The use of dependence-producing drugs involves a complex interaction between the properties of the drug taken, the characteristics of the drug taker and his socio-cultural environment.

The capacity to induce psychic dependence is the only characteristic shared by all dependence-producing drugs. Not all persons who experiment with, or even use, these drugs develop psychic dependence. Some persons are more prone than others to develop such dependence, and some drugs are more liable than others to induce it. Psychic dependence may be said to exist when the use of dependence-producing drugs becomes an important life-organizing factor or a stereotyped response to a wide variety of internal and external stimuli. Drug-taking becomes an important life-organizing factor when substantial amounts of time and energy are devoted to obtaining, thinking about, using or discussing the drug or drugs in question; it is a stereotyped response when a person tends to deal with all problems and joys by taking drugs.

Among the more important motives that often appear to be associated with the use of drugs are (1) to escape from something, (2) to have a new, pleasurable or thrilling experience, (3) to achieve improved "understanding" or "insight," (4) to achieve a sense of belonging, and (5) to express independence and sometimes hostility.

In settings where a particular drug is socially acceptable, moderate use tends to be widespread. However, when large numbers of persons use a drug, and attitudes towards intoxication are lenient or ambivalent, a significant proportion of users tend to become dependent. Where the use of a drug is not culturally accepted, such individual use as does occur tends to be excessive though not widespread in the population. The deviant use of drugs often appears to be associated with rapid socio-economic change and may be related to a weakening of cultural controls as old patterns of living are replaced by new. Also, the extent and rapidity of mass communication and transportation now enables many persons in one part of the world to learn quickly of the doings of others far away. The sensational manner in which news of drug use and users is sometimes presented, rumours and misinformation about alleged benefits of such use may stimulate some persons to seek out and experiment with drugs. Looking at some of the so-called news reports on drugs, I am sometimes reminded of a perhaps apocryphal entrepreneur, active in the United States during the prohibition era, who marketed, at least temporarily, a packet containing sugar and a fruit flavour. The label read somewhat as follows: "Instructions: Use only for the preparation of syrup! Warning: Do *not* place in an earthenware container with yeast and cover with two gallons of water. To do so might result in the production of an alcoholic beverage, which is unlawful."

HELEN H. NOWLIS

Prevention of Drug Abuse Through Education

This paper is a transcript of a speech given by Dr. Nowlis at a conference on drug abuse. The audience consisted of members of the military who were concerned with learning about drug abuse and techniques that might help them to deal with the growing problems of drug abuse among military personnel. Because of its focus on education as a vehicle to the control of drug abuse, it is relevant to the sections on psychotherapeutic approaches and community psychology. No miracle techniques are suggested as, indeed, none exist. However, the enormous complexity of the problem and its many ramifications are well spelled out.

Prevention of drug abuse through education seems a rather straightforward endeavor. You have invited me here to tell you how to prevent people from doing something which an increasing number of them are doing despite strenuous, if not sometimes frantic, efforts to dissuade them. Some of you have traveled half way around the world to seek answers. This would suggest that the task may not be quite as simple as it sounds, and I detect both a hope and a challenge.

During the past few years innumerable films have been produced, TV campaigns have been launched, lectures have been given. Millions of pamphlets have been distributed, dozens of curricula have been developed, classes have been taught, but drug abuse keeps rolling along. Can education prevent drug abuse? The challenge is a serious one and I intend to accept it. But before doing so I would like to speak to the hope because it becomes part of the challenge.

Since 1914 our society's response to drug abuse has been criminalization and imprisonment with the assumption that the threat of either or both would deter a type of behavior which the majority within our society has declared unacceptable. Not everyone has been happy with this response or accepted the assumption of deterrence. A widely but by no means universally accepted alternative has been to define drug abuse as an illness which requires treatment rather than punishment and to rely on the assumption that the

Paper presented at the Army World-Wide Drug Abuse Conference, September 1971, and reprinted with the permission of Dr. Nowlis.

prospect of illness will deter. We are presently being forced at least to question both sets of assumptions.

Drug abuse is no longer an activity confined to socially distant and unfamiliar minorities—Chinese on the West Coast, Blacks and Puerto Ricans in the ghettoes of our large cities, or jazz musicians or Bohemians in New Orleans, Chicago, or New York. It now involves us, our children, our friends, our troops, and we are being forced finally to take seriously what we managed to ignore for so many years. But an increasing number of middle class parents are having great difficulty in perceiving their sons and daughters who have been or they fear may be "busted" as felons, as desperate criminals who deserve to be shackled, finger-printed, tried, convicted, and perhaps imprisoned. Nor are they very comfortable with the idea that their apparently healthy though sometimes maddening offspring are suddenly mentally ill and in need of psychiatric treatment. Some of these sons and daughters are convinced that the only purpose of treatment is to help them adapt to a society which they reject. I would imagine that you may have had equal difficulty in so perceiving many of the men with whom you have lived and fought.

Faced with this uneasiness and the all too human reluctance to grapple with difficult and complex problems which resonate with deeply held beliefs and attitudes, not only about drugs and drug use but about the nature of man and of the good life, many are searching for a more comfortable and acceptable means of doing what threats of punishment and predictions of great physical and psychological harm do not seem to have accomplished. They hope that education will succeed where other means have not. Is education equal to the task? Herein lies the challenge. My answer must be a very frustrating, if not maddening, "That depends." It depends on how you define drug, drug abuse, education, and, curiously enough, man and what makes him tick.

Each of us defines all of these terms, even drug, from the perspective of his own background, training, experience, and personal investment. This applies to me as well. I hope that to be aware of it mitigates its influence. I am a psychologist and erstwhile psychopharmacologist whose major concern as student, teacher, researcher, and administrator has been with understanding and facilitating optimal growth and development of young people of all ages. I was trained as a behavioral scientist and have functioned as one for many years. It is almost instinctive for me to insist that definitions be objective and descriptive and not based on value judgments. I am convinced that the first step in seeking the solution to a problem is to understand and carefully analyze that problem, to make explicit and examine any implicit assumptions about the nature of the problem to the end that we can at least agree on why we disagree, and to define clearly what goals we are seeking. Only then can we search for appropriate tools with which to reach those goals. A scalpel is a powerful tool in the hands of a surgeon who, on the basis of examinations and tests, thoroughly understands his patient and knows exactly what he wishes to accomplish. It would be of little use to a lumberjack whose goal is to fell a tree.

Education is many things to many people. Currently it is increasingly equated with dispensing information with the somewhat dubious assumption that the "right" information will change behavior in some desired direction. In its broadest sense it is a process, the goal of which is some clearly specified change in behavior. Education so defined has an arsenal of powerful tools at its disposal, but they are effective only if they are carefully chosen to accomplish clearly defined purposes with adequately described individuals or groups of individuals. We know how to control unacceptable behavior such as drug abuse with punishment, but the conditions necessary for punishment to be effective are both impossible and unacceptable in a society with a value system such as ours. It would cost far more money than we are willing to pay, would violate too many values we hold dear, and would have consequences which would be less acceptable than the behavior we wished to change. When we compromise the method to avoid its unacceptable consequences it cannot possibly be effective. One cannot eliminate the use of marihuana by punishment or threat of punishment when the chances of that punishment actually occurring, whether it be legal, psychological, or social, are "guesstimated" to be significantly less than one in a thousand.

There are other highly sophisticated tools which have been used with great effectiveness in advertising and in politics. Madison Avenue has persuaded millions of us to believe that we cannot be happy or bring up healthy, happy children unless we purchase products that generations have survived without. Political science has successfully put many of these tools to work to influence the voting behavior of thousands. They are based on very sophisticated analyses of the meaning and function of the behavior to be modified. They are carefully tailored to well-defined target groups. Many of them seem on the surface to have little to do with the actual behavior they are intended to influence.

Before we can discuss the tools available for modifying drug-using behavior, whether they be direct or devious, we must understand thoroughly the behavior we wish to modify, the individuals we wish to influence, and why and how we wish to change them. This is a tall order. We cannot do it in the time available to us this afternoon. I propose, therefore, to throw you a number of curves, not to catch you off balance, although they may, but to give you an understanding of why some of our present educational efforts may not only be ineffective but counterproductive and to suggest to you that, for reasons which should become obvious, we have not given good education a chance.

First, some definitions. A drug is a substance which by its chemical nature affects the structure or function of the living organism. It will take only a moment's thought to realize that this definition covers a wide spectrum of substances—medicines, over-the-counter drugs, illegal drugs, drugs which we are used to thinking of as beverages or cigarettes, food additives, agricultural chemicals, industrial chemicals, even food. From some points of view it is not a very useful definition but it is the one with which we must start. It should remind us that a drug is a drug no matter why we use it or what we call it; that all drugs interact with the organism according to the same basic principles; and that we must specify the reasons why we select out any group of these substances and call them medicine, narcotic, beverage, or industrial chemical. When we do this we find that the reasons have more to do with the purposes for which we use them than with any characteristic of the substance itself.

Drug abuse is an amount and pattern and frequency of use which interferes with the physical, psychological, social, or vocational functioning of a given individual. You should have no difficulty in applying this definition to abuse of alcohol, but we do not call alcohol a drug. When we apply it to drugs ordinarily used for medically approved reasons we call it misuse. We do not apply it at all to illegal drug use. Socially and legally drug abuse is any use, even possession, of substances which have no approved medical use or the use of medically approved substances for non-medical reasons—if, that is, the substance is called a drug. It is essentially abuse of society's controls on drugs. Either definition is acceptable but a definition must represent consensus if it is to be useful. We have to make up our minds or at least recognize that in the one case we are dealing with destructive behavior and in the other with socially deviant behavior. They are not interchangeable if you wish to modify either.

There is no such thing as the effect of any drug. All drugs have multiple effects and these vary from dose level to dose level, from individual to individual, from time to time in the same individual. For every drug there is an effective dose (ED50), a toxic dose (TD50) and, at least theoretically, a lethal dose (LD50). Each of these is a statistical abstraction, that dose by which 50% of a given group show whatever effect is sought, whatever effect is defined as toxic, or die.

At low and moderate dose levels non-drug factors such as physiological and psychological characteristics of the individual, the reasons why he takes the drug, what he expects the effect will be, the physical and social setting in which he takes it, are often more important in determining effects than the drug itself. Think for a moment about alcohol. Sociable, talkative, withdrawn, depressed, gay, sleepy, abusive, destructive, uninhibited—it all depends on who and where.

Let's turn briefly from drugs to people. People are all different. All behavior is multiply determined. There are no simple one-to-one relationships between cause and effect. Human behavior always occurs in a social and cultural context, and it is often this context which gives it its meaning and significance. Percept is more important than precept in influencing behavior. Do as I say, not as I do is comforting but not very effective. Behavior is influenced by what one believes and how one perceives, regardless of whether it is judged to be true by others. Individuals seldom continue to do something which does not fulfill some need, real or imagined. Man is seldom completely rational; most decisions of most individuals are determined more by feeling, belief, and attitude than information, no matter how good that information is. (Cigarette smoking increased appreciably last year and the nicotine content of cigarettes is up, not down.)

While keeping in mind these facts from pharmacology and psychology, what can we add from communication and persuation? The perceived source of a message must be judged both expert and trustworthy. It helps if that source is liked and is perceived as similar to or at least understanding of those to be informed. Scare techniques are effective only under certain very limited conditions. Mere repeated exposure of an unfamiliar situation, regardless of whether it is presented positively or negatively, may be enough to increase the attractiveness of the situation. Information must be appropriate to developmental differences, differences in knowledge and experience, differences in exposure to risk. When bombarded by more stimuli than he can process, man tends to insulate himself from that stimulation, to turn off. When level of anxiety is raised to a sufficiently high level and no way to deal with it is provided, it tends to be denied. These are only a few of the conclusions of twenty-five years of research.

Essentially we have been ignoring or violating most of what we know as we have plunged ahead with more and more of what we have been doing in the past, more reliance on information, more use of media directed to unknown and undifferentiated audiences, more information about drugs which does not take into account basic pharmacological principles or the actual experience of the majority of those who have tried, more ignoring age and social differences, of level of exposure to risk.

There are, however, significant trends toward attempts to take into account what we know about drugs and how they act, about people and what makes them tick, about the factors that make for successful communication and persuasion. This involves less emphasis on information about the possible dangers of specific drugs, more emphasis on the possible risks involved in all drug use, more emphasis on the individual and the meaning and function of his drug use, on effective communication, on the involvement of youth and of the total community, and an attempt to put drug use and abuse in the perspective of the myriad problems faced by young people as they live and learn and grow toward maturity.

Whenever one departs from traditional and widely accepted approaches to any problem, particularly to drug abuse education, and challenges deeply held beliefs and attitudes about drugs and drug users and wishful thinking about controlling behavior, he finds himself in the "damned if you do and damned if you don't" situation not too different from that which Nevitt Sanford describes in relation to the teacher in alcohol education: "Should it be explained to young people that according to the modern view alcoholism results from a complex interplay of physiological, psychological, and social processes, and should they then be offered a few of the theories that have been put forward to explain this largely still obscure condition? . . . If he confronts the issues he is bound to make some parents unhappy and will probably receive suggestions from the principal that he not rock the boat; but if he stays on safe ground the students are likely to be bored." If this is true of alcohol education forty years after prohibition, we would have to substitute furious parents, charges of promoting drug use, getting fired and not only bored but at least some disdainful students in the above quote in the heat of the present prohibition.

Richard Blum has suggested that the necessary factors for initiation of drug use are access to the drug and a setting for drug use which is perceived as relatively safe, but that beyond these such factors as personality and interests, peer groups, school atmosphere, mass media information, social class and family background, parent-child interaction styles, and the culture's use of and attitude toward drug use are all important determinants of the decision to use or not to use and of the pattern and extent of use. "Drug initiation and use, however 'strange' they seem to outsiders or 'not like him' to parents, is very much like him after all, for it is in keeping with his social, psychological, and physiological apparatus. If it doesn't 'fit' him, he will stop, otherwise we may presume that his continued drug use serves a variety of functions at many levels."

Some of the functions which drug use may serve are described in research studies. Blumer, on the basis of studies of adolescents chiefly from under-privileged minority groups, concludes: "Youngsters who are growing up in an adolescent milieu that places a premium on being 'cool,' and who aspire to acceptance and recognition as being cool will move over into drug use (if channels are open to them) not as a retreat from reality, but as a positive effort to get into the major stream as they see it." Feldman, on the basis of studies of ghetto street gangs in New York City and Boston, concludes that, for these individuals, "The user turns to drugs not as a result of anomie, but rather to capitalize on a new mode of enhancing his status and prestige within a social system where the highest prizes go to the persons who demonstrate toughness, daring, and adventure. Within the life of the stand-up cat, movement into heroin use is one route to becoming somebody in the eyes of important people who comprise the slum network." Blum concludes on the basis of his studies of high school and college students, that: "The more daring the deed in terms of social attitudes and the more daring the drug in terms of biochemical effects, the more significance it is likely to serve both as symptom and as sign. . . ." We must at least ask the question, "How did drug use come to be defined as being "cool," become synonymous with toughness, daring, and adventure?" Why only recently? These drugs have been around and available for a long time.

I wish I could confidently assure you that there is a recipe for successful effort. I would be stupid if I did and you would be more stupid if you believed me. I can assure you with great confidence that there are no simple prescriptions. All behavior is complex. Drug abuse, however you choose to define it, is among the more complex. It involves complex and highly variable interaction between organisms and chemicals which we are only beginning to understand. It involves changes in cells, and systems of cells, which technically are all that drugs as drugs actually do, and changes in complex behavior. We are on the frontier in understanding of these relationships. All we can do is hypothesize. Hypotheses are fine if they are tested and evaluated; they are disastrous if they are believed to be true. Beyond this, and perhaps more important, it involves perceptions and deeply held beliefs and attitudes; it involves value judgment about different groups of substances, about the people who use them, about the reasons why they use them or why we believe they use them. It involves the way in which a society defines all kinds of drug use and how it responds to them.

This may seem more a recipe for pessimism than for preventing drug abuse through education, but I am not pessimistic, at least not enough to quit.

There are beginning to be some programs which are brave enough to specify their goals, however limited, to analyze and tackle *their* problem, not *the* problem, to make use of carefully selected educational tools, to bear up under the charge that they are not fighting drug abuse just because they are not doing it as we always have. Most of them are more involved with people than with drugs. They accept the fact that throughout history man has used drugs to modify mood, feeling, and perception, that drug use would not persist unless it served some purpose, and that at least one way to change it may be to modify the need or the conditions which support the need, or to provide other and varied ways of responding to the need which involve less potential risk to the individual and are more acceptable to society.

The results are not all in. Preliminary evaluations are encouraging. With each success and each failure we learn a little more. We are actually engaged in a problem-solving venture. We can shorten the process by adopting a real problem-solving attitude. Define the problem objectively, search for possible tools which are appropriate to that problem anywhere we can find them, test, adapt, modify. After all, that is what living and growing is all about. We should never be too old to grow, never too sure to learn.

References

BLUM, R. H. (1969). *Drugs II: Students and Drugs.* San Francisco: Jossey-Bass.

BLUMER, H. (1967). *The World of Youthful Drug Use.* Berkeley: School of Criminology, University of California (mimeographed).

FELDMAN, H. W. (1968). Ideological supports to becoming and remaining a heroin addict. *J. Health and Soc. Behav.*, **9** (2), 131–139.

SANFORD, N. (1967). *Where Colleges Fail.* San Francisco: Jossey-Bass.

MORRIS E. CHAFETZ

Clinical Studies in Alcoholism

This paper was prepared by Ms. Antoinette A. Gattozzi to describe an innovative clinical research program directed by Dr. Chafetz. In our concern with problems of drug abuse, it is easy to lose sight of the fact that the abuse of alcohol continues to be the most prevalent and costly drug problem in our country. This paper, too, could easily be placed in other sections of the book, since it describes an approach to treatment that depends upon a modification of the medical model by requiring a change in the traditional role of the therapist. When the therapist abandoned his customary passive role and took active responsibility for the establishment of an effective working relationship, sharp improvement was shown in therapeutic progress. Additionally, interesting comments are made about the use of alcoholism as a diagnostic category.

Perhaps the cruelest of the myths surrounding the myth-ridden subject of alcoholism is that alcoholics really do not want to be helped. Among the general public the idea is backed by an essentially moralistic line of thought that starts from the fact that drinking is an act of volition, then proceeds with the observation that a person who drinks too much not only consistently lies and denies it but compounds his callous self-indulgence by ignoring the pleas of family and the advice of friends that he see a doctor. A great many medical professionals also believe in the myth although their reasons for doing so are quite different. Most recognize that alcoholism is a severe behavior disorder for which there are certain treatments—specifically, psychotherapy and drug therapy. But, they say, rarely do alcoholics present themselves for treatment, and those who do come or are coerced into coming do not stay in treatment. The typical alcoholic is just not sufficiently motivated, the therapists say, by which they mean "alcoholics really do not want to be helped."

This view has now been effectively challenged by Dr. Morris E. Chafetz and his colleagues at the Massachusetts General Hospital. In a series of studies and demonstrations made over the past 10 years, Doctor Chafetz has shown that alcoholics are as motivated to seek help as are patients in other

---

Reprinted from the *Mental Health Program Reports*, **4** (1970), 107–125, with the permission of Dr. Chafetz.

diagnostic classifications of psychiatric disorder, and that they will indeed enter and stay in treatment programs tailored to their needs. The fault, the investigators discovered, lay not in an absence of motivation in the patients but in misunderstanding and antipathy in the caretakers.

The investigators began their systematic work on this question as a consequence of uncovering the dismaying fact that less than 1 percent of the alcoholic patients seen in the MGH emergency ward made even one contact with the hospital's Alcohol Clinic. At first glance, Doctor Chafetz recalled, this evidence seemed to confirm the old notion that most alcoholics, even when given the opportunity for rehabilitation, simply do not choose to get expert help. But Doctor Chafetz and his associates were disposed to look more closely into the causes of failure to seek treatment. Specifically, the investigators began by asking themselves two questions: What are the characteristic personality traits of alcoholics that may decisively influence their willingness to make a therapeutic alliance; what is the impact on these traits of encounters actually experienced in the initial therapeutic setting, that is, in the hospital's emergency ward?

The consensus of workers in the field today is that excessive, uncontrolled, self-destructive drinking is a behavioral symptom manifesting a wide range of disorders. Although every alcoholic is, of course, a unique personality, certain psychodynamic features are thought to be more or less common to all. From these, students of alcoholism have constructed a theoretical psychodynamic formulation of the disorder, which may be summarized briefly as follows. The three outstanding features, as Doctor Chafetz has noted them, are deprivation, depression, and denial. Early childhood deprivation of a critical emotional relationship—most frequently involving the mother—is found very often in the histories of alcoholics. This loss, in turn, is conceived as the root cause of the prevailing emotional state of alcoholism—depression—against which the alcoholic uses denial as the primary defense strategy. Alcoholism is thus seen as a symptom of a primitive personality disorder that originated in the preverbal stage of an individual's emotional development. The characteristics typically associated with such disorders are low self-esteem, minimal tolerance for frustration, marked dependency, and a great difficulty in relating to other people coupled with a supersensitivity about being rejected by others.

"Most primitive disorders," Doctor Chafetz noted, "are treated within the protective and supportive confines of an institution [e.g., schizophrenia]. Not only does the addicted alcoholic suffer from a primitive psychological disorder, but there is a great tendency to act out conflict situations. Hence the attempt to treat him psychotherapeutically on an ambulatory basis can be fraught with danger."

A significant source of the danger rises from the therapist's rather rigidly held concept of his proper role and behavior vis-a-vis a patient. He sits back and waits for the patient to come to him, to talk to him, to reveal himself, to gain insight while he, the therapist, maintains a posture of patient, passive sagacity and tempers his readiness to understand with a sharp lookout for signs that he is being manipulated into abetting the patient's illness. During the initial contact, particularly, he is likely to be silent and watchful with an air of, at most, friendly impartiality.

But, Doctor Chafetz has asserted, with an alcoholic patient a therapist must be prepared to step outside the safe bounds of this traditional, nondirective role. As with all patients suffering primitive personality disorders, prompt establishment of an unmistakably positive relationship is critically important. From the very first meeting the therapist must be openly and warmly interested in the patient's well-being. He must reach out to the patient. Moreover, he must make his concern explicit by taking an active hand in helping the patient solve urgent problems of daily living.

"It is not what we say to the alcoholic but what we really feel and do that will determine the outcome," Doctor Chafetz noted. "Alcoholism, as a preverbal disorder, must be treated by action—by 'doing for' the patient. For example, if the patient requires physical treatment then hospitalization and medical care should be readily provided." For many, the sorest needs are quite rudimentary—a bath and shave, a meal, a room to live in, a pair of shoes, or a set of dentures.

The incessant, insatiable demands of alcoholics and the fundamental hostility that colors all their relations can quickly become points of rupture and failure. Few people can be expected to endure this kind of emotional barrage regularly and not respond with anger. To sustain the ideal treatment ambience of warmth and acceptance, then, Doctor Chafetz has recommended a team approach in which the emotional burden that the alcoholic patient presents can be spread out, as it were, over more than one caretaker.

In sum, this was what the investigators regarded as a sort of minimum basis on which the alcoholic could begin the arduous task of rehabilitation: A continuous relationship with a team of caretakers who are accepting of him, warm and supportive from the first and throughout all subsequent meetings, and who will give him all reasonable help with his immediate problems of living. The Boston researchers then turned to examine in detail the actual conditions experienced by alcoholic patients when they enter the treatment scene through the doors of the MGH emergency ward. They did not have to look very far to discover why it was that so few alcoholics followed through on the referral from emergency ward to Alcohol Clinic.

The patient entering the emergency ward must be seen by six or more people including the admitting clerk, the chief medical officer, and the discharge officer who talks about finances. Once his immediate medical or surgical problem has been attended to, the patient who has been diagnosed as alcoholic will be referred to the Clinic. Only if he has not been disheartened by the waiting and the questions and has not decided that he is being shuffled about like an unwelcome parcel—big *ifs* for someone with a low tolerance for frustration and little self-esteem—will he actually go upstairs to the Clinic. There he finds that six or seven other people want to see and question him. Eventually he can make an appointment to meet the resident psychiatrist for evaluation. If he comes to this meeting and is accepted for treatment, he is placed on a 4 to 6 weeks' waiting list, after which time he will finally meet his permanent therapist.

In addition to having to endure this protracted procedure, which might well daunt the stoutest motivation, the alcoholic patient, especially if he is either intoxicated or in alcoholic withdrawal, is likely to be dirty, unkempt, and odorous. He is sick and suffering, but this is too often interpreted by the caretakers as the justly deserved outcome of his having indulged in the supposed pleasures of drink. Any one of the several people he meets in the caretaking setting may reveal their distate at his appearance and their indifference to his distress; any of them may react with outright anger and hostility.

"We found, on the one hand, that the alcoholic needs a continuous nonfragmented, accepting relationship," Doctor Chafetz said. "And we saw, on the other hand, that he was actually experiencing the exact opposite at just that point in time when his motivation for treatment may be strongest, that is, when he is in the crisis that brought him to the emergency ward."

With this evidence in hand, the investigator and his associates decided to work out a new and rational approach to alcoholic patients, one that would specifically avoid the circumstances that seemed to be blocking the patient's path to treatment. The development of their program rested on certain fundamental premises. First, an explicit conception of the disorder was needed. The researchers employed a widely accepted definition in which alcoholism is regarded as a chronic behavioral disorder manifested in drinking that is excessive in relation to the norms prevailing in the drinker's culture and that interferes with his physical well-being or with his social and economic functioning.

Second, the researchers employed a concept of crisis developed by Dr. Erich Lindemann. The implications of this concept for their own program were, first, that when a person initially makes a medical contact, his act springs from a situation of physical, psychological, or social crisis in his life; and second, that motivation for treatment is higher at a time of crisis than at other times. Thus, the investigators were prepared to assume not only that there is motivation to seek help for the immediate complaint, but also for the basic problem which generated the complaint. For example, if an alcoholic entered the emergency ward complaining of severe gastrointestinal upset, the investigators would assume that thc patient's motivation to get help for the upset is strong and, further, that the patient is also more motivated than he has been to accept help for the underlying problem with drinking. "The mere fact of admission to the emergency ward," they noted, "furnishes the opportunity to effect a rehabilitative relationship with the alcoholic with a more-than-usual chance of success."

Finally, a logical extension of these concepts suggested a specific set of general caretaking conditions, which are as follows. The alcoholic's low self-esteem must always be borne in mind, and caretakers must explicitly accord him ample respect and treat him with dignity. His extreme dependency needs must be recognized and constructively utilized as a means to gain his trust. The patient's standing in his primary social network and in the larger community are key elements in his condition; help with this aspect of his life must be rapidly mobilized. The same team of caretakers must initiate and follow an individual patient through treatment; one or another should always be available when the patient asks for help. As much as possible, help should be offered in the form of action rather than words.

Would an approach based on these conditions of care be more effective than customary approaches in getting alcoholic patients to enter a therapeutic alliance? Doctor Chafetz and his colleagues designed a clinical research study to find the answer. At the same time, they took the opportunity to study the sociocultural characteristics of a group of alcoholics.

In a small preliminary study the investigators discussed their ideas with the caretaking personnel that would be involved with alcoholic patients and, with 15 patients as pilot cases, worked out practical methods of treatment and data collection. An important task accomplished during the pilot period was the compilation of completely accurate, up-to-date information about the community resources available for referral and the establishment of good liaison with these agencies.

In the main study, 200 alcoholic patients were selected as subjects; half were experimental and the other half were controls. The first 20 patients diagnosed as alcoholic by the chief medical officer in the emergency ward at the beginning of each month were assigned, alternately, to the experimental and control groups. Each experimental patient was then assigned to a treatment team that would be putting the investigators' ideas into practice, while control patients simply received the care routinely given alcoholic patients entering the emergency ward. At the end of 1 year all subjects were followed up to determine whether they had made at least one visit to the Alcohol Clinic and, if so, whether they had formed a successful therapeutic alliance. This, in turn, was defined operationally as five or more visits to the Alcohol Clinic (in other clinical research of this sort, a criterion of three or more visits to a therapist is generally accepted as evidence of a therapeutic alliance.) Patient contact during the course of the study was assessed by making a note of every self-initiated face-to-face meeting between caretakers and patient in the clinic, for example, scheduled interviews and attendance at group therapy meetings. The investigators predicted that there would be greater incidences of initial visits and of five or more visits to the Alcohol Clinic among subjects in the experimental group compared to control subjects.

The heart of the new approach was the treatment-catalyst teams, each consisting of a resident psychiatrist and a psychiatric social worker. These caretakers met the alcoholic patient as quickly as possible after his arrival in the emergency ward. They let him know they were *his* psychiatrist and *his* social worker, and followed him closely throughout his stay in the ward. If he had to wait, they saw to it he was made comfortable and was offered coffee.

They smoothed his way with other hospital personnel and, by their own evident concern, attempted to forestall attitudes of indifference or hostility.

Once the patient's medical complications had been attended to, psychiatrist and social worker concentrated on an evaluation of the patient and his primary social network—getting information from family, friends, employer, and others who could help—and worked out a long-term treatment plan. Because the MGH has very limited inpatient facilities for acute alcoholic patients, those who need inpatient care must be referred to one or another of the State institutions that provide such care for voluntary patients. When this was required for their patient, the team made the telephone arrangements that cleared the patient's entry, and he was strongly urged to come back to the MGH after discharge. Most patients needed a variety of social or welfare services that were available outside the hospital, and the social workers saw to it that the patient got the right referrals. Advance telephone calls made certain the patient could be helped and was expected. Followup calls not only ensured that the patient would not be forgotten but built a sound working relationship between the MGH and the network of community agencies.

In short, the main thrust of this experimental clinical method reflected a new approach in medicine, namely, that primary responsibility for establishing a treatment relation rests with the caretakers rather than with the patient. Moreover, the kind and quality of the care given in the *initial* contact is deemed critical; it is at this point that ultimate therapeutic success may be gained or forfeited.

The results of the study were quite conclusive. Sixty-five percent of the experimental group made one visit to the Alcohol Clinic as compared to 5.4 percent of the control group. Similarly, 42 percent of the experimental group, compared to 1 percent of the controls, made five or more visits to the Clinic. Moreover, 23 percent of the experimental subjects made one to four visits compared to 4.3 percent of controls

The researchers were also interested in knowing how sustained the treatment relationship became among subjects who visited the Clinic at least five times. They found that of the total 42 patients, 25 made five to nine visits, 11 made 10 to 19 visits, and 6 patients came to the Clinic more than 20 times. This was a remarkable accomplishment when it is recalled that, prior to the initiation of the new approach, virtually no patients came to the Clinic on referral from the emergency ward. Further, when the investigators compared their results with results obtained by researchers working with other types of psychiatric patients, they found that their clinical approach was about as effective in establishing treatment alliances with chronic alcoholics as traditional approaches have been with general psychiatric cases.

The success achieved with the alcoholic population was even more impressive when the subjects' social histories were taken into account. The researchers had compiled detailed social histories on each patient admitted to the study. These inventories included information on such items as marital stability, occupational history, the use the patient and his family made of public welfare and other social agencies, and arrest history.

The men were found to be middle-aged, on the average, and eight out of ten were either single, separated, divorced, or widowed. Less than half reported being employed, and more than half were brought into the emergency ward by police. Only 17 percent reported subscribing to any sort of medical insurance. It was perhaps most revealing that 29 of the 100 experimental subjects were homeless at the time of admission (one man gave his address as the Boston Commons, a public park in the center of the city). Another 40 lived alone or in social institutions.

The study population, then, consisted largely of men existing outside the social fabric of the community, most of them shifting haphazardly along with no roots in family life or in meaningful work. As a group they fit the classic description of skid row alcoholics. To have achieved such good results with these supposedly hopeless cases was indeed a convincing demonstration of the validity of the new approach to alcoholics.

Who Is Labeled "Alcoholic"

In addition to demonstrating the effectiveness of their rational approach to fostering treatment relations with alcoholic patients, the study gave the investigators an unexpected opportunity to explore certain complex issues related to the diagnosis of alcoholism. Not long after the study began with the monthly selection of patient-subjects in the emergency ward, it appeared to the investigators that many patients who could be considered alcoholic were not being diagnosed as such and not being assigned to the study by the chief medical officer. This was an intriguing observation, so when the study was completed they decided to look into it more closely.

The researchers went back to the emergency ward daily logbook to examine the records of all patients seen during each of the 10 subject-selection periods. Then they called in for review some 3,000 medical records, one for every male aged 16 or more who had come through the emergency ward during the relevant periods. Using the same criteria for alcoholism that the chief medical officers had employed to guide them, and referring only to the original admission notes, the investigators found that a total of 238 cases of alcoholism had been missed. Their impression was now confirmed; next they attempted to discover why. What consistent differences were there between the group of 200 alcoholic men who had been assigned to the alcohol treatment project and the group of 238 alcoholic men who had not been assigned? How did the attitudes of physicians toward alcoholism influence their judgments?

The investigators focused on certain characteristics of the patients—all of which had been noted in the original admission record—and on two sets of attitudes believed to be held by physicians. One set encompasses the physician's predilection for a medical-surgical diagnosis as opposed to one indicating social or psychological disorder. The other set embraces the physician's tendency to regard alcoholism as a disorder occurring principally among the impoverished and socially deteriorated. They hypothesized that, first, the missed alcoholic patients would show a higher incidence of medical characteristics associated with physical disorders than assigned alcoholics would; and second, missed patients would possess fewer of the social characteristics associated with a skid row life than would assigned patients.

Both hypotheses were confirmed. First, compared to assigned patients, the missed cases were more often referred by a physician; they more frequently complained of a medical or surgical problem, more often received a medical diagnosis, and more frequently were hospitalized after emergency ward treatment. The investigators concluded that "the alcoholic who presents himself at the emergency ward in a manner consistent with the physician's preference for a diagnosis involving systemic disorder . . . will receive specific treatment for physical pathology but not necessarily for the alcoholic context in which the physical disorder occurs." Second, the missed alcoholics were found to be more socially integrated and more often possessed stable psychological attachments than did the assigned patients.

The researchers also constructed a combined social-medical index, consisting of 11 statistically significant social and medical variables. They found that the power of this combined index to discriminate between assigned and missed alcoholic patients was greater than that of either a social index or a medical index alone. From this they inferred that the medical and social characteristics a patient possesses tend to interact with one another in the physician's decisionmaking process. Still, it appeared that the physician's preference for a medical-surgical diagnosis took precedence over his view of alcoholics as derelicts. "From the physician's viewpoint," the investigators commented, "an alcoholic is an alcoholic only if he is relatively well physically and if he is a derelict."

The investigators' findings about the relationship between alcoholism and social isolation are relevant in this context. Although the differences between the groups of assigned and missed cases were indeed significant, the fact was the groups shared certain broad sociocultural characteristics. It was the researchers' impression that the men in both groups were more socially isolated than normal.

To test this impression they undertook a study in which the groups of missed and assigned alcoholics were each compared to a third control group of emergency ward patients. The control group was selected randomly and matched with the two alcoholic groups for age and time of admission (during subject-selection periods). Again, information about social integration and psychological attachments was obtained retrospectively from admission records. Three aspects were measured: social contact (especially with people psychologically important to the patient), social stability, and use of social resources such as medical insurance. When all patients were rated on these three measures, both assigned and missed alcoholics were found to be far more socially isolated than the men in the nonalcoholic control group. These findings suggested that some of the problems commonly associated with alcoholism may be, instead, problems of social isolation which, in turn, point to a need for clarifying the nature of alcoholism. Further, so long as the diagnosis of alcoholism relies heavily on the presence of severe social isolation, alcoholic individuals who are socially integrated only marginally will not usually be diagnosed as alcoholic and thus will not receive treatment for the disorder.

The investigators confirmed this important point again in their study of physician's attitudes toward the diagnosis of alcoholism. The physicians who had served as chief medical officers in the emergency ward during the subject-selection periods were interviewed a year later. They answered a series of open-end questions about alcoholism, which were recorded on tape for later analysis.

The comments of these physicians made it clear that they thought the alcoholics coming to the emergency ward were almost exclusively drawn from the skid row population. As the investigators pointed out, this was literally a half-truth—the physicians had missed at least as many alcoholics as they had diagnosed. On the other hand, no physician came right out and said that alcoholism was a disorder of derelicts. On the contrary, they all agreed that alcoholism could and did occur in every social stratum, and the alcoholic-as-derelict was only one type of alcoholic patient. Their comments indicated, however, that they would be hesitant to diagnose alcoholism in patients who seemed to be socially intact.

The investigators suspected that the wide gap between the physicians' intellectual understanding of alcoholism and their actual diagnostic behavior resulted from certain subtle emotional perceptions and prejudgments. They also thought that social class identifications may have been in play; thus, a middle-class physician confronted by an alcoholic who is clearly middle class in background may simply not perceive the symptoms of the disorder and, if he does, may be uncomfortable about making a diagnosis of alcoholism.

The taped interviews also yielded information confirming the physicians' predilections for a medical-surgical diagnosis. The physicians were simply more interested in physical ailments and considered psychosocial problems to be secondary, if they considered them at all.

The work of other investigators reported over the past several years strongly indicates that the attitudes of the MGH physicians are not uncommon. One may safely conclude that most physicians harbor such complex and contradictory attitudes about alcoholism and its diagnosis. The situation is tragic in implication because physicians are least likely to refer socially intact alcoholic patients to specialized treatment resources. These patients have a more favorable prognosis than do the late-stage, socially deteriorated alcoholics. A followup study by the Boston group did, in fact, demonstrate that alcoholics who were more socially intact than the original sample of patients showed even higher proportions than did the original sample of those making initial visits (78 percent) and of those making five or more visits to the Alcohol Clinic (56 percent).

What has actually been happening, then, is that the most advanced cases of alcoholism—patients suffering what Dr. Chafetz has called "the metastasis of alcoholism"—are the alcoholics most likely to be referred to treatment. Yet these are precisely the cases that are most difficult and costly to treat and least likely to achieve significant recovery. Thus the myth that alcoholics are hopeless is sustained. It has been estimated that derelict alcoholics make up some 3 to 5 percent of the total population of alcoholics in the Nation. The tragedy is that unless physicians and the general public can be made to alter their perceptions and forego their prejudices, the 95 percent will struggle along without treatment unless they, too, end up in skid row.

Doctor Chafetz has proposed one way to begin halting this human waste—by getting rid altogether of the label "alcoholic." Whether one speaks of alcoholism, alcohol-related problems, or alcoholic excess, he pointed out, one is referring to a symptom of a highly complex disorder produced by myriad factors. "There is really no such thing as an alcoholic," Dr. Chafetz said. "Just as there is no headache-ic, no fever-ic, no pain-ic, there is no alcoholic. I am strongly proposing that to free ourselves from the bondage of subjective statements and dogmatic pronouncements, we must begin to examine the use and nonuse, the meaning and significance, and the implications of alcohol problems as they relate to the total individual and his society. . . ."

Doctor Chafetz repeatedly emphasized the importance of broadening current efforts in the field of alcoholism to include secondary prevention—that is, early diagnosis—and primary prevention—steps to prevent the disorder from starting. "No effort in social and medical problems can hope to succeed if it is directed solely to treatment of the late stages of condition," he noted. "Treatment at best can only slow the flood waters, because the production of ill people far outruns the production of treaters." Under his direction, the Boston group has been active in these areas also; the researchers are now carrying out studies designed to explore various approaches to early case-finding.

Evaluating Treatment of Alcoholics

The treatment-catalyst team approach developed by the Boston group has been shown to be very effective in getting alcoholic patients into rehabilitation programs. What happens then? Just how efficacious are treatment methods generally in restoring victims of alcoholism to healthy useful lives? The answer is that no one knows; at least, there are no scientifically rigorous answers available.

Recently Doctors Hill and Blane reviewed the literature evaluating psychotherapy with alcoholic patients. They looked at a total of 49 papers published in the years 1952–63 and found that almost all were descriptive surveys rather than reports of research programs. Most authors did not attempt to devise a systematic methodology or to use statistical techniques for analyses. Only two of the 49 were prospective studies. Methods of control, of subject selection and the selection and definition of criterion variables, and of measuring change were found to be mainly inadequate and unreliable. Doctors Hill and Blane concluded that the summary offered 25 years earlier by the authors of the same sort of critical review was still accurate: "We are unable to form a conclusive opinion as to the value of psychotherapeutic methods in the treatment of alcoholism."

This situation is not unique to alcoholism treatment. There are no definitive answers about the efficacy of treatment for the whole range of psychoneurotic disturbances, character disorders, and social deviances. "Evaluation of psychotherapeutic treatment is the hardest research problem of all," Doctor Chafetz said. "The methodology is unsound and hard data are lacking. What we have got to do is set up an adequate model. We load the dice against ourselves when we use the acute infectious model. In that model you see symptoms, give specific medication, and the symptoms go away never to return. But with alcoholism we are dealing with a chronic illness. We can arrest and control but we cannot cure in the sense that we can cure an infection. People ask—'is he dry?'—and think that's all the answer they need. But that is not all. It is a clinical myth that recovered alcoholics cannot be social drinkers. We don't know; we simply do not have the facts. In our work we use a rating scale with multiple points including overall functioning, interpersonal relationships, and internalized feelings. We get base points on these measures when a patient first comes to us, then check again at various points in treatment. We may end an active phase of treatment but we know you can't discharge a chronic patient. They need to be able to come back, and they do."

Doctor Hill is just beginning a study that takes a very pragmatic approach to the problem of an adequate model of therapeutic success. In her view, one way to get at success is to define it in terms of what the patient wants from treatment and what the therapist wants. The researcher is interviewing patients at the beginning of treatment and finding out what goals he has. So far, most have responded immediately that they want "to quit drinking"; but Doctor Hill urges them to name other goals they may wish to reach. Then, after a therapist has seen an individual patient three or four times, Doctor Hill asks him about his goals for the patient during the coming 3 months. Patients and therapists will be interviewed again at the end of 6 months, when a therapist will be asked to *predict* what goals his patient named. It will be interesting to know how congruent patient and therapist goals are, "success" may have disparate meaning to the patient and the therapist.

The design of this study will also make it possible to learn something about behavioral correlates of moderation and abstinence. In other words, how else does the patient's behavior change as his drinking habits change?

There is no lack of opinion on this question, but there are almost no factual answers. Abstinence has traditionally been the major, often the exclusive, goal of treatment efforts. Yet when consumption drops to zero or is significantly moderated, the patient may develop ulcers or suffer anxiety attacks or lose every friend he has. Abstinence as a goal may be unrealistic on other counts as well. This is the heart of the issue that Doctor Chafetz raises when he stresses the importance of seeing, and treating, the total individual in his total social system.

References

BLANE, H. T. (1966). Attitudes, treatment, and prevention. *International Psychiatry Clinics*, **3** (2), 103–126.

BLANE, H. T. (1968). Trends in the prevention of alcoholism. *Psychiatric Research Report*, **24**, 1–9, March.

BLANE, H. T., & HILL, M. J. (1964). Public health nurses speak up about alcoholism. *Nursing Outlook*, **12**, 5.

BLANE, H. T., MULLER, J. J., & CHAFETZ, M. E. (1957). Acute psychiatric services in the general hospital. II. Current status of emergency psychiatric services. *American Journal of Psychiatry*, **124** (4), 37–45, October (Supplement).

BLANE, H. T., OVERTON, W. F., Jr., & CHAFETZ, M. E. (1963). Social factors in the diagnosis of alcoholism. I. Characteristics of patients. *Quarterly Journal of Hospital News*, **222**, 1–3, May.

CHAFETZ, M. E. (1959). Practical and theoretical considerations in the psychotherapy of alcoholism. *Quarterly Journal of Studies on Alcohol*, **20**, 281–291.

CHAFETZ, M. E. (1963). Acute psychiatric services in the emergency ward. *Massachusetts General Hospital News*, **222**, 1–3, May.

CHAFETZ, M. E. (1965). The effect of a psychiatric evaluation service on motivation for psychiatric treatment. *Journal of Nervous and Mental Disease*, **140** (6), 442–448.

CHAFETZ, M. E. (1966). Alcohol excess. *Annals of the New York Academy of Sciences*, **133**, 808–813.

CHAFETZ, M. E. (1966). Management of the alcoholic patient in an acute treatment facility. *International Psychiatric Clinics*, **3** (2), 127–141.

CHAFETZ, M. E. (1967). Motivation for recovery in alcoholism. In Fox, R., ed., *Alcoholism—Behavioral Research, Therapeutic Approaches*, New York, Springer, 110–117.

CHAFETZ, M. E. (1968). Research in the alcoholic clinic and around-the-clock psychiatric service of the Massachusetts General Hospital. American Journal of Psychiatry, **124**, 96–101, June.

CHAFETZ, M. E., BLANE, H. T., ABRAM, H. S., CLARK, E., GOLNER, J. H., HASTIE, E. L., & MCCOURT, W. F. (1964). Establishing treatment relations with alcoholics: a supplemental report. *Journal of Nervous and Mental Disease*, **138** (4), 390–393.

CHAFETZ, M. E., BLANE, H. T., ABRAM, H. S., GOLNER, J., LACY, E., MCCOURT, W. F., CLARK, E., & MYERS, W. (1962). Establishing treatment relations with alcoholics. *Journal of Nervous and Mental Disease*, **134** (5), 395–409.

CHAFETZ, M. E., BLANE, H. T., and MULLER, J. J. (1966). Acute psychiatric services in the general hospital. I. Implications for psychiatry in emergency admissions. *American Journal of Psychiatry*, **123** (6), 664–670.

CHAFETZ, M. E., DEMONE, W. H., Jr., & SOLOMON, H. C. (1962). Alcoholism: its cause and prevention. *New York State Journal of Medicine*, **62** (10), 1614–1625.

CLARK, E. (1963). Round-the-clock emergency psychiatric services. In Meier, E. G., Kassius, C., & Ray, F., (eds.), *Social Work Practice*. 1963 National Conference on Social Welfare. New York: Columbia University Press, 44–57.

HILL, M. J., & BLANE, H. T. (1967). Evaluation of psychotherapy with alcoholics: a critical review. *Quarterly Journal of Studies on Alcohol*, **28** (1), 76–104.

MENDELSON, J. H., & CHAFETZ, M. E. (1959). Alcoholism as an emergency ward problem. *Quarterly Journal of Studies on Alcohol*, **20**, 270–275.

MULLER, J. J., CHAFETZ, M. E., & BLANE, H. T. (1967). Acute psychiatric services in the general hospital. III. Statistical survey. *American Journal of Psychiatry*, **124** (4), 46–57, October (Supplement).

SINGER, E., BLANE, H. T., & KASSCHAU, R. (1964). Alcoholism and social isolation. *Journal of Abnormal and Social Psychology*, **69** (6), 681–685.

WOLF, I., CHAFETZ, M. E., BLANE, H. T., & HILL, M. J. (1965). Social factors in the diagnosis of alcoholism. II. Attitudes of physicians. *Quarterly Journal of Studies on Alcohol*, **26** (1), 72–79.

RAY B. EVANS

Childhood Parental Relationships of Homosexual Men

One of the major studies of homosexuality was by Bieber and his associates, and it highlighted some difficulties in the early histories of homosexual men. The generality of the conclusions of that study were questioned because all the subjects were in therapy, and all the data were derived from the analysts rather than from the patients themselves. In this study, Dr. Evans extended Bieber's findings to a group of homosexual men who were not in treatment and who responded directly to questionnaire items. Many of the original findings were replicated, but the difficulties inherent in drawing retrospective causal conclusions from data of this sort were discussed. When this paper was originally published it was accompanied by invited discussions written by Drs. Ralph Gundlach and Evelyn Hooker. The interested reader is referred to them.

A major conclusion of a study comparing homosexual and heterosexual men who were all in psychoanalytic therapy was that parental roles are paramount in the etiology of homosexuality (Bieber, Dain, Dince, Drellich, Grand, Gundlach, Kremer, Rifkin, Wilbur, & Bieber, 1962). Those authors described the "classical" pattern as one where the mother is close-binding and intimate with her son and is dominant and minimizing toward her husband, who is a detached (particularly a hostile-detached) father to the son. They concluded that any son exposed to that parental combination will likely develop severe

---

Reprinted from the *Journal of Consulting and Clinical Psychology*, **33** (1969), 129–135, with the permission of the American Psychological Association and Dr. Evans.

homosexual problems. The Bieber study was based on extensive questionnaires completed by the analysts for each patient; the patients themselves were not aware of the study. Two series of questions proved especially useful in differentiating the homosexual and heterosexual groups, a Developmental Six Score (concerning childhood fears and activities) and a Twenty Questions Score (relating to interparental and parent-child relationships).

There is an obvious risk in generalizing findings from patients in psychotherapy to a non-patient population. The purpose of the present study was to determine whether questionnaire items adapted from Bieber et al. would differentiate samples of heterosexual and homosexual men who had never sought psychotherapy.

Method

Subjects

The sample consisted of 185 American-born, Caucasian men between the ages of 22 and 47, who had at least a high school education, had never sought psychotherapy, and were living in the Los Angeles metropolitan area. All *S*s were volunteers in a study of cardiovascular disease, but only the 43 homosexuals knew that aspects of homosexuality were also being studied. The latter volunteered, as homosexuals, through the cooperation of a Los Angeles based organization; they did not constitute a representative group of homosexuals. The 142 "heterosexual" *S*s volunteered for the cardiac study through a number of sources, and there was no opportunity to develop the kind of rapport needed to elicit information about their sexual preferences and behavior. For purposes of this study, it was assumed they were all heterosexual, though there may have been homosexuals among them, which would tend to attenuate group differences.

The homosexual men ranged in age from 22 to 46, with a mean of 33.8 years ($SD = 7.1$); the heterosexuals ranged from 25 to 47, with an average of 39.3 ($SD = 4.4$), and the difference was significant ($t = 4.84$, $p < .001$). They were reasonably similar to patients in the Bieber study, where the homosexuals averaged approximately 35 and the heterosexuals approximately 38 years of age.

In education, the homosexuals ranged from 12 to 19 years, with a mean of 14.4 ($SD = 2.2$); and the heterosexuals ranged from 12 to 20 years, with a mean of 15.1 ($SD = 2.1$), with the difference approaching statistical significance ($t = 1.87$, $p < .10$). Again, they were relatively similar to the Bieber patients, who averaged approximately 15 years of education.

There was an obvious and expected difference between the two groups in marital status. Among the heterosexuals, 5% were single, 87% married, and 8% separated or divorced; 86% of the homosexuals were single, 5% married, and 9% divorced. In the Bieber et al. study, 8% of the homosexuals and 51% of the heterosexuals were married.

As to sibling constellations, there were 12%, 35%, 14%, and 40%, respectively, only, oldest, middle, and youngest children among the homosexuals; comparable figures for the heterosexuals were 8%, 28%, 27%, and 37%. Those distributions were not significantly different. Bieber et al. reported 10% of their homosexuals and 22% of their heterosexuals were only children, which difference was significant at the .05 level.

Proportionately more of the homosexuals were employed in clerical work and in the arts, and fewer of them in other professions, management, and sales work. The difference in hetero-sexual-homosexual occupational distributions was significant ($\chi^2 = 42.88$, $df = 5$, $p < .001$). The occupational classifications of the present *S*s and the Bieber patients were fairly comparable.

The homosexual volunteers rated their sexual experiences on a 7-point scale adapted from Kinsey, Pomeroy, and Gebhard (1948), which ranged from entirely heterosexual to entirely homosexual. Of the 43 *S*s, 58% described their experience as having been exclusively homosexual, 35% as predominantly homosexual with incidental heterosexual, and 7% as predominantly homosexual but more than incidental heterosexual experience. For their homosexual patients, Bieber et al. reported 68% as exclusively homosexual, 28% as having some heterosexual experience, and 4% as inactive, so that the proportion of exclusive homosexuals in the two studies was similar ($\chi^2 = .89$, $p = .50$).

The homosexual *S*s also completed an 11-item questionnaire designed to determine their sexual identification. In their overall feelings, 40 *S*s (93%) considered themselves moderately or strongly masculine, and responses to the other 10 items also indicated essentially masculine identification. Bieber et al. reported that approximately 2% of their homosexual patients were "markedly effeminate," so that seemingly *S*s from the two studies were similar in this regard.

Procedure

Each *S* completed a 27-item questionnaire adapted from Bieber et al. so as to be as nearly comparable as possible. The essential content of the questionnaire appears in Table 1. Included were the Developmental Six (Items 2–7) and Twenty Questions (Items 8–27) scores, and one additional question regarding physical make-up in childhood (Item 1), which had also differentiated the Bieber groups. Four possible choices were provided for each item, whereas the Bieber study used a yes-no dichotomy for all except three items. Following is an example from Bieber et al. completed by the analysts: "Was patient excessively fearful of physical injury in childhood? (yes/no)." The corresponding item modified for the present study, for completion by *S* himself, was: "During childhood, were you fearful of physical injury? (seldom/sometimes/often/always)."

Questionnaires were used in the analysis only where all 27 items had been answered, which eliminated 11 potential *S*s, one homosexual and 10 heterosexual. Differences between groups were calculated by means of chi-square, with twofold classifications corrected for continuity.

TABLE 1 *Parental relationships of homosexual men. Questionnaire content and item responses*

Questionnaire item	Bieber study				Present study			
	Response	Homo-sexual	Hetero-sexual	*p*	Response	Homo-sexual	Hetero-sexual	*p*
Physical make-up as a child	Frail	50	17		Frail	37	11	
	Clumsy	24	08		Clumsy	14	06	
	Athletic	13	33		Athletic	05	45	
	Well coordinated	13	42	.001	Coordinated	44	38	.001
Fearful of physical injury as a child	Yes	75	46		Seldom	23	49	
	No	25	54	.001	Sometimes	51	46	
					Often	19	04	
					Always	07	01	.001
Avoided physical fights	Yes	90	56		Always	56	12	
	No	10	44	.001	Often	30	35	
					Sometimes	14	46	
					Never	00	07	.001
Played with girls before adolescence	Yes	34	10		Never	09	03	
	No	66	90	.001	Sometimes	49	83	
					Often	40	14	
					Always	02	00	.001
"Lone wolf" in childhood	Yes	61	27		Never	12	38	
	No	39	73	.001	Sometimes	35	51	
					Often	42	11	
					Always	12	01	.001
Played competitive group games	Yes	17	64		Never	09	01	
	No	83	36	.001	Sometimes	65	15	
					Often	23	52	
					Very often	02	32	.001
Played baseball	Yes	16	64		Never	19	05	
	No	84	36	.001	Sometimes	70	29	
					Often	09	35	
					Very often	02	32	.001
Father and mother spent time together	Great deal	01	13		Great deal	16	28	
	Average	42	50		Considerable	53	39	
	Little	36	24		Little	26	23	
	Very little	21	13	.002	Very little	05	09	.23
Parents shared similar interests	Yes	20	38		Great many	21	30	
	No	80	62	.01	Several	37	32	
					Few	35	33	
					None	07	05	.70
Mother insisted on being center of son's attention	Yes	64	36		Never	30	18	
	No	36	64	.001	Seldom	37	63	
					Often	16	17	
					Always	16	01	.001
Mother "seductive" toward son as a child	Yes	57	34		Highly	07	00	
	No	43	66	.002	Moderately	07	03	
					Slightly	09	13	
					No	77	85	.02
Mother discouraged masculine attitudes/activities	Yes	39	17		Often	05	02	
	No	61	83	.002	Sometimes	21	07	
					Seldom	30	14	
					Never	44	77	.001
Mother encouraged feminine attitudes/activities	Yes	36	12		Never	53	87	
	No	64	88	.001	Seldom	21	11	
					Sometimes	21	02	
					Often	05	01	.001

Questionnaire item	Bieber study				Present study			
	Response	Homo-sexual	Hetero-sexual	p	Response	Homo-sexual	Hetero-sexual	p
Mother considered puritanical	Yes	67	51		Strongly	28	11	
	No	33	49	.05	Moderately	33	35	
					Mildly	23	23	
					No	16	30	.04
Mother's relationships with father/other men	Frigid	72	56		Frigid	12	00	
	Not frigid	28	44	.04	Cold	26	23	
					Warm	63	77	.10
Mother allied with son against father	Yes	63	40		Often	33	06	
	No	37	60	.002	Sometimes	21	18	
					Seldom	16	35	
					Never	30	42	.001
Mother openly preferred son to father	Yes	59	38		Always	12	01	
	No	41	62	.005	Often	14	06	
					Seldom	21	31	
					Never	53	62	.004
Mother interfered with heterosexual activities	Yes	37	25		Often	12	00	
	No	63	75	.08	Sometimes	16	08	
					Seldom	19	20	
					Never	53	71	.004
Son was mother's confidant	Yes	52	36		Never	30	27	
	No	48	64	.03	Seldom	19	32	
					Sometimes	23	36	
					Often	28	05	.001
Son was father's favorite	Yes	08	29		Strongly	09	09	
	No	92	71	.001	Moderately	16	40	
					Mildly	40	37	
					No	35	14	.005
Felt accepted by father	Yes	23	48		Strongly	23	42	
	No	77	52	.001	Moderately	35	42	
					Mildly	23	11	
					No	19	06	.006
Son spent time with father	Great deal	03	03		Great deal	02	08	
	Average	12	39		Considerable	09	39	
	Little	37	31		Little	53	32	
	Very little	48	27	.001	Very little	35	21	.001
Father encouraged masculine attitudes/activities	Yes	48	61		Often	26	41	
	No	52	39	.07	Sometimes	26	32	
					Seldom	23	21	
					Never	26	06	.002
Aware of hating father as a child	Yes	61	37		Never	28	59	
	No	39	63	.002	Seldom	19	20	
					Sometimes	37	18	
					Often	16	03	.001
Afraid father might physically harm him	Yes	57	43		Often	14	04	
	No	43	57	.06	Sometimes	19	23	
					Seldom	30	13	
					Never	37	60	.003
Accepted father	Yes	21	51		Strongly	26	51	
	No	79	49	.001	Moderately	28	37	
					Mildly	33	09	
					No	14	03	.001
Respected father	Yes	30	49		Strongly	37	56	
	No	70	51	.01	Moderately	21	32	
					Mildly	21	08	
					No	21	03	.001

Note.—Significance levels based on chi-square, with twofold classifications corrected for continuity. Decimals omitted.

Results

The content of each questionnaire item is given in Table 1, together with the proportion of *S*s responding in each category, and the significance of differences between the homosexual and heterosexual groups. Comparable figures from the Bieber study are also included, with the significance values calculated from figures in Appendix A (Bieber et al., (1962) using only *S*s for whom definite response was available. Differences between the Bieber groups reached at least the .05 level of significance for 24 of the 27 items, and the other three approached significance. (Bieber et al. reported all items significant, and the discrepancy may be due to the method used here of ignoring "No Answer" and "Not Applicable" categories in the calculation of chi-square.)

In the present study, homosexual-heterosexual differences were significant at the .05 level or less for 24 items, one other approached significance, and for two items no difference was found. Thus, despite the very different method of collecting data, the non-patient status of the *S*s, and (perhaps minor) differences due to geographical location, the results were remarkably similar to those reported by Bieber et al.

Specifically, in retrospect, the homosexuals more often described themselves as frail or clumsy as children and less often as athletic. More of them were fearful of physical injury, avoided physical fights, played with girls, and were loners who seldom played baseball and other competitive games. Their mothers more often were considered puritanical, cold toward men, insisted on being the center of the son's attention, made him her confidant, were "seductive" toward him, allied with him against the father, openly preferred him to the father, interfered with his heterosexual activities during adolescence, discouraged masculine attitudes, and encouraged feminine ones. The fathers of the homosexuals were retrospectively considered as less likely to encourage masculine attitudes and activities, and *S*s spent little time with their fathers, were more often aware of hating him and afraid he might physically harm them, less often were the father's favorite, felt less accepted by him, and in turn less frequently accepted or respected the father. Unlike Bieber's patients, these homosexuals were no different from the heterosexuals in amount of time they estimated their parents spent together or in the interests shared by their parents.

In addition, a total score on the 27-item questionnaire was obtained for each *S* by weighting each item from 0 to 3 points, with the higher weighting at the "masculine" end, so there was a maximum possible score of 81. The scores of the homosexuals ranged from 9 to 64, with a mean of 42.9 ($SD = 11.6$); those of the heterosexuals from 36 to 77, with a mean of 57.3 ($SD = 9.2$). Though there was considerable overlap in scores for the two groups, the difference was highly significant ($t = 7.50$, $p < .001$).

Discussion

The results could not be accounted for on the basis of sample characteristics other than sexual orientation; no relationship was found between age and questionnaire scores, and the same was true of marital status, occupational classification, and sibling constellation. The fact that the homosexuals knew homosexuality was being studied might have affected the results, but if there was any tendency to distort in the direction of "normal," it was not sufficient to obscure group differences.

As to preponderance of homosexual experience, no relationship was observed between Kinsey-type ratings (completed only by homosexual *S*s) and questionnaire scores ($\chi^2 = 0.0$), perhaps because of the limited variation in proportion of homosexual experience. However, a product-moment correlation of .47 ($t = 3.41$, $p < .01$) was found between the 27-item questionnaire and the 11-item sexual identity questionnaire; the homosexuals with more "desirable" family backgrounds tended to consider themselves as more masculine.

It may be noteworthy that the present results were so similar to those obtained by the Bieber group despite a major difference in the level of observation. In the present study, the data were based on retrospective self-reports of how they now view their childhood, by *S*s who had never been in psychotherapy. The Bieber data, on the other hand, were based on psychoanalysts' reconstructions of patients' early life circumstances, derived from impressions during psychotherapy. Arguments could be advanced for the superiority of one method over the other, and certainly both have limitations. The agreement in results could be interpreted as evidence of validity in both methods, or perhaps as an indication that the two methods are not essentially different.

The results strongly suggested poor parental relationships during childhood for the homosexual men, at least as seen in retrospect; however, the etiological significance of such relationships, or even the etiology of the relationships themselves, is another matter. Bieber et al. considered the chances high that any son exposed to the parental combination of maternal close-binding intimacy and paternal detachment-hostility will develop severe homosexual problems. Nevertheless, only 28% of their homosexual patients had such a parental combination, and the 11% of their control patients who had such parents did not become homosexual. Furthermore, Bieber et al. very much underemphasized one-third of the "triad," the son himself. They reported that "each parent had a specific type of relationship with the homosexual son which generally did not occur with other siblings," and that son was the "focal point for the most profound parental psychopathology." As to why a particular son is singled out, Bieber et al. proposed that son is unconsciously identified by the mother with her own father or brothers, and the son thereby becomes the recipient of sexual feelings carried over from the mother's own early life. Similarly, the father transfers to that son his unresolved hostility and rivalry with his own father/brothers. The above is an oversimplified summary of the Bieber formulation, but it does not exaggerate the neglect of the son's contribution to the triadic relationship, beyond eliciting parental transference feelings.

The personalities and behavior of parents undoubtedly affect a child's personality, but some consideration must be given to the notion that the child's innate characteristics at least partially determine parental reactions and attitudes toward him. For instance, that the father of a homosexual son becomes detached and/or hostile because he does not understand or is disappointed in the son is just as tenable as that the son becomes homosexual because of the father's rejection. Similarly, that a mother may be more intimate with and bind her homosexual son more closely because of the kind of person he is, is just as reasonable as the idea that he becomes homosexual because she is too binding and intimate. Bieber et al. did question whether paternal rejection and hostility were stimulated out of feelings of disappointment and failure because of the son's homosexuality, but concluded that was not likely since only 17% of the fathers were reported to have been aware of the son's homosexuality. Surely most parental reactions crucially affecting the child's personality occur when the child is far too young to be labeled homosexual or heterosexual. The Bieber group also concluded that the father's attitudes were not traceable to the fact that the sons were inadequate and unattractive children, since the mothers did not find them so. That the mothers did not find these sons unattractive is no indication the fathers did not; the evidence suggests the fathers did find them unappealing.

Judging from experience with adult homosexual males, O'Connor (1964) also refuted the idea that lack of a good father relationship was a consequence rather than a cause of homosexuality, on the grounds that would make it difficult to account for the many homosexuals whose fathers were physically absent. Bene (1965) rejected the notion that the lack of a positive father relationship might be due to the son repulsing the father rather than the father repulsing the son, and she cited O'Connor's reasoning. That homosexuality occurs in sons whose fathers are physically absent is irrelevant to the fact that when the father is physically present the relationship with the homosexual son is often a poor one. Furthermore, that homosexuality occurs in the absence of a father not only detracts from the etiological significance of a poor paternal relationship but in fact supports the importance of other causal factors (possibly such as innate physical/personality characteristics of the son).

Information was obtained relevant to another conclusion of Bieber and colleagues, who stated: "We have come to the conclusion that a constructive, supportive, warmly related father *precludes* the possibility of a homosexual son; he acts as a neutralizing, protective agent should the mother make seductive or close-binding attempts [p. 311]." The questionnaire responses gave no full and complete answer as to whether these fathers were constructive, supportive, and warmly related, but there was evidence that the father relationship of some homosexuals was as good as that of many heterosexuals. A score was calculated for each *S* based on Items 20–27 in Table 1, all of which concern the father-son relationship. With 0–3 points possible for each item, the total scores for the homosexuals ranged from 0 to 22, with a mean of 11.7; and scores for heterosexuals ranged from 3 to 23, with a mean of 16.5. While the difference was significant ($t = 5.95$, $p < .001$), 16% of the homosexuals scored above the heterosexual mean, and 16% of the heterosexuals scored below the homosexual mean. Therefore, it would seem that a moderately good relationship, at least as reflected in the above questionnaire items, does not preclude the appearance of homosexuality, even though it is well established that a poor father relationship is common among homosexual sons. The responses for the Bieber homosexuals on the corresponding questionnaire items suggested their father relationships were poorer than those of the present homosexual *S*s, which could merely reflect methodological differences, but more likely is related to the fact that the Bieber *S*s had all sought psychotherapy, whereas none of the present *S*s had done so.

In a similar fashion, two other questionnaire scores were calculated, one regarding mother-son relationships (Items 10–19) and the other pertaining to development (Items 1–7). With a maximum score of 30 on the 10 mother items, the homosexuals ranged from 4 to 29, with a mean of 18.8; the heterosexuals ranged from 13 to 29, mean 22.9. Although the difference was significant ($t = 5.39$, $p < .001$), 30% of the homosexuals scored above the heterosexual mean, and 12% of the heterosexuals scored below the homosexual mean. As to the seven developmental items, with a possible score of 21, the homosexuals ranged from 1 to 15, with a mean of 8.9; and the heterosexuals ranged from 6 to 19, mean of 14.3. That difference was most significant ($t = 10.39$, $p < .001$), and only 2% of the homosexuals exceeded the heterosexual mean, with 4% of the heterosexuals scoring below the homosexual mean. Of the three content areas, then, the developmental items clearly differentiated *S*s best, with the father and mother items similar in their differentiation. The childhood behavior reflected in some of the developmental items, of course, is not unaffected by parents, but the findings suggest the possibility of something more fundamental in homosexuality than a poor father relationship.

The results of the present study agreed closely with those obtained by Bieber et al. but they neither supported nor refuted the Bieber conclusions as to causal relationships. The complicated problem of the etiology of homosexuality probably could be more productively investigated with a prospective study.

References

BENE, E. (1965). On the genesis of male homosexuality: an attempt at clarifying the role of the parents. *British Journal of Psychiatry*, **111**, 803–813.

BIEBER, I., DAIN, H. J., DINCE, P. R., DRELLICH, M. G., GRAND, H. G., GUNDLACH, R. H., KREMER, M. W., RIFKIN, A. H., WILBUR, C. B., & BIEBER, T. B. (1962). *Homosexuality: A Psychoanalytic Study*. New York: Basic Books.

KINSEY, A., POMEROY, W. B., & GEBHARD, P. H. (1948). *Sexual Behavior in the Human Male*. Philadelphia: Saunders.

O'CONNOR, J. (1964). Aetiological factors in homosexuality as seen in Royal Air Force psychiatric practice. *British Journal of Psychiatry*, **110**, 381–399.

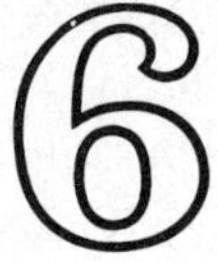

Children's Disorders

There are many reasons why it is important to study the disorders of children apart from their adult counterparts. First of all, many workers feel that at least some disorders of childhood are unique to that period of life and could not appear at a later time. Furthermore, many events in childhood potentially can be expressed in adult behavior patterns. Lastly, those theorists who subscribe to a developmental personality theory feel that an understanding of childhood is essential to a full understanding of the adult.

JEAN W. MacFARLANE and JOHN A. CLAUSEN

Childhood Influences upon Intelligence, Personality, and Mental Health

This paper was prepared by Herbert Yahraes to describe a portion of the findings of an extensive longitudinal study that is still in progress, and has been conducted by the Institute of Human Development in Berkeley, California, for over forty years. Drs. MacFarlane and Clausen are among a group of distinguished project directors. Most field research in psychology suffers because data are only collected at one point in time, and it is unwise to draw retrospective conclusions about possible antecedent factors that contributed to the issue under study. This is precisely the point Evans makes in his discussion of Bieber's data. The solution to this problem is the longitudinal study, which provides data over an extended period of time.

Reprinted from Julius Segal (ed.), *The Mental Health of the Child.* Washington, D.C.: U.S. Government Printing Office, 1971, pp. 131–154. Reprinted by permission of the U.S. Government Printing Office, Publishers, and Dr. MacFarlane.

Unfortunately, these studies, of necessity, take a great deal of time and administrative skill. The Berkeley studies are among the best examples of such an approach, and this partial report of their findings has been abridged to focus on issues of personality and mental health. There are references in the text to books that are being prepared and also a bibliography listing of some of the articles that have reported project results. These should be of value to the interested reader.

Introduction and Summary

The usual way of studying how the circumstances of childhood affect the characteristics of adulthood is to start with the grown person and try to work back. So-called longitudinal studies, though, begin with the child. Three of these, directed by the Institute of Human Development of the University of California, Berkeley, and supported recently with NIMH help, are now approximately 40 years old and probably offer the richest collection of data ever assembled on human beings over a long period.

The projects have attempted to answer such questions as:

- Do personality and intelligence change during the years or remain constant? To what extent are they related to a person's very early experiences?
- How is the mental health of an adult related to his life at home and to other influences during childhood and adolescence?
- What factors contribute to an adult's attitudes, achievement, psychological health?

In the beginning each study had its own set of objectives:

The Guidance Study was primarily interested in personality development. It began studying its subjects as infants. There were 252 of them—every third child born in Berkeley over an 18-month period beginning January 1928. The children were weighed, measured, tested, interviewed, and observed at various times through their eighteenth year. Special attention was given to their life at home during the preschool years. Information about them was obtained also from their parents, brothers and sisters, teachers, and classmates. At 30, when they were rearing children of their own, 167 of them were studied again. (The project got its name from one of the original objectives: to learn whether or not psychological guidance offered to parents would lead to better mental health for their children as adults.) The project's director until recently was Jean Walker MacFarlane, Ph.D., who is now Professor of Psychology and Research Psychologist, emeritus, at the Institute of Human Development and is still working on the study. The present director is Marjorie P. Honzik, Ph.D., Research Psychologist and Lecturer in Psychology.

The Berkeley Growth Study, which also began in 1928, has been particularly interested in physical and mental growth. Its original sample comprised 61 healthy hospital-born babies, who were studied while they were still in the hospital and then every month until they were 15 months old. After that, they were studied every 3 months until they were 3 years old, then every 6 months until they were 18. They were examined and interviewed again when they were 21, 26, and 36 years old. The sample now numbers 54. The project's director is Nancy Bayley, Ph.D., research psychologist.

The Oakland Growth Study has been concerned with the effect of adolescence —the physical and psychological changes occurring then, and the accompanying attitudes and behavior—upon later life. The study began in 1931 with the fifth grade pupils of five Oakland, California, schools who would be entering the same junior high school. There were 200 of these. They were studied intensively—through measurements, tests, observation, self-reports, ratings by classmates and teachers, and other means—through the six years of junior and senior high school. At graduation, 165 were still in the group. Follow-up studies made 15, 20, and 26 years later have reached as many as 123. The study began under the direction of Harold E. Jones, Ph.D., and Herbert R. Stolz, M.D. Its director since 1960 has been John A. Clausen, Ph.D., professor of sociology and research sociologist.

Almost all of the subjects were white. In the Guidance Study, though, 3 percent were Negro, a proportion representative of the community's Negro population in 1928. Though all socioeconomic levels were represented, the families of the subjects were predominantly middle class.

In some respects—in anthropometrics, intelligence tests, certain personality measures—the three studies overlapped, making it possible for one set of findings to be compared to another. In some of the analyses now being made, data from more than one study are used. All the subjects, it is planned, will be followed through life, with the principal research interest from now on being factors connected with the aging process.

Intelligence as Related to Behavior and Personality

The follow-up of the people in the Berkeley Growth Study when they were 36 included a detailed personality assessment made on the basis of the 100-item Block Q-sort. (In a Q-sort, characteristics noted during an interview are given numerical weight by scoring each item on a scale. The interviewer thus can say that the given quality was absent, present to a very high degree, or present to one of the several degrees in between. In this study the transcribed interviews were Q-sorted by the interviewer and by two clinical psychologists.) Bayley has now analyzed the findings and compared them with the scores made on IQ tests during the same follow-up.

The men who had been scored high on such items as impatient, negativistic, self-pitying, and hostile were found to be those who in general had the lowest IQ's. The men described as critical, introspective, socially perceptive, and having wide interests were those in general with the highest IQ's. Little or no relationship was found between IQ scores on the one hand, and on the other hand, characteristics described as either distant and avoiding or warm, calm, and gregarious.

"The men in this sample with high intelligence," Bayley reports, "are best characterized as introspective, thoughtful, and concerned with problems, meanings, and values; they are men who are perceptive and have a wide range of interests. The least intelligent are most often found to be impatient, prone to vent their hostilities and to project them onto others."

The correlations between the women's IQ's and various personality attributes are much weaker but similar in pattern. Again it is the thoughtful, insightful person with wide interests who is more likely to score high on the IQ tests. Women described as bland, conventional, or anxious are much less likely to rate high on the tests; so are women described as cheerful, poised, and gregarious.

Another measure of personality styles and psychological attitudes administered during this follow-up was the California Psychological Inventory, a questionnaire designed to measure such characteristics as sociability, self-acceptance, sense of well-being, tolerance, and responsibility. It has 17 scales. Bayley has compared the scores made on each of these at the age of 36 with the IQ scores at that age and also at 16, 18, 21, and 26 years.

Certain of these characteristics appear to be significantly associated with a high order of intelligence at all the ages studied. For men, the clearest and most consistent associations with IQ's are socialization (referring to social maturity, integrity, rectitude); the ability to make a good impression; potential for achievement, whether by conforming with the group or acting independently; and intellectual efficiency. For women, the clearest and most consistent associations are with tolerance, potential for achievement by acting independently, and flexibility.

Ratings on self-acceptance and self-control, qualities usually associated with mental health, were not significantly related to intelligence in either men or women.

When Bayley used the scores on the subscales of the intelligence test, she found some other provocative patterns. Little or no sex difference appeared in the correlations between scores on the verbal-academic scales of the IQ tests and the ratings for achievement potential, intellectual efficiency, and interest in intellectual pursuits. But the other scales pointed to marked differences. With men but not with women, for example, the score on the picture-completion test correlated strongly with the score on socialization; with women but not with men it correlated with flexibility. Scores on the object-assembly test correlated with flexibility, achievement potential, and intellectual efficiency with the women but not with the men. The highest scores in arithmetic were made by the women rating highest in feminine qualities and by the men rating lowest in them. The highest scores in the digit-span test were made by the men ranking high in sociability, well-being, and interest in making a good impression and by the women ranking low in these characteristics.

In short, for this small sample at least, there seems to be a relationship between intellectual processes and personality as manifested in various social attitudes, interests, and motivations. The relationship remains fairly stable over the years between 16 and 36, but differs both with the nature of the intellectual process and with the personality characteristic being considered. It often differs widely between the sexes as well.

In the case of males, the investigators have also found some relations between mental test scores throughout the 36-year period and the behavior and personality characteristics of the subjects during their first three years. Boys who were calm, responding, and happy, and who were active after 15 months rather than before, were more likely than the others to have high IQ's (determined in this case only from the verbal scale). Girls showed no clear pattern.

With females through the years, considerably fewer significant correlations between IQ scores and personality ratings were noted than for males. Bayley suggests that a girl's intellectual potential is less affected than a man's by social and emotional factors. A girl comes into life physiologically tougher, it has been shown; perhaps she is by nature psychologically tougher as well.

Psychological Mechanisms and the IQ

After the subjects in the Oakland Growth Survey had been interviewed at 37, Norma Haan, a psychologist, rated them for the presence of coping and defense mechanisms. Among the coping mechanisms she includes objectivity, logical analysis, empathy, sublimation, and tolerance of ambiguity. Among the defense mechanisms are repression, doubt and indecision, and denial of facts and feelings that would be unpleasant or self-threatening to acknowledge. The coping and defense mechanisms are counterparts. For example, the coping partner of denial, says Haan, is concentration—the ability to set aside disturbing feelings or thoughts in order to get on with necessary tasks at hand.

In general, the adults who tended to make use of coping rather than defense mechanisms had the highest IQ's. Further, they were the persons whose IQ's between adolescence and adulthood were most likely to have risen. Coping, the investigator suggests, leads to the development of one's intelligence; defensiveness interferes with one's intelligence as well as one's effectiveness.

Persistence of Personality Traits

Dr. Wanda C. Bronson, a psychologist, has begun to analyze the attitudes and characteristics of subjects in the Guidance Study to learn if these become set very early or change with the years.

Between the ages of 5 and 16, the period covered by the analysis so far, she finds two persistent "behavioral dimensions." One is behavior characterized at one end of the dimension as reserved, somber, shy, and at the other end as expressive, gay, socially easy. The second dimension is a contrast between reactive, explosive, resistive behavior at one end—calm, phlegmatic, compliant behavior at the other end.

If a child was either reserved (somber, shy) or expressive (gay, socially easy) at the age of five, he was likely to be the same at 16. If he was either reactive (explosive, resistive) or calm (phlegmatic, compliant) at five, he was likely to be the same at 16.

The reserved individual tended also to be introspective and, to a lesser extent, anxious and socially withdrawn. In early childhood, he was likely to be inactive and a poor eater; at 16, uncertain and uncompetitive. The expressive boy was the extrovert. Girls showed only one marked difference from the boys on this behavior measure. The reserved girl tended to be cautious and unadventurous at all ages whereas the reserved boy was cautious and unadventurous only between the ages of 8 and 10.

In the case of the other behavior grouping, the reactive and explosive boy tended also to be emotionally unstable, quarrelsome, and complaining. In adolescence but not earlier he was also likely to be rated active and adventurous. Girls showed some differences. The correlation between reactiveness and emotional instability was not significantly strong except during early childhood; the correlations between reactiveness and the activity level, strong between the ages of 8 and 13. The reactive girls tended to be finicky about their food at all ages and to be exhibitionistic at 16.

Both of these attitude patterns—reserve v. expressiveness and reactivity v. placidity—describe characteristics that the individual brings with him to every situation and that affect the environment's impact upon him. An expressive child, for example, would be more ready to initiate or be drawn into an intensive relation with his mother than a withdrawn child. A reactive child, more than a placid one, would be affected by an anxious, intrusive mother.

To what extent and through the mediation of what mechanisms these persistent personality traits are inherited, affected by the environment, and developed in the interaction between heredity and environment is not clear. Bronson does find that the children tend to take after the parent of the same sex and to reject or be unaffected by the characteristics of the other parent. Expressive boys, for example, tended to have fathers of expressive and even aggressive temperament; expressive girls, mothers of the same type. More information on this question is expected to come from an analysis of the children of the subjects in the study.

In another of the Berkeley studies, the boys with the loving mothers—these were the boys most likely to have high IQ's later on—tended as babies to be happy, inactive, and slow. Beginning about the age of 4, though, these boys were consistently rated as independent, social, and friendly.

Personality as Related to Speed of Development

Some of the personality traits noted in preceding sections seem to be related to the rate at which the people developed—began talking, began walking, reached adolescence. The early talkers, Dr. MacFarlane reports, tended to be the late walkers. And those who matured late, as indicated by the age they reached pubescence, differed considerably in some respects during adolescence and young adulthood from those who matured early. This was true of boys in particular.

As an example of how the rate of physical development in youth can influence a person's life for years afterward, this investigator tells of two boys who differed mainly in speed of maturation. The early maturer (who reached adult sexual status before he was 13) excelled in athletics and enjoyed the accompanying rewards. He showed interest in girls at 13 and they in him. The late maturer (who reached adult sexual status after he was 17) avoided girls, and they him, till he was 20. The first boy got a summer job at 14; the second went to Boy Scout camp. After college, the early maturer joined a firm in another city, married, and by 30 had reached a responsible position that takes him and his family to all parts of the world. The late maturer married a girl he had known since grade school, got a promising job with her father's help, and established a home in the neighborhood where they had been born and raised. At 30 he had yet to reach the administrative level in his firm. "I'm too young, they tell me," he reported. "I've always been too young."

Though the details differ from person to person, the early maturing male has been found by the Guidance Study to have an easier time during adolescence and to show more confidence both then and later. This was to have been expected, MacFarlane thinks, because the boy who matured early was also likely to have begun early getting into things and exploring the environment. His interests were outward because there's where the excitement lay. On the other hand, the late maturer was typically the early talker, and introverted fellow who was apparently more fascinated from the start by thinking processes than by action.

At 30, the early maturer was likely to have advanced farther in his work than the late maturer, more likely to be married, and likely to have more children.

Findings by Dr. Mary Cover Jones, Professor of Education, emeritus, from her study of a different sample—early and late maturing boys in the Oakland Growth Study—confirm those results, add some interesting details, and carry the comparison a little farther along. At 33, the men who had matured early rated significantly higher in both sociability and responsibility. They were also more conventional in their attitudes and thinking. Five years later the differences were less marked, but the man who had matured early still appeared to be more assured and somewhat less fearful, and also less insightful and independent. More of the early maturing men have attained executive, status-conferring vocational goals.

The boy who most rapidly approaches physical manhood, Jones suggests, is the one who is first recognized by the adult community and who therefore is most likely to take on—if he doesn't have them already—the personality traits likely to be most valued by that community. Dr. Harvey Peskin, a psychologist, thinks the difference found in both studies may well have a deep psychological basis. The early maturer, he suggests, is less prepared for the changes of adolescence. So he may experience them as less tolerable and therefore less acceptable. He flees, therefore, into adulthood and makes an early and rewarding commitment to the values of his culture. So he is "naturally" more sociable and conforming. On the other hand, the late maturer, not having to deal with the hormonal-inspired drives till later, has more time to look around, expand his skills, and develop a variety of psychological mechanisms for regulating crises. So when puberty comes, he tolerates it better and has less need of outside supports and rewards. This would explain his greater insightfulness.

Here again an apparent sex difference has been found. Girls who reached maturity early, MacFarlane reports, were usually less confident as adults. In school they seem to have felt out of things. These girls are described by Mary Jones, on the basis of observational ratings, as "socially disadvantaged." However, their responses on the Thermatic Apperception Test and their self-report scores indicate adequate self-concepts.

Dr. Louis Stewart adds this finding: Among males, at least, the firstborn tends to mature earlier than an only child or a lastborn child. This psychologist thinks the earlier maturation is somehow associated with the events attendant on the arrival of a new baby, for when a mother was pregnant with her second child, and for a year or two after its birth, the firstborn showed an unusual spurt in growth. Numerous experiments with animals and some studies of people show that stimulation in infancy, even painful stimulation, makes for growth, and separation from the mother appears to be an important form of such stimulation. The mother's pregnancy and the arrival of a new child, the investigator suggests, constitute painful, development-spurring stimulation for the firstborn.

Incidentally, other work on birth order by Dr. William T. Smelser, also a psychologist, throws new light on the recurrent finding that firstborn children get more education than those born last. In two-child families where both children are of the same sex, Smelser finds, there is no significant difference in the number of years they go to school. But where one child is a boy and the other is a girl, the firstborn, of whichever sex, goes to school significantly longer. And there is a greater proportion of these cross-sex (girl-boy or boy-girl) families. In studying the effects of birth order on years of schooling, then, it is important to ascertain not only a person's birth position but also the sex of the child next to him.

Early talkers v. late. Analyzing the records of men in the Guidance Study,

Dr. Kenwood Bartelme finds that the early talkers and the late show significant personality difference both as children and as adults. The same findings seem to apply to women, too, but in a less clear-cut fashion.

The early talkers were taken to be those who had said at least five words before they were 12 months old; the late talkers, those who had not done so until after 15 months. The boys in this second group talked well enough once they got started, but they had a different personality style.

Through adolescence, at least, the early talkers were on the restrained and somber side. Their IQ's were consistently higher than those of the later talkers but largely because of the difference in scores on the verbal factor tests. In high school, the early talkers were known as eggheads; at 30, they still valued intellectual matters and were inclined to intellectualize about a subject, even to the point of splitting hairs. They were also at 30 more practical, prudent, and conservative. The late talkers were active, relatively uninhibited, and even rebellious. "The late-talker," Bartelme remarks, "is the social non-conformist."

The middle group, who began talking between 12 and 15 months, turned out to be the most conventional.

Why one person starts talking exceptionally early and another exceptionally late, even in the same family, is not known, but Bartelme has found one environmental difference. The early talker had received more than the usual amount of attention from his parents, particularly from his mother; the mother, in fact, had seemed to be more involved with him during infancy than with her husband.

Predicting Adult Psychological Health

When the subjects of one of the longitudinal studies (Oakland Growth) were 36, Stewart divided a sample of them into three groups:

1. Those with psychosomatic disorders. Of the 20 afflicted persons in this group, most had either stomach ulcer or hypertension. The others suffered from migraine headaches, spastic colitis, asthma, or arthritis.
2. Those with behavioral maladjustments. Two of the 21 persons here were alcoholic, six had had repeated divorces, another six had failed to make a satisfactory social adjustment, and seven had been treated for mental illness.
3. Those who were symptom-free: 25.

Then he went back to the data showing the social and emotional adjustments of these individuals when they had been adolescents. (The data came from the University of California Social and Adjustment Inventory, which had been administered each year between 11 and 17.) He found some important differences.

The people with psychosomatic ailments as adults were reporting a poorer-than-average adjustment to life when they were only 11 years old, which was from 15 to 20 years before the diagnosis of the illness. On scales measuring such characteristics as attitudes toward family, feelings about their own worth, and ability to get along with other people, these persons had rated themselves toward the low end. So had the individuals with behavioral maladjustments as adults. During late adolescence, however, the scores on family and social adjustment had improved among the psychosomatic group but not among the behavioral maladjustment group. During the same period, those who were later to be afflicted with a psychosomatic disorder also expressed a number of vague physical complaints.

Members of the psychosomatic group had been marked, too, by an underlying tendency toward depression, as indicated by feelings of worthlessness, lack of energy, sleep disturbance, and the loss—actual or feared—of parental attention and love. On all such traits there had been during adolescence highly significant differences between the psychosomatic group and the normal. The group with behavioral maladjustments had fallen in between. The results suggest to Stewart that a basic depressive tendency is an important factor in the onset of psychosomatic disorder. And he is inclined to agree with some other investigators that virtually all illness is caused by psychic as well as somatic factors.

To try to find the basis of the maladjustments noted during adolescence, Stewart is now analyzing the records of another study (Guidance) which go back to infancy. His preliminary findings confirm that adults with psychosomatic ailments or with psychological problems worse than usual had been poorly adjusted adolescents. Further, the new findings indicate that (1) members of both groups came from families where, very early in the children's life, there had been more disturbance, and less satisfaction and security, than usual; (2) members of both groups tended to be those who had matured either very early or very late.

This second finding does not imply that early and late maturers are inevitably bound for trouble. The processes associated with either extreme of the maturation rate do seem to produce not only differences in personality, as noted earlier, but also a higher than average potential for illness and psychological difficulties. Stewart is now trying to find early family and childhood patterns that distinguish the two groups—the ill and the maladjusted. He is also looking for childhood factors that distinguish people with one type of ailment from those with another.

In related work, Drs. Norman Livson and Harvey Peskin have been trying to determine which, if any, specific characteristics of a child, displayed at which particular age, can be used to predict his psychological health as an adult. The subjects were 64 young adults, from the Guidance Study, who had been rated for psychological health at 30 by comparing their scores on a personality appraisal with theoretically ideal scores. (The ideal scores were a composite of those made by four clinical psychologists as they attempted to define a fully healthy person.) The adults' ratings were then compared with their ratings as children, from the ages of five through 16, on numerous behavior and personality scales.

High scores on certain characteristics during the years from 11 to 13, but only during those years, were found to be significantly related to adult psychological health. The healthiest men were those who as boys of 11–13 had been relatively extroverted, cheerful, relaxed, and expressive, and relatively immune to irritability. The women had been relatively independent, confident, and inquiring—and had shown a hearty attitude toward food.

The 11–13 age period proved significant, the investigators speculate, because it encompassed the transitional period from elementary school to junior high. Now once again, as when he had left the family to enter school, the child had to take an important step toward maturity. "The demands and opportunities of the junior high school, for both boys and girls," the investigators suggest, "may represent so profound a difference from elementary school as to constitute a qualitatively new experience. The manner in which the child responds to the transition—actively inviting or passively withdrawing from the new experience—tells us something about how healthy an adult he will be."

The psychological health of these subjects will be assessed again during the 40-year follow-up. The investigators plan also to look for factors in the family environment during childhood that may portend good or poor psychological health in later life.

Children Who Turned Out Better or Worse Than Expected

Because of the work reported in the preceding section and of the research under way at Berkeley and other centers, the investigators think we shall be better able to predict while a person is still in school the probable state of his mental health as an adult—and, if the outlook is poor, to take steps to alter it. They emphasize, however, that the relationships reported are based on group averages and that in every group studied there were individuals who did not conform.

More than 20 years ago, when the children in the Guidance Study were 18, MacFarlane and her associates made predictions about them as adults—their personalities, their success in marriage and work, their ability to cope with the problems of life: in short, their mental health. Though the investigators had had few scientific guides, they were surprised by the results of the analysis after the subjects were followed up at the age of 30. In many cases, the predictions turned out to have been wrong. The reasons ought to be helpful for parents, teachers, doctors, and everyone else associated with children.

Many of the most mature adults—integrated, competent, clear about their values, and accepting of themselves and others—were found to have been those who as youngsters had been faced with difficult situations and whose characteristic responses had seemed to compound their problems. They included chronic rebels who had been expelled from school, MacFarlane reports, highly intelligent students who were nevertheless academic failures, children filled with hostility, and unhappy, withdrawn schizoids. But the behavior regarded by the investigators as disruptive to growth and maturity seemed in these cases to have led directly or indirectly to adult strength. One of the former rebels recalled that he had desperately needed approval "even if it was from kids as maladjusted as I was." To maintain his rebel status, he said, he had had to commit all of his intelligence and stamina, a circumstance he believed had contributed to his adult strength in tackling difficult problems. "I hope my children find less wasteful ways to mature," he remarked, "—but who knows?"

Close to half of the subjects fell into the group for whom crippled or inadequate personalities had been predicted. But as adults almost all of them were better than had been expected, and some of them far better.

One man, for example, held back three times in elementary school, had not graduated from high school until he was 21. His IQ over the years had averaged less than 100. He had shown little interest in studies, school activities, or people. The school had not recommended that he go to college. The staff thought he'd always be a misfit, a sideliner. But 12 years later he was a talented environmental designer, a good father, and an active worker in community affairs. "Obviously," says MacFarlane. "his tested IQ's were no measure of his true ability."

One girl, who early was suspicious of and even hostile to members of the study staff, lived with a rejecting mother and a poorly adjusted aunt. She hated home and she hated school, partly because of her poor clothes. To escape, she married while still in high school a boy as erratic and immature as she. They soon separated. At 30, with the investigators dreading the impending interview, in came a personable, well-groomed, gracious woman with two buoyant but well-mannered children. She had married again and was living a stable, contented life.

Why were the predictions wrong in such cases?

For one thing, MacFarlane answers, the investigators gave too much weight to the troublesome and pathogenic elements in a child's life—quite naturally, in view of the studies that have traced neuroses and psychoses to such elements—and too little weight to the healthful, maturity-inducing elements. (The latter were present even in the case of the girl who sought escape through marriage at 17. She always remembered that another aunt had given her affection and happiness—had helped her plant seeds that grew into flowers, had given her a kitten to love, had taught her to bake, and one year had been able to help her buy clothes "so I could finally risk being friendly.")

The investigators also overestimated the durability of certain "undesirable" behaviors and attitudes shown habitually over a long period. These frequently turned out to have been devices for achieving some desired end. As an example, MacFarlane cites hurt feelings, in both boys and girls, as "a very successful parent-manipulation tool." In changed situations, such early useful devices lost their effectiveness, and the big majority of the young people then dropped or modified them, sometimes not without difficulty. With a number of girls, the game of getting their feelings hurt was carried over into marriage.

Sometimes the undesirable but long-continued patterns were converted, to the investigators' surprise, into almost the opposite characteristics. For example, it was predicted that overdependent boys with energetic and dominant mothers would pick wives like the mothers and continue the pattern of overdependence. Instead, nearly all such boys chose girls who were lacking in confidence. The boys thus won themselves a role as the proud male protector and giver of support, and in this role, says the investigator, they thrived.

Along the same line, a number of those in the study who were socially inept and insecure as children and adolescents became, again to everyone's surprise, highly successful salesmen. Looking back, MacFarlane sees this as a quite natural transformation. The boys did not have easy, intimate relationships growing up because they did not have them at home. As adults they still fear intimate relationships but have an unconscious desire for social intercourse. Selling gives them the needed contacts without the feared intimacy. (She could be wrong, she adds. The director of sales training for a large firm told her he deliberately picked shy people, because they would concentrate on selling the product instead of themselves.)

One man, who is remembered with special pride, is the highly successful manager of a large business concern. Years ago he had been a shy little boy without friends. Though he had dropped in from time to time to see members of the Guidance Study Staff, his communications had often been limited to hello and goodbye. After high school he enlisted and, since he had taken some shop courses, he was asked to help with the building and repair work at his Army post. First he was flattered that anyone should think he could do anything; then he was proud that he could actually do it. After his service, he went to business school, where he got all A's, as compared to C's in high school. Now he says the most interesting part of his job is to give people "something to do that is a little harder than what they have done or think they can do—but not something they would fail at—and then to watch them expand. Nothing is more exciting to me than to see people get confidence"—which he himself had lacked for so long.

A number of other subjects had had similar experiences. They did not achieve "ego identity"—did not find themselves—until they had been forced into or been given an opportunity to take on a responsible role that gave them the sense of worth they had missed at home. Often these people did not find this new and satisfying role until they had left both their childhood homes and their home towns.

"Don't give up on our present generation of adolescents," MacFarlane urges. "Many of ours came through bad times and developed into mature, stable adults in spite of our fears."

In a speech before The American Academy of Pediatrics recently, the investigator quoted comments made spontaneously by a number of the Guidance Study subjects at 30. Some examples:

> "When I was confused and worried, the Institute was the only place I could talk out loud to myself and find out what I thought and felt."
>
> "I sensed your respect for me, even when I knew I wasn't acting very sensibly and knew you wouldn't have had respect for me if there wasn't something there to respect because, believe me, I can tell a phony in a split second—because at times I'm a phony myself."
>
> "You asked questions, you listened, but you were the only grown-ups who didn't give advice. You helped me to ferret things out for myself, to make my own decisions. I try to carry this on in the raising of my children."

The investigator then pled with the doctors to take a similar role with their patients. "You pediatricians are the only professional groups," she said, "that can furnish continuity and interest over the long age-span of growth from babyhood to maturity, provided, of course, you have the temperament to be sympathetically interested in the vagaries of the human struggle for competence and maturity. Provided, too, you can accept the fact that you can't play God or believe you know all the answers, because one thing we have learned is how little we know. Provided, too, that you can train yourselves to look for strengths in individuals and their situations and not just for pathology. If you don't furnish this function, what professional will? If teaching departments don't incite interest, who will?"

About 20 percent of the cases turned out worse than expected. These included many of the persons who as children and adolescents had had easy, confidence-inducing lives, free of severe strains and marked by academic, social, or athletic success. Prominent among these were a high proportion of the men who had been outstanding athletes in high school and of the women who as girls had been pretty and exceptionally popular. At 30, many of these people had failed to live up to their potentialities and were puzzled and discontented.

MacFarlane gives several possible explanations. Early success may have led to unreal expectations and to a draining of energies into maintaining an image. It may have sidetracked the development of patterns and attitudes that would have made adult life more rewarding. Perhaps there wasn't enough stress in these youngsters' lives to foster development. She thinks some of the people in this group will work free from their dissatisfactions as young adults and will yet live up to their predictions for them; others will go through life wondering what happened and where they slipped.

About 30 percent of the people turned out as predicted. Among the two main groups here were the overcontrolled, who had built a psychological shield against the dangers to be found in other people and in life in general. As young adults they still had the shield. It seems to have protected them,

MacFarlane reports, but it also—by denying them access to many kinds of learning experience—has impoverished them. The second main group includes the youngsters who had been subjected to marked variability in family treatment, being handled indulgently one day and slapped down the next. Neither as adolescents nor young adults had they developed stable patterns of behavior. Of the nine adults in this study who were found to be compulsive drinkers at the age of 30, all but one came from this group. Perhaps significantly, the compulsive drinkers had manifested physical vulnerability, too—acute allergies, beginning in infancy.

The Effects of Guidance

The parents of half of the children in the Guidance Study were encouraged to turn to the staff psychologists for discussion of problems whenever they wished. Many did no. Through these discussions, they were helped to a better understanding not only of their children's behaviors and attitudes but also of their own and their spouses'. The control families were not intensively interviewed and discussions were avoided or kept to a minimum. The subjects in the guidance and control groups—the children who have grown up and become parents themselves—are now being compared in order to help explain why they grew up to be the kind of parents they are and have the kind of children they have.

So far, only hard fact has emerged: The group whose parents received little or no opportunity for discussion of interpersonal relations and children's problems has had about four times as many divorces as the guidance group. Dr. Ann Stout, the psychologist who is handling the parent-child study, finds other evidence pointing to the conclusion that when parents are encouraged to discuss family problems with professional workers, their children tend as adults to have more flexible qualities and a better ability to cope with situations. As she puts it, the guidance seems to have tempered some of the negative factors influencing the children's development. For example, there are persons in both groups who were ebullient as youngsters but who for some reason, at some point, took on a rather depressive attitude. They are not getting the satisfaction out of life that they should. However, the depressive subjects in the guidance group show more resilience than those in the control group, and a tendency to find more satisfaction.

Antecedents of Drinking

As another example of using a longitudinal study to answer questions almost impossible to answer in any other way, Mary Jones has been studying the personalities of drinkers and nondrinkers. Her question was: Do personality characteristics associated with a given drinking pattern show up early in life, before the pattern has been established? The tentative answer is that they do.

In the work to date, 68 men and 70 women in the Oakland Growth Study were classified according to their drinking habits and their reasons for drinking. The subjects were in their middle forties. Then their personalities were assessed, through the use of California Q Sort, for three age levels: junior high school, senior high school, and adulthood.

More than half of the behavioral items that differentiated problem drinkers from moderate drinkers (typically, a drink or two before dinner, three or four at a party) and abstainers in adulthood were found to have differentiated them also in junior high school. For example, the men problem drinkers, compared with the other men studied, were found to be rebellious, self-indulgent, gregarious, unpredictable, and disorganized. They were less dependable, less considerate, less fastidious, and less moralistic. As junior high students, these men had been marked by the same characteristics. And they had been more concerned than the others to demonstrate their masculinity. Behavior during the junior high school years proved to be a better predictor of adult drinking patterns than behavior during later adolescence.

On the rating that distinguished the three groups both as adults and junior high students, the men who were problem drinkers as adults usually stood at one end of the scale, the abstainers at the other, and the moderate drinkers in between.

Preliminary findings indicate that women problem drinkers resemble their male counterparts in respect to instability, unpredictableness and impulsiveness. However, they tend to be introversive and more marked by feelings of depression, self-doubt, and distrust than the men.

Looking Ahead

When the longitudinal studies began at Berkeley, there was little documented knowledge about factors that helped shape intelligence, personality, and mental health from childhood onward. Now there is a good deal, thanks not only to these pioneering investigations but also to numerous other studies undertaken more recently.

Because of man's complexity and the great variety of the influences pressing upon him, much remains to be learned—a statement that may always be true. But the body of our knowledge is being steadily increased. Among the continuing investigations at Berkeley, two seem especially important: the attempt to identify those factors in infancy and childhood that predispose to psychosomatic illness and psychological maladjustment, and the attempt to ferret out the influence of heredity on certain abilities, and characteristics.

Other important work under way includes research on:

- The relationship of physical factors, such as body build, to specific types of intellectual function, such as mathematical ability.

- The ethical, religious, political, and other values held by a person's family as he grew up; the values he took with him into marriage; the values that now dominate his home.
- What difference it makes if one parent is the disciplinarian rather than the other, or both.
- The value of the Rorschach test, which was administered to Guidance Study members for 7 years during adolescence and again at 30, in predicting psychological health.
- The relationship between a person's interest and satisfactions during childhood to his personality and psychological health as an adult.

Staff members are also busy fitting together and interpreting the findings so that these can be of the widest use. Important books coming up include (1) "Ways of Personality Development: Continuity and Change from Adolescence to Adulthood," by Jack Block and Norma Haan, which uses data from both the Oakland Growth and the Guidance studies; (2) "Children of the Depression," an analysis by Dr. Glen H. Elder, Jr., of the immediate and long-term effects of the depression on the subjects in the Oakland Growth Study; and (3) "The Course of Human Development," a collection of major papers from, and new essays about three studies, edited by Drs. Mary Jones, Bayley, Honzik, and MacFarlane. Also Dr. Clausen is working on a major "life careers" monograph based on information from the Oakland Growth Study. It seeks to answer: What are the major influences upon a person's performance in the most salient roles of adulthood—those of worker, spouse, parent and community participant?

In the near future, Berkeley's Institute of Human Development hopes to establish a program of Intergenerational Studies of Development and Aging that will use the people who have been participating in the present studies—the original subjects, their surviving parents, and the subjects' children. The questions to be investigated include the patterns and processes of aging, the heritability of traits and abilities, and the similarities and differences in family patterns and styles of life from one generation to another.

References

BAYLEY, N. (1963). The life span as a frame of reference in psychological research. *Vita Humana*, **6**, 125.

BAYLEY, N. (1964). Consistency of maternal and child behaviors in the Berkeley Growth Study. *Vita Humana*, **7**, 73.

BAYLEY, N. (1965). Research in child development: a longitudinal perspective. *Merrill Palmer Quarterly of Behavior and Development*, **11**, 3.

BAYLEY, N. (1966). Age-trends in mental scores: ages 16 to 36 years. Paper for American Psychological Association.

BAYLEY, N. (1966). Learning in adulthood: the role of intelligence. In *Analyses of Concept Learning*. New York: Academic Press.

BAYLEY, N. (1967). Cognition. Paper for University of West Virginia Conference on Theory and Methods of Research and Aging.

BAYLEY, N. (1967). Behavioral correlates of mental growth: birth to 36 years. Paper for American Psychological Association.

BAYLEY, N., and SCHAEFER, E. S. (1964). Correlations of maternal and child behaviors with the development of mental abilities: data from the Berkeley Growth Study. Monographs of the Society for Research in Child Development, **29**:6,1-80.

BRONSON, W. C. (1966). Early antecedents of emotional expressiveness and reactivity control. *Child Development*, **37**, 793–810.

BRONSON, W. C. (1966). Central orientations: a study of behavior organization from childhood to adolescence. *Child Development*, **37**, 1.

CAMERON, J., LIVSON, N., and BAYLEY, N. (1967). Infant vocalizations and their relationship to mature intelligence. *Science*, **157**, 3786.

CLAUSEN, J. A. (1968). Adolescent antecedents of cigarette smoking: data from Oakland Growth Study. *Social Science and Medicine*, **1**, 4.

HAAN, N. (1963). Proposed model of ego functioning: coping and defense mechanisms in relationship to IQ change. *Psychological Monographs: General and Applied*, **77**, 8.

HONZIK, M. P. (1963). A sex difference in the age of onset of the parent-child resemblance in intelligence. *Journal of Educational Psychology*, **54**, 5.

HONZIK, M. P. (1966). The environment and mental growth from 21 months to 30 years. Paper for International Congress of Psychology.

HONZIK, M. P. (1967). Environmental correlates of mental growth: prediction from the family setting at 21 months. *Child Development*, **38**, 337–363.

JONES, M. C. (1965). Psychological correlates of somatic development. *Child Development*, **36**, 4.

JONES, M. C. (1968). Personality correlates and antecedents of drinking patterns in adult males. *Journal of Consulting and Clinical Psychology*, **32**, 1.

LIVSON, N., and PESKIN, H. (1967). The prediction of adult psychological health in a longitudinal study. *Journal of Abnormal Psychology*, **72**, 509–518.

MACFARLANE, J. (1963). From infancy to adulthood. *Childhood Education*, **39**, 336–342.

MACFARLANE, J. (1964). Perspectives on personality consistency and change from the Guidance Study. *Vita Humana*, **7**, 115.

MACFARLANE, J. (1967). The dilemmas of adolescents. Paper for American Academy of Pediatrics.

PESKIN, H. (1967). Pubertal onset and ego functioning: a psychoanalytic approach. *Journal of Abnormal Psychology*, **72**, 1–15.

STEWART, L., and LIVSON, N. (1966). Smoking and rebelliousness: a longitudinal study from childhood to maturity. *Journal of Consulting Psychology*, **30**, 325–329.

The Hyperactive Child: A Guide for Parents

This material was taken from a pamphlet prepared for the parents of hyperactive children. It is in the form of questions and answers concerning the syndrome, with the questions those that might be raised by concerned parents, and the answers providing much basic information about hyperactivity. This

Reprinted from *The Hyperactive Child: A Guide for Parents* (1969), 4–30, with the permission of Smith, Kline and French Laboratories.

disorder is also known as a hyperkinetic reaction or as minimal brain damage, and attention to this neurological basis of some behavior problems in young children is relatively recent.

The Nature of Hyperactivity

Hyperactivity is a general term that means different things to different people. When a physician uses the term, he is describing behavior relative to other children of the same age. To the parent, the term is used to describe behavior that often seems to demand excessive discipline in the home. To the teacher, a hyperactive child is one that creates problems in the classroom. In all cases hyperactivity refers to behavior that is different from the behavior of the average child of the same age.

The following questions and answers will help to pinpoint the nature of hyperactivity in a child.

Q. What exactly does a child do and how does he behave to warrant diagnosis as hyperactive?

A. He is generally irritable, easily frustrated and quick to anger—in an explosive and unpredictable way. At home or in school, his attention shifts rapidly and he cannot concentrate on any activity for any reasonable length of time. He fidgets or squirms when he sits. His scholastic performance is poor, especially in arithmetic, reading and writing. He tends to take an independent tack—in school, for example, by asking totally irrelevant questions, pulling another child's hair, walking around during rest period, etc. At home, he has little patience and may not sit still for meals, TV, or even a bedtime story that spellbinds his brothers and sisters. He runs when he should walk or, perversely, walks when everybody's running. He seems to never sleep and may even get out of bed in the middle of the night and roam around the house.

Q. What causes hyperactivity?

A. A number of theories have been advanced. The explanation most widely accepted at present is that hyperactivity occurs when the control centers of the brain have not developed as rapidly as those centers that cause mechanical function. Intelligence is not impaired though emotional immaturity is common.

Q. Is hyperactivity a sign of brain damage?

A. While brain damage may cause similar symptoms in some children, most hyperactive children do not have histories of brain damage.

Q. Does hyperactivity run in families?

A. Usually not. More boys than girls and more first-born than later children are hyperactive, according to available statistics.

Q. At what age is hyperactivity first apparent?

A. Usually it is discovered and diagnosed when the child begins nursery school, somewhere between three and four years of age.

Q. How long does it last?

A. In the majority of children who receive treatment, hyperactivity diminishes gradually as the child matures and usually is no longer a problem by the time the child reaches adolescence.

Q. Are there any early-warning signals that a child may be hyperactive?

A. Some early indications may appear in infancy. Head-bangers and crib-rockers may be hyperactive. Later on, teeth-grinding and temper tantrums can be symptoms.

Q. Is hyperactivity rare among children?

A. Not at all. For example, in the public schools of New York City, it is estimated that about 4% of the total enrollment (that's 44,000 children) have been diagnosed as hyperactive. And conservative estimates of the entire elementary school enrollment of the United States indicates that over a million children are hyperactive.

Q. Some doctors use the word "hyperkinetic" to describe the overactive, impulsive and occasionally belligerent child. What does the word mean?

A. It is another medical term for "hyperactive." The child's symptoms taken together are sometimes called "the hyperactive or hyperkinetic syndrome."

How Medicine Helps

There are several different kinds of drugs used today to help treat the hyperactive child. If your physician has prescribed one of these it is very likely either a member of the tranquilizer group or one of the stimulating drugs. Some hyperactive children respond best to one type; others respond better to the other.

Q. What can drugs do for the hyperactive child?

A. They can make his condition more normal. *Tranquilizing drugs* tend to slow him down and make him more manageable. In addition they help a child control his emotions. *Stimulating drugs*, such as the amphetamines, are currently the most frequently prescribed agents for the hyperactive child—both as treatment and as an aid in diagnosis. As mentioned earlier, it is believed that in the hyperactive child the control centers in the brain have not developed as rapidly as the motor centers. So, by stimulating the control centers, these drugs enable the child to have more control over his behavior and therefore to function more normally.

Q. How soon will I see results?

A. As a rule, the hyperactive child will respond to drug therapy within a few days.

Q. What should I do if the medicine doesn't help?

A. If no improvement is noted in two or three days, call your physician for advice. Probably all that's needed is an adjustment in dosage. However, do not attempt to change the dosage yourself.

Q. But aren't stimulant drugs harmful and habit-forming?

A. Stimulant drugs have been used successfully to treat hyperactive children for over 30 years. This experience has shown no tendency toward habituation or addiction in children.

Q. Are there any side effects with this type of medication?

A. Occasionally, a few children taking stimulant drugs may develop a pale, anxious expression. However, the most common side effects are insomnia and reduced appetite. These are not usually a problem if the drug is given just before breakfast and before lunch. But except for individual sensitivity, which your doctor has probably mentioned, experience has shown that hyperactive children usually tolerate stimulating drugs better than adults.

Q. If a side effect occurs, what should be done?

A. If you notice a side effect—or no effect—notify your doctor immediately. A change in dosage may be needed. Or a change in medication. In any event, do not attempt to make such changes yourself. Call your doctor for advice.

Helping the Hyperactive Child: At Home

There are many ways in which you can help your hyperactive child to slow down. Your goal is to eliminate as many frustrations as possible by helping him to re-channel his energies contructively. Begin by asking yourself a question. Are you expecting too much of your child? It's natural for parents to want their children to excel. But perhaps your sights are prematurely high. Don't push. Relax. Try not to be tense. A child is quick to sense impatience and your attitude or actions may aggravate his behavior.

Anger is a normal and frequent by-product of hyperactivity—both in your child and in yourself. So be prepared! Expect your child to be angry when frustrated and remember that his frustration level is abnormally low. Let this foreknowledge help you to handle his outbursts sympathetically while keeping your own anger under control.

Next take a look at the physical surroundings of your home. See whether the environment or organization can be improved to eliminate potential trouble spots of needless worry or friction.

Q. Should the physical set-up of the home be changed to accomodate the hyperactive child?

A. Not necessarily. With small children in the home, you would normally child-proof medicine cabinets, tool closets and other areas where youngsters might accidentally harm themselves. And with normally-active children around, you would not leave fragile objects within their reach. Put valuable breakables away and avoid the constant tension of his waiting for your next "Don't touch."

At the same time, it's important to provide your child with a room or area to call his own. This provides him with a focus of activity, a feeling of importance and helps to keep him out of harm's way.

Q. Should the routine in the home be changed?

A. The hyperactive child is more comfortable on a fixed routine so that he can expect certain things to happen at a certain time—mealtimes, naptime, playtime, TV-time, storytime, bedtime, etc. He will also need forewarning of even the expected events. If it's playtime, say "Now we will play with this," And play with him, giving him your attention. If your attention wanders, he'll wander. Though he may not show it, or be as responsive as you might like, he needs a little extra love and extra attention. Order and regulate your home life so that you can give him the attention he needs.

Q. What if that carefully-planned routine has to be varied now and then?

A. Obviously, no family's activities can or should be inflexible. If, for example, you have agreed to watch television with him at a specific time and then find you must go to a PTA meeting, explain to him why you can't and offer him an extra bit of time the next day.

Q. How should a violent temper tantrum be handled?

A. In the same way as with any other child. At its peak, restrain him quietly but firmly and prevent him from doing damage or harming himself. When his anger subsides, point out what he has done and offer comfort and soothing attention. Frequently you will find that he is ashamed for having lost control, and needs your comfort and reassurance.

Q. How can his older brothers and/or sisters help him?

A. His problem should be explained to them so that they will understand and be able to help in minimizing tension and frustration. However, very young children quite naturally may poke fun at him, even scoff and sneer.

Q. What about grandparents, close relatives and friends?

A. Their patience and understanding should also be encouraged. Grandparents, however, tend to be difficult, and their attention may stimulate the child to greater hyperactivity. If this is the case, keep calm and if necessary enlist their cooperation in limiting the length and frequency of their visits.

Q. What kinds of play activities are best for the hyperactive child?

A. These depend on his age and his abilities. What is important in any activity is that it must hold his attention and usually this will require the help of another person. To given the hyperactive child paper and fingerpaints and expect him to play at this alone is unreasonable. Make a game of it. Do it with him. Teach his older brother or sister how to help hold his attention. *Supervision means that you care about him.* And that he needs to know. Choose playthings and activities that are right for his age, that are non-competitive and that do not require concentration or skills that are beyond him. Build his confidence by giving ample time—and praise—for things he seems to do particularly well. Remember, he becomes bored very easily. So games that lend themselves to numerous variations are particularly desirable.

Q. What *are* those magic games and playthings?

A. Ball games, for one. The variations possible from infancy to adulthood are almost endless. (Check any good child development book for what game at what age.) Or simple jig-saw puzzles. The hyperactive child usually has good coordination and learns physical activities faster than other children. Swimming and other non-competitive sports provide an excellent way of letting him throw off a lot of steam.

Q. Why shouldn't he play competitive games with children his own age?

A. Until his hyperactivity levels off he is in enough competition with himself. Games involving groups of children or waiting his turn may overstimulate him or increase the chance of frustration compared to those that can be played with fewer children or enjoyed individually. Later, as he gains more self-control and as frustrations diminish in frequency, he may be encouraged—gradually—to join his peers in competition.

Helping the Hyperactive Child: At School

It is in the classroom, usually, that the first clues of disruptive behavior are uncovered. But today's overworked teachers have little time, too many students, too many pressures and, as a result, may have too little patience to cope with hyperactive children. And the day may come, usually after a preliminary warning, that your hyperactive youngster will be sent home—perhaps for an extended period.

Q. What kind of cooperation may you expect from your child's teacher?

A. In many public schools today, you will be invited to meet with your child's teacher or the school psychologist. (If not, you should request such a meeting.) When you meet, listen and then ask for her recommendations. If your child is seriously disruptive, chances are he will be shifted to a special class.

Q. What about the school guidance department?

A. A good guidance department can be helpful, as can the school psychologist. In some cases, the recommendations made by the school, in combination with your physician's advice, and specially-supervised classes within the school can be of great value in appraising your hyperactive child's particular problems.

Q. If the child who has been suspended temporarily responds to treatment, can he comfortably re-enter school?

A. Yes. However, to ease the transition, it's best to meet with the guidance counselor, principal or teacher beforehand. If possible, arrange for your child to be placed in another division or section so that he does not immediately return to the same group of children as before. Assure him that you and his teacher love him and know that he's trying. Ask his teacher to reassure him herself.

The Hyperactive Child's Future

With proper guidance and treatment, the prognosis for the hyperactive child's future is a good one. Close yet relaxed supervision on the part of the parent, working together with the physician, will help channel and direct the resources of the hyperactive child and to provide suitable outlets for his excess energy until he is able to assume responsibility for his actions.

As with any process of maturation and growing up, the time this takes will vary from one child to another. With treatment, hyperactivity usually ceases to be a problem during adolescence.

Some Useful Do's and Don'ts

- Don't push the hyperactive child beyond his capability.
- Do follow a regimen and program his activities so that he usually knows what to expect and when to expect it.
- Build his confidence by giving ample time—and praise—for things he seems to do particularly well.
- Don't be oversolicitous. Encourage your child to be a participating member of the family to the extent that he is able—not an "it" sitting on the sidelines.

- Allow for flexibility in your daily routine but give adequate warning if a major change is required—particularly if it involves cancellation of a favored activity or event, in which case encourage his participation in the selection of an alternative.
- Don't panic in the face of his disruptive behavior. Try to keep calm and on top of the situation.
- Avoid constant nagging. Be willing to overlook small breaches of discipline so that you can concentrate on the big ones.
- If you are normally a somewhat energetic person, try to slow down a bit when you're with your child. If you are less active, he'll be less active.
- Don't let the other children in the family feel that your hyperactive child gets all the attention. It is important for the others not to tease him—a difficult, if not impossible restraint for children—but don't encourage them.
- Do move in and stop extreme disruptiveness. The hyperactive child is inwardly begging to be stopped and your calm intervention is reassuring that you do care.
- Don't think you're alone and don't despair. You are in vastly numbered company. You are not to blame and lots of disruptive youngsters have grown up to be healthy, happy citizens.

O. IVAR LOVAAS, BENSON SCHAEFFER, and JAMES Q. SIMMONS

Building Social Behavior in Autistic Children by Use of Electric Shock

The autistic child, as described by Eisenberg and Kanner (American Journal of Orthopsychiatry, 26 (1956), 556–566), is characterized by a number of distinct features: (1) extreme detachment from human relationships seemingly from birth; (2) failure to use speech to communicate; (3) little or no spontaneity and a preference for obsessive rituals; (4) an intense fascination for certain objects and many details about them; and (5) apparently high intellectual potential as judged from either the language they had managed to acquire or from motor facility. As can be imagined, such children are extraordinarily

---

Reprinted from *Journal of Experimental Research in Personality*, **1** (1965), 99–109, with the permission of Academic Press and Dr. Lovaas.

difficult to do therapy with since they are so encapsulated that the outsider can barely make a dent on them. This study by Lovaas, Schaeffer, and Simmons has received a great deal of attention and comment because it utilized pain associated with electric shock in order to "get through" to autistic children in an effort to begin shaping their behavior along desired lines. This approach is in keeping with many recently introduced therapeutic techniques based on laboratory studies of the learning process among animals.

Psychological or physical pain is perhaps as characteristic in human relationships as is pleasure. The extensive presence of pain in everyday life may suggest that it is necessary for the establishment and maintenance of normal human interactions.

Despite the pervasiveness of pain in daily functioning, and its possible necessity for maintaining some behaviors, psychology and related professions have shied away from, and often condemned, the use of pain for therapeutic purposes. We agree with Solomon (1964) that such objections to the use of pain have a moral rather than a scientific basis. Recent research, as reviewed by Solomon, indicated that the scientific premises offered by psychologists for the rejection of punishment are not tenable. Rather, punishment can be a very useful tool for effecting behavior change.

There are three ways pain can be used therapeutically. First, it can be used directly as punishment, i.e., it can be presented contingent upon certain undesirable behaviors, so as to suppress them. This is perhaps the most obvious use of pain. Second, pain can be removed or withheld contingent upon certain behaviors. That is, certain behaviors can be established and maintained because they terminate pain, or avoid it altogether. Escape and avoidance learning exemplify this. The third way in which pain can be used is the least well known, and perhaps the most intriguing. Any stimulus which is associated with or discriminative of pain reduction acquires *positive* reinforcing (rewarding) properties (Bijou and Baer, 1961), i.e., an organism will work to "obtain" those stimuli which have been associated with pain reduction. The action of such stimuli is analogous to that of stimuli whose positive reinforcing properties derive from primary positive reinforcers.

These three aspects of the use of pain can be illustrated by observations on parent-child relationships. The first two are obvious; a parent will punish his child to suppress specific behaviors, and his child will learn to behave so as to escape or avoid punishment. The third aspect of the use of pain is more subtle, but more typical. In this case, a parent "rescues" his child from discomfort. In reinforcement theory terms, the parent becomes discriminative for the reduction or removal of negative reinforcers or noxious stimuli. During the first year of life many of the interactions a parent has with his children may be of this nature. An infant will fuss, cry, and give signs indicative of pain or distress many times during the day, whereupon most parents will pick him up and attempt to remove the discomfort. Such situations must contribute a basis for subsequent meaningful relationships between people; individuals are seen as important to each other if they have faced and worked through a stressful experience together. It may well be that much of a child's love for his parents develops in situations which pair parents with stress reductions. Later in life, the normal child does turn to his parent when he is frightened or hurt by nightmares, by threat of punishment from his peers, by fears of failure in school, and so on.

In view of these considerations, it was considered appropriate to investigate the usefulness of pain in modifying the behaviors of autistic children. Autistic children were selected for two reasons: (1) because they show no improvement with conventional psychiatric treatment; and (2) because they are largely unresponsive to everyday interpersonal events.

In the present study, pain was induced by means of an electrified grid on the floor upon which the children stood. The shock was turned on immediately following pathological behaviors. It was turned off or withheld when the children came to the adults who were present. Thus, these adults "saved" the children from a dangerous situation; they were the only "safe" objects in a painful environment.

Study 1

The objectives of Study 1 were (1) to train the children to avoid electric shock by coming to *E* when so requested; (2) to follow the onset of self-stimulatory and tantrum behaviors by electric shock so as to decrease their frequency; and (3) to pair the word "no" with electric shock and test its acquisition of behavior-suppressing properties.

Method

Subjects. The studies were carried out on two identical twins. They were five-years old when the study was initiated and were diagnosed as schizophrenics. They evidenced no social responsiveness; they did not respond in any manner to speech, nor did they speak; they did not recognize each other or recognize adults even after isolation from people; they were not toilet trained; their handling of physical objects (toys, etc.) was inappropriate and stereotyped, being restricted to "fiddling" and spinning. They were greatly involved in self-stimulatory behavior, spending 70 to 80 per cent of their day rocking, fondling themselves, and moving hands and arms in repetitive, stereotyped manners. They engaged in a fair amount of tantrum behaviors, such as screaming, throwing objects, and hitting themselves.

It is important to note, in view of the moral and ethical reasons which might preclude the use of electric shock, that their future was certain institutionalization. They had been intensively treated in a residential setting by conventional psychiatric techniques for one year prior to the present study without any observable modification in their behaviors. This failure in treatment is consistent with reports of other similar efforts with such children (Eisenberg, 1957; Brown, 1960), which have suggested that if a schizophrenic child does not have language and does not play appropriately with physical objects by the age of three to five, then he will not improve, despite traditional psychiatric treatment, including psychotherapy, of the child and/or his family.

Apparatus. The research was conducted in a 12 × 12-foot experimental room with an adjoining observation room connected by one-way mirrors and sound equipment. The floor of the experimental room was covered by one-half inch wide metal tapes with adhesive backing (Scotch Tape). They were laid one-half inch apart so that when the child stepped on the floor he would be in contact with at least two strips, thereby closing the circuit and receiving an electric shock. A six-volt battery was wired to the strips of tape via a Harvard Inductorium. The shock was set at a level at which each of three *E*s standing barefoot on the floor agreed that it was definitely painful and frightening.

The *S*s' behavior and the experimental events were recorded on an Esterline Angus pen recorder by procedures more fully described in an earlier paper (Lovaas *et al.*, 1965). The observer could reliably record both frequency and duration of several behaviors simultaneously on a panel of pushbuttons. A given observer recorded at randomly selected periods.

Pre-shock Sessions. The *S*s were placed barefoot in the experimental room with two *E*s, but were not shocked. There were two such pre-experimental sessions, each lasting for about 20 minutes. The *E*s would invite the *S*s to "come here" about five times a minute, giving a total of approximately 100 trials per session. The observers recorded the amount of physical contact (defined as *S*'s touching *E* with his hands), self-stimulatory and tantrum behavior, the verbal command "come here," and positive responses to the command (coming to within one foot of *E* within five seconds).

First Shock Sessions. The two pre-experimental sessions were followed by three shock sessions distributed over three consecutive days during which *S*s were trained, in an escape-avoidance paradigm, to avoid shock by responding to *E*'s verbal command according to the pre-established criterion. In the escape phase of the training, consisting of fifty trials, the two *E*s faced each other, about three feet apart, with *S* standing (held, if necessary) between them so that he faced one of the *E*s, who would lean forward, stretch his arms out, and say "come here." At the same time shock was turned on and remained on until *S* moved in the direction of this *E*, or, if *S* had not moved within three seconds, until the second *E* pushed *S* in the direction of the inviting *E*. Either type of movement of *S* toward the inviting *E* immediately terminated the shock. The *S* had to walk alternately from one *E* to the other.

In the avoidance sessions which followed, shock was withheld provided *S* approached *E* within five seconds. If *S* did not start his approach to the inviting *E* within five seconds, or if he was not within one foot of *E* within seven seconds, the shock was turned on and the escape procedure was reinstated for that trial.

During these avoidance sessions *E*s gradually increased their distance from each other until they were standing at opposite sides of the room. At the same time they gradually decreased the number of cues signaling *S* to approach them. In the final trials, *E*s merely emitted the command "come here," without turning toward or otherwise signaling *S*.

Shock was also turned on if *S* at any time engaged in self-stimulatory and/or tantrum behaviors. Whenever possible, shock was administered at the onset of such behaviors. Shock was never given except on the feet; no shock was given if *S* touched the floor with other parts of his body. In order to keep *S* on his feet, shock was given for any behavior which might have enabled him to avoid shock, such as beginning to sit down, moving toward the window to climb on its ledge, etc.

Extinction Sessions. The three shock sessions were followed by eleven extinction sessions distributed over a ten-month period. These sessions were the same as those in the previous sessions, except that shock and the command "no" were never delivered during this period.

The Second Shock Sessions. Three additional sessions terminated Study 1. In the first of these, *S* was brought into the experimental room and given a two-second shock not contingent upon any behavior of *S* or *E*. This was the only shock given. In all other respects these final sessions were similar to the preceding extinction sessions.

Procedure for Establishing and Testing "No" as a Secondary Negative Reinforcer. During the first shock sessions, shock had been delivered contingent upon self-stimulatory and/or tantrum behaviors. Simultaneous with the onset of shock *E*s would say "no," thereby pairing the word "no" and shock. The test for any suppressing power which the word "no" had acquired during these pairings was carried out in the following manner. Prior to the shock sessions, *S*s were trained to press a lever (wired to a cumulative recorder) for M & M candy on a fixed ratio 20 schedule. The sessions lasted for ten minutes daily. A stable rate of lever-pressing was achieved by the twelfth session, at which *E*s tested the word "no" for suppressing effects on the lever-pressing rate. The *E* delivered the "no" contingent upon lever-pressing toward the middle of each session, during three sessions *prior* to the shock sessions, and during three sessions *subsequent* to the shock sessions, i.e., after "no" had been paired with shock.

Results and discussion

Figure 1 gives the proportion of time *S*s responded to *E*s' commands (proportion of Rs to S^Ds). As can be seen, in the two pre-shock sessions *S*s did not respond to *E*s' commands. During the first three shock sessions (Shock I), *S*s learned to respond to *E*s' requests within the prescribed time interval and thus avoided shock. This changed responsiveness of *S*s to *E*s' requests was maintained for the subsequent nine months (no shock sessions). There was a relatively sudden decrease in *S*s' responsiveness after nine months, i.e., the social behavior of coming to *E* extinguished. One non-contingent shock, however, immediately reinstated the social responsiveness (Shock II), suggesting that *S*s responded to it as a discriminative stimulus for social behavior.

The data on *S*s' pathological behaviors (self-stimulation and tantrums) and other social behaviors (physical contacts) are presented in Fig. 2. Prior

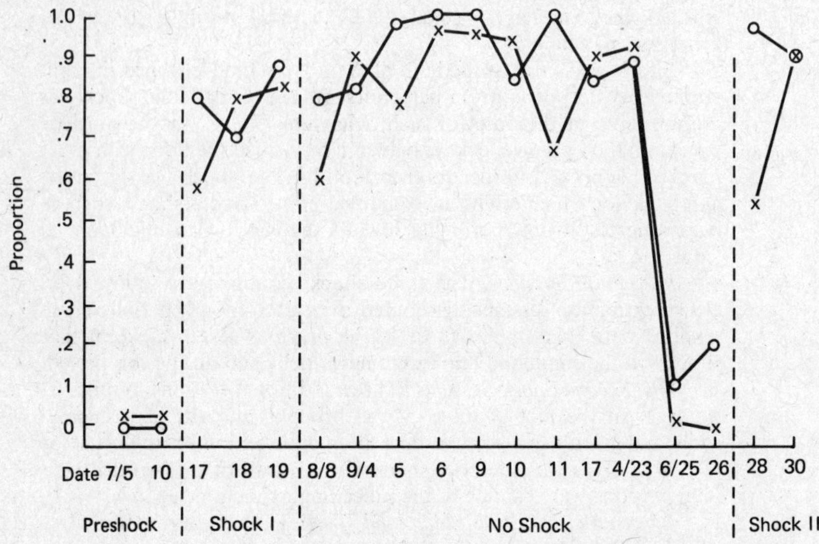

Fig. 1. *Proportion of time* Ss *responded to* Es *commands—proportion of* Rs *to* S^Ds.

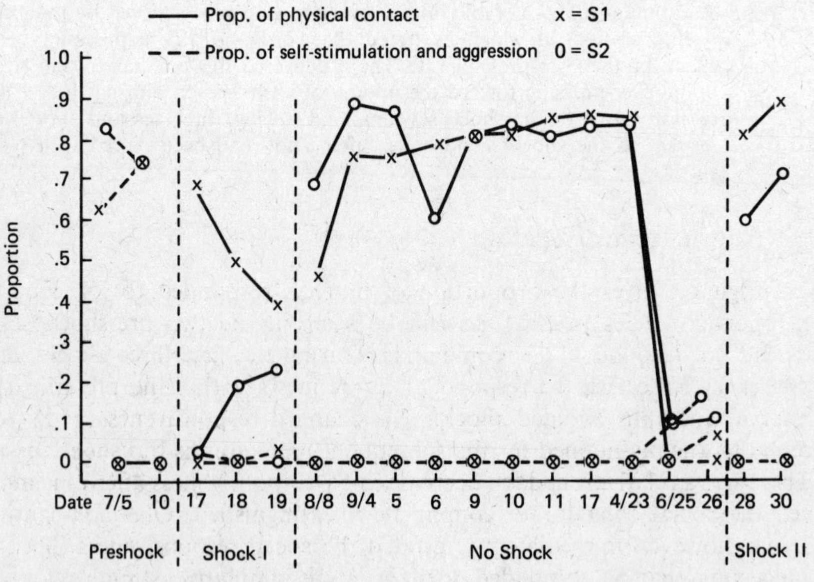

Fig. 2. *Proportion of self-stimulation and tantrums (pathological behaviors) and physical contact (social behavior).*

to shock pathological behaviors occurred 65–85 per cent of the time; physical contacts were absent. Shock I suppressed the pathological behaviors immediately, and they remained suppressed during the following eleven months. In addition, social behaviors replaced the pathological behaviors. This change was very durable (ten to eleven months), but did eventually extinguish. One non-contingent shock reinstated the social responsiveness and suppressed the pathological behaviors.

The data on the acquisition of "no" as a negative reinforcer are presented in Fig. 3. The records of bar-pressing for candy are presented as cumulative curves. The word "no" was presented contingent upon a bar-pressing response three sessions before and three sessions subsequent to shock, i.e., before and after the pairing of "no" with shock. The cumulative curves of the session immediately preceding and the session following shock to *S*1 is presented. The curves for the other sessions, both for *S*1 and *S*2, show the same effects. It is apparent upon inspection of Fig. 3 that the word "no" had no effect upon *S*1's performance prior to its pairing with shock, but that after such pairing it suppressed the bar-pressing response.

Observations of *S*s' behaviors in the experimental room indicated that the shock training had a generalized effect; it altered several behaviors which were not recorded. Some of these changes took place within minutes after the *S*s had been introduced to shock. In particular, they seemed more alert, affectionate, and seeking of *E*'s company. And surprisingly, during successful shock avoidance they appeared happy. These alterations in behavior were only partially generalized to the environment outside the experimental room. The changes in behaviors outside were most noticeable during the first fourteen days of the shock training, after which *S*s apparently discriminated between situations in which they would be shocked and those in which they would not. According to their nurse's notes, certain behaviors, such as *S*s' responsiveness to "come here" and "no" were maintained for several months, while others, such as physical contact, soon extinguished.

These observations formed the basis for the subsequent two studies. In

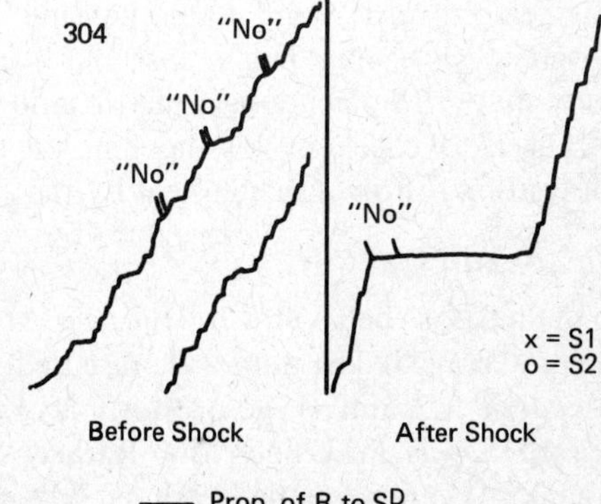

Fig. 3. *Lever-pressing for candy as cumulative response curves: effect of "no" on lever-pressings by* S1 *before and after "no" was paired with shock.*

Study 2 a more objective assessment of the changes in *S*s' affectionate behavior toward adults was made, and a technique for extending these effects from the experimental room to the ward was explored. In Study 3 a test was made of any reinforcing power adults might have acquired as a function of their association with the termination of shock.

Study 2

Study 2 involved two observations. One attempted to assess changes in *S*s' affectionate behavior to *E* who invited them to kiss and hug him. The other observation was conducted by nurses who rated *S*s on behavior change in seven areas (given below). Both observations incorporated measures of transfer of behavior changes to new situations brought about by the use of the remote control shock apparatus. Both observations were conducted immediately following the completion of Study 1.

The "Kiss and Hug" Observations. These observations consisted of six daily sessions. Three of the sessions (3, 5, and 6) are referred to as shock-relevant sessions. Sessions 3 and 5 were conducted in the experimental room where *S*s had received shock during avoidance training. Three sessions (1, 2, and 4) are labeled control sessions. They took place in a room sufficiently different from the experimental room to minimize generalization of the shock effect. The last shock-relevant session (session 6) was conducted to test the changes produced by remotely controlled shock. This session was conducted in the same room as the previous control sessions. However, immediately preceding the session *S*s received five shock-escape trials, similar to those of Study 1. The shock was delivered from a Lee-Lectronic Trainer.[1] The *S* wore the eight-ounce receiver (about the size of a cigarette pack) strapped on his back with a belt. Shock was delivered at "medium" level over two electrodes strapped to *S*'s buttock.

In order to minimize the effects of a particular observer's recording bias, two observers alternated in recording *S*s' behavior. Each observer recorded at least one shock session. The sessions lasted for six minutes each. Every five seconds *E* would face *S*, hold him by the waist with outstretched arms, bow his head toward *S*, and state "hug me" or "kiss me." The *E* would alternate his requests ("hug me," "kiss me") every minute. The observer recorded (1) embrace (*S* placing his arms around *E*'s neck), (2) hug and kiss (*S* hugging *E* cheek to cheek or kissing him on the mouth), (3) active physical withdrawal by *S* from *E* when held by the waist, and (4) *E*'s requests.

Results

Since *S*s' behaviors on the test were virtually identical, their behaviors were averaged. The data are presented in Fig. 4. During the control sessions (sessions 1, 2, and 4) the proportion of time that *S*s embraced, or hugged and kissed *E* was extremely low. Rather, they withdrew from him. During the shock-relevant sessions (sessions 3, 5, and 6) *S*s' behavior changed markedly

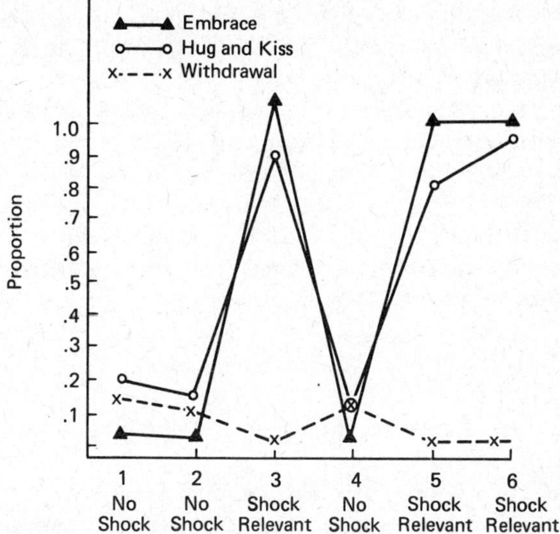

Fig. 4. *Social reactions of* Ss *as a function of shock presentations. The "no shock" sessions (1, 2, 4) were run in a room where* Ss *had not been shocked. ("Shock" sessions (3, 5) were conducted in a room in which* Ss *had received shock-avoidance training. The last "shock" session (6) was conducted in the same room as the "no shock" sessions, but* Ss *had received remote controlled shock.)*

toward increased affection. In a situation where they had received shock-avoidance training they responded with affection to *E* and did not withdraw from him. The fact that this affectionate behavior maintained itself in session 6 demonstrates that the remotely controlled shock can produce transfer of behavior change to a wide variety of situations.

NURSES' RATINGS. The nurses' ratings were initiated at the completion of the "kiss and hug" sessions. Four nurses who were familiar with *S*s but unfamiliar with the experiment, and did not know that shock had been used, were asked to complete a rating scale pertaining to seven behaviors: (1) dependency on adults, (2) responsiveness to adults, (3) affection seeking, (4) pathological behaviors, (5) happiness and contentment, (6) anxiety and fear, and (7) overall clinical improvement. The scale was comprised of nine points, with the mid-point indicating no change. The nurses were asked to indicate whether they considered *S* to have changed (increased or decreased) in any of these behaviors as compared to *S*'s behaviors the preceding day or morning. The ratings were obtained under two conditions: (1) an experimental condition in which *S*, wearing the remote control unit on his belt underneath his clothing, was introduced to the nurses who "casually" interacted with him for ten minutes. *S* was not shocked while with the nurses, but he had been given a one-second, non-contingent shock immediately prior to his interaction with the nurses; (2) a control condition, which was run in the same manner as the experimental condition, except that *S* had no shock prior to the ratings.

The nurses rated changes in *S*s under both conditions. They were not counter-balanced. The ratings from the control conditions were subtracted from the ratings based on the experimental conditions. The difference shows an increase in the ratings of all behaviors following the shock treatment, except for pathological behaviors and happiness-contentment, which both decreased. Only the ratings on dependency and affection seeking behaviors increased more than one point.

Study 3

Study 3 showed the degree to which the association of an adult with shock reduction (contingent upon an approach response of the children) would establish the adult as a positive secondary reinforcer for the children. Increased resistance to extinction of a lever-pressing response producing the sight of the adult was used to measure the acquired reinforcing power of the adult.

The study was conducted in two parts. The first part constituted a "pre-training" phase. During this period the children were trained to press a lever to receive M & Ms and simultaneously see *E*'s face. Once this response was acquired, extinction of the response was begun by removing the candy reinforcement, *S* being exposed only to *E*'s face. The second part of the study constituted a test of the reinforcing power *E* had acquired as a result of having been associated with shock reduction. This association occurred when, immediately preceding several of the extinction sessions of the lever-press, *S*s were trained to come to *E* to escape shock. The change in rate of responding to obtain a view of *E* during these sessions was used as a measure of *E*'s acquired reinforcing power.

Method

Study 3 was initiated after the completion of Study 2. It was conducted in an enclosed cubicle, four feet square, in which *E* and *S* sat separated by a removable screen. A lever protruded from a box at *S*'s side. Lever-pressings were recorded on a cumulative recorder. An observer (O) looking through a one-way screen recorded the following behaviors of *S* as they occurred: (1) vocalizations (any sound emitted by *S*), and (2) standing on the chair or ledge in the booth. The latter measures were taken in a manner similar to that described in Study 1. These additional measures were obtained in an attempt to check on the possibility that an eventual increase in lever-pressing for *E* might be due to a conceivable "energizing" effect of shock, rather than to the secondary reinforcing power associated with shock reduction. This rationale will be discussed more fully below.

The first ten were labeled *pre-training* sessions. In each, a fifteen-minute acquisition preceded a twenty-minute extinction of the lever-pressing response.

During acquisition *S* received a small piece of candy and a five-second exposure to *E* (the screen was removed momentarily, placing *E*'s face within *S*'s view) on a fixed ratio 10 schedule. During extinction, *S* received only the five-second exposure to *E* on the same schedule as before. Both *S*s reached a stable rate of about 500 responses during the first acquisition session.

The ten pre-training sessions were followed for *S*1 by nine *experimental* sessions. In these experimental sessions *S* never received candy. The sessions consisted only of a twenty-minute extinction period. An *S*'s performance during the last extinction session of pre-training labeled Session 1 in Fig. 5, served as a measure of the pre-experimental rate of lever-pressing. Electric shock was administered before the 2nd, 7th, and 9th experimental sessions, as follows: *S* was placed facing *E* in the room outside the cubicle. Shock was administered for two to four seconds, at which point *E* would tell *S* to "come here." *S* would invariably approach *E* and shock would be terminated. The *E* would then comfort *S* (fondle and stroke him) for one minute. This procedure was repeated four times. Immediately following this procedure, *S* was placed within his cubicle. *E* would repeat *S*'s name every five seconds. On the fixed ratio 10 schedule, the screen would open and *E* would praise *S* ("good boy") and stroke him.

The experimental treatment of *S*2 was identical to that of *S*1 with the following exceptions: (1) *S*2 received only seven experimental sessions; (2) shock preceded session 2, 6, and 8; (3) *E* did not call *S*2's name while he was in the cubicle; and (4) *E* was only visually exposed to *S*2 (*E* did not stroke or praise *S*2).

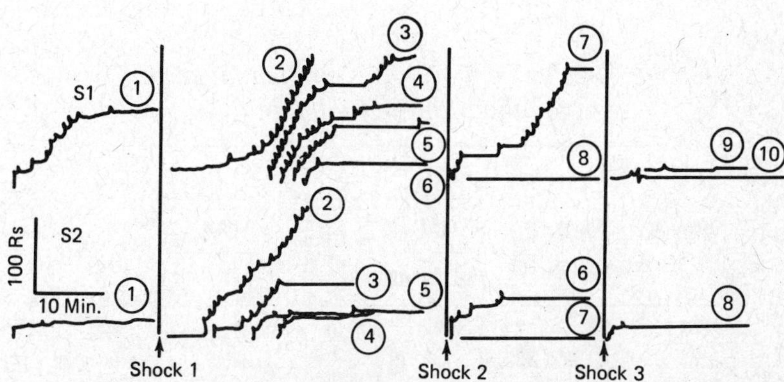

Fig. 5. *The* Ss' *lever-pressing behavior for* E *as function of* E's *association with shock reduction. (Curve labelled "1" is the last extinction curve from the pretraining. Shock preceded sessions 2, 7, and 9 for* S1, *and sessions 2, 6, and 8 for* S2. *The upward moving hatchmarks on the curves indicate occasions at which* E *was visually presented to* S.)

Results and discussion

The *S*'s lever-pressing behavior is presented in Fig. 5 as cumulative curves. The last extinction curve from the pre-training is labeled one. This curve gives the rate of lever-pressing in the last extinction session preceding *E*'s association with shock reduction. The upward moving hatchmarks on the curves show the occasions on which *E* was visually presented to *S*. The heavy vertical lines labeled shock, show shock-escape training preceding sessions 2, 7, and 9 for *S*1, and sessions 2, 6, and 8 for *S*2.

There was a substantial increase in rate of lever-pressing accompanying shock-escape training for both *S*s. The curves also show the extinction of this response. The extinction is apparent in the falling rate between shock sessions (e.g., sessions 2 through 6 for *S*1 show a gradual decrease in rate of responding). A similar extinction is also manifested over the various shock sessions, i.e., the highest rate was observed after the first shock training, the next highest after the second shock training, and so on. The *S*s' performances were very systematic and orderly.

Data based on the two additional measures, vocalization and standing on the chair or ledge, are presented in Table 1. The entries in the column labeled *0*1 can be compared to those in column *0*2. These data indicate that there was a high degree of agreement between the two observers rating amount of vocalizations of *S*s. The *0*2's ratings were based on tape recordings taken from *S*s while in the booth. It was physically impossible to have a second *O* assess the reliability of *O*1's ratings of climbing. However, because of the ease of recording such behavior it was judged unnecessary to check on its reliability. The agreement between *O*s on vocalizations was judged adequate for the purposes of this study.

TABLE 1 *Per cent of total time engaged in vocalization and climbing*

Session	Shock	*S*1 Vocal 01	*S*1 Vocal 02	*S*1 Climb 01	*S*2 Vocal 01	*S*2 Vocal 02	*S*2 Climb 01
1		49		0	27		96
2	*S*1 and *S*2	19	19	0	27		0
3		47		0	20		20
4		25		32	23		0
5		18		65	26	29	0
6	*S*2	22	23	97	22		0
7	*S*1	22	23	33	23	23	0
8	*S*2	22		83	22		0
9	*S*1	11		0			
10		13		75			

If the increase in lever-pressing behavior was correlated with an increase in the two additional behaviors, then it might not be that shock-escape training had led to an increase in behavior toward people *per se*. Rather, it might have led to an "arousal" of many behaviors, asocial as well as social. As Table 1 shows, the two additional measures showed no systematic relationship to the shock-escape sessions for *S*2. In the case of *S*1 there is some possibility of *suppression* of vocalization and climbing subsequent to shock-escape sessions (sessions 2, 7, and 9). It is unlikely, then, that shock-escape training involving other people can be viewed simply as activating many behaviors; rather, such training selectively raised behavior which yielded a social consequence.

Thus it is concluded that this increase in behavior toward *E* subsequent to shock-escape training came about because *E* was paired with shock reduction, thereby acquiring reinforcing powers. This conceptualization is consistent with the findings of Studies 1 and 2, both of which demonstrated an increase in social and affectionate behaviors. The findings are similar to those reported by Risley (1964) who observed an increase in acceptable social behavior (eye-to-eye contact) in an autistic child to whom *E* had administered electric shock for suppression of behaviors dangerous to the child. The data are also consistent with the results of studies by Mowrer and Aiken (1954) and Smith and Buchanen (1954) on animals which demonstrated that stimuli which are discriminative for shock reduction take on secondary positive reinforcing properties. It is to be noted, however, that the data from the studies reported here also fit a number of other conceptual frameworks.

An apparent limitation in these data pertains to the highly situational and often short-lived nature of the effects of shock. This had definite drawbacks when one considers the therapeutic implications of shock. It is considered, however, that the effects of shock can be made much more durable and general by making the situation in which shock is delivered less discriminable from situations in which it is not. The purpose of the present studies was to explore certain aspects of shock for possible therapeutic use. Therefore, only the minimal amount of shock considered necessary for observing reliable behavior changes was employed. It is quite possible that the children's responsiveness to adults would have been drastically reduced if shock had been employed too frequently. It is worth making the point explicitly: a certain use of shock can, as in these studies, contribute toward beneficial, even therapeutic, effects; but it does not at all follow that a more widespread use of the same techniques in each case will lead to even better outcomes. Indeed, the reverse may be true. Recent studies with schizophrenic children in our laboratory have shown, tentatively, that non-contingent shock facilitates performance of a well-learned task; however, such shock interferes with learning during early stages of the acquisition of new behaviors.

Certain more generalized effects of shock training, even though not recorded objectively, were noticed by *E*s and ward staff. First of all, *S*s had to be trained (shaped) to come to *E* to escape shock. When shock was first presented to *S*2, for example, he remained immobile, even though adults were in the immediate vicinity (there was no way in which *S*s could have "known" that *E*s presented the shock). This immobility when hurt is consistent with observations of *S*s when they were hurt in the play-yard, e.g., by another child. But after *S*s had been trained to avoid shock successfully in the experimental room, their nurses' notes state that *S*s would come to the nurses when hurt in other settings.

*E*s had expected considerable expression of fear by *S*s when they were shocked. Such fearful behavior was present only in the beginning of training. On the other hand, once *S*s had been trained to avoid shock, they often smiled and laughed, and gave other signs of happiness or comfort. For example, they would "mold" or "cup" to *E*'s body as small infants do with parents. Such behaviors were unobserved prior to these experiments. Perhaps avoidance of pain generated contentment.

In their day-to-day living, extremely regressed schizophrenic children such as these *S*s rarely show signs of fear or anxiety. The staff who dealt with these children in their usual environments expressed concern about the children's lack of worry or anxiety. There are probably several reasons why children such as these fail to demonstrate anxiety. It is possible that their social and emotional development has been so curtailed and limited that they are unaffected by the fear-eliciting situations acting upon a normal child. For example, they do not appear to be afraid of intellectual or social inadequacies, nor are they known to experience nightmares. Furthermore, by the age of three or four, like normal children, these children appear less bothered by physiological stimuli, and unlike the small infant, are rather free of physiological discomforts. Finally, when these children are brought to treatment, for example in a residential setting, there is much effort made to make their existence maximally comfortable.

If it is the case, as most writers on psychological treatment have stated, that the person's experience of discomfort is a basic condition for improvement, then perhaps the failure of severely retarded schizophrenic children to improve in treatment can be attributed partly to their failure to fulfill this hypothesized basic condition of anxiety or fear. This was one of the considerations which formed the basis for the present studies on electric shock. It is important to note that the choice of electric shock was made after several alternatives for the inducement of pain or fear were tested and found wanting. For example, in the early work with these children we employed loud noise. Even at noise levels well above 100 decibels we found that the children remained unperturbed particularly after the first two or three presentations.

It seems likely that the most therapeutic use of shock will not lie primarily in the suppression of specific responses or the shaping of behavior through escape-avoidance training. Rather, it would seem more efficient to use shock reduction as a way of establishing social reinforcers, i.e., as a way of making adults meaningful in the sense of becoming rewarding to the child. The failure of autistic children to acquire social reinforcers has been hypothesized as basic to their inadequate behavioral development (Ferster, 1961). Once social stimuli acquire reinforcing properties, one of the basic conditions for the acquisition of social behaviors has been met. A more complete argument supporting this thesis has been presented elsewhere (Lovaas et al., 1964). A basic question, then, is whether it is necessary to employ shock in accomplishing such an end or whether less drastic methods might not suffice. In a previous study (Lovaas et al., 1964) autistic children did acquire social reinforcers on the basis of food delivery. However, the necessary conditions for the acquisition of social reinforcers by the use of food were both time-consuming and laborious, and by no means as simple as the conditions which were necessary when we employed shock reduction.

References

BIJOU, S. W., & BAER, D. M. (1961). *Child Development: A Systematic and Empirical Theory.* New York: Appleton-Century-Crofts.

BROWN, JANET L. (1960). Prognosis from presenting symptoms of preschool children with atypical development. *American Journal of Orthopsychiatry*, **30**, 382–390.

EISENBERG, L. (1957). The course of childhood schizophrenia. *American Medical Association Archives for Neurology and Psychiatry*, **78**, 69–83.

FERSTER, C. B. (1961). Positive reinforcement and behavioral deficits of autistic children. *Child Development*, **32**, 437–456.

LOVAAS, O. I., FREITAG, G., GOLD, V. J., & KASSORLA, I. C. (1965). A recording method and observations of behaviors of normal and autistic children in free play settings. *Journal of Experimental Child Psychology*, **2**, 108–120.

LOVAAS, O. I., FREITAG, G., KINDER, M. I., RUBENSTEIN, D. B., SCHAEFFER, B., & SIMMONS, J. Q. (1964). Experimental studies in childhood schizophrenia—Establishment of social reinforcers. Paper delivered at Western Psychological Association, Portland, April.

MOWRER, O. H., & AIKEN, E. G. (1954). Contiguity vs. drive-reduction in conditioned fear: temporal variations in conditioned and unconditioned stimulus. *American Journal of Psychology*, **67**, 26–38.

RISLEY, TODD (1964). The effects and "side effects" of the use of punishment with an autistic child. Unpublished manuscript, Florida State University.

SMITH, M. P., & BUCHANEN, G. (1954). Acquisition of secondary reward by cues associated with shock reduction. *Journal of Experimental Psychology*, **48**, 123–126.

SOLOMON, R. L. (1964). Punishment. *American Psychologist*, **19**, 239–253.

DAVID ELKIND

Middle-Class Delinquency

Juvenile delinquency has always been a vexing problem involving, as it does, young people on the threshold of adulthood whose entire future may well be shaped by the way their adolescent acting-out problems are dealt with. It is an even more vexing problem when it arises among youngsters who have grown up in homes offering comforts and advantages that would seem to make delinquent behavior unnecessary. When a boy with a deprived background goes wrong we can readily relate it to unfulfilled needs and the frustrations offered by the circumstances of his life. When the delinquency occurs among the middle-class person, we are upset by both the antisocial nature of the behavior and our own inability to understand how it could come about. In this paper, Elkind, who has worked with such problems, offers an excellent discussion of the subtle interpersonal factors within the middle-class family which actually provoke such delinquency.

The research literature on juvenile delinquency is already vast and continues to grow at an increasing pace (1). By and large, however, this research tends to deal with lower-class children living in slum areas of large cities. Much less is known about the young people from suburban, middle-class homes who also get into trouble with the law.

Some writers (2, 3) have suggested that delinquent youngsters from "respectable homes" are acting out the parents' repressed antisocial impulses and are subtly encouraged by the parents in this regard. Although this explanation probably holds true in a certain number of cases, my own experience (as consulting psychologist to a suburban juvenile court) suggests that the vicarious satisfaction of needs is but one of many forms of parental exploitation that can lead to delinquent behavior on the part of children. In what follows I shall elaborate on some of the forms of parental exploitation and some of the possible adolescent reactions to such exploitation.

Before proceeding, however, it is necessary to distinguish among three quite distinct groups of middle-class delinquents. There are, first of all, those adolescents whose delinquency is a direct manifestation of a long-standing emotional disturbance and for whom the remedy is usually psychiatric rather

Reprinted from *Mental Hygiene*, **51** (1967), 80–84, with the permission of the National Association for Mental Health and Dr. Elkind.

than probationary. Secondly, there are those young people who came before the court almost by accident—quite often for pulling some prank that turned out to be more serious than they had anticipated—and who are seldom, if ever, adjudicated for a second time. By far the largest group, however, are those adolescents who get into trouble more or less regularly and who have a series of past charges filed against them. Although these young people do not appear to have serious internalized conflicts, they are usually in quite open conflict with their parents.

It is with the etiology of delinquent behavior in this third group of young people that the present paper is primarily concerned.

The Contract

The concept of parental exploitation makes sense only if there is an implicit contract between parents and their offspring. In middle-class families such a contract does exist. For their part, the parents agree to provide for the physical and emotional well-being of their children, who, in return, agree to abide by the norms of middle-class society. Although minor infractions of this contract on the part of both parents and children are to be found in most middle-class families, they tend to be temporary. For the most part, the contract is honored on both sides.

This appears not to be true in the families of the delinquent children under discussion. If one inquires deeply enough into the family relationships of these children, one finds that the contract has been broken by one or both parents *over a prolonged period of time*. More particularly, that part of the contract is broken which ensures that the parent will take responsibility for the emotional well-being of his child. What one finds in these cases is that the parent not only puts his own needs before those of the child, but, more significantly, attempts to use the child as an instrument in the satisfaction of those needs. It is because the parent violates the contract with his child while demanding that the child hold to his end of the bargain that such violations are legitimately called "parental exploitation."

Forms of Parental Exploitation

Although particular instances of parental exploitation are almost infinite in their variety, they can nonetheless be grouped under a few reasonably comprehensive headings. We have already noted that the *vicarious satisfaction of parental needs* is one frequent form of exploitation.

This form of exploitation is illustrated by a case in which a sexually frustrated mother encouraged her daughter to act out sexually. When the daughter returned from a date, the mother would demand a kiss-by-kiss description of the affair and end by calling the girl a tramp. When I saw the girl, who was being adjudicated for sexual vagrancy, she told me, "I have the name so I might as well play the role." When she left my office, her mother, who had been waiting outside, teasingly asked her how far she had gotten with the "cute psychologist."

A somewhat different form of parental exploitation might be called *ego bolstering*. In this category fall those parents who demand academic or athletic achievement far beyond what the young person is able, or has the capacity, to produce. This form of exploitation has an element of vicarious satisfaction in it, but the dominant affect seems to be the need to bolster flagging parental self-esteem. Although it is normal to want to take pride in one's child's achievements, it becomes pathologic when the parents' own needs to bask in reflected glory take precedence over the emotional welfare of the child.

A somewhat different variety of this form of exploitation is illustrated by the father who encouraged his 17-year-old son to drink, frequent prostitutes, and generally "raise hell." This particular father was awakened late one night by the police who had caught his son in a raid on a so-called "massage" parlor. The father's reaction was, "Why aren't you guys out catching crooks?" This same father would boast to his co-workers that his son was "all boy" and a "chip off the old block."

Still another form of parental exploitation occurs when parents use their youngsters as *slave labor*. In one instance, a father who owned a motel demanded that his son do all the lawn work and help to clean up the rooms and make the beds. To top it off, he insisted that the boy take the lids off all the cans in the trash barrels and then flatten the cans so that the volume of trash, and hence the cost of disposal, would be lessened. The boy barely had time to do his homework, much less to visit with his friends. Mothers who get their teenage daughters to do more of the housework and the baby-sitting than is reasonable or equitable provide another example of slave labor exploitation.

A fourth form of parental exploitation is frequently encountered in broken homes in which the mother, who usually retains custody of the children, is relatively young and attractive. In one case a mother took a lover, much younger than herself, into her home over the protestations of her teenage daughter, who had to cope with the curiosity of friends and the indignation of neighbors. Another young divorcee had a baby out of wedlock whom she kept in the home without any explanation to her teenage children. Still another mother, who had lost her husband under tragic circumstances, took to drinking away her afternoons with a younger man, to whom she gave large sums of money. She could not understand why her teenage son ran off to Mexico.

In all such cases, the mothers demand not only that their children accept the situation, but that they condone it. By demanding that their children accept and condone their behavior, these mothers hope to use their children to *assuage their own consciences*.

One of the saddest forms of parental exploitation is engaged in by parents who are very much in the public eye, particularly school principals, clergymen (of whatever faith), and judges. If a parent in one of these professions see his child's behavior primarily in terms of what it means to his career, he may demand a degree of conformity to middle-class mores that is quite unreasonable from the young person's point of view. When young people of this kind get into trouble, it is not because the parents are too strict, but rather because the parents are using their children to *proclaim their own moral rectitude.* As in all cases of parental exploitation, the dominant affect in such children is not so much the feeling of being restricted as it is the feeling of being *used.*

Reactions to Parental Exploitation

When a worker is exploited he has at least four courses of action open to him. He can either quit, go out on strike, sabotage the plant, or passively submit to the exploitation.

Parallel types of reaction are found in middle-class delinquents. Some young people literally quit the scene. They may quit school and become truant, quit the home and become runaways, or quit the family psychologically and become incorrigible. Other adolescents go on strike. They continue to go to school, but refuse to perform; they stay in the home, but refuse to do their fair share of the chores; they stay out late, and they go with a group of whom the parents don't approve. In short, they defy parental authority generally. More serious reactions are observed in young people who wish to sabotage their parents. These kids get pregnant, steal cars, vandalize schools, get drunk, sniff glue, or take drugs. Such reactions cost the parents plenty in worry, time, money, and bad publicity. The saddest reaction of all is that of the youngsters who passively submit to parental exploitation in the hope of winning or regaining parental love.

Despite the variety of these reactions, they all have one feature in common: parental exploitation is essentially private and is seldom recognized by anyone outside the home. Whereas the worker often has a union to voice his grievances and to stand up for his rights, there are no unions for children. Consequently, the delinquent behavior of adolescents who are being exploited by their parents often serves as a kind of "cry for help." Put differently, delinquent behavior often has as one of its components the desire to make the exploitation public, to let the world know what is happening behind the drawn drapes and closed doors. The sad thing about such cries for help is that they are as injurious to the young person as they are to the parents.

Treatment

To say that middle-class delinquency is difficult to treat psychotherapeutically is a gross understatement. The major reason for this is the fact that, *although the pathology exists in the parents, the symptoms appear in the children.* Since it is the children who are in trouble, the parents find it hard, except on a superficial basis, to accept their responsibility in the matter. Blind to their own violation of the parent-child contract, they insist that the young person live up to his side of the bargain. For his part, the young person feels that he has been used and abused and generally will not take responsibility for his actions.

With both parents and children blaming each other for the difficulty, there is little motivation for change on either side. Usually, however, the children are more tractable than the parents on this score. In many cases all that one can do is either remove the young person from the home, or help him to understand and deal with the exploitation in a more effective and less self-injurious way.

Summary and Implications

In the foregoing discussion, I have argued that middle-class delinquency is essentially a reaction to parental exploitation and have tried to enumerate some of the forms of exploitation as well as some of the reactions to it. Such a position clearly places the burden of blame for middle-class delinquency upon the parents. To some extent, this is perhaps unjust, since children may encourage exploitation on their own behalf and may well exploit their parents in return. In many cases the exploitation is as likely to be circular as it is to be unidirectional. And yet, my impression is that in the majority of cases the parents are much more to blame than are their children.

It should be said, too, that I don't offer the notion of parental exploitation as a complete explanation of middle-class delinquency. It is probably true that many of these young people have ego and superego defects of long standing. It is also true that we don't know why one form of exploitation will lead to a particular kind of delinquency and not another. In some cases, the connections seem direct and clear-cut, whereas in others they remain obscure. Unknown, too, is how prolonged the exploitation must be and how much of it is needed to incite an adolescent to delinquent acting-out. Such threshold values are probably a joint function of the child's personality and the quality of parental exploitation.

In short, a detailed understanding of any particular case of middle-class delinquency will have to involve a psychodynamic evaluation of the personalities of both parent and child. On the other hand (or so it seems to me), a psychodynamic evaluation of the parent-child interaction, although providing an explanation in a particular case, may well miss the common theme that seems to run through all cases of middle-class delinquency, namely, parental exploitation. Taken together, however, the concept of parental exploitation and psychodynamic evaluations may well provide a general, as well as a specific, explanation for middle-class delinquency.

The value of such a general explanation of delinquency as parental exploitation is shown in the way it helps to make plausible why certain familial conditions are regularly associated with delinquent behavior. Broken homes, for example, have routinely contributed more than their fair share to the delinquent population (4–7). It seems reasonable to assume that in broken homes one is more likely to find unmet parental needs than would be the case in intact families. Under these conditions, the temptation to put one's own needs ahead of those of the child and to use the child as an instrument in the satisfaction of those needs would probably be greatly enhanced. In short, the concept of parental exploitation might allow one to predict, or at least hypothesize, the kinds of family constellations that would be most likely to produce delinquent behavior.

Before closing, I want to take up one more point that has been raised by those who attribute middle-class delinquency to the antisocial impulses of parents that are vicariously satisfied through the child. It has already been noted that the vicarious satisfaction of parental needs is indeed one form of parental exploitation. Where I disagree with this position is in the implication that middle-class delinquency is antisocial, regardless of whether or not this is true of the parental need. If antisocial means the intent to harm or injure society in general, then I do not believe middle-class delinquency is antisocial. I do believe it is antifamilial. Looked at from the point of view of the adolescent, and not necessarily from the point of view of society, delinquent behavior may be the most psychologically adaptive action a young person can take in the face of parental exploitation. Delinquent behavior not only calls attention to his plight, but also may remove him from the home on temporary or permanent basis.

Although I have limited the application of the concept of exploitation to the question of middle-class delinquency, it is possible that all delinquency is, at least in part, a reaction to exploitation and that society, as well as parents, can be culpable in this regard.

References

1. QUAY, H. C. (ed.) (1965). *Juvenile Delinquency*. Princeton: Von Nostrand.
2. GIFFIN, M. E., JOHNSON, A. M., & LITIN, E. M. (1954). *American Journal of Orthopsychiatry*, **24**, 668.
3. JOHNSON, A. M., & BURKE, E. C. (1955). Proceedings of the Staff Meetings of the Mayo Clinic, **30**, 557.
4. BURT, C. (1929). *The Young Delinquent*. New York: Appleton.
5. GLUECK, S., & GLUECK, E. T. (1950). *Unraveling Juvenile Delinquency*. New York: Commonwealth Fund.
6. MONAHAN, T. P. (1957). *Social Forces*, **35**, 250.
7. NYE, F. I. (1958). *Family Relationships and Delinquent Behavior*. New York: Wiley.

Section III

Psychotherapy

Any study of abnormality would seem incomplete without some mention of the means by which pathological patterns may be altered. This is essentially the business of psychotherapy, a procedure that had its beginnings in the work of Freud, but one that has come, over the years, to be viewed differently by different theorists. Such diversity has probably stemmed from experiences with varying types of patients and the continued growth of our understanding about the forces that shape the individual's behavior. This section samples a number of diverse approaches to psychotherapy, ranging from classical psychoanalytic thinking to current developments in behavior modification and existential therapy. Because of the current popularity of a number of group approaches, papers reviewing sensitivity and encounter techniques are included. Finally, a review of research findings is also presented.

7 Approaches and Research in Psychotherapy

This chapter includes many different approaches to psychotherapy, both of a clinical and a research nature. This diversity should give some indication of the controversy and current state of flux that typifies current developments in this area.

ROBERT P. KNIGHT

A Critique of the Present Status of the Psychotherapies

Dr. Knight presents a summary of a wide variety of approaches to psychotherapy. Most of these approaches have in common the fact that basically they are varieties of some form of psychoanalysis. When Knight refers to dynamic psychology, he is describing classical Freudian theory, and he sees good therapy as essentially developing from a Freudian framework. A number of radically different frameworks will be presented in later papers. Dr. Knight was a medically trained psychoanalyst, and it is interesting to note that he implies that the analyst must initially be a psychiatrist, and does not give very much attention to lay, or nonmedically trained, analysts. However, in describing the personal qualities that he feels are necessary for an analyst, he clearly argues that psychiatry is different from other medical specialties such as surgery, and describes characteristics, such as personal integrity, which clearly are not restricted to physicians.

Before one can write a meaningful critical evaluation of the psychotherapies of today, he must attempt to define the types of treatment methods which are commonly assumed to be distinguishable varieties of psychotherapy. This

---

Reproduced by permission from: Knight, R. P.: "A Critique of the Present Status of the Psychotherapies." *Bull. N.Y. Acad. Med.* **25**:100–14, 1949.

is no easy task, for there exists no such generally accepted classified listing of the psychotherapies. A motley array of adjectives is found to designate brands of psychotherapy which are supposedly different from each other but which actually overlap each other in manifold ways. It will be a necessary preliminary task for us to review the terms commonly used in psychiatric literature and in ordinary professional parlance to designate various types of psychotherapy.

In a survey of usages which probably falls short of being exhaustive, I have noted that the type of psychotherapy may be characterized from any one of a number of frames of reference:

1. With regard to the preponderant attitude taken or influence attempted by the therapist; e.g., suggestion, persuasion, exhortation, intimidation, counselling, interpretation, re-education, retraining, etc.
2. With regard to the general aim of the therapy; e.g., supportive, suppressive, expressive, cathartic, ventilative, etc.
3. With regard to the supposed "depth" of the therapy—superficial psychotherapy and deep psychotherapy.
4. With regard to the duration—brief psychotherapy and prolonged psychotherapy.
5. With regard to its supposed relationship to Freudian psychoanalysis, as, for example, orthodox, standard, classical, or regular psychoanalysis, modified psychoanalysis, wild analysis, direct psychoanalysis, psychoanalytic psychotherapy, psychoanalytically oriented psychotherapy, psychodynamic psychotherapy, psychotherapy using the dynamic approach, and psychotherapy based on psychoanalytic principles.
6. With regard to the ex-Freudian dissident who started a new school of psychotherapy. Thus we have Adler's individual psychology with its Adlerian "analysis," Jung's analytical psychology with its Jungian "analysis," the Rankian analysis, the Stekelian analysis, and the Horney modifications.
7. With regard to whether patients are treated singly or in groups—individual psychotherapy and group psychotherapy.
8. With regard to whether the psychotherapy is "directive" or "non-directive," an issue emphasized strongly by the Rogers group of psychologists.
9. With regard to the adjunctive technique which is coupled with psychotherapy; e.g., narcotherapy (narcoanalysis, narcosynthesis), and hypnotherapy (hypnoanalysis), the first using drugs and the second hypnosis for technical reasons to be discussed later.

It is not surprising that both physicians and the lay public regard this welter of terminology as something less than scientific, and that patients seeking help for emotional distress are often confused as to where to find that help and as to what type of psychotherapy to trust. In defense of the present confusion one can remind himself that although psychotherapy is said to be the oldest form of medical treatment, it is also one of the very latest to achieve a scientific, rational basis, i.e., to rest on a basic science of dynamic psychology. Because of its partial derivation from many unscientific and extra-scientific sources—primitive magical practices of tribal medicine men, religious rites, parental exhortations and commands, mysticism, commonsense advice and intuitive insights of friends, and downright quackery, to mention but a few—psychotherapy has among its practitioners today not only many lay fakirs but also a good many physicians whose training in dynamic psychology is grossly inadequate. Also, even among the best trained psychiatrists there exist some honest differences of opinion regarding principles and techniques of psychotherapy. However, research and experimentation continue to expand, and slowly the phenomena of artful and intuitive psychotherapeutic influences are translated into scientific principles and techniques.

It is impossible to overstate the importance of dynamic psychology as a basic science on which all competent psychotherapy must rest. Without an underlying structure of psychodynamics and psychopathology, in which the psychotherapist must be well trained, all psychotherapy is at best empirical, at the worst the blind leading the blind. No valid critique of the psychotherapies is possible except in relation to the penetrating understanding of human personality and behavior provided by dynamic psychology, the chief contributions to which have been made by psychoanalysis.

It seems necessary, therefore, to review for an essentially nonpsychiatric medical audience the theoretical essentials in modern dynamic psychology. The cornerstone of dynamic psychology is the concept of repression. As the psychic structure of the human personality develops in infancy and childhood, the primitive erotic and aggressive impulses come to be opposed by counter-impulses deriving from the child's training and adaptive experiences. The chief counter-impulse is repression, which banishes from consciousness—but not from continued active existence in the unconscious—those impulses, some native and some stimulated by specific experiences, which the child discovers are condemned and forbidden expression by its upbringers. Both the strength of the alien impulses and the child's capacity to oppose them are partially determined by his native constitution, partly by the nature of his early experiences, and partly by the character and upbringing methods of those adults who rear him. Some condemned impulses are simply repressed, along with their associated fantasies and affects; others are modified in partial expression and partial repression assisted by other defense mechanisms. Topographically the unconscious is regarded as the repository of repressed impulses and forgotten memories, the preconscious as that part of the mind in which reside the rememberable but currently unattended-to memories, and the conscious mind as the aware, focusing, thinking portion of the psychic structure. Viewed dynamically, the primitive impulses arise out of biological and psychological drives identified collectively as the Id, while the opposing, defensive forces arise from Ego, or organized part of the personality, and the

Super-ego—roughly the conscience. The sum total of these dynamic internal and external interactions, plus constitution and native intellectual endowment, equals the developing personality in all of its individual uniqueness. While the major battle between opposing internal forces appears to be settled at about age five or six, thus forming the basic personality structure, there is a continuous internal interaction and a constant external adaptive attempt throughout life, with special crises during adolescence and in reaction to the Protean forms that stressful life experiences can take. Also, each individual, however healthy his adaption appears to be, has his own particular psychological areas of vulnerability to stress, and he may be precipitated into clinical neurotic or psychotic illness by experiences whose qualitative or quantitative nature exceed his capacity to master them through healthy adaptive methods.

This highly condensed exposition of dynamic psychology with its emphasis on the uniqueness of the individual will, I hope, be sufficient to serve as a background for the following proposition, namely, that competent treatment of a patient by psychotherapeutic means requires of the psychotherapist:

1. That he be thoroughly grounded in the basic science of dynamic psychology.
2. That he be well trained in clinical methods of evaluating the individual patient, not only in terms of general comparison with others presenting similar clinical pictures, but also in terms of the uniquely individual forces and factors in each individual patient.
3. That he then utilize, from among the available psychotherapeutic approaches and techniques, those particular ones which, according to his best clinical judgment, are most appropriate in a given case.
4. A fourth prerequisite does not follow logically from the previous argument but is of an importance at least equal to the other three, namely, that the psychotherapist be a person of integrity, objectivity, and sincere interest in people, and that he be relatively free from personal conflicts, anxieties, biases, emotional blind spots, rigidities of manner, and settled convictions as to how people should properly behave.

This last prerequisite for psychotherapeutic work requires some amplification. Unlike the situation in other fields of medical therapy, the man well grounded in the basic science underlying his therapy, well trained in diagnostic methods, and possessing technical competence to use the indicated therapy may still, in psychotherapy, be a poor practitioner if he is personally anxious, rigid, or full of moral convictions. Other therapies in medicine can be competently performed, with good results on patients, without these personal qualities, largely because a great deal of medical and surgical treatment consists of doing something *to* the patient. To be sure the personal qualities in a physician which cause his patients to love and trust him are exactly the ones which make him a real physician rather than a mechanical artisan; but far greater emotional demands are made on the psychotherapist. The nature of the subject material in psychotherapy, the intense personal give and take in the patient-therapist relationship, the enormously increased possibilities of anti-therapeutic personal involvement, the self knowledge in the therapist required both to understand his patients and to steer a sound therapeutic course with them, all require of the psychotherapist certain personal qualities not essential to other medical specialists. It is not particularly difficult for physicians to acquire protective attitudes of detachment in respect to those bodily elements and products—blood, pus, urine, diseased tissue, mucus, feces, guts—which so upset the squeamish layman, and this detachment serves the physician in good stead as he works coolly and efficiently at his therapeutic task. But this sort of detachment in a psychotherapist is not only no protection against the psychological products of his patients, it actually hampers and distorts his therapeutic work and, if extreme, even disqualifies him from undertaking to deal with psychopathology and psychotherapy. The counterphobic attitude may be sufficient for competent work in physiology, pathology, and surgery; it is a poor and brittle defense for work in psychiatry and psychotherapy.

Such personal considerations with regard to the psychotherapist raise important questions regarding selection of candidates for psychiatric training, and regarding the importance of personal psychoanalysis as a part of psychoanalytic and psychiatric training. Certainly every psychiatrist who wishes to do psychoanalytic therapy should have full psychoanalytic training, including, of course, the personal analysis. It might also be said that every psychiatrist who expects to practice major psychotherapy of any kind should have full psychoanalytic training, just as every physician who plans to do major surgery should have full surgical training.

I have so far attempted to show that the terminology designating supposed varieties of psychotherapy is very confusing because of the many frames of reference in which identifying adjectives were applied, and to indicate that a critique of these psychotherapies is not possible until a valid frame of reference is established. I then tried to show that familiarity with the basic science of dynamic psychology, and the clinical techniques derived from it is necessary to provide a valid frame of reference for a critique. This led to the collateral but vital point of the psychotherapist's personal suitability. It is necessary to establish one more phase of this frame of reference. This has to do with the nature and vicissitudes of the patient-physician relationship in psychotherapy.

Most physicians are not much concerned about the attitudes, emotions, and fantasies their patients have about them as long as the patients are co-operative, don't go to other physicians, and pay their bills for professional services. Occasionally physicians are startled to encounter outbursts of un-provoked hostility or professions of love or jealousy, or suspicion from their patients. I suppose the usual result is that the patient is then discharged by that physician in the event the physician cannot "talk him out of his nonsense." Many psychiatrists of the past (and some in the present) have been more concerned about emotional reactions of patients to them, but have thought of them in terms of "good rapport" or the lack of it, without paying much attention to the exact nature of these reactions, whether friendly or hostile. Sigmund Freud, picking up a cue noted but abandoned by Josef Breuer, had the genius to follow through to a penetrating study of patients' emotional attitudes toward their doctors and to bring this group of phenomena into both the theoretical framework of dynamic psychology and the clinical framework of psychotherapy. He saw that whereas the various emotional reactions of the individual patient appeared at first to be irrational and unprovoked, actually these attitudes could be understood the same as other psychological phenomena in the patient could be understood, such as recovered memories, dreams, fantasies, and so on, and could, instead of being emotionally reacted to by the therapist, provide him with material for fresh insights into his patient. Freud called these reactions "transference" because of his understanding of them as emotions originally felt toward other significant persons in the patient's past experience, and now transferred to the doctor. He discovered that their nature could be interpreted to the patient, and that such interpretations, when correctly timed and accurately expressed, had significant therapeutic effect on the patient. Thus the theoretical understanding and clinical use of transference phenomena became one of the significant contributions of psychoanalysis to the field of psychiatry, and, indeed, to the practice of medicine in general, for transference reactions by patients are by no means limited to those being treated psychotherapeutically.

Freud also had the objectivity to observe and analyze his own reactions to patients, and concluded that all psychotherapists would have their own particular tendencies to react inappropriately (that is, inappropriately from the standpoint of correct therapeutic technique) to the material, or behavior, or persons of their patients. He called such reactions and reaction tendencies "counter-transference," and bade all analysts to be acutely observant of themselves in this regard so that they might analyze and dissipate these counter-transference reactions without letting themselves be unwittingly influenced by them to the detriment of their therapeutic efforts. Again, such counter-transference reactions are not confined to psychiatrists, psychoanalysts, or psychotherapists, but are present in all physicians toward their patients, albeit with considerably less significance, for the most part, in therapy other than psychotherapy. Once more, then, we see the importance for the psychotherapist of those personal qualities of integrity, objectivity, sincerity, and relative freedom from emotional blind spots.

I have now used almost half of my time to develop the background frame of reference in which any psychotherapy may properly be critically evaluated. The following elements have been emphasized:

1. The theoretical understanding of human personality provided by dynamic psychology.
2. The clinical evaluation of each individual patient—the nature and intensity of his internal and external conflicts, the genetic history of

those conflicts, his particular defenses against anxiety, his strengths as shown by past adaptations and achievements, his vulnerabilities and weaknesses as shown by the extent of his decompensation, his way of relating initially to the therapist, his intelligence and its possible impairments, the intactness of his concept formation, his loyalty to reality, his capacity for introspection and selfconfrontation, and so on.

3. The utilization of psychotherapeutic techniques based on sufficient knowledge of dynamic psychology and applied appropriately to the individual case in the light of the clinical evaluation.
4. The personal qualifications and suitability of the psychotherapist, and, we may now add, his capacity to recognize and deal with transference manifestations in his patients and counter-transference tendencies in himself.

If these four criteria provide a valid frame of reference in which to evaluate psychotherapy, it is readily seen that those psychotherapists who have a fixed system of treatment for all patients who come to them are practicing poor psychotherapy. This is true whether it refers to those therapists who treat all patients with such banal exhortations as "Buck up," "Go home and forget it," "Stop worrying about that," "Pull yourself together," "Don't cross bridges until you come to them," and so on; to therapists who treat all patients by assigning reading for subsequent interview discussions in prepared booklets on how to live; to psychoanalysts who put all patients on the couch and tell them to free-associate; or to therapists who keep the syringe loaded with sodium pentothal for each patient, or who routinely start their hypnotic maneuvers promptly. One may give insulin to every diabetic, or operate every acute appendix, with, of course, some judgment as to dosage, timing, and collateral measures, but psychotherapy is, or should be, a highly individual matter for each patient. Far too often in current practice the type of psychotherapy used with the patient is determined solely by the limited training and ability of the psychotherapist rather than by either the type of illness the patient has or the type of patient that has the illness.

Of the various possible ways of classifying psychotherapeutic attempts, most psychiatrists would agree that two large groups could be identified—those which aim primarily at support of the patient, with suppression of his symptoms and his erupting psychological material, and those which aim primarily at expression. It is actually more appropriate to speak of a group of techniques utilized to accomplish suppression or expression than to speak of sub-groups of psychotherapies under each major heading. Suppressive or supportive psychotherapy, also called superficial psychotherapy, utilizes such devices as inspiration, reassurance, suggestion, persuasion, counselling, re-education, and the like and avoids investigative and exploratory measures. Such measures may be indicated, even though the psychotherapist is well trained and experienced in expressive techniques, where the clinical evaluation of the patient leads to the conclusion that he is too fragile psychologically to be tampered with, or too inflexible to be capable of real personality alteration, or too defensive to be able to achieve insight. Certain recovering schizophrenics or agitated depressions or children might illustrate the fragility; rigid character disorders, certain manics and hypomanics, and elderly patients might illustrate the inflexibility; and some paranoid states might illustrate the defensiveness. The decision to use suppressive measures is made actually because of contraindications to using exploratory devices. One can say, then, that supportive or suppressive psychotherapy, with its variety of techniques and devices for accomplishing support and suppression, is a valid psychotherapy provided it is applied on the basis of sound indications and not indiscriminately to all or most patients simply because the particular psychotherapist does not know how to do anything else with the patient, and provided the psychotherapist realizes that transference and counter-transference manifestations can and do occur, and need to be handled, even in such superficial psychotherapy. Supportive psychotherapy may be brief or prolonged, as indicated, and may be carried out with individuals or with groups.

It is in the group of psychotherapies intended to be expressive that one encounters the various schools of thought, the adjunctive devices, the more frequent conflicts in theory, and the more significant question of personal suitability of the therapist. Expressive psychotherapies utilize such devices as exploratory probing through questioning, free-association, abreaction, confession, relating of dreams, catharsis, interpretation and the like, all with the purpose of uncovering and ventilating preconscious and unconscious pathogenic psychological material. Elements of support, reassurance, suggestion, advice, and direction are not necessarily excluded, and may, in fact, be consciously utilized. Expressive psychotherapy may be brief and intensive or prolonged, depending on the aims of the therapist and the response of the patient. Expressive psychotherapy is major psychotherapy and should not be undertaken without thorough grounding in dynamic psychology, adequate experience in clinical evaluation, practice under supervision, and personal suitability. Lacking this background, the psychotherapist is extremely likely to get into difficulties. He introduces topics for the patient to discuss without being aware that they are irrelevant to the matters pressing for expression within the patient, or that the patient cannot tackle a given topic until certain defenses are first pointed out and removed. He gives long and sententious theoretical explanations which he regards as interpretations, but which are either then learned as intellectual defenses by the patient or their content ignored while the patient basks in this verbal bath at the hands of the therapist. He permits himself unwittingly to be drawn into an active role as an ally in the patient's external interpersonal struggles, while remaining oblivious to the provocative shenanigans of the patient which keep these struggles going on. He pounces on dreams or slips of the tongue with ready and pat interpretations which miss the point. He focusses his attention on symptoms, and tries to treat them by interpretation, or special investigatory questioning. He becomes embroiled in transference-counter-transference jams and does not know how to extricate himself except by discontinuing the interviews for a while. I cite these common errors as illustrations of what may happen if the inadequately trained psychotherapist undertakes expressive psychotherapy. Needless to say such mishandling complicates the patient's illness exceedingly and renders more difficult the task of the inevitable subsequent psychotherapist.

Competent expressive psychotherapy may have goals which vary considerably. In cases where there has been an acute onset of neurotic symptoms in reaction to a discoverable precipitating event, and the patient's history shows a comparatively healthy course, the therapy may properly consist of thorough ventilation of the reaction to the upsetting event, with the therapist pointing out connections, relationships, and hidden motivations in the limited life area of the setting prior to the event, of the event itself, and of the patient's immediate and later reactions to the event. In skillful hands this is a most rewarding type of expressive psychotherapy. Recovery may be achieved in a very few interviews and the patient is restored to his previous good functioning with insights he would not otherwise have achieved. In such instances there is no therapeutic aim of exhaustive investigation, recovery of infantile memories, or altered ego structure. In other cases which may at first seem similar, the early clinical evaluation uncovers more neurotic difficulties than were at first apparent, and it becomes clear that the patient's adjustment prior to the precipitating event was a precarious one at best. The therapeutic aim may now change to one of more thoroughgoing alteration of the neurotic personality structure, and the expressive techniques lead into psychoanalysis. If the psychotherapist is competent to conduct psychoanalysis as well as the shorter expressive therapies with limited aim, he will have so handled the early therapy that the analytic techniques are a logical continuation of his early therapeutic work. If he is not so trained, he should at this point refer the patient to a suitable analyst.

Freudian psychoanalysis—and psychoanalysis actually implies "Freudian"—is a major, time-consuming, and therefore expensive, type of psychotherapy. It is by no means a panacea, and its most competent practitioners would readily concede that as a method of therapy it has limited application in the vast field of human psychological distress. (As a dynamic psychology and as a method of investigation it is, of course, invaluable, and possesses almost unlimited applicability.) Its limitations as a method of therapy do not depend merely on such factors as its duration (twelve to eighteen months as a minimum; four to five years as a maximum), its cost to the patient, and the availability of analysts (approximately 500 in the United States, with one-fourth of these in New York City). There is also a considerable list of special indications and contraindications, as, for example:

1. The patient should be of at least bright normal intelligence on the Bellevue-Wechsler scale (115 to 120 IQ).
2. The suitable age range for adults is about 20 to 50, with certain exceptions to be made at either end of this range.

3. There must be some capacity for introspection, and some awareness of nuances of feeling in himself and in others.
4. There must be sufficient motivation in terms of initial distress and strong desire to change.
5. The patient must possess sufficient intactness of personality so that this intact portion may become allied with the analyst in the analytic work.
6. In general, patients with unalterable physical handicaps are not suitable subjects for psychoanalysis.
7. The general field for psychoanalytic therapy includes the psychoneuroses, character disorders, some of the perversions, neurotic depressions, anxiety states, and some of the psychoses. Patients in the midst of acute external turmoil should not begin psychoanalysis as such until their life situations are more stable.

With all of its limitations, however, psychoanalytic therapy is, in well-trained hands, a highly effective procedure for achieving in patients a profound alteration in their neurotic personality structure and developing otherwise latent potentialities for achievement and responsible living.

The Freudian school of psychoanalysis is the main stream of the psychoanalytic movement. There have, in the past, been several split-offs from the main stream which resulted in transient and minor developments of non-Freudian schools. The school of the late Alfred Adler took one aspect of psychoanalysis, namely, the methods of the ego in dealing with external forces, and attempted to develop it into a system called individual psychology. The central theme of this psychology was that of inferiority feelings and the drive for power. This psychology and system of therapy died out with its leader. Carl Jung, also an early pupil and associate of Freud, split with him and developed a school of "analytical psychology" which emphasized symbolism and religious beliefs and which explained mental disorders, especially those of middle life and after, in terms of regressions to a collective unconscious, or racial heritage. His school still persists but his incorporation of Nazi racial ideology into his psychological theories has caused him to be severely criticized. The late Otto Rank, also an early pupil of Freud's, developed a system of therapy which emphasized the transference and the uncovering and working through of birth anxiety in a three months' period of treatment. There were many short Rankian analyses in the 1920's, but this system is now also extinct. The late Wilhelm Stekel, a remarkably intuitive man and a prolific writer, attracted a few followers to his technique of rapid and early deep interpretations of symbolic and unconscious meanings. His influence has now become almost nil. Karen Horney, originally a Freudian with many fine contributions to the literature, has led a movement in the last decade to eliminate a number of the fundamental concepts of psychoanalysis and to focus attention on current cultural conflicts as the main source of personality disorders. She rejects the libido theory, the significance of early psychosexual development, and in general takes a stand against genetic psychology in favor of culturalism.

There are other deviations from orthodox psychoanalytic techniques which are not represented by their practitioners nor regarded by others as separate dissident schools of psychoanalysis, but which are modifications of technique to meet the therapeutic problems in patients who are too ill to cooperate in the usual analytic procedure. These modifications are used chiefly with psychotics and involve approaches by the analyst which actively cultivate a treatment relationship, communication with the sick patient being established on whatever level is possible in the individual case. The success of such attempts depends on the resourcefulness of the analyst in coping with the patient's inaccessibility and his capacity for empathy and intuition in understanding what is communicated by the patient's verbalizations, behavior, and attitudes. Long periods of careful therapeutic work are required but the results are often very rewarding. As the patient improves the treatment may merge into a more regular psychoanalytic procedure.

A special type of analytic psychotherapy developed by Rosen, for which the designation "direct psychoanalysis" has been made, deserves some comment. Rosen has reported a striking series of recoveries of severe and chronic schizophrenias. His method consists of repeated, prolonged sessions with the patient in which deep interpretative activity is carried out fearlessly and relentlessly. Interpretations are based on psychoanalytic theory, and sometimes on insights provided by other schizophrenics. The usual cautions and tentative approaches which have characterized others' work with psychotics are abandoned, and direct, deep interpretations are made promptly when the therapist believes he understands. The therapist also, when necessary to make contact, takes the roles of powerful figures in the patient's delusions and shouts denials, reassurances, and interpretations. Remarkable results are reported, and this work is now undergoing study under research conditions. It promises much but is at present difficult to evaluate.

The school of Adolf Meyer, identified as psychobiology, emphasized the sound concept of all-embracing study of man in his totality. He developed a new system of nomenclature which did not achieve significant acceptance, and termed his treatment "distributive analysis and synthesis." This psychotherapy aimed at exhaustive collecting of data regarding the patient's life, past and present, utilized diagrams to depict life influences, and assigned to the therapist the role of educator and explainer of the experiences and reactions in the patient's life. This procedure may be criticized as being far too theoretical and intellectual to influence many patients, and as having almost totally ignored the elements of transference and counter-transference in the relationship between therapist and patient. As a school of psychotherapy, it probably has a diminishing number of adherents.

All of the major psychotherapies—i.e., those which aim at significant alterations in personality structure rather than at symptomatic relief—have encountered the phenomenon discovered by Freud and termed by him "resistance." This refers to those partly conscious and partly unconscious tendencies in patients to resist self-knowledge and change, as manifested in their inability to remember the past or to capture for therapeutic use the current unconscious content. Resistance produces a marked slowing down of progress, often approaching stalemate, while symptoms continue unaltered. Technical problems of resistance are among the most difficult to solve, and the long duration of major psychotherapy is attributable chiefly to this phenomenon.

In order to shorten the duration of therapy many attempts have been made to circumvent resistance. Chief among these techniques have been the use of hypnosis and certain sedative drugs. Under hypnosis or narcosis (also mild elation or light anesthesia) some patients are able to gain access to and to verbalize with affect otherwise unconscious memories, and to profit from the ventilation and abreaction and the interpretations of the therapist associated with this therapeutic experience. During World War II there was widespread use of intravenous sodium amytal and sodium pentothal as well as of hypnosis to produce dissolution of the resistance barriers against recalling overwhelming traumatic experiences. There often resulted clear recall and reliving of the traumatic experiences, with associated assimilation of the over-stressful event and great diminution or relief of the symptoms. It was found that early treatment was essential, delay resulting in the building of stronger barriers against recall and fixing of the symptomatology, to which was then added the exploitation of secondary gains. These psychotherapeutic procedures had enormous significance in military psychiatry, but, as sole treatment attempts, have proved to be disappointing in civilian psychiatry except with early traumatic neuroses in civil life. Such techniques of reducing resistance through hypnosis or narcosis do not constitute separate systems of psychotherapy, so that it is incorrect to speak of narcoanalysis, narcosynthesis, hypnotherapy, and hypnoanalysis as psychotherapies. They are adjuvant techniques to be used as a preliminary step in overcoming an initial impasse, or as devices to be introduced during psychotherapy when strong resistance blocks further progress.

The attempts to shorten the duration of psychotherapy have led to other techniques which make use of psychoanalytic principles but which try to achieve faster results especially through manipulation of the transference, role-taking by the therapist in order to provide a corrective emotional experience, and interruptions of treatment to avoid a difficult dependent transference. Alexander, French, and others who report this work maintain that their therapy is entitled to be called psychoanalysis—psychoanalysis with more flexible utilization of techniques. Many critics insist that the techniques as reported represent abandonment of fundamental analytic principles and that the goals of such therapy have become relief of symptoms and conventional social adaptation instead of the goals of structural personality alterations of psychoanalysis. Many other studies of short psychotherapy using psychoanalytic principles have been reported in the literature, and it seems well established that the whole field of psychotherapy has been greatly enriched by contributions from psychoanalysis.

In the last analysis there is only one psychotherapy, with many techniques. This one psychotherapy must rest on a basic science of dynamic psychology, and those techniques should be used which are clinically indicated for each individual patient—certain appropriate techniques for the initial stages and others later as the continuous clinical evaluation proceeds pari passu with therapy, and the goals and potentialities for the patient become more clearly delineated through his responses to therapy. And, finally, it is important to recognize that techniques as such are hardly separable from the individual who uses them. Psychotherapy is an enormously complex intercommunication and emotional interaction between two individuals, one of whom seeks help from the other. What is done and said by the one who tries to give help is inevitably his personal version of technique. Beyond all knowledge of dynamic psychology and training in techniques is his own individual personality, with its inevitable variables as to sex, physical appearance, depth of understanding, ability to communicate ideas, tone of voice, set of values, and all of the other highly individual elements which differentiate one therapist from another. The utmost impersonality and analytic incognito cannot exclude the effect of such individual elements. Hence we may say that in addition to a critique of psychotherapy one must also make a critique of the psychotherapist.

ALBERT BANDURA

Psychotherapy as a Learning Process

A radically different approach to psychotherapy is embodied in a school known as behavior modification. This school seeks to apply scientifically established laws of learning in the psychotherapy session, so that attempts to modify the patient's behavior are based on principles of broad generality and sound evidence. In this paper, Bandura reviews a number of the principles that are utilized by behavior therapists. The counter-conditioning approach is most closely identified with the work of Dr. Joseph Wolpe, and the technique of systematic desensitization is its leading application. Many of the other

---

Reprinted from the *Psychological Bulletin*, **58** (1961), 143–159, with the permission of the American Psychological Association and Dr. Bandura.

principles are outgrowths of the approach taken in the laboratory by Dr. B. F. Skinner, and are more closely related to operant conditioning than to classical conditioning.

While it is customary to conceptualize psychotherapy as a learning process, few therapists accept the full implications of this position. Indeed, this is best illustrated by the writings of the learning theorists themselves. Most of our current methods of psychotherapy represent an accumulation of more or less uncontrolled clinical experiences and, in many instances, those who have written about psychotherapy in terms of learning theory have merely substituted a new language; the practice remains essentially unchanged (Dollard, Auld, & White, 1954; Dollard & Miller, 1950; Shoben, 1949).

If one seriously subscribes to the view that psychotherapy is a learning process, the methods of treatment should be derived from our knowledge of learning and motivation. Such an orientation is likely to yield new techniques of treatment which, in many respects, may differ markedly from the procedures currently in use.

Psychotherapy rests on a very simple but fundamental assumption, i.e., human behavior is modifiable through psychological procedures. When skeptics raise the question, "Does psychotherapy work?" they may be responding in part to the mysticism that has come to surround the term. Perhaps the more meaningful question, and one which avoids the surplus meaning associated with the term "psychotherapy," is as follows: Can human behavior be modified through psychological means and if so, what are the learning mechanisms that mediate behavior change?

In the sections that follow, some of these learning mechanisms will be discussed, and studies in which systematic attempts have been made to apply these principles of learning to the area of psychotherapy will be reviewed. Since learning theory itself is still somewhat incomplete, the list of psychological processes by which changes in behavior can occur should not be regarded as exhaustive, nor are they necessarily without overlap.

Counterconditioning

Of the various treatment methods derived from learning theory, those based on the principle of counterconditioning have been elaborated in greatest detail. Wolpe (1954, 1958, 1959) gives a thorough account of this method, and additional examples of cases treated in this manner are provided by Jones (1956), Lazarus and Rachman (1957), Meyer (1957), and Rachman (1959). Briefly, the principle involved is as follows: if strong responses which are incompatable with anxiety reactions can be made to occur in the presence of anxiety evoking cues, the incompatible responses will become attached to these cues and thereby weaken or eliminate the anxiety responses.

The first systematic psychotherapeutic application of this method was reported by Jones (1924b) in the treatment of Peter, a boy who showed severe phobic reactions to animals, fur objects, cotton, hair, and mechanical toys. Counterconditioning was achieved by feeding the child in the presence of initially small but gradually increasing anxiety-arousing stimuli. A rabbit in a cage was placed in the room at some distance so as not to disturb the boy's eating. Each day the rabbit was brought nearer to the table and eventually removed from the cage. During the final stage of treatment, the rabbit was placed on the feeding table and even in Peter's lap. Tests of generalization revealed that the fear responses had been effectively eliminated, not only toward the rabbit, but toward the previously feared furry objects as well.

In this connection, it would be interesting to speculate on the diagnosis and treatment Peter would have received had he been seen by Melanie Klein (1949) rather than by Mary Cover Jones!

It is interesting to note that while both Shoben (1949) and Wolpe (1958) propose a therapy based on the principle of counterconditioning, their treatment methods are radically different. According to Shoben, the patient discusses and thinks about stimulus situations that are anxiety provoking in the context of an interpersonal situation which simultaneously elicits positive affective responses from the patient. The therapeutic process consists in connecting the anxiety provoking stimuli, which are symbolically reproduced, with the comfort reaction made to the therapeutic relationship.

Shoben's paper represents primarily a counterconditioning interpretation of the behavior changes brought about through conventional forms of psychotherapy since, apart from highlighting the role of positive emotional reactions in the treatment process, no new techniques deliberately designed to facilitate relearning through counterconditioning are proposed.

This is not the case with Wolpe, who has made a radical departure from tradition. In his treatment, which he calls reciprocal inhibition, Wolpe makes systematic use of three types of responses which are antagonistic to, and therefore inhibitory of, anxiety. These are: assertive or approach responses, sexual responses, and relaxation responses.

On the basis of historical information, interview data, and psychological test responses, the therapist constructs an anxiety hierarchy, a ranked list of stimuli to which the patient reacts with anxiety. In the case of desensitization based on relaxation, the patient is hypnotized and given relaxation suggestions. He is then asked to imagine a scene representing the weakest item on the anxiety hierarchy and, if the relaxation is unimpaired, this is followed by having the patient imagine the next item on the list, and so on. Thus, the anxiety cues are gradually increased from session to session until the last phobic stimulus can be presented without impairing the relaxed state. Through this procedure, relaxation responses eventually come to be attached to the anxiety evoking stimuli.

Wolpe reports remarkable therapeutic success with a wide range of neurotic reactions treated on this counterconditioning principle. He also contends that the favorable outcomes achieved by the more conventional psychotherapeutic methods may result from the reciprocal inhibition of anxiety by strong positive responses evoked in the patient-therapist relationship.

Although the counterconditioning method has been employed most extensively in eliminating anxiety-motivated avoidance reactions and inhibitions, it has been used with some success in reducing maladaptive approach responses as well. In the latter case, the goal object is repeatedly associated with some form of aversive stimulus.

Raymond (1956), for example, used nausea as the aversion experience in the treatment of a patient who presented a fetish for handbags and perambulators which brought him into frequent contact with the law in that he repeatedly smeared mucus on ladies' handbags and destroyed perambulators by running into them with his motorcyle. Though the patient had undergone psychoanalytic treatment, and was fully aware of the origin and the sexual significance of his behavior, nevertheless, the fetish persisted.

The treatment consisted of showing the patient a collection of handbags, perambulators, and colored illustrations just before the onset of nausea produced by injections of apomorphine. The conditioning was repeated every 2 hours day and night for 1 week plus additional sessions 8 days and 6 months later.

Raymond reports that, not only was the fetish successfully eliminated, but also the patient showed a vast improvement in his social (and legal) relationships, was promoted to a more responsible position in his work, and no longer required the fetish fantasies to enable him to have sexual intercourse.

Nauseant drugs, especially emetine, have also been utilized as the unconditioned stimulus in the aversion treatment of alcoholism (Thirmann, 1949; Thompson & Bielinski, 1953; Voegtlen, 1940; Wallace, 1949). Usually 8 to 10 treatments in which the sight, smell, and taste of alcohol is associated with the onset of nausea is sufficient to produce abstinence. Of 1,000 or more cases on whom adequate follow-up data are reported, approximately 60% of the patients have been totally abstinent following the treatment. Voegtlen (1940) suggests that a few preventive treatments given at an interval of about 6 months may further improve the results yielded by this method.

Despite these encouraging findings, most psychotherapists are unlikely to be impressed since, in their opinion, the underlying causes for the alcoholism have in no way been modified by the conditioning procedure and, if anything, the mere removal of the alcoholism would tend to produce symptom substitution or other adverse effects. A full discussion of this issue will be presented later. In this particular context, however, several aspects of the Thompson and Bielinski (1953) data are worth noting. Among the alcoholic patients whom they treated, six "suffered from mental disorders not due to alcohol or associated deficiency states." It was planned, by the authors, to follow up the aversion treatment with psychotherapy for the underlying psychosis. This, however, proved unnecessary since all but one of the patients, a case of chronic mental deterioration, showed marked improvement and were in a state of remission.

Max (1935) employed a strong electric shock as the aversive stimulus in treating a patient who tended to display homosexual behavior following exposure to a fetishistic stimulus. Both the fetish and the homosexual behavior were removed through a series of avoidance conditioning sessions in which the patient was administered shock in the presence of the fetishistic object.

Wolpe (1958) has also reported favorable results with a similar procedure in the treatment of obsessions.

A further variation of the counterconditioning procedure has been developed by Mowrer and Mowrer (1938) for use with enuretic patients. The device consists of a wired bed pad which sets off a loud buzzer and awakens the child as soon as micturition begins. Bladder tension thus becomes a cue for waking up which, in turn, is followed by sphincter contraction. Once bladder pressure becomes a stimulus for the more remote sphincter control response, the child is able to remain dry for relatively long periods of time without wakening.

Mowrer and Mowrer (1938) report complete success with 30 children treated by this method; similarly, Davidson and Douglass (1950) achieved highly successful results with 20 chronic enuretic children (15 cured, 5 markedly improved); of 5 cases treated by Morgan and Witmer (1939), 4 of the children not only gained full sphincter control, but also made a significant improvement in their social behavior. The one child with whom the conditioning approach had failed was later found to have bladder difficulties which required medical attention.

Some additional evidence for the efficacy of this method is provided by Martin and Kubly (1955) who obtained follow-up information from 118 of 220 parents who had treated their children at home with this type of conditioning apparatus. In 74% of the cases, according to the parents' replies, the treatment was successful.

Extinction

"When a learned response is repeated without reinforcement the strength of the tendency to perform that response undergoes a progressive decrease" (Dollard & Miller, 1950). Extinction involves the development of inhibitory potential which is composed of two components. The evocation of any reaction generates reactive inhibition (I_r) which presumably dissipates with time. When reactive inhibition (fatigue, etc.) reaches a high point, the cessation of activity alleviates this negative motivational state and any stimuli associated with the cessation of the response become conditioned inhibitors (${}_sI_r$).

One factor that has been shown to influence the rate of extinction of maladaptive and anxiety-motivated behavior is the interval between extinction trials. In general, there tends to be little diminution in the strength of fear-motivated behavior when extinction trials are widely distributed, whereas under massed trials, reactive inhibition builds up rapidly and consequently extinction is accelerated (Calvin, Clifford, Clifford, Bolden, & Harvey, 1956; Edmonson & Amsel, 1954).

An illustration of the application of this principle is provided by Yates (1958) in the treatment of tics. Yates demonstrated, in line with the findings from laboratory studies of extinction under massed and distributed practice, that massed sessions in which the patient performed tics voluntarily followed by prolonged rest to allow for the dissipation of reactive inhibition was the most effective procedure for extinguishing the tics.

It should be noted that the extinction procedure employed by Yates is very similar to Dunlap's method of negative practice, in which the subject reproduces the negative behaviors voluntarily without reinforcement (Dunlap, 1932; Lehner, 1954). This method has been applied most frequently, with varying degrees of success, to the treatment of speech disorders (Fishman, 1937; Meissner, 1946; Rutherford, 1940; Sheehan, 1951; Sheehan & Voas, 1957). If the effectiveness of this psychotherapeutic technique is due primarily to extinction, as suggested by Yates' study, the usual practice of terminating a treatment session before the subject becomes fatigued (Lehner, 1954), would have the effect of reducing the rate of extinction, and may in part account for the divergent results yielded by this method.

Additional examples of the therapeutic application of extinction procedures are provided by Jones (1955), and most recently by C. D. Williams (1959).

Most of the conventional forms of psychotherapy rely heavily on extinction effects although the therapist may not label these as such. For example, many therapists consider *permissiveness* to be a necessary condition of therapeutic change (Alexander, 1956; Dollard & Miller, 1950; Rogers, 1951). It is expected that when a patient expresses thoughts or feelings that provoke anxiety or guilt and the therapist does not disapprove, criticize, or withdraw interest, the fear or guilt will be gradually weakened or extinguished. The extinction effects are believed to generalize to thoughts concerning related topics that were originally inhibited, and to verbal and physical forms of behavior as well (Dollard & Miller, 1950).

Some evidence for the relationship between permissiveness and the extinction of anxiety is provided in two studies recently reported by Dittes (1957a, 1957b). In one study (1957b) involving an analysis of patient-therapist interaction sequences, Dittes found that permissive responses on the part of the therapist were followed by a corresponding decrease in the patient's anxiety (as measured by the GSR) and the occurrence of avoidance behaviors. A sequential analysis of the therapeutic sessions (Dittes, 1957a), revealed that, at the onset of treatment, sex expressions were accompanied by strong anxiety reactions; under the cumulative effects of permissiveness, the anxiety gradually extinguished.

In contrast to counterconditioning, extinction is likely to be less effective and a more time consuming method for eliminating maladaptive behavior (Jones, 1924a; Dollard & Miller, 1950); in the case of conventional interview therapy, the relatively long intervals between interview sessions, and the ritualistic adherence to the 50-minute hour may further reduce the occurrence of extinction effects.

Discrimination Learning

Human functioning would be extremely difficult and inefficient if a person had to learn appropriate behavior for every specific situation he encountered. Fortunately, patterns of behavior learned in one situation will transfer or generalize to other similar situations. On the other hand, if a person overgeneralizes from one situation to another, or if the generalization is based on superficial or irrelevant cues, behavior becomes inappropriate and maladaptive.

In most theories of psychotherapy, therefore, discrimination learning, believed to be accomplished through the gaining of awareness or insight, receives emphasis (Dollard & Miller, 1950; Fenichel, 1941; Rogers, 1951; Sullivan, 1953). It is generally assumed that if a patient is aware of the cues producing his behavior, of the responses he is making, and of the reasons that he responds the way he does, his behavior will become more susceptible to verbally-mediated control. Voluntarily guided, discriminative behavior will replace the automatic, overgeneralized reactions.

While this view is widely accepted, as evidenced in the almost exclusive reliance on interview procedures and on interpretative or labeling techniques, a few therapists (Alexander & French, 1946) have questioned the importance attached to awareness in producing modifications in behavior. Whereas most psychoanalysts (Fenichel, 1941), as well as therapists representing other points of view (Fromm-Reichmann, 1950; Sullivan, 1953) consider insight a precondition of behavior change, Alexander and French consider insight or awareness a result of change rather than its cause. That is, as the patient's anxieties are gradually reduced through the permissive conditions of treatment, formerly inhibited thoughts are gradually restored to awareness.

Evidence obtained through controlled laboratory studies concerning the value of awareness in increasing the precision of discrimination has so far been largely negative or at least equivocal (Adams, 1957; Erikson, 1958; Razran, 1949). A study by Lacy and Smith (1954), in which they found aware subjects generalized anxiety reactions less extensively than did subjects who were unaware of the conditioned stimulus provides evidence that awareness may aid discrimination. However, other aspects of their findings (e.g., the magnitude of the anxiety reactions to the generalization stimuli were greater than they were to the conditioned stimulus itself) indicate the need for replication.

If future research continues to demonstrate that awareness exerts little influence on the acquisition, generalization, and modification of behavior, such negative results would cast serious doubt on the value of currently popular psychotherapeutic procedures whose primary aim is the development of insight.

Methods of Reward

Most theories of psychotherapy are based on the assumption that the patient has a repertoire of previously learned positive habits available to him, but that these adaptive patterns are inhibited or blocked by competing responses motivated by anxiety or guilt. The goal of therapy, then, is to reduce the severity of the internal inhibitory controls, thus allowing the healthy patterns of behavior to emerge. Hence, the role of the therapist is to create permissive conditions under which the patient's "normal growth potentialities" are set free (Rogers, 1951). The fact that most of our theories of personality and therapeutic procedures have been developed primarily through work with oversocialized, neurotic patients may account in part for the prevalence of this view.

There is a large class of disorders (the undersocialized, antisocial personalities whose behavior reflects a failure of the socialization process) for whom this model of personality and accompanying techniques of treatment are quite inappropriate (Bandura & Walters, 1959; Schmidberg, 1959). Such antisocial personalities are likely to present *learning deficits*, consequently the goal of therapy is the acquisition of secondary motives and the development of internal restraint habits. That antisocial patients prove unresponsive to psychotherapeutic methods developed for the treatment of oversocialized neurotics has been demonstrated in a number of studies comparing patients who remain in treatment with those who terminate treatment prematurely (Rubenstein & Lorr, 1956). It is for this class of patients that the greatest departures from traditional treatment methods is needed.

While counterconditioning, extinction, and discrimination learning may be effective ways of removing neurotic inhibitions, these methods may be of relatively little value in developing new positive habits. Primary and secondary rewards in the form of the therapist's interest and approval may play an important, if not indispensable, role in the treatment process. Once the patient has learned to want the interest and approval of the therapist, these rewards may then be used to promote the acquisition of new patterns of behavior. For certain classes of patients such as schizophrenics (Atkinson, 1957; Peters, 1953; Robinson, 1957) and delinquents (Cairns, 1959), who are either unresponsive to, or fearful of, social rewards, the therapist may have to rely initially on primary rewards in the treatment process.

An ingenious study by Peters and Jenkins (1954) illustrates the application of this principle in the treatment of schizophrenic patients. Chronic patients from closed wards were administered subshock injections of insulin designed to induce the hunger drive. The patients were then encouraged to solve a series of graded problem tasks with fudge as the reward. This program was followed 5 days a week for 3 months.

Initially the tasks involved simple mazes and obstruction problems in which the patients obtained the food reward directly upon successful completion of the problem. Tasks of gradually increasing difficulty were then administered involving multiple-choice learning and verbal-reasoning problems in which the experimenter personally mediated the primary rewards. After several weeks of such problem solving activities the insulin injections were discontinued and social rewards, which by this time had become more effective, were used in solving interpersonal problems that the patients were likely to encounter in their daily activities both inside and outside the hospital setting.

Comparison of the treated group with control groups, designed to isolate the effects of insulin and special attention, revealed that the patients in the reward group improved significantly in their social relationships in the hospital, whereas the patients in the control groups showed no such change.

King and Armitage (1958) report a somewhat similar study in which severely withdrawn schizophrenic patients were treated with operant conditioning methods; candy and cigarettes served as the primary rewards for eliciting and maintaining increasingly complex forms of behavior, i.e., psychomotor, verbal, and interpersonal responses. Unlike the Peters and Jenkins study, no attempt was made to manipulate the level of primary motivation.

An interesting feature of the experimental design was the inclusion of a group of patients who were treated with conventional interview therapy, as well as a recreational therapy and a no-therapy control group. It was found that the operant group, in relation to similar patients in the three control groups, made significantly more clinical improvement.

Skinner (1956b) and Lindsley (1956) working with adult psychotics, and Ferster (1959) working with autistic children, have been successful in developing substantial amounts of reality-oriented behavior in their patients through the use of reward. So far their work has been concerned primarily with the effect of schedules of reinforcement on the rate of evocation of simple impersonal reactions. There is every indication, however, that by varying the contingency of the reward (e.g., the patient must respond in certain specified ways to the behavior of another individual in order to produce the reward) adaptive interpersonal behaviors can be developed as well (Azran & Lindsley, 1956).

The effectiveness of social reinforcers in modifying behavior has been demonstrated repeatedly in verbal conditioning experiments (Krasner, 1958; Salzinger, 1959). Encouraged by these findings, several therapists have begun to experiment with operant conditioning as a method of treatment in its own right (Tilton, 1956; Ullman, Krasner, & Collins, 1961; R. I. Williams, 1959); the operant conditioning studies cited earlier are also illustrative of this trend.

So far the study of generalization and permanence of behavior changes brought about through operant conditioning methods has received relatively little attention and the scanty data available are equivocal (Rogers, 1960; Sarason, 1957; Weide, 1959). The lack of consistency in results is hardly surprising considering that the experimental manipulations in many of the conditioning studies are barely sufficient to demonstrate conditioning effects, let alone generalization of changes to new situations. On the other hand, investigators who have conducted more intensive reinforcement sessions, in an effort to test the efficacy of operant conditioning methods as a therapeutic technique, have found significant changes in patients' interpersonal behavior in extra-experimental situations (King & Armitage, 1958; Peters & Jenkins, 1954; Ullman et al., 1961). These findings are particularly noteworthy since the response classes involved are similar to those psychotherapists are primarily concerned in modifying through interview forms of treatment. If the favorable results yielded by these studies are replicated in future investigations, it is likely that the next few years will witness an increasing reliance on conditioning forms of psychotherapy, particularly in the treatment of psychotic patients.

At this point it might also be noted that, consistent with the results from verbal conditioning experiments, content analyses of psychotherapeutic interviews (Bandura, Lipsher, & Miller, 1960; Murray, 1956) suggest that many of the changes observed in psychotherapy, at least insofar as the patients' verbal behavior is concerned, can be accounted for in terms of the therapists' direct, although usually unwitting, reward and punishment of the patients' expressions.

Punishment

While positive habits can be readily developed through reward, the elimination of socially disapproved habits, which becomes very much an issue in the treatment of antisocial personalities, poses a far more complex problem.

The elimination of socially disapproved behaviors can be accomplished in several ways. They may be consistently unrewarded and thus extinguished. However, antisocial behavior, particularly of an extreme form, cannot simply be ignored in the hope that it will gradually extinguish. Furthermore, since the successful execution of antisocial acts may bring substantial material rewards as well as the approval and admiration of associates, it is extremely unlikely that such behavior would ever extinguish.

Although punishment may lead to the rapid disappearance of socially disapproved behavior, its effects are far more complex (Estes, 1944; Solomon, Kamin, & Wynne, 1953). If a person is punished for some socially disapproved habit, the impulse to perform that act becomes, through its association with punishment, a stimulus for anxiety. This anxiety then motivates competing responses which, if sufficiently strong, prevent the occurrence of, or inhibit, the disapproved behavior. Inhibited responses may not, however, thereby lose their strength, and may reappear in situations where the threat of punishment is weaker. Punishment may, in fact, prevent the extinction of a habit; if a habit is completely inhibited, it cannot occur and therefore cannot go unrewarded.

Several other factors point to the futility of punishment as a means of correcting many antisocial patterns. The threat of punishment is very likely to elicit conformity; indeed, the patient may obligingly do whatever he is told to do in order to avoid immediate difficulties. This does not mean, however, that he has acquired a set of sanctions that will be of service to him once he is outside the treatment situation. In fact, rather than leading to the development of internal controls, such methods are likely only to increase the patient's reliance on external restraints. Moreover, under these conditions, the majority of patients will develop the attitude that they will do only what they are told to do—and then often only half-heartedly—and that they will do as they please once they are free from the therapist's supervision (Bandura & Walters, 1959).

In addition, punishment may serve only to intensify hostility and other negative motivations and thus may further instigate the antisocial person to display the very behaviors that the punishment was intended to bring under control.

Mild aversive stimuli have been utilized, of course, in the treatment of voluntary patients who express a desire to rid themselves of specific debilitating conditions.

Liversedge and Sylvester (1955), for example, successfully treated seven cases of writer's cramp by means of a retraining procedure involving electric shock. In order to remove tremors, one component of the motor disorder, the patients were required to insert a stylus into a series of progressively smaller holes; each time the stylus made contact with the side of the hole the patients received a mild shock. The removal of the spasm component of the disorder was obtained in two ways. First, the patients traced various line patterns (similar to the movements required in writing) on a metal plate with a stylus, and any deviation from the path produced a shock. Following training on the apparatus, the subjects then wrote with an electrified pen which delivered a shock whenever excessive thumb pressure was applied.

Liversedge and Sylvester report that following the retraining the patients were able to resume work; a follow-up several months later indicated that the improvement was being maintained.

The aversive forms of therapy, described earlier in the section on counterconditioning procedures, also make use of mild punishment.

Social Imitation

Although a certain amount of learning takes place through direct training and reward, a good deal of a person's behavior repertoire may be acquired through imitation of what he observes in others. If this is the case, social imitation may serve as an effective vehicle for the transmission of prosocial behavior patterns in the treatment of antisocial patients.

Merely providing a model for imitation is not, however, sufficient. Even though the therapist exhibits the kinds of behaviors that he wants the patient to learn, this is likely to have little influence on him if he rejects the therapist as a model. Affectional nurturance is believed to be an important precondition for imitative learning to occur, in that affectional rewards increase the secondary reinforcing properties of the model, and thus predispose the imitator to pattern his behavior after the rewarding person (Mowrer, 1950;

Sears, 1957; Whiting, 1954). Some positive evidence for the influence of social rewards on imitation is provided by Bandura and Huston (1961) in a recent study of identification as a process of incidental imitation.

In this investigation preschool children performed an orienting task but, unlike most incidental learning studies, the experimenter performed the diverting task as well, and the extent to which the subjects patterned their behavior after that of the experimenter-model was measured.

A two-choice discrimination problem similar to the one employed by Miller and Dollard (1941) in their experiments of social imitation was used as the diverting task. On each trial, one of two boxes was loaded with two rewards (small multicolor pictures of animals) and the object of the game was to guess which box contained the stickers. The experimenter-model (*M*) always had her turn first and in each instance chose the reward box. During *M*'s trial, the subject remained at the starting point where he could observe the *M*'s behavior. On each discrimination trial *M* exhibited certain verbal, motor, and aggressive patterns of behavior that were totally irrelevant to the task to which the subject's attention was directed. At the starting point, for example, *M* made a verbal response and then marched slowly toward the box containing the stickers, repeating, "March, march, march." On the lid of each box was a rubber doll which *M* knocked off aggressively when she reached the designated box. She then paused briefly, remarked, "Open the box," removed one sticker, and pasted it on a pastoral scene which hung on the wall immediately behind the boxes. The subject then took his turn and the number of *M*'s behaviors performed by the subject was recorded.

A control group was included in order to, (*a*) provide a check on whether the subjects' performances reflected genuine imitative learning or merely the chance occurrence of behaviors high in the subjects' response hierarchies, and (*b*) to determine whether subjects would adopt certain aspects of *M*'s behavior which involved considerable delay in reward. With the controls, therefore, *M* walked to the box, choosing a highly circuitous route along the sides of the experimental room; instead of aggressing toward the doll, she lifted it gently off the container.

The results of this study indicate that, insofar as preschool children are concerned, a good deal of incidental imitation of the behaviors displayed by an adult model does occur. Of the subjects in the experimental group, 88% adopted the *M*'s aggressive behavior, 44% imitated the marching, and 28% reproduced *M*'s verbalizations. In contrast, none of the control subjects behaved aggressively, marched, or verbalized, while 75% of the controls imitated the circuitous route to the containers.

In order to test the hypothesis that children who experience a rewarding relationship with an adult model adopt more of the model's behavior than do children who experience a relatively distant and cold relationship, half the subjects in the experiment were assigned to a nurturant condition; the other half of the subjects to a nonnurturant condition. During the nurturant sessions, which preceded the incidental learning, *M* played with subject, she responded readily to the subject's bids for attention, and in other ways fostered a consistently warm and rewarding interaction with the child. In contrast, during the nonnurturant sessions, the subject played alone while *M* busied herself with paperwork at a desk in the far corner of the room.

Consistent with the hypothesis, it was found that subjects who experienced the rewarding interaction with *M* adopted significantly more of *M*'s behavior than did subjects who were in the nonnurturance condition.

A more crucial test of the transmission of behavior patterns through the process of social imitation involves the delayed generalization of imitative responses to new situations in which the model is absent. A study of this type just completed, provides strong evidence that observation of the cues produced by the behavior of others is an effective means of eliciting responses for which the original probability is very low (Bandura, Ross, & Ross, 1961).

Empirical studies of the correlates of strong and weak identification with parents, lend additional support to the theory that rewards promote imitative learning. Boys whose fathers are highly rewarding and affectionate have been found to adopt the father-role in doll-play activities (Sears, 1953), to show father-son similarity in response to items on a personality questionnaire (Payne & Mussen, 1956), and to display masculine behaviors (Mussen & Distler, 1956, 1960) to a greater extent than boys whose fathers are relatively cold and nonrewarding.

The treatment of older unsocialized delinquents is a difficult task, since they are relatively self-sufficient and do not readily seek involvement with a therapist. In many cases, socialization can be accomplished only through residential care and treatment. In the treatment home, the therapist can personally administer many of the primary rewards and mediate between the boys' needs and gratifications. Through the repeated association with rewarding experiences for the boy, many of the therapist's attitudes and actions will acquire secondary reward value, and thus the patient will be motivated to reproduce these attitudes and actions in himself. Once these attitudes and values have been thus accepted, the boy's inhibition of antisocial tendencies will function independently of the therapist.

While treatment through social imitation has been suggested as a method for modifying antisocial patterns, it can be an effective procedure for the treatment of other forms of disorders as well. Jones (1924a), for example, found that the social example of children reacting normally to stimuli feared by another child was effective, in some instances, in eliminating such phobic reactions. In fact, next to counterconditioning, the method of social imitation proved to be most effective in eliminating inappropriate fears.

There is some suggestive evidence that by providing high prestige models and thus increasing the reinforcement value of the imitatee's behavior, the effectiveness of this method in promoting favorable adjustive patterns of behavior may be further increased (Jones, 1924a; Mausner, 1953, 1954; Miller & Dollard, 1941).

During the course of conventional psychotherapy, the patient is exposed to many incidental cues involving the therapist's values, attitudes, and patterns of behavior. They are incidental only because they are usually considered secondary or irrelevant to the task of resolving the patient's problems. Nevertheless, some of the changes observed in the patient's behavior may result, not so much from the intentional interaction between the patient and the therapist, but rather from active learning by the patient of the therapist's attitudes and values which the therapist never directly attempted to transmit. This is partially corroborated by Rosenthal (1955) who found that, in spite of the usual precautions taken by therapists to avoid imposing their values on their clients, the patients who were judged as showing the greatest improvement changed their moral values (in the areas of sex, aggression, and authority) in the direction of the values of their therapists, whereas patients who were unimproved became less like the therapist in values.

Factors Impeding Integration

In reviewing the literature on psychotherapy, it becomes clearly evident that learning theory and general psychology have exerted a remarkably minor influence on the practice of psychotherapy and, apart from the recent interest in Skinner's operant conditioning methods (Krasner, 1955; Skinner, 1953), most of the recent serious attempts to apply learning principles to clinical practice have been made by European psychotherapists (Jones, 1956; Lazarus & Rachman, 1957; Liversedge & Sylvester, 1955; Meyer, 1957; Rachman, 1959; Raymond, 1956; Wolpe, 1958; Yates, 1958). This isolation of the methods of treatment from our knowledge of learning and motivation will continue to exist for some time since there are several prevalent attitudes that impede adequate integration.

In the first place, the deliberate use of the principles of learning in the modification of human behavior implies, for most psychotherapists, manipulation and control of the patient, and control is seen by them as antihumanistic and, therefore, bad. Thus, advocates of a learning approach to psychotherapy are often charged with treating human beings as though they were rats or pigeons and of leading on the road to Orwell's *1984*.

This does not mean that psychotherapists do not influence and control their patients' behavior. On the contrary. In any interpersonal interaction, and psychotherapy is no exception, people influence and control one another (Frank, 1959; Skinner, 1956a). Although the patient's control of the therapist has not as yet been studied (such control is evident when patients subtly reward the therapist with interesting historical material and thereby avoid the discussion of their current interpersonal problems), there is considerable evidence that the therapist exercises personal control over his patients. A brief examination of interview protocols of patients treated by therapists representing differing theoretical orientations, clearly reveals that the patients have been thoroughly conditioned in their therapists' idiosyncratic languages. Client-centered patients, for example, tend to produce the client-centered terminology, theory, and goals, and their interview content shows little or no overlap with that of patients seen in psychoanalysis who, in turn, tend to speak the language of psychoanalytic theory (Heine, 1950). Even more direct evidence of the therapists' controlling influence is provided in studies of patient-therapist interactions (Bandura et al., 1960; Murray, 1956; Rogers, 1960). The results of these studies show that the therapist not only controls the patient by rewarding him with interest and approval when the patient behaves in a fashion the therapist desires, but that he also controls through punishment, in the form of mild disapproval and withdrawal of interest, when the patient behaves in ways that are threatening to the therapist or run counter to his goals.

One difficulty in understanding the changes that occur in the course of psychotherapy is that the independent variable, i.e., the therapist's behavior, is often vaguely or only partially defined. In an effort to minimize or to deny the therapist's directive influence on the patient, the therapist is typically depicted as a "catalyst" who, in some mysterious way, sets free positive adjustive patterns of behavior or similar outcomes usually described in very general and highly socially desirable terms.

It has been suggested, in the material presented in the preceding sections, that many of the changes that occur in psychotherapy derive from the unwitting application of well-known principles of learning. However, the occurrence of the necessary conditions for learning is more by accident than by intent and, perhaps, a more deliberate application of our knowledge of the learning process to psychotherapy would yield far more effective results.

The predominant approach in the development of psychotherapeutic procedures has been the "school" approach. A similar trend is noted in the treatment methods being derived from learning theory. Wolpe, for example, has selected the principle of counterconditioning and built a "school" of psychotherapy around it; Dollard and Miller have focused on extinction and discrimination learning; and the followers of Skinner rely almost entirely on methods of reward. This stress on a few learning principles at the expense of neglecting other relevant ones will serve only to limit the effectiveness of psychotherapy.

A second factor that may account for the discontinuity between general psychology and psychotherapeutic practice is that the model of personality to which most therapists subscribe is somewhat dissonant with the currently developing principles of behavior.

In their formulations of personality functioning, psychotherapists are inclined to appeal to a variety of inner explanatory processes. In contrast, learning theorists view the organism as a far more mechanistic and simpler system, and consequently their formulations tend to be expressed for the most part in terms of antecedent-consequent relationships without reference to inner states.

> Symptoms are learned S-R connections; once they are extinguished or deconditioned treatment is complete. Such treatment is based exclusively on present factors; like Lewin's theory, this one is a-historical. Non-verbal methods are favored over verbal ones, although a minor place is reserved for verbal methods of extinction and reconditioning. Concern is with *function*, not with *content*. The main difference between the two theories arises over the question of "symptomatic" treatment. According to orthodox theory, this is useless unless the underlying complexes are attacked. According to the present theory, there is no evidence for these putative complexes, and symptomatic treatment is all that is required (Eysenck, 1957, pp. 267–268). (Quoted by permission of Frederick A. Praeger, Inc.)

Changes in behavior brought about through such methods as counter-conditioning are apt to be viewed by the "dynamically-oriented" therapist, as being not only superficial, "symptomatic" treatment, in that the basic underlying instigators of the behavior remain unchanged, but also potentially dangerous, since the direct elimination of a symptom may precipitate more seriously disturbed behavior.

This expectation receives little support from the generally favorable outcomes reported in the studies reviewed in this paper. In most cases where follow-up data were available to assess the long-term effects of the therapy, the patients, many of whom had been treated by conventional methods with little benefit, had evidently become considerably more effective in their social, vocational, and psychosexual adjustment. On the whole the evidence, while open to error, suggests that no matter what the origin of the maladaptive behavior may be, a change in behavior brought about through learning procedures may be all that is necessary for the alleviation of most forms of emotional disorders.

As Mowrer (1950) very aptly points out, the "symptom-underlying cause" formulation may represent inappropriate medical analogizing. Whether or not a given behavior will be considered normal or a symptom of an underlying disturbance will depend on whether or not somebody objects to the behavior. For example, aggressiveness on the part of children may be encouraged and considered a sign of healthy development by the parents, while the same behavior is viewed by school authorities and society as a symptom of a personality disorder (Bandura & Walters, 1959). Furthermore, behavior considered to be normal at one stage in development may be regarded as a "symptom of a personality disturbance" at a later period. In this connection it is very appropriate to repeat Mowrer's (1950) query: "And when does persisting behavior of this kind suddenly cease to be normal and become a symptom" (p. 474).

Thus, while a high fever is generally considered a sign of an underlying disease process regardless of when or where it occurs, whether a specific behavior will be viewed as normal or as a symptom of an underlying pathology is not independent of who makes the judgement, the social context in which the behavior occurs, the age of the person, as well as many other factors.

Another important difference between physical pathology and behavior pathology usually overlooked is that, in the case of most behavior disorders, it is not the underlying motivations that need to be altered or removed, but rather the ways in which the patient has learned to gratify his needs (Rotter, 1954). Thus, for example, if a patient displays deviant sexual behavior, the goal is not the removal of the underlying causes, i.e., sexual motivation, but rather the substitution of more socially approved instrumental and goal responses.

It might also be mentioned in passing, that, in the currently popular forms of psychotherapy, the role assumed by the therapist may bring him a good many direct or fantasied personal gratifications. In the course of treatment the patient may express considerable affection and admiration for the therapist, he may assign the therapist an omniscient status, and the reconstruction of the patient's history may be an intellectually stimulating activity. On the other hand, the methods derived from learning theory place the therapist in a less glamorous role, and this in itself may create some reluctance on the part of psychotherapists to part with the procedures currently in use.

Which of the two conceptual theories of personality—the psychodynamic or the social learning theory—is the more useful in generating effective procedures for the modification of human behavior remains to be demonstrated. While it is possible to present logical arguments and impressive clinical evidence for the efficiency of either approach, the best proving ground is the laboratory.

In evaluating psychotherapeutic methods, the common practice is to compare changes in a treated group with those of a nontreated control group. One drawback of this approach is that, while it answers the question as to whether or not a particular treatment is more effective than no intervention in producing changes along specific dimensions for certain classes of patients, it does not provide evidence concerning the relative effectiveness of alternative forms of psychotherapy.

It would be far more informative if, in future psychotherapy research, radically different forms of treatment were compared (King & Armitage, 1958; Rogers, 1959), since this approach would lead to a more rapid discarding of those of our cherished psychotherapeutic rituals that prove to be ineffective in, or even a handicap to, the successful treatment of emotional disorders.

References

Adams, J. K. (1957). Laboratory studies of behavior without awareness. *Psychol. Bull.*, **54**, 393–405.

Alexander, F. (1956). *Psychoanalysis and Psychotherapy*. New York: Norton.

Alexander, F., & French, M. T. (1946). *Psychoanalytic Therapy*. New York: Ronald.

Section III: Psychotherapy

Atkinson, Rita L. (1957). Paired-associate learning by schizophrenic and normal subjects under conditions of verbal reward and verbal punishment. Unpublished doctoral dissertation, Indiana University.

Azran, N. H., & Lindsley, O. R. (1956). The reinforcement of cooperation between children. *J. Abnorm. Soc. Psychol.*, **52**, 100–102.

Bandura, A., & Huston, Aletha C. (1961). Identification as a process of incidental learning. *J. Abnorm. Soc. Psychol.*, **63**, 311–318.

Bandura, A., Lipsher, D. H., & Miller, Paula E. (1960). Psychotherapists' approach-avoidance reactions to patient's expressions of hostility. *J. Consult. Psychol.*, **24**, 1–8.

Bandura, A., Ross, Dorothea, & Ross, Sheila A. (1961). Transmission of aggression through imitation of aggressive models. *J. Abnorm. Soc. Psychol.*, **63**, 575–582.

Bandura, A., & Walters, R. H. (1959). *Adolescent Aggression.* New York: Ronald.

Cairns, R. B. (1959). The influence of dependency-anxiety on the effectiveness of social reinforcers. Unpublished doctoral dissertation, Stanford University.

Calvin, A. D., Clifford, L. T., Clifford, B., Bolden, L., & Harvey, J. (1956). Experimental validation of conditioned inhibition. *Psychol. Rep.*, **2**, 51–56.

Davidson, J. R., & Douglass, E. (1950). Nocturnal enuresis: A special approach to treatment. *British Med. J.*, **1**, 1345–1347.

Dittes, J. E. (1957). Extinction during psychotherapy of GSR accompanying "embarrassing" statements. *J. Abnorm. Soc. Psychol.*, **54**, 187–191. (a)

Dittes, J. E. (1957). Galvanic skin responses as a measure of patient's reaction to therapist's permissiveness. *J. Abnorm. Soc. Psychol.*, **55**, 295–303. (b)

Dollard, J., Auld, F., & White, A. M. (1954). *Steps in Psychotherapy.* New York: Macmillan.

Dollard, J., & Miller, N. E. (1950). *Personality and Psychotherapy.* New York: McGraw-Hill.

Dunlap, K. (1932). *Habits, Their Making and Unmaking.* New York: Liveright.

Edmondson, B. W., & Amsel, A. (1954). The effects of massing and distribution of extinction trials on the persistence of a fear-motivated instrumental response. *J. Comp. Physiol. Psychol.*, **47**, 117–123.

Erickson, C. W. (1958). Unconscious processes. In M. R. Jones (ed.), *Nebraska Symposium on Motivation.* Lincoln: Univer. Nebraska Press.

Estes, W. K. (1944). An experimental study of punishment. *Psychol. Monogr.*, **57** (3, Whole No. 363).

Eysenck, H. J. (1957). *The Dynamics of Anxiety and Hysteria.* New York: Praeger.

Fenichel, O. (1941). *Problems of Psychoanalytic Technique.* (Trans. by D. Brunswick) New York: Psychoanalytic Quarterly.

Ferster, C. B. (1959). Development of normal behavioral processes in autistic children. *Res. Relat. Child.*, No. 9, 30. (Abstract)

Fishman, H. C. (1937). A study of the efficiency of negative practice as a corrective for stammering. *J. Speech Dis.*, **2**, 67–72.

Frank, J. D. (1959). The dynamics of the psychotherapeutic relationship. *Psychiatry*, **22**, 17–39.

Fromm-Reichmann, Frieda (1950). *Principle of Intensive Psychotherapy.* Chicago: Univer. Chicago Press.

Heine, R. W. (1950). An investigation of the relationship between change in personality from psychotherapy as reported by patients and the factors seen by patients as producing change. Unpublished doctoral dissertation, University of Chicago.

Jones, E. L. (1955). Exploration of experimental extinction and spontaneous recovery in stuttering. In W. Johnson (ed.), *Stuttering in Children and Adults.* Minneapolis: Univer. Minnesota Press.

Jones, H. G. (1956). The application of conditioning and learning techniques to the treatment of a psychiatric patient. *J. Abnorm. Soc. Psychol.*, **52**, 414–419.

Jones, Mary C. (1924). The elimination of childrens' fears. *J. Exp. Psychol.*, **7**, 382–390. (a)

Jones, Mary C. (1924). A laboratory study of fear: The case of Peter. *J. Genet. Psychol.*, **31**, 308–315. (b)

King, G. F., & Armitage, S. G. (1958). An operant-interpersonal therapeutical approach to schizophrenics of extreme pathology. *Amer. Psychologist*, **13**, 358. (Abstract)

KLEIN, MELANIE (1949). *The Psycho-analysis of Children.* London: Hogarth.

KRASNER, L. (1955). The use of generalized reinforcers in psychotherapy research. *Psychol. Rep.*, **1**, 19–25.

KRASNER, L. (1958). Studies of the conditioning of verbal behavior. *Psychol. Bull.*, **55**, 148–170.

LACEY, J. I., & SMITH, R. I. (1954). Conditioning and generalization of unconscious anxiety. *Science*, **120**, 1–8.

LAZARUS, A. A., & RACHMAN, S. (1957). The use of systematic desentization in psychotherapy. *S. Afr. Med. J.*, **32**, 934–937.

LEHNER, G. F. J. (1954). Negative practice as a psychotherapeutic technique. *J. Gen. Psychol.*, **51**, 69–82.

LINDSLEY, O. R. (1956). Operant conditioning methods applied to research in chronic schizophrenia. *Psychiat. Res. Rep.*, **5**, 118–138.

LIVERSEDGE, L. A., & SYLVESTER, J. D. (1955). Conditioning techniques in the treatment of writer's cramp. *Lancet* **1**, 1147–1149.

MARTIN, B., & KUBLY, DELORES (1955). Results of treatment of enuresis by a conditioned response method. *J. Consult. Psychol.*, **19**, 71–73.

MAUSNER, B. (1953). Studies in social interaction: III. The effect of variation in one partner's prestige on the interaction of observer pairs. *J. Appl. Psychol.*, **37**, 391–393.

MAUSNER, B. (1954). The effect of one partner's success in a relevant task on the interaction of observer pairs. *J. Abnorm. Soc. Psychol.*, **49**, 557–560.

MAX, L. W. (1935). Breaking up a homosexual fixation by the conditioned reaction technique: A case study. *Psychol. Bull.*, **32**, 734.

MEISSNER, J. H. (1946). The relationship between voluntary nonfluency and stuttering. *J. speech Dis.*, **11**, 13–33.

MEYER, V. (1957). The treatment of two phobic patients on the basis of learning principles: Case report. *J. Abnorm. Soc. Psychol.*, **55**, 261–266.

MILLER, N. E., & DOLLARD, J. (1941). *Social Learning and Imitation.* New Haven: Yale Univer. Press.

MORGAN, J. J. B., & WITMER, F. J. (1939). The treatment of enuresis by the conditioned reaction technique. *J. Genet. Psychol.*, **55**, 59–65.

MOWRER, O. H. (1950). *Learning Theory and Personality Dynamics.* New York: Ronald.

MOWRER, O. H., & MOWRER, W. M. (1938). Enuresis—a method for its study and treatment. *Amer. J. Orthopsychiat.*, **8**, 436–459.

MURRAY, E. J. (1956). The content-analysis method of studying psychotherapy. *Psychol. Monogr.*, **70**(13, Whole No. 420).

MUSSEN, P., & DISTLER, L. M. (1959). Masculinity, identification, and father-son relationships. *J. Abnorm. Soc. Psychol.*, **59**, 350–356.

MUSSEN, P., & DISTLER, L. M. (1960). Child-rearing antecedents of masculine identification in kindergarten boys. *Child Develpm.*, **31**, 89–100.

PAYNE, D. E., & MUSSEN, P. H. (1956). Parent-child relationships and father identification among adolescent boys. *J. Abnorm. Soc. Psychol.*, **52**, 358–362.

PETERS, H. N. (1953). Multiple choice learning in the chronic schizophrenic. *J. Clin. Psychol.*, **9**, 328–333.

PETERS, H. N., & JENKINS, R. L. (1954). Improvement of chronic schizophrenic patients with guided problem-solving motivated by hunger. *Psychiat. Quart. Suppl.*, **28**, 84–101.

RACHMAN, S. (1959). The treatment of anxiety and phobic reactions by systematic desensitization psychotherapy. *J. Abnorm. Soc. Psychol.*, **58**, 259–263.

RAYMOND, M. S. (1956). Case of fetishism treated by aversion therapy. *Brit. Med. J.*, **2**, 854–857.

RAZRAN, G. (1949). Stimulus generalization of conditioned responses. *Psychol. Bull.*, **46**, 337–365.

ROBINSON, NANCY M. (1957). Paired-associate learning by schizophrenic subjects under conditions of personal and impersonal reward and punishment. Unpublished doctoral dissertation, Stanford University.

ROGER, C. R. (1951). *Client-centered Therapy.* Boston: Houghton Mifflin.

ROGERS, C. R. (1959). Group discussion: Problems of controls. In E. H. Rubinstein & M. B. Parloff (eds.), *Research in Psychotherapy*. Washington, D.C.: American Psychological Association.

ROGERS, J. M. (1960). Operant conditioning in a quasi-therapy setting. *J. Abnorm. Soc. Psychol.*, **60**, 247–252.

ROSENTHAL, D. (1955). Changes in some moral values following psychotherapy. *J. consult. Psychol.*, **19**, 431–436.

ROTTER, J. B. (1954). *Social Learning and Clinical Psychology*. Englewood Cliffs, N.J.: Prentice-Hall.

RUBENSTEIN, E. A., & LORR, M. (1956). A comparison of terminators and remainers in outpatient psychotherapy. *J. clin. Psychol.*, **12**, 345–349.

RUTHERFORD, B. R. (1940). The use of negative practice in speech therapy with children handicapped by cerebral palsy, athetoid type. *J. Speech Dis.*, **5**, 259–264.

SALZINGER, K. (1959). Experimental manipulation of verbal behavior: A review. *J. Gen. Psychol.*, **61**, 65–94.

SARASON, BARBARA R. (1957). The effects of verbally conditioned response classes on post-conditioning tasks. *Dissertation Abstr.*, **12**, 679.

SCHMIDBERG, MELITTA (1959). Psychotherapy of juvenile delinquents. *Int. Ment. Hlth. Res. Newsltr.*, **1**, 1–2.

SEARS, PAULINE S. (1953). Child-rearing factors related to playing of sex-typed roles. *Amer. Psychologist*, **8**, 431. (Abstract)

SEARS, R. R. (1957). Identification as a form of behavioral development. In D. B. Harris (ed.), *The Concept of Development: An Issue in the Study of Human Behavior*. Minneapolis: Univer. Minnesota Press.

SHEEHAN, J. G. (1951). The modification of stuttering through non-reinforcement. *J. Abnorm. Soc. Psychol.*, **46**, 51–63.

SHEEHAN, J. G., & VOAS, R. B. (1957). Stuttering as conflict: I. Comparison of therapy techniques involving approach and avoidance. *J. Speech Dis.*, **22**, 714–723.

SHOBEN, E. J. (1949). Psychotherapy as a problem in learning theory. *Psychol. Bull.*, **46**, 366–392.

SKINNER, B. F. (1953). *Science and Human Behavior*. New York: Macmillan.

SKINNER, B. F. (1956). Some issues concerning the control of human behavior. *Science*, **124**, 1057–1066. (a)

SKINNER, B. F. (1956). What is psychotic behavior? In, *Theory and Treatment of Psychosis: Some Newer Aspects*. St. Louis: Washington Univer. Stud. (b)

SOLOMON, R. L., KAMIN, L. J., & WYNNE, L. C. (1953). Traumatic avoidance learning: The outcomes of several extinction procedures with dogs. *J. Abnorm. Soc. Psychol.*, **48**, 291–302.

SULLIVAN, H. S. (1953). *The Interpersonal Theory of Psychiatry*. New York: Norton.

THIRMANN, J. (1949). Conditioned-reflex treatment of alcoholism. *New Engl. J. Med.*, **241**, 368–370, 406–410.

THOMPSON, G. N., & BIELINSKI, B. (1953). Improvement in psychosis following conditioned reflex treatment in alcoholism. *J. Nerv. Ment. Dis.*, **117**, 537–543.

TILTON, J. R. (1956). The use of instrumental motor and verbal learning techniques in the treatment of chronic schizophrenics. Unpublished doctoral dissertation, Michigan State University.

ULLMAN, L. P., KRASNER, L., & COLLINS, BEVERLY J. (1961). Modification of behavior through verbal conditioning: effects in group therapy. *J. Abnorm. Soc. Psychol.*, **62**, 128–132.

VOEGTLEN, W. L. (1940). The treatment of alcoholism by establishing a conditioned reflex. *Amer. J. Med. Sci.*, **119**, 802–810.

WALLACE, J. A. (1949). The treatment of alcoholics by the conditioned reflex method. *J. Tenn. Med. Ass.*, **42**, 125–128.

WEIDE, T. N. (1959). Conditioning and generalization of the use of affect-relevant words. Unpublished doctoral dissertation, Stanford University.

WHITING, J. W. M. (1954). The research program of the Laboratory of Human Development: The development of self-control. Cambridge: Harvard University. (Mimeo)

WILLIAMS, C. D. (1959). The elimination of tantrum behaviors by extinction procedures. *J. Abnorm. Soc. Psychol.*, **59**, 269.

WILLIAMS, R. I. (1959). Verbal conditioning in psychotherapy. *Amer. Psychologist*, **14**, 388. (Abstract)

WOLPE, J. (1954). Reciprocal inhibition as the main basis of psychotherapeutic effects. *AMA Arch. Neurol. Psychiat.*, **72**, 205–226.

WOLPE, J. (1958). *Psychotherapy by Reciprocal Inhibition.* Stanford: Stanford Univer. Press.

WOLPE, J. (1959). Psychotherapy based on the principle of reciprocal inhibition. In A. Burton (ed.), *Case Studies in Counseling and Psychotherapy*. Englewood Cliffs, N.J.: Prentice-Hall.

YATES, A. J. (1958). The application of learning theory to the treatment of tics. *J. Abnorm. Soc. Psychol.*, **56**, 175–182.

ROLLO MAY

Existential Bases of Psychotherapy

Along with the traditional, deterministic psychoanalytic approaches and the newly developed, scientifically based, equally deterministic behavior modification approach, the last few years have seen the emergence of what has come to be known as a "third force." This is the humanistic, existential influence on psychotherapy. This school has been a very popular one for a long period of time in Europe, but its influence in the United States is quite recent, and rapidly growing. Its emphasis on immediacy of experience makes it a very exciting and compelling approach to a large number of therapists. However, others have criticized it as lacking in adequate theoretical or research underpinnings and, although not of necessity, tending to attract a number of undisciplined and antiscientific practitioners. In his paper, Dr. May gives a well-balanced presentation of the basic tenets of an existential approach, indicating areas of convergence and contrasts with more traditional approaches, and illustrating his remarks with appropriate case material.

Though the existential approach has been the most prominent in European psychiatry and psychoanalysis for two decades, it was practically unknown in America until a year ago. Since then, some of us have been worried that it might become *too* popular in some quarters, particularly in national

Reprinted from *American Journal of Orthopsychiatry*, **30** (1960), 685–695.

magazines. But we have been comforted by a saying of Nietzsche's, "The first adherents of a movement are no argument against it."

We have no interest whatever in importing from Europe a ready-made system. I am, indeed, very dubious about the usefulness of the much-discussed and much-maligned term "Existentialism." But many of us in this country have for years shared this approach, long before we even knew the meaning of that confused term.

On the one hand this approach has a deep underlying affinity for our American character and thought. It is very close, for example, to William James' emphases on the immediacy of experience, the unity of thought and action, and the importance of decision and commitment. On the other hand, there is among some psychologists and psychoanalysts in this country a great deal of hostility and outright anger against this approach. I shall not here go into the reasons for this paradox.

I wish, rather, to *be* existentialist, and to speak directly from my own experience as a person and as a practicing psychoanalytic psychotherapist. Some fifteen years ago, when I was working on my book *The Meaning of Anxiety*, I spent a year and a half in bed in a tuberculosis sanatorium. I had a great deal of time to ponder the meaning of anxiety—and plenty of firsthand data in myself and my fellow patients. In the course of this time I studied the two books written on anxiety up till our day, the one by Freud, *The Problem of Anxiety*, and the one by Kierkegaard, *The Concept of Dread*. I valued highly Freud's formulations: namely, his first theory, that anxiety is the reemergence of repressed libido, and his second, that anxiety is the ego's reaction to the threat of the loss of the loved object. Kierkegaard, on the other hand, described anxiety as the struggle of the living being against non-being which I could immediately experience there in my struggle with death or the prospect of being a lifelong invalid. He went on to point out that the real terror in anxiety is not this death as such but the fact that each of us within himself is on both sides of the fight, that "anxiety is a desire for what one dreads," as he put it; thus like an "alien power it lays hold of an individual, and yet one cannot tear one's self away."

What powerfully struck me then was that Kierkegaard was writing about *exactly what my fellow patients and I were going through.* Freud was not; he was writing on a different level, giving formulations of the psychic mechanisms by which anxiety comes about. Kierkegaard was portraying what is immediately experienced by human beings in crisis—the crisis specifically of life against death which was completely real to us patients, but a crisis which I believe is not in its essential form different from the various crises of people who come for therapy, or the crises all of us experience in much more minute form a dozen times a day even though we push the ultimate prospect of death far from our minds. Freud was writing on the technical level, where his genius was supreme; perhaps more than any man up to his time, he *knew about* anxiety. Kierkegaard, a genius of a different order, was writing on the existential, ontological level; he *knew anxiety.*

This is not a value dichotomy; obviously both are necessary. Our real problem, rather, is given us by our cultural-historical situation. We in the Western world are the heirs of four centuries of technical achievement in power over nature, and now over ourselves; this is our greatness and, at the same time, it is also our greatest peril. We are not in danger of repressing the technical emphasis (of which Freud's tremendous popularity in this country were proof if any were necessary). But rather we repress the opposite. If I may use terms which I shall be discussing more fully presently, we repress the *sense of being*, the ontological sense. One consequence of this repression of the sense of being is that modern man's image of himself, his experience of himself as a responsible individual, his experience of his own humanity, have likewise disintegrated.

The existential approach, as I understand it, does not have the aim of ruling out the technical discoveries of Freud or those from any other branch of psychology or science. It does, however, seek to place these discoveries on a new basis, a new understanding or rediscovery, if you will, of the nature and image of man.

I make no apologies in admitting that I take very seriously the dehumanizing dangers in our tendency in modern science to make man over into the image of the machine, into the image of the techniques by which we study him. This tendency is not the fault of any "dangerous" men or "vicious" schools; it is rather a crisis brought upon us by our particular historical predicament. Karl Jaspers, both psychiatrist and existentialist philosopher, holds that we in the Western world are actually in process of losing self-consciousness and that we may be in the last age of historical man. William Whyte in his *Organization Man* cautions that modern man's enemies may turn out to be a "mild-looking group of therapists, who . . . would be doing what they did to help you." He refers here to the tendency to use the social sciences in support of the social ethic of our historical period; and thus the process of helping people may actually make them conformist and tend toward the destruction of individuality. We cannot brush aside the cautions of such men as unintelligent or antiscientific; to try to do so would make *us* the obscurantists.

You may agree with my sentiments here but cavil at the terms "being" and "non-being"; and many of you may already have concluded that your suspicion was only too right, that this so-called existential approach in psychology is hopelessly vague and muddled. Carl Rogers remarked in his paper at the American Psychological Association convention last September in Cincinnati that many American psychologists must find these terms abhorrent because they sound so general, so philosophical, so untestable. Rogers went on to point out, however, that he had no difficulty at all in putting the existential principles in therapy into empirically testable hypotheses.

But I would go further and hold that *without* some concepts of "being" and "non-being," we cannot even understand our most commonly used psychological mechanisms. Take for example, *repression*, *resistance* and *transference*.

The usual discussions of these terms hang in mid-air, without convincingness or psychological reality, precisely because we have lacked an underlying structure on which to base them. The term "repression," for example, obviously refers to a phenomenon we observe all the time, a dynamism which Freud clearly described in many forms. We generally explain the mechanism by saying that the child represses into unconsciousness certain impulses, such as sex and hostility, because the culture in the form of parental figures disapproves, and the child must protect his own security with these figures. But this culture which assumedly disapproves is made up of the very same people who do the repressing. Is it not an illusion, therefore, and much too simple, to speak of the culture over against the individual in such fashion and make it our whipping boy? Furthermore, where did we get the ideas that child or adult are so much concerned with security and libidinal satisfactions? Are these not a carry-over from our work with the *neurotic, anxious* child and adult?

Certainly the neurotic, anxious child is compulsively concerned with security, for example; and certainly the neurotic adult, and we who study him, read our later formulations back into the unsuspecting mind of the child. But is not the normal child just as truly interested in moving out into the world, exploring, following his curiosity and sense of adventure—going out "to learn to shiver and to shake," as the nursery rhyme puts it? And if you block these needs of the child, you get a traumatic reaction from him just as you do when you take away his security. I, for one, believe we vastly overemphasize the human being's concern with security and survival satisfactions because they so neatly fit our cause-and-effect way of thinking. I believe Nietzsche and Kierkegaard were more accurate when they described man as the organism who makes certain values—prestige, power, tenderness—more important than pleasure and even more important than survival itself.

My implication here is that we can understand repression, for example, only on the deeper level of the meaning of the human being's potentialities. In this respect, "being" is to be defined as the individual's pattern of potentialities." These potentialities will be partly shared with other persons but will in every case form a unique pattern in each individual. We must ask the questions: What is this person's relation to his own potentialities? What goes on that he chooses or is forced to choose to block off from his awareness something which he knows, and on another level *knows that he knows?* In my work in psychotherapy there appears more and more evidence that anxiety in our day arises not so much out of fear of lack of libidinal satisfactions or security, but rather out of the patient's fear of his own powers, and the conflicts that arise from that fear. This may be the particular "neurotic personality of our time"—the neurotic pattern of contemporary "outer-directed," organizational man.

The "unconscious," then, is not to be thought of as a reservoir of impulses, thoughts, wishes which are culturally unacceptable; I define it rather as *those potentialities for knowing and experiencing which the individual cannot or will not actualize.* On this level we shall find that the simple mechanism of repression is infinitely less simple than it looks; that it involves a complex struggle of the individual's *being* against the possibility of *non-being*; that it cannot be adequately comprehended in "ego" and "not-ego" terms, or even "self" and "not-self"; and that it inescapably raises the question of the human being's margin of freedom with respect to his potentialities, a margin in which resides his reponsibility for himself which even the therapist cannot take away.

Let us now come back from theory to more practical matters. For a number of years as a practicing therapist and teacher of therapists, I have been struck by how often our concern with trying to understand the patient in terms of the mechanisms by which his behavior takes place blocks our understanding of what he really is experiencing. Here is a patient, Mrs. Hutchens (about whom I shall center some of my remarks this morning) who comes into my office for the first time, a suburban woman in her middle thirties who tries to keep her expression poised and sophisticated. But no one could fail to see in her eyes something of the terror of a frightened animal or a lost child. I know, from what her neurological specialists have already told me, that her presenting problem is hysterical tenseness of the larynx, as a result of which she can talk only with a perpetual hoarseness. I have been given the hypothesis from her Rorschach that she has felt all her life, "If I say what I really feel, I'll be rejected; under these conditions it is better not to talk at all." During this first hour, also, I get some hints of the genetic *why* of her problem as she tells me of her authoritarian relation with her mother and grandmother, and how she learned to guard firmly against telling any secrets at all. But if as I sit here I am chiefly thinking of these *why's* and *how's* concerning the way the problem came about, I will grasp everything except the most important thing of all (indeed the only real source of data I have), namely, this person now existing, becoming, emerging, this experiencing human being immediately in the room with me.

There are at present in this country several undertakings to systematize psychoanalytic theory in terms of forces, dynamisms and energies. The approach I propose is the exact opposite of this. I hold that our science must be relevant to the distinctive characteristics of what we seek to study, in this case the human being. We do not deny dynamisms and forces—that would be nonsense—but we hold that they have meaning only in the context of the existing, living person; that is to say, in the *ontological* context.

I propose, thus, that we take the one real datum we have in the therapeutic situation, namely, the *existing person* sitting in a consulting room with a therapist. (The term "existing person" is used here as our European colleagues use *Dasein.*) Note that I do not say simply "individual" or "person"; if you take individuals as units in a group for the purposes of statistical prediction—certainly a legitimate use of psychological science—you are exactly *defining out of the picture* the characteristics which make this individual an existing person. Or when you take him as a composite of drives and deterministic forces, you have defined for study everything except *the one to whom these experiences happen*, everything except the existing person himself. Therapy is one activity, so far as I can see, in which we cannot escape the necessity of taking the subject as an existing person.

Let us therefore ask, What are the essential characteristics which constitute this patient as an existing person in the consulting room? I wish to propose six characteristics which I shall call principles,[1] which I find in my work as a psychotherapist. Though these principles are the product of a good deal of thought and experience with many cases, I shall illustrate them with episodes from the case of Mrs. Hutchens.

First, Mrs. Hutchens like every existing person *is centered in herself*, and an attack on this center is an attack on her existence itself. This is a characteristic which we share with all living beings; it is self-evident in animals and plants. I never cease to marvel how, whenever we cut the top off a pine tree on our farm in New Hampshire, the tree sends up a new branch from heaven knows where to become a new center. But this principle has a particular relevance to human beings and gives a basis for the understanding of sickness and health, neurosis and mental health. Neurosis is not to be seen as a deviation from our particular theories of what a person should be. *Is not neurosis, rather, precisely the method the individual uses to preserve his own center, his own existence?* His symptoms are ways of shrinking the range of his world (so graphically shown in Mrs. Hutchens' inability to let herself talk) in order that the centeredness of his existence may be protected from threat; a way of blocking off aspects of the environment that he may then be adequate to the remainder. Mrs. Hutchens had gone to another therapist for half a dozen sessions a month before she came to me. He told her, in an apparently ill-advised effort to reassure her, that she was too proper, too controlled. She reacted with great upset and immediately broke off the treatment. Now technically he was entirely correct; existentially he was entirely wrong. What he did not see, in my judgment, was that this very properness, this over-control, far from being things Mrs. Hutchens wanted to get over, were part of her desperate attempt to preserve what precarious center she had. As though she were saying, "If I opened up, if I communicated, I would lose what little space in life I have." We see here, incidentally, how inadequate is the definition of neurosis as a failure of adjustment. *An adjustment is exactly what neurosis is; and that is just its trouble.* It is a necessary adjustment by which centeredness can be preserved; a way of accepting *non-being*, if I may use this term, in order that some little *being* may be preserved. And in most cases it is a boon when this adjustment breaks down.

This is the only thing we can assume about Mrs. Hutchens, or about any patient, when she comes in: that she, like all living beings, requires centeredness, and that this has broken down. At a cost of considerable turmoil she has taken steps, that is, come for help. Our second principle thus, is: *every existing person has the character of self-affirmation, the need to preserve its*

[1] From a philosophical point of view, these are to be termed "ontological principles."

centeredness. The particular name we give this self-affirmation in human beings is "courage." Paul Tillich's emphasis on the "courage to be" is very cogent and fertile for psychotherapy at this point. He insists that in man being is never given automatically but depends upon the individual's courage, and without courage one loses being. *This makes courage itself a necessary ontological corollary.* By this token, I as a therapist place great importance upon expressions of the patients which have to do with willing, decisions, choice. I never let little remarks the patient may make such as "maybe I can," "perhaps I can try," and so on slip by without my making sure he knows I have heard him. It is only a half truth that the will is the product of the wish; I wish to emphasize rather the truth that the wish can never come out in its real power except with will.

Now as Mrs. Hutchens talks hoarsely, she looks at me with an expression of mingled fear and hope. Obviously a relation exists between us not only here but already in anticipation in the waiting room and ever since she thought of coming. She is struggling with the possibility of participating with me. Our third principle is, thus: *all existing persons have the need and possibility of going out from their centeredness to participate in other beings.* This always involves risk; if the organism goes out too far, it loses its own centeredness—its identity—a phenomenon which can easily be seen in the biological world. If the neurotic is so afraid of loss of his own conflicted center that he refuses to go out but holds back in rigidity and lives in narrowed reactions and shrunken world space, his growth and development are blocked. This is the pattern in neurotic repressions and inhibitions, the common neurotic forms in Freud's day. But it may well be in our day of conformism and the outer-directed man, that the most common neurotic pattern takes the opposite form, namely, the dispersing of one's self in participation and identification with others until one's own being is emptied. At this point we see the rightful emphasis of Martin Buber in one sense and Harry Stack Sullivan in another, that the human being cannot be understood as a self if participation is omitted. Indeed, if we are successful in our search for these ontological principles of the existing person, it should be true that the omission of any one of the six would mean we do not then have a human being.

Our fourth principle is: *the subjective side of centeredness is awareness.* The paleontologist Pierre Teilhard de Chardin has recently described brilliantly how this awareness is present in ascending degrees in all forms of life from amoeba to man. It is certainly present in animals. Howard Liddell has pointed out how the seal in its natural habitat lifts its head every ten seconds even during sleep to survey the horizon lest an Eskimo hunter with poised bow and arrow sneak up on it. This awareness of threats to being in animals Liddell calls *vigilance,* and he identifies it as the primitive, simple counterpart in animals of what in human beings becomes anxiety.

Our first four characteristic principles are shared by our existing person with all living beings; they are biological levels in which human beings participate. The fifth principle refers now to a distinctively human characteristic, self-consciousness. *The uniquely human form of awareness is self-consciousness.* We do not identify awareness and consciousness. We associate awareness, as Liddell indicates above, with vigilance. This is supported by the derivation of the term—it comes from the Anglo-Saxon *gewaer*, *waer*, meaning knowledge of external dangers and threats. Its cognates are *beware* and *wary*. Awareness certainly is what is going on in an individual's neurotic reaction to threat, in Mrs. Hutchens' experience in the first hours, for example, that I am also a threat to her. Consciousness, in contrast, we define as not simply my awareness of threat from the world, but *my capacity to know myself as the one being threatened*, my experience of myself as the subject who has a world. Consciousness, as Kurt Goldstein puts it, is man's capacity to transcend the immediate concrete situation, to live in terms of the possible; and it underlies the human capacity to use abstractions and universals, to have language and symbols. This capacity for consciousness underlies the wide-range of possibility which man has in relating to his world, and it constitutes the foundation of psychological freedom. Thus human freedom has its ontological base and I believe must be assumed in all psychotherapy.

In his book, *The Phenomenon of Man*, Pierre Teilhard de Chardin, as we have mentioned, describes awareness in all forms of evolutionary life. But in man, a new function arises, namely, this self-consciousness. Teilhard de Chardin undertakes to demonstrate something I have always believed, that when a new function emerges the whole previous pattern, the total gestalt of the organism, changes. Thereafter the organism can be understood only in terms of the new function. That is to say, it is only a half truth to hold that the organism is to be understood in terms of the simpler elements below it on the evolutionary scale; it is just as true that every new function forms a new complexity which conditions all the simpler elements in the organism. *In this sense, the simple can be understood only in terms of the more complex.*

This is what self-consciousness does in man. All the simpler biological functions must now be understood in terms of the new function. No one would, of course, deny for a moment the old functions, nor anything in biology which man shares with less complex organisms. Take sexuality for example, which we obviously share with all mammals. But given self-consciousness, sex becomes a new gestalt as is demonstrated in therapy all the time. Sexual impulses are now conditioned by the *person* of the partner; what we think of the other male or female, in reality or fantasy or even repressed fantasy, can never be ruled out. The fact that the subjective person of the other to whom we relate sexually makes least difference in *neurotic* sexuality, say in patterns of compulsive sex or prostitution, only proves the point the more firmly; for such requires precisely the blocking off, the checking out, the distorting of self-consciousness. Thus when we talk of sexuality in terms of sexual *objects*, as Kinsey does, we may garner interesting and useful statistics; but we simply are not talking about human sexuality.

Nothing in what I am saying here should be taken as antibiological in the slightest; on the contrary, I think it is only from this approach that we *can* understand human biology without distorting it. As Kierkegaard aptly put it, "The natural law is as valid as ever." I argue only against the uncritical acceptance of the assumption that the organism is to be understood solely in terms of those elements below it on the evolutionary scale, an assumption which has led us to overlook the self-evident truth that makes a horse a horse is not the elements it shares with the organisms below it but what constitutes distinctively "horse." Now *what we are dealing with in neurosis are those characteristics and functions which are distinctively human.* It is these that have gone awry in our disturbed patients. The condition for these functions is self-consciousness—which accounts for what Freud rightly discovered, that the neurotic pattern is characterized by repression and blocking off of consciousness.

It is the task of the therapist, therefore, not only to help the patient become aware; but even more significantly to help him to *transmute this awareness into consciousness.* Awareness is his knowing that something is threatening from outside in his world—a condition which may, as in paranoids and their neurotic equivalents, be correlated with a good deal of acting-out behavior. But self-consciousness puts this awareness on a quite different level; it is the patient's seeing that *he is the one who is threatened*, that he is the being who stands in this world which threatens, he is the subject who *has* a world. And this gives him the possibility of *in-sight*, of "inward sight," of seeing the world and its problems in relation to himself. And thus it gives him the possibility of doing something about the problems.

To come back to our too-long silent patient: After about 25 hours of therapy Mrs. Hutchens had the following dream. She was searching room by room for a baby in an unfinished house at an airport. She thought the baby belonged to someone else, but the other person might let her take it. Now it seemed that she had put the baby in a pocket of her robe (or her mother's robe) and she was seized with anxiety that it would be smothered. Much to her joy, she found that the baby was still alive. Then she had a strange thought, "Shall I kill it?"

The house was at the airport where she at about the age of 20 had learned to fly solo, a very important act of self-affirmation and independence from her parents. The baby was associated with her youngest son, whom she regularly identified with herself. Permit me to omit the ample associative evidence that convinced both her and me that the baby stood for herself. The dream is an expression of the emergence and growth of self-consciousness, a consciousness she is not sure is hers yet, and a consciousness which she considers killing in the dream.

About six years before her therapy, Mrs. Hutchens had left the religious faith of her parents, to which she had had a very authoritarian relation. She had then joined a church of her own belief. But she had never dared tell her parents of this. Instead, when they came to visit, she attended their church in great tension lest one of her children let the secret out. After about 35 sessions, when she was considering writing her parents to tell them of this change of faith, she had over a period of two weeks spells of partially fainting in my office. She would become suddenly weak, her face would go white, she would feel empty and "like water inside," and would have to lie down for a few moments on the couch. In retrospect she called these spells "grasping for oblivion."

She then wrote her parents informing them once and for all of her change in faith and assuring them it would do no good to try to dominate her. In the following session she asked in considerable anxiety whether I thought she would go psychotic. I responded that whereas anyone of us might at some time have such an episode, I saw no more reason why she should than any of the rest of us; and I asked whether her fear of going psychotic was not rather anxiety coming out of her standing against her parents, as though genuinely being herself she felt to be tantamount to going crazy. I have, it may be remarked, several times noted this anxiety at being one's self experienced by the patient as tantamount to psychosis. This is not surprising, for consciousness of one's own desires and affirming them involves accepting one's originality and uniqueness, and it implies that one must be prepared to be isolated not only from those parental figures upon whom one has been dependent, but at that instant to stand alone in the entire psychic universe as well.

We see the profound conflicts of the emergence of self-consciousness in three vivid ways in Mrs. Hutchens, whose chief symptom, interestingly enough, was the denial of that uniquely human capacity based on consciousness, namely, talking: 1) the temptation to kill the baby; 2) the grasping at oblivion by fainting, as though she were saying, "If only I did not have to be conscious, I would escape this terrible problem of telling my parents"; and 3) the psychosis anxiety.

We now come to the sixth and last ontological characteristic, *anxiety*. Anxiety is the state of the human being in the struggle against what would destroy his being. It is, in Tillich's phrase, the state of being in conflict with nonbeing, a conflict which Freud mythologically pictured in his powerful and important symbol of the death instinct. One wing of this struggle will always be against something outside one's self; but even more portentous and significant for psychotherapy is the inner side of the battle, which we saw in Mrs. Hutchens, namely, the conflict within the person as he confronts the choice of whether and how far he will stand against his own being, his own potentialities.

From an existential viewpoint we take very seriously this temptation to kill the baby, or kill her own consciousness, as expressed in these forms by Mrs. Hutchens. We neither water it down by calling it "neurotic" and the product merely of sickness, nor do we slough over it by reassuring her, "O.K., but you don't need to do it." If we did these, we would be helping her adjust at the price of surrendering a portion of her existence, that is, her opportunity for fuller independence. The self-confrontation which is involved in the acceptance of self-consciousness is anything but simple: it involves, to identify some of the elements, accepting the hatred of the past, her mother's against her and hers of her mother; accepting her present motives of hatred and destruction; cutting through rationalizations and illusions about her behavior and motives, and the acceptance of the responsibility and aloneness which this implies; the giving up of childhood omnipotence, and acceptance of the fact that though she can never have absolute certainty of choices, she must choose anyway. But all of these specific points, easy enough to understand in themselves, must be seen in the light of the fact that *consciousness itself implies always the possibility of turning against one's self, denying one's self.* The tragic nature of human existence inheres in the fact that consciousness itself involves the possibility and temptation at every instant of killing itself. Dostoevski and our other existential forebears were not indulging in poetic hyperbole or expressing the aftereffects of immoderate vodka when they wrote of the agonizing burden of freedom.

I trust that the fact that existential psychotherapy places emphasis on these tragic aspects of life does not at all imply it is pessimistic. Quite the contrary. The confronting of genuine tragedy is a highly cathartic experience psychically, as Aristotle and others through history have reminded us. Tragedy is inseparably connected with man's dignity and grandeur, and is the accompaniment, as illustrated in the dramas of Oedipus and Orestes *ad infinitum*, of the human being's moments of greatest insight.

I hope that this analysis of ontological characteristics in the human being, this search for the basic principles which constitute the existing person, may give us a structural basis for our psychotherapy. Thus the way may be opened for the developing of sciences of psychology and psychoanalysis which do not fragmentize man while they seek to study him, and do not undermine his humanity while they seek to help him.

FRANZ G. ALEXANDER and SHELDON T. SELESNICK

The Organic Approach

Most of the therapeutic approaches that we have described are equally well practiced by well-trained therapists with backgrounds in psychiatry or psychology. There is one approach that is legally restricted to men with medical training, and that is the organic approach. Earlier versions of this were dramatic in their violent manner of dealing with the patient, with techniques such

---

Reprinted from *The History of Psychiatry*, by Franz G. Alexander and Sheldon T. Selesnick (New York: Harper & Row, 1966), pp. 279–296.

as shock therapy and psychosurgery common. Electric shock therapy, particularly with depressive patients, is still widely used. However, the major thrust of contemporary organic approaches is to replace these gross physical treatments with drugs. One of the major developments of the past decade has been in psychopharmacology, and the use of drugs, either as a method of treatment or as an adjunct to more traditional methods, has had enormous impact on the mental health field. It should be clear that drugs are frequently used along with psychotherapy, as a method of making the patient more comfortable and more accessible to psychotherapy. Drs. Alexander and Selesnick have written a comprehensive book detailing the history of developments in psychiatry. The selection presented here is that portion of the book discussing the organic approaches, but the reader is referred to the original volume for a fuller picture of historical developments in this area.

Shock Treatments and Psychosurgery

The isolation, in 1922, of insulin by Frederick Banting, C. H. Best, and J. R. MacLeod brought diabetes, one of man's most dread diseases, under control. It also inaugurated the first systematized biological approach to a somatic treatment for schizophrenia. It so happened that small dosages of insulin were often used to stimulate appetite in patients with chronic illnesses, including those who were hospitalized with severe mental illnesses. Although such physicians as H. Steck in Switzerland, C. Munn in America, and H. Haack in Germany had noted beneficial effects of these insulin doses on the moods of excited psychotic patients, the idea of using insulin in the treatment of psychotics was developed by Manfred Sakel (1900–1957). Sakel had treated patients recovering from morphine addiction at the Lichterfelde Hospital, Berlin, from 1927 to 1933 and had observed that morphine abstainers became overly excited. He considered this excitement to be caused by overactivity of the adrenal-thyroid endocrine systems and reasoned that a drug antagonistic to this system would also decrease the tone of the sympathetic nervous system, which enhances overactivity of this endocrine system. He experimented with insulin and found that high dosages did indeed appear to diminish the overactive states. Sakel then decided to try using insulin in high enough dosages to produce coma in excited patients, especially those who had been diagnosed as schizophrenic. Late in 1933 Sakel reported his first experimental findings of beneficial results in schizophrenia following insulin shock.

Sakel's therapeutic endeavors were not unanimously accepted by the medical profession, in part because the theoretical rationale of his treatment method was vague. Although schizophrenic patients, especially those who had recently become ill, appeared to benefit by the treatment, it has been increasingly recognized over the years that schizophrenics in their early stage of illness respond to most treatments with benefit. Insulin, as well as other therapies, is less effective in the chronic stages of the illness. Because it was not an easy therapeutic regimen, the technique of the treatment came under attack. For maximum effect at least thirty to fifty hours of coma had to be produced; patients required continuous nursing care, and physicians had to be highly skilled in insulin administration in order to avoid such hazards as irreversible coma and circulatory and respiratory collapse. Exactly how insulin-shock treatment benefits the schizophrenic is still an open question. Recent speculations hold that the nucleoproteins in the neuron may be affected by the reduction in blood sugar caused by insulin or that the brain's enzyme systems are brought into better equilibrium, thus making the brain better able to utilize beneficial minerals circulating in the blood. These physiological hypotheses are, however, as yet unconfirmed.

Another explanation for the benefits of insulin shock depends on the idea that the reduced blood-sugar supply also reduces the amount of oxygen present in the bloodstream. If the highest brain centers require the greatest amount of oxygen, then the function of the cortex will be impaired first by any diminishment in the glucose supply, and the lower centers of the brain will thus be released from the inhibition of the cerebral cortex. In essence, then, insulin treatment encourages the individual to regress to lower and more primitive levels of adaptation. Viewed from a psychological standpoint, the patient awakens from an insulin coma in a regressed psychological state. He has to be fed intravenously or with a stomach tube and is extremely dependent on external help. This continuing physiological and psychological regression, it is presumed, gradually leads to a reshaping of higher physiological and psychological patterns as the patient responds to the great amount of attention and the hopefulness of the psychiatric team administering the insulin.

Because of its dangers, unreliable results, and high cost, insulin therapy was largely superseded during the 1940's by other forms of shocking the nervous system. The next phase in shock treatment developed as a result of investigations of epilepsy, the "sacred disease" of the ancients. In the late 1920's Ladislaus Joseph von Meduna (1896–1964), then the superintendent of the Royal State Mental Hospital in Budapest, observed that the glial tissue, which connects the cell structures of the cortex, had thickened in epileptic patients. When he compared their brains with those of deceased schizophrenic patients he noted that the latter showed a deficiency of glial structure. On the basis of these findings (which have not been subsequently confirmed) Meduna became convinced that schizophrenia and epilepsy were incompatible diseases and that a convulsive agent administered to schizophrenics would therefore cure them.[1]

[1] In the late 1920's and early 1930's Meduna had read of statistical clinical studies purporting that schizophrenia and epilepsy rarely, if ever, occur in the same patient. These reports claimed that should a schizophrenic develop epilepsy, his psychosis could be cured.

This technique was not original with Meduna, for convulsive agents had been used by previous investigators to treat severe mental states.[2] Not knowing of these earlier experiments, he decided in 1933 to test camphor and soon thereafter began to use a less toxic synthetic camphor preparation, Metrazol (also called Cardiazol). Metrazol had several practical shortcomings, among them an unpredictable time lag between injection and convulsion, during which the patient was fearful and uncooperative. Also, the convulsions frequently were severe enough to cause fractures.

In 1932 Ugo Cerletti (1877–1963), at the Neuropsychiatric Clinic in Genoa, was autopsying bodies of those who had died from epilepsy; he noted a hardening in a sector of the brain known as Ammon's horn. Cerletti decided to find out whether this hardening caused or was the result of epileptic attacks. Because he assumed that drugs used to produce experimental convulsions might have produced the hardening in the brain, he decided to use electrical stimulation instead.[3]

Later, in Rome, in 1935, Cerletti began collaborating with L. Bini. Cerletti learned that hogs were killed at a Roman slaughterhouse after they had been stupefied by an electrical current; Bini used these hogs to establish a safe dosage of electricity, and on April 15, 1938, Cerletti and Bini administered their first electroshock treatment to a schizophrenic patient. It soon became evident that electroshock was superior to Metrazol, since it was less dangerous, less expensive, and produced a milder convulsion. Because of its simplicity of procedure and favorable results, electroshock had, by the 1940's, also widely replaced insulin-shock treatments in schizophrenia.

Shock treatment today consists of passing seventy to one hundred and thirty volts for one tenth to five tenths of a second through electrodes attached to the patient's head. Usually three treatments a week are given; anywhere from five to thirty-five treatments may be considered optimal. For such a relatively violent procedure the side effects are mild, and the patient experiences no pain. The danger of bone fractures has been minimized by the use of curare-like drugs (by A. E. Bennet in 1941) that inhibit the production

[2] Dr. William Oliver in 1785 reported in a London medical journal that he had cured a case of mania by giving camphor. Dr. G. Burrows made a similar claim in a book. *Commentaries on the Causes, Forms, Symptoms, Treatment, Moral and Medical, of Insanity*, published in 1828. And in the eighteenth century, Auenbrugger, the discoverer of auscultation, and a Dr. Weickhardt has also recommended camphor for the treatment of mental diseases.

[3] The use of nonconvulsive electrotherapy as a method for alleviating symptoms through suggestion dates back to Scribonius Largus (*c.* A.D. 47), who treated the headaches of the Roman emperor with an electric eel. Nonconvulsive electrotherapy was in widespread use in the late nineteenth century, advocated by the German neurologist W. H. Erb and the French neurologist G. B. Duchenne. Probably the first electroconvulsive treatment for mental illness was administered by the French physician J. B. LeRoy in 1755 on a patient with a psychogenic blindness; almost a half century later F. L. Augustin of Germany reported a similar case. These were isolated experiments and were not followed up; the exact amount of electricity that produced convulsions without fatality was unknown. Cerletti was unfamiliar with these reports, but he did know that experimental convulsions had been produced in animals and that humans too had seizures after accidental electrical exposure.

of acetylcholine at the neuromuscular junction and thus reduce muscular spasm. The patient loses consciousness immediately after the shock is administered and therefore resistance to further treatment is not connected with a recollection of physical trauma. The most striking feature of the post-treatment period is that the patient has a memory loss of a varying degree for recent events. This amnesia may last for several weeks or months following the treatment, but eventually memory is restored. Whatever brain changes do occur are reversible, and persisting brain damage is very rare.

Electroshock treatment has been proved a particularly effective measure for the severe depression—involutional melancholia—that appears in late middle age. On the other hand, shock treatments effect only a relief of symptoms. They do not reach the basic psychological disturbance underlying the illness, and patients who receive electroshock without psychotherapy—which reaches the source of the illness—frequently relapse, even those who have psychotic depressions, for which electroshock is most effective. Despite this drawback, it must be recognized that electroshock may be imperative in cases where symptoms must be alleviated immediately in order to protect the life of a suicidal patient or the lives of others exposed to an excessively aggressive patient.

Speculations about the mode of action of electroshock treatment fall roughly into two sets of theories, one set based on possible psychological reactions to the treatment, the other on possible physiological reactions. One psychological theory maintains that the patient is so fearful of the treatment that he "escapes into health" rather than face another treatment; another proposes that the treatment satisfies the patient's need for punishment. If this were true, however, beating or chaining the patients—as practiced in the Middle Ages—would more readily cure them. Metrazol produced a much more violent reaction and was more painful to the patient, yet its effects were inferior to electroshock. A third psychological theory holds that the patient releases his pent-up aggressive and hostile impulses through the violent muscular convulsions; but if this were true, running around the block or doing push-ups to the point of exhaustion should be equally effective. Still another psychological theory proposes that the patient experiences the electroshock as a threat to his life, against which his body mobilizes all its defenses. But if this theory were true, then psychotic patients in the analogous circumstances of facing death from cancer or other terminal illness should inevitably show signs of remission of their psychotic illness. Occasionally this does occur, but it is by no means frequent. Another theory holds that the patient's family, fearful of the treatment, gives the patient more attention and thus helps him to get better. But there are families who are consciously or unconsciously hostile to the sick person in their group and therefore would not be influenced by any such threat at all. In general it may be said that all these psychological theories may be applicable to individual patients but that they cannot hold true for all individuals.

The physiological theories about electroshock are just as speculative.

Claims that electroshock stimulates the hypothalamus and therefore the sympathetic nervous system or that it stimulates adaptive responses from the adrenal cortex suffer from the observation that specific sympathetic stimulators or adrenal-cortical hormones do not cure psychotic conditions. Perhaps a plausible explanation for the efficacy of shock is that it produces a slight brain damage and thus erases the most recent neurohistological changes in the highest brain area, which stores as memories those experiences which precipitated the psychosis. In other words, as the result of shock treatment the patient completely forgets the events leading up to his symptoms and thus is put back into a predepression psychological state. The best-substantiated facts of electroshock therapy are that amnesia occurs during this period and that when the temporary memory defect based on the patient's reversible brain damage is restored, illness is apt to reoccur. The exceptions are those lucky patients whose external-life situations fortuitously improve after the shock therapy.

One speculation about the way shock treatment operates involves the concepts of feedback and reverberating circuits. After Hans Berger's discovery of the electrical potentials of the brain and his inauguration of electroencephalography, some scientists began to view the brain as a series of electrical circuits. Norbert Wiener (1894–1964) compared the brain to an electrical computer governed by mechanisms—that is, self-regulating and self-corrective devices—that allow a machine to operate according to prearranged patterns. Negative feedback keeps a machine in a state of stability; positive feedback acts to increase instability of whatever system it governs and in effect causes a machine to develop what is called a reverberating cycle in which internal control is lost. Some psychiatrists have therefore suggested that electroshock therapy breaks up a reverberating circuit in the brain that is caused by positive feedback and thereby clears the brain. The question of how far the "neurotic machines" of Norbert Wiener can be compared with a neurotic personality offers interesting areas for further research. As of the moment, the positive-feedback theory must remain in the realm of speculation.

The idea of a vicious cycle in which morbid ideas become intensified if they are not checked predated the concepts of cybernetics and was one of the theoretical concepts that led to the development of psychosurgery. Egas Moniz (1874–1955), clinical professor of neurology at the University of Lisbon, believed that "morbid" ideas stimulate and restimulate the neuron. Although no pathological changes could be detected in the synapses or in the nerve cells of patients suffering from functional psychoses, nevertheless Moniz "was particularly struck by the circumstance that certain mental patients as a type—I had in mind obsessive and melancholic cases—have a circumscribed mental existence confined to a limited cycle of ideas which, dominating all others, constantly revolved in the patient's diseased brain." Moniz believed that if the frontal area of the brain were to be altered, this recurrence of unhealthy thoughts would be interrupted. He decided that the connection of the thalamus and the frontal lobes would be the most logical to work with because the thalamus is the relay center ol impressions, while the prefrontal lobe is concerned with interpreting se experiences and rendering them conscious.

Two studies influenced Moniz' interest in the prefrontal lobes. The function of the frontal lobes had been studied at Yale by Fulton and Jacobson, who noted that monkeys whose prefrontal-lobe fibers had been severed seemed to accept frustration better and were easier to manage. Richard Brickner had removed parts of frontal lobes while removing a tumor and reported that the patient subsequently seemed less worried and less inhibited and did not appear intellectually deteriorated. A Swiss psychiatrist, Burckhardt, in 1890 had also removed part of the frontal lobe in a mental patient, but the work was not followed up, probably because of ethical pressure, and Moniz was thus the first to operate on a large number of patients.

Moniz' first frontal lobotomy on a psychiatric patient was performed in 1935 with the aid of Almeida Lima, a Portuguese neurosurgeon; during the 1940's psychosurgery was often advocated for patients with irretractable psychoses resistant to shock treatments. Although mortality from prefrontal operations was only one or two percent, loud protests were raised against its use. Patients who had this kind of surgery were not merely calmer—much of the time they were reduced to being placid "zombies." Many postoperative patients lacked ambition, tact, and imagination; although the patients themselves may have felt more comfortable, their families did not. Anxiety was relieved, but at the price of a loss of self-respect and of empathy with others. Furthermore, patients with recurrent severely morbid thoughts—that is, with obsessional psychoses—were not relieved of their symptoms. A major difficulty was that psychosurgery, which mutilated irrevocably a part of the brain, was final. Not a dispensable part, such as the appendix, is removed, but an area essential to the human being—his personality—is forever destroyed. Fortunately, before the brains of too many unapproachable psychotics could be operated upon, another approach was discovered to relieve insufferable anxiety and tension—psychopharmacology.

Psychopharmacology

Primitive medicine men often used dry leaves, roots of plants, and fermented fruits to produce transient psychotic states as a way to heighten and intensify the experiences of religious ceremonials. However, only one of these naturally occurring drugs—opium, the product of poppy seeds—has been deliberately used throughout the centuries to reduce emotional stress. Theophrastus, the Greek physician-botanist, mentions opium's pain-relieving qualities; Paracelsus stored a bit of it in his walking cane; and Sydenham claimed that he could not practice medicine without it.

The drugs that have been used in medicinal therapy for disturbed emotional states can be categorized into five very general classes.

1. Drugs that do not act upon the central nervous system and do not

ior, but that do act through suggestion—otherwise " Doctors of all periods have had their favorite a doctor's belief that the drug will be helpful is

ect a deficiency or combat an infection that has led to central nervous system. Thyroxin, for example, helps the mental ardation occurring in myxedema and cretinism; and states of severe confusion caused by a vitamin-B deficiency have been corrected by proper administration of vitamins. Syphilis of the central nervous system has been cited as an infectious disease that can be cured by drug therapy. Drugs that are given for these specific causes are, however, ineffective for any other mental disorder.

3. Sedatives administered to convert excited states into quiescent ones and stimulants used to produce increased activity in depressed patients. Sedatives like chloral hydrate were first synthesized about 1870 and were used in psychiatric disorders, bromides were also prescribed extensively during the nineteenth century to produce heavy sedation, and in the early twentieth century barbiturates came into use for the same purpose. As for stimulants, the effects of alcoholic beverages and of caffeine have been known for centuries. Synthetic drugs used extensively during the 1930's to treat depression were the amphetamine derivatives (Benzedrine and Dexedrine), but their disagreeable side effects—they caused loss of appetite, palpitations, and an increase in heart rate and blood pressure—interfered with widespread acceptance. Stimulants, like sedatives, act for a limited period of time; they do not produce permanent changes of mood. In the first years of this century, on the assumption that excitement interferes with clear thinking, prolonged administration of barbiturates in excited states was proposed. In 1922 Jacob Klasi recommended prolonged sedative-induced sleep, on the basis that excitement was a result of an inflammatory process in the brain that could be relieved through rest, as other inflammatory conditions were. Prolonged-sleep treatment preceded insulin therapy and may be considered a forerunner of the shock treatments.

4. Drugs that facilitate verbal expression of emotions, often called narcotherapy. World War II patients suffering from traumatic war neuroses were given intravenous injections of barbiturates to help them relate the sensations they had experienced during combat. Enough of the barbiturate was given to enable a patient to speak freely without putting him to sleep. Variants of this technique continued to be used throughout the 1940's, but it is generally conceded today that this kind of treatment helps the patient to express repressed feelings and has some value in relieving acute hysterical symptoms but that it is not suited to resolving underlying conflicts. Another drug used in narcotherapy is carbon dioxide, which has also proved to have the same kind of limited value.

5. Drugs used to test pet theories about mental illness. A list of all these would fill volumes, and indeed textbooks of psychiatry used to recommend

many drugs, enzymes, concoctions, extracts, hormones, and vitamins for use in mental disorders. Many of them represent desperate attempts to validate an organic explanation for psychoses, and some of them should, of course, also be considered as drugs that work by suggestion.

In general the pattern of drug therapy for mental illness has been one of initial enthusiasm followed by disappointment. Twenty years after Balard discovered bromides (1826) they were widely used in psychiatric illnesses. During the latter part of the nineteenth century and in the early years of the twentieth, physicians found that uncontrollable states of excitement could be markedly relieved by the administration of bromides. By the mid-twenties, even some psychiatrists writing in the official journal of the American Psychiatric Association were claiming that finally a drug—bromide—had been discovered that could alleviate serious symptoms of disturbed behavior. The American public, following the lead of physicians, so desired bromides that by 1928 one out of every five prescriptions was for bromides. As is usual when drugs are hailed as the solution to mental illness, disillusionment gradually set in. Patients had to be continuously maintained on bromides in order to show improvement. Nonetheless, despite the repeated shattering of the drug dream, physicians still hope eventually to alleviate man's inner strife by chemical means.

Since antiquity men have desired a state of perfect tranquility—what the Epicureans called "ataraxia," a serene calmness. The Greeks used alcoholic beverages or narcotics to dull their senses into a state of relative peacefulness; but then, as now, they suffered eventually from confusion and hangover. In the tropical areas of the Orient, however, one drug was said to produce contentment without cloudiness. It was derived from a red-blossomed plant, about eighteen inches high, whose roots zigzagged along the ground like snakes. This plant's many names reflect its use both as an antidote for snakebite ("snakeroot plant," "serpentina," and "sarpagandha," or snake repellent) and as a treatment for moonsickness or insanity ("chabdra," or moon, and "pagla-ka-dawa," or insanity herb).

The snakeroot plant was unknown to the Western world until early in the seventeenth century, when Plumier, a French botanist, first described it. He named it *Rauwolfia serpentina* after the German physician-botanist Leonard Rauwolf, who had, between 1573 and 1574, explored the medicinal plants of the orient. It was not until the 1930's however, that any serious scientific interest was given to its medical potential. In 1931 two Indian doctors, S. Siddiqui and Rafat Siddiqui, isolated five alkaloids from the snakeroot plant, and two other Indian scientists, Ganneth Sen and Katrick Bose, described the use of *Rauwolfia serpentina* in cases of high blood pressure and also in psychoses. By the 1950's *Rauwolfia's* ability to lower blood pressure and to calm excited patients without producing a state of confusion was known to Western physicians as well, and medication incorporating the alkaloids from its roots was being prescribed throughout the world (under many trade names, some of which are Moderil, Sandril, Serpasil, Reserpine, and Harmonyl).

Another group of potent tranquilizers, the phenothiazine derivatives, evolved as the product of meticulous laboratory investigation. One of these derivatives was used to combat parasitic worms in cattle; it also proved effective against malaria and trypanosomiasis—a form of sleeping sickness caused by a parasite in humans. Further investigation revealed that other phenothiazines were effective against some forms of allergies. In 1952 a French psychiatrist, Jean Delay, along with his coworker, Pierre Deniker, reported the beneficial results of using chlorpromazine, a phenothiazine, for treating psychotic patients. In the 1950's the derivatives of the snakeroot plant of ancient India and chemical compounds of this new drug (sold under the trade names Thorazine, Sparine, Compazine, Stelazine, etc.) seemed to combat everything from allergy to psychosis and competed for dominance in the medical journals. Then a third drug was introduced that was to challenge the other tranquilizers in sales as a psychopharmacological panacea. Mephenesin, a glycerol derivative, was known to have a marked muscle-relaxing effect and was used extensively in the treatment of muscle spasm in acute excited conditions like delirium tremens. F. M. Berger, medical director of Wallace Laboratories, realized that Mephenesin's action was of too short a duration and in the early 1950's synthetized a related chemical compound, meprobamate, that had a more lasting effect. Meprobamate (Miltown, Equanil) had in its favor few side effects, and yet mildly tranquilized the patient.

Because these tranquilizing drugs do not significantly impair consciousness, memory, or intellectual functioning, the conclusion has been drawn that the cerebral cortex must be more or less unaffected and that the subcortical areas must be most implicated, in particular the hypothalamus, the limbic system, and the reticular-activating system.

The phenothiazines appear to inhibit significantly the alerting r.a.s., thereby diminishing awareness of disturbing stimuli. If a phenothiazine is given to a patient in a state of severe pain, for example, the patient continues to feel pain but is not as attentive to it, not as aware of it, and consequently not as troubled by it. For this reason the phenothiazines are widely used in obstetrics and surgery. These drugs are not merely effective against physical pain, however; they also reduce mental anguish and anxiety, so that individuals who usually would be driven by their inner impulses to excessive activity and excitement quiet down remarkably well after taking a phenothiazine derivative. The *Rauwolfia* compounds are less sedative than the phenothiazine derivatives and apparently have their most crucial effect upon the hypothalamus and the autonomic nervous system. They seem both to inhibit the sympathetic nervous system and stimulate the parasympathetic nervous system, which would account for some of their annoying side effects, such as pupillary constriction, increased motility of the gastrointestinal tract, and lowering of the blood pressure. Their most untoward side effect is that in many cases they produce depression.

The mildest tranquilizers, the meprobamates, seem to act in completely dissimilar fashion from both the *Rauwolfia* and the phenothiazines. They do not affect the hypothalamus or the r.a.s., but instead apparently slow down transmission of sensory impulses from the thalamus to the cortex. The exact manner of this inhibition is uncertain, and the suppression of impulses appears to be incomplete, since if it were complete the effect would be equivalent to a chemical lobotomy, which it is not. In general the tranquilizers, with a few exceptions, have proved to be safe with relatively few side effects.

The tranquilizers have proved least effective for cases of depression, which is not surprising. Any drug that tranquilizes or inhibits alertness to stimuli could scarcely have much value for patients who are already hypertranquilized, inattentive, and excessively limited in their activity. However, a group of stimulating drugs, the amine-oxidase inhibitors, have proved promising for lifting the spirits of depressed patients. Amphetamines had been used during the 1930's as antidepressants, but their undesirable side effects brought them into some disfavor. Then, in the 1950's, it was observed that a drug, Iproniazid, used in the treatment of tuberculosis appeared to elate the depressed tubercular patients who took it, and research work began on using similar compounds that were less toxic than Iproniazid in the treatment of depressions. These drugs, which do not have the same undesirable side effects as the amphetamines, apparently act by inhibiting an enzyme called amine-oxidase, which seems to destroy serotonin; consequently the body is able to store up reserves of serotonin in the body. In addition to the amine-oxidase inhibitors, there are several other classes of antidepressants that are presently under full-scale investigation.

The use of the new psychotropic drugs—tranquilizers and antidepressants—has opened up new horizons for psychiatry. They have the practical advantages that they neither affect the state of consciousness to the same degree as the traditional sedatives nor have the unpleasant side effects of the amphetamines; they offer physicians the opportunity to influence specific psychic functions and shift the equilibrium between inhibitions and excitations in the desired direction. Retarded depressive patients can be stimulated; excited manic patients can be tranquilized.

Although the mode of action of these drugs is not yet fully understood, it is well established that tranquilizing drugs act primarily on the midbrain, the reticular formation, and the vegetative centers. They do not interfere with cortical functions, nor do they induce excessive drowsiness like the barbiturates. The fact that they act on the lower centers renders them therapeutically more useful than drugs that have a direct effect upon the higher centers of the nervous system: they leave integrative and cognitive functions unaffected and thus allow drug treatment to be combined with psychotherapy, which of necessity has to rely on the integrative functions of the highest centers. The very limited therapeutic usefulness of hypnotherapy and narcotherapy has shown that a genuine reconstruction of a neurotic personality cannot be achieved without involvement of these integrative functions.

Used with psychotic patients, tranquilizers reduce anxiety, restlessness, hallucinations, and delusions, which are the outward manifestations of underlying disturbances that seriously interfere with the patient's human relationships, with his functioning in life, and with psychotherapy. The manifest florid symptoms, particularly anxiety, impair the higher integrative functions. Moreover, hallucinations and delusions make contact with others more difficult and induce further withdrawal from reality. This vicious cycle is broken when drug treatment is successful. Symptomatic improvements from drugs allow for further spontaneous ego development. However, since the drug does not change the underlying personality disturbance and merely reduces its secondary manifestations, psychotherapy remains still the most incisive tool. It is still not clear, though, how far systematic and expert psychotherapy can go with psychotic patients, even when drugs have made them more accessible to intensive psychological treatment.

Whether or not psychotropic drugs should be used in cases of neurosis is a controversial issue. The secondary symptoms, such as the disturbance of the sensorium and of the thought processes that makes the psychological approach to psychotics often impossible, are much less common in neurotic patients. Reduction of extreme anxiety remains a real indication for the use of drugs in the psychoneurotic, but treatment should focus on its essential target, the underlying personality disturbance. Some psychoanalysts combine their treatment with a judicious administration of psychotropic drugs, trying to create by the reduction of disturbing excessive anxiety more favorable conditions for the psychological approach; other psychoanalysts, more fundamentalistic in their approach, believe, for technical reasons, that the use of drugs seriously interferes with their therapeutic work. These psychoanalysts maintain that to give drugs is to play the role of the magician who is trying to relieve symptoms quickly, thereby hampering his role as a psychotherapist who is trying to help the patient reveal and understand himself.

There can be no question that the psychotropic drugs have great practical value. Their use has markedly shortened the hospital stay of severely disturbed patients and has also simplified the hospital management of these patients by making them more tractable. And what is most important, the more drastic methods of treating psychotics—electroshock, insulin therapy, and psychosurgery—are less frequently used. Unfortunately most severely depressed patients respond less rapidly to the antidepressant drugs than to electroshock; nonetheless, these drugs have made it possible to humanize the hospital treatment of psychotic patients by substituting chemical for corporal restraint.

It is most tempting for a person to get relief from the unavoidable burdens and anxieties of everyday life by taking a drug rather than by facing his actual problems realistically. However, psychological habituation to a chemically induced oblivion is an unrealistic solution and a basically unreliable crutch that only compounds the problems encountered in day-to-day living. Concern about real problems induces a person to plan and strive realistically. Anxiety mobilizes both biological and psychological defenses to ensure survival. Unquestionably, under certain extremely stressful life conditions and also in pathological states of mind, tension and anxiety may hamper effectual planning and concentration. Relief by tranquilizers, even temporary relief, in such conditions may allow the person to face more realistically his internal and external problems. Only an expert psychological evaluation of the situation can lead to the correct decision whether or not administration of drugs is indicated in an individual case. Meanwhile, indiscriminate use of psychotropic drugs constitutes a definite danger for proper psychiatric care as well as for mental hygiene in general.

New drugs will come to take over for older ones, and there will be many new drug trials. It does not seem foreseeable that one drug will solve the dilemma of mental illness, but the experimentation into how drugs act on the nervous system will aid us inestimably to understand better the functioning of the brain. As we learn more about the reticular-activating system, the limbic system, and the hypothalamus, and the enzymes and the neurohormones active in the nervous system, the gap between the mind and brain becomes narrowed. Already we suspect that the cerebral cortex can block through inhibitory discharges unpleasant stimuli reaching it from other neuronal centers. We call this psychological repression. We have noted that interruption of thalamic-cortical circuits, inhibition of the r.a.s. system, or reverberations set up in the limbic lobe are not dissimilar and occur with drug intervention. The day will arrive when the mind will come to its intended resting place, not as a structure of the brain, but as a function of it. How disturbing thoughts, feelings, and sensations, the psychological phenomenon called mind, are transmitted, stored as memories, and reacted to at a later time in life will be the legacy left by what appeared at one time to be psychopharmacological fads. Nevertheless, in the future we must be cautious lest we overevaluate valuable neurological data and claim from it more than is justified. In the final analysis, the situations that provoke emotional upsets and the subjective experience of psychic pain cannot be explained in terms of the nervous system but must be described in psychological language.

The Hallucinogens and Experimental Psychosis

The rediscovery of hallucinogens, drugs that produce transient psychotic states, has in recent years aroused the hope that chemical compounds may be found that will terminate not only experimentally induced psychoses, but other psychotic states as well. Man's attempt to produce states in himself in which he would have vivid and fantastic experiences long outdates man's attempt to cure psychosis. Over the ages men have looked for agents that would allow escape from life's pressures: opium, for instance, is such a drug, and so are alcohol and hashish. Marihuana, cohoba seed, mushrooms, and the buttons from the peyote cactus are others.

In the late nineteenth century an alkaloid isolated from the peyote cactus, mescaline, was found to produce intense perceptual disturbances, which have often been described by those who have taken it. During the 1950's mescaline was used experimentally to induce psychotic states; but also another compound, dissimilar in structure and ten thousand times more potent, lysergic acid diethylamide (LSD), has also been so used.

Lysergic acid is the active ingredient of ergot, a fungus that causes the rye cereal plant to decay. Its hallucinogenic quality was discovered by accident in 1943, when, working on the derivatives of the rye ergot, a Swiss chemist, Dr. A. Hofmann, accidentally sniffed one of the synthetic products he was using. He later wrote: "I was seized in the laboratory by a peculiar sensation of vertigo and restlessness. Objects in my vicinity and also the shape of my co-workers in the laboratory appeared to undergo optical changes. . . . In a dreamlike state I left the laboratory and went home where I was seized by an irresistible urge to lie down and sleep. Daylight was felt as being unpleasantly intense. I drew the curtains and immediately fell into a peculiar state of 'drunkenness,' characterized by an exaggerated imagination. With closed eyes, fantastic pictures of extraordinary plasticity and intensive kaleidoscopic colorfulness seemed to surge towards me. After two hours this state gradually subsided." Further investigations in the 1940's and 1950's brought reports of perceptual distortions, mood modulations multicolored illusionary and hallucinatory patterns made up of glowing and beautiful geometrical designs.

Investigators have so far been unable to establish the causes of the vivid experiences that mescaline and LSD produce; both compounds appear to have similar psychological effects in man and animals. It has been theorized but not confirmed that mescaline, which is similar in structure to adrenalin, becomes converted in the body to one of the breakdown products of adrenalin, adrenochrome, which produces hallucinogenic states. The entire problem of how adrenalin is metabolized in the body has been a major concern of biological research in the past several years.

LSD on the other hand, has an indole nucleus also present in serotonin and the *Rauwolfia* compounds; LSD seems to be antagonistic to serotonin, which perhaps may underlie its psychotomimetic qualities. However, we still do not know how abnormal quantities of serotonin are related to mental illness. Some investigators postulate that by combining LSD with psychotherapy, repression might be overcome so that unconscious conflicts would reach consciousness and be communicated. The use of LSD at this time is, however, in the experimental stage, and the neurophysiological and psychological phenomena produced by these drugs remain enigmatic.

LESTER LUBORSKY, MICHAEL CHANDLER,
ARTHUR H. AUERBACH, JACOB COHEN,
and HENRY M. BACHRACH

Factors Influencing the Outcome of Psychotherapy: Review of Quantitative Research

The enormous amount of attention that has been given to case studies and to theoretical speculations about psychotherapy has not been matched in volume by substantial research into the process and outcome of treatment. However, sufficient research has been done to allow a number of conclusions to be solidly established. In this paper, Luborsky and his colleagues review the body of research and indicate areas where such conclusions are justified. The conclusions, accompanied by extensive comments on the methodology of these studies, is valuable for any reader who wishes a quick review of the status of psychotherapy research at the present time. For such a reader, it should also be noted that this article was orginally accompanied by an extensive Appendix listing each of the 166 studies included in the review along with a brief summary of its findings.

When a patient and psychotherapist agree to meet, is what follows largely an unpredictable venture? Most psychotherapists believe it is predictable because patients, *as a group*, will improve; it is unpredictable because only a few of the factors influencing the fate of the *individual* patient in psychotherapy can be discerned, even after a thorough initial evaluation and even after the early sessions. All psychotherapists agree on this one fact: Some patients seem to improve; others do not. Responsibility for such differences could theoretically be traced to a variety of sources—the qualities of the patient and therapist, the mode of treatment, or some higher order interaction of these factors.

Digging through past research does not unearth an easy path to the relative influences of those factors. The line of inquiry with the deepest roots in practice is that of clinical research. Through this route Freud (1913)

Reprinted from the *Psychological Bulletin*, **75** (1971), 145–185, with the permission of the American Psychological Association and Dr. Luborsky.

concluded, in terms of his well-known analogy between chess and psychotherapy, that we know only some of the opening and closing moves; for the rest we have only intuitively applied guidelines. Therefore, "this gap in instruction can only be filled by a diligent study of games fought out by masters [p. 123]." This kind of tutorial exercise or apprenticeship training, coupled with self-scrutiny, has been one of the primary means of ferreting out factors governing the outcome of treatment. Among the attempts to map out the area, three classical clinical papers serve as landmarks: Freud (1937), Rogers (1957), and Rosenzweig (1936). Qualities of the therapist thought to influence the course of psychotherapy were catalogued by Holt and Luborsky (1958); a similar series of patient qualities was enumerated by Wallerstein, Robbins, Sargent, and Luborsky (1956). Also available are several comprehensive reviews, for instance, Wolberg (1967).

The relatively newer and fewer quantitative studies need more systematic reviews. Some of them are part of surveys of prediction of change in mental patients regardless of type of treatment (Fulkerson & Barry, 1961; Windle, 1952), some are in a review of issues and trends in psychotherapy research (Strupp & Bergin, 1969a), and some are part of a book in preparation (Bergin & Garfield, 1970). The impact of the quantitative research on the practice of psychotherapy has been negligible (Luborsky, 1969). Clinical research and quantitative research have tended to stay distant from each other; those who know one tend not to know the other. The scattered studies which may come to a therapist's attention often have contradictory findings and lack clinical sophistication in their conception and interpretation. Whether or not a skeptical attitude is justified on the basis of the existing quantitative research can only be judged from a thorough overview—which is the primary goal of this survey.

Our present review of the quantitative research is intended to serve several specific purposes:

1. To offer guidelines to clinicians in the form of lists of qualities of patient, therapist, and patient-therapist interaction which have been shown to relate to various criteria of outcome. The lists are being developed into an easily applied prognostic index. These guidelines may eventually suggest modifications to psychotherapy in the interest of improving therapeutic results. For example, if it turns out that the therapist's empathy leads to benefits for the patient, therapists who have or can develop that quality will be in demand.

2. To systematically compare the clinical and quantitative lists of factors. What should be investigated by quantitative research will be highlighted when we find clinical areas with no quantitative exploration.

3. To provide a methodological evaluation of the research as a guide to future investigation.

Limits of the literature search

To accomplish these aims, all *quantitative* studies of the factors which influence outcome of *individual psychotherapy* for *adult* patients were examined. They were included if there was at least some attempt to provide reasonably controlled comparisons, and the conclusions were passably supported. This meant including all relevant quantitative studies except for a few poorly conceived or ambiguous ones.

For the definition of psychotherapy, we followed the lead of Zax and Klein (1960) in their review of the types of changes that occur via psychotherapy. They put limits on the scope of their search by following Snyder's (1947) definition of psychotherapy, which rules out research primarily on educational and guidance activities emphasizing the giving of information. Also excluded were occupational therapy, shock therapy, chemotherapy, behavior therapy, and laboratory analogues of psychotherapy unless these latter were compared with psychotherapy. Excluded from the main body of the review were articles predicting only the length of the treatment, or only the patient's remaining or leaving, rather than the gains made by the patient. Most studies were omitted that were available only in the form of unpublished theses or in foreign language journals. Governed by these delimitations, 166 studies were finally included in our review, and form the substrate for our conclusions. They cover a period of 23 years of research—from 1946 through 1969. Most of our eligible 166 are from Strupp and Bergin's (1969b) bibliography of all types of individual psychotherapy research through 1967 in which there are listed approximately 2,700 publications. Obviously, quantitative prognostic studies of factors influencing change in individual psychotherapy have been relatively scarce.

Main factors influencing outcome of psychotherapy

The main factors can be organized within the model presented by Sanford (1962). It is a diagram applicable to any social system designed to change the person who passes through it (Figure 1).

Patient 1 (P-1) refers to the patient before he begins treatment; Therapist 1 (T-1) to the therapist before he begins interacting with the patient; the P-T Interaction rectangle refers to the period of treatment; Patient 2 (P-2) to the patient at termination of treatment; and Patient 3 (P-3) to the patient one year after the treatment has ended. The model suggested the divisions under which we classified results of each study: I: Patient Factors (before Treatment and Judged from the Sessions); II: Therapist Factors (before Treatment and Judged from the Sessions); III: The Match between Patient and Therapist (Patient and Therapist Assessed Apart from Treatment); IV: Treatment Factors.

We should note that there is a distinct asymmetry in the weights to be attached to significant and nonsignificant findings—the latter receiving much less weight. Obviously, a nonsignificant result does not warrant the positive conclusion of no relationship, but merely the absence of evidence sufficient to conclude that a relationship exists. Given the likely poor statistical power of

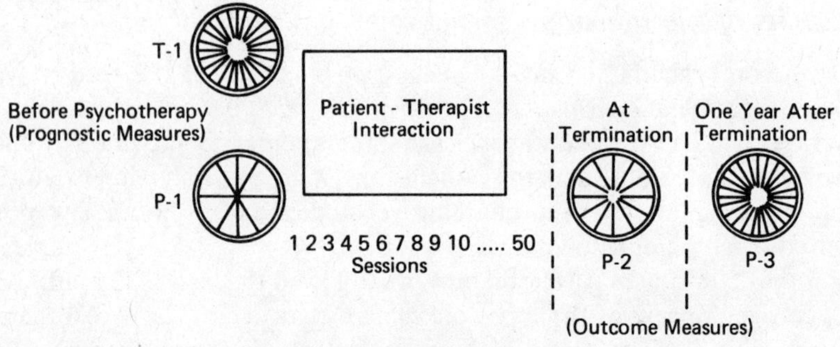

Fig. 1. *Plan assessment of the patient and therapist (cf. Sanford & Luborsky, 1962, p. 155) before, during, and after going through the psychotherapy change system.*

much of this research (small samples, measurement-error attenuated relationships), this point takes on particular force (Cohen, 1962; 1965, pp. 95–101).

A few qualities remain significantly predictive across several studies, despite different patients, different forms of treatment, and different criteria of outcome. Only a few of them manage this feat, but by accomplishing it become more worthy of our attention. These qualities are listed in Table 1 and then are reviewed in more detail.

I: Patient Factors

Adequacy of general personality functioning

We have included terms from a variety of psychological languages—mental health versus sickness, pathology, psychotic tendencies, integration, ego strength, adjustment, and dysfunction. Probably all arrive at similar global estimates of adequacy of general personality functioning. Of the 28 studies that fall within this category, 15 show a significant relationship between the level of initial personality functioning and outcome of treatment; of these, 14 are in the positive direction. They indicate that the healthier the patient is to begin with, the better the outcome—or the converse—the sicker he is to begin with, the poorer the outcome. Only one study indicates a significant negative relationship—the sicker the patient, the better the outcome. Gottschalk, Mayerson, and Gottlieb (1967) showed that the patients with the higher psychiatric morbidity scale ratings fared the best in the six-session, short-term treatment. The remaining 13 studies are nonsignificant.

Many diverse studies contributed to our findings. It was our hope to discern differences in methods or samples for the 14 positively significant versus the 13 nonsignificant. Several types of interstudy differences were examined: (*a*) The severity of illness in the sample for each study: No obvious differences appear. (*b*) The use of difference scores versus improvement ratings

TABLE 1 *Condensed summary of main trends—number of quantitative studies with significant versus nonsignificant relationship between predictor and outcome measures*

Main trend	Number of studies	
	Significant[a]	Nonsignificant
Patient Factors before Treatment		
Adequacy of Personality Functioning:		
Integration, mental health, etc.	15 { 6; 1−	8 } 13
Miscellaneous test findings	2	0
Ego strength	4	5
TAT adequacy	2	0
Rorschach Prognostic Rating Scale	6	3
Rorschach (general)	11	7
Diagnosis, especially absence of psychotic trends	7	0
Motivation	4	1
Expectation	3	2
Intelligence	7	2
Other Intellectual Skills	3	1
Anxiety	$5\frac{1}{2}$	$3\frac{1}{2}$
Presence of other affects	5	0
Human relations interest	4	0
Age	4; 2−	5
Social class	2; 1−	2
Education	5	2
Student status	3	1
Previous psychotherapy	0	3
Patient Factors as Judged from the Treatment		
Likability	2	0
Experiencing	6	0
Therapist Factors Before Treatment		
Experience	8	4
Skill	3	2
Interest pattern and attitudes	6; 1−	2
Therapist Factors Judged from the Treatment		
Empathy (judged from tape recordings)	3	3
Other empathy measures	4	2
The Match between Patient and Therapist		
Similarities between patient and therapist	10; 1−; 1 curvilinear	3
Treatment Factors		
Time-limited versus unlimited treatment	2; 1−	5
Number of sessions	20	2
Waiting time before beginning psychotherapy	3	0

[a] Minus sign indicates number of negatively significant studies.

as a criterion: Difference scores *may* make positive findings less likely (see section entitled Evaluation of Criteria, Item 5). Three of the four studies using difference scores are in the nonsignificant group (Cartwright & Roth, 1957; Klein, 1960; Luborsky, 1962); one just reaches significance (Fiske, Cartwright, & Kirtner, 1964). (*c*) The type of initial assessment in the predictors: The Appendix studies are grouped according to the type of assessment—observer ratings (14), miscellaneous (2), Barron Ego Strength (9), TAT (2). No obvious differences appear within those subgroups.

The Rorschach test results were summarized separately because of the difficulty of knowing exactly what was being measured. Among the prognostic tests, the Rorschach Prognostic Rating Scale (RPRS) of Klopfer, Kirkner, Wisham, and Baker (1951) turned out to be a big surprise. In nine studies the RPRS had been applied before therapy; in six of the nine, a significant positive relationship emerged; high RPRS is associated with improvement in psychotherapy. These Rorschach scores are weighted combinations of six variables thought to be related to adequacy of personality functioning. This result, therefore, is consistent with the significant studies under the heading of General Personality Functioning (described previously). Of 18 other studies in which the Rorschach test had been used less systematically (i.e., conceptual relationship of variables to initial personality functioning and to outcome of treatment was not considered), 11 were found where test signs predicted outcome. Since the Rorschach test can yield many different scores, these results are less impressive than those of the single RPRS.

Two main conclusions emerge. First, the initial level of the patient's illness is a crucial factor: *Initially sicker patients do not improve as much with psychotherapy as the initially healthier do.* (Possibly, as Astrup believes—Astrup and Noreik, 1966—the patient's qualities are even more important for his improvement than the psychotherapy or other treatment he receives.) Second, *some improvement is shown by patients, whatever their initial level of functioning* (e.g., Klein, 1960; Luborsky, 1962). A safe prediction, therefore, is that any method of psychotherapy in which one person tries to help another will usually yield gains for the one designated to be the patient. (A story with a similar point has been persistently retold with glee around the Menninger Hospital: A visitor once asked the receptionist, "How can you tell the patients from the doctors? They all look alike." The receptionist replied, "The patients get better.")

Diagnosis (*especially absence of psychotic trends*)

The implications here are similar to the findings under the section Personality Functioning. In various samples, the more serious diagnoses (involving the terms schizophrenia, psychotic trends, or psychosis) are associated with less improvement in psychotherapy (Gottschalk et al., 1967; Hamburg, Bibring, Fisher, Stanton, Wallerstein, Weinstock, & Haggard, 1967; Harris & Christiansen, 1946; Karush, Daniels, O'Connor, & Stern, 1968;

Katz, Lorr, & Rubinstein, 1958; Stephens & Astrup, 1963; Tolman & Mayer, 1957). Within the schizophrenic groups, the severity distinction of process versus nonprocess has a similar predictive power for the outcome of psychotherapy (Stephens & Astrup, 1963).

Motivation and/or expectation

The common clinical opinion of the value of good motivation for treatment is upheld by four out of five studies (R. Cartwright & Lerner, 1963; Conrad, 1952; Schroeder, 1960; Strupp, Wallach, Jenkins, & Wogan, 1963). The nonsignificant study is by Siegel and Fink (1962). Patient's expectation of change is similarly predictive in three out of five studies (Goldstein & Shipman, 1961; Lipkin, 1954; Uhlenhuth & Duncan, 1968); two are nonsignificant (Brady, Reznikoff, & Zeller, 1960; Goldstein, 1960).

Although *amount* of motivation and/or expectation tends to be positively related to outcome, type of motivation is not predictive (Gliedman, Stone, Frank, Nash, & Imber, 1957); surprisingly, patients with congruent motives for treatment do not fare better than those with noncongruent motives (e.g., treatment should change their life situation, rather than themselves). Similarly, *type* of transference expectation is not predictive (Apfelbaum, 1958).

In two studies (Goodman, 1960; Rosenbaum, Friedlander, & Kaplan, 1956), payment of a fee is related to gains. Motivation may be implicated—payment of a fee may (*a*) increase motivation, or (*b*) presuppose good motivation. Another condition may hold: Those who are able to pay a fee may have other social assets which make treatment for them more auspicious (see section entitled Social Achievements).

Intelligence

Seven of the nine studies using different ways of estimating intelligence show that *patients with higher initial intelligence performed better in psychotherapy*. All but two of the nine studies are based on the Wechsler Intelligence Tests—either full-scale or four subtests. The significant studies are by Barron (1953a); Casner (1950); Fiske et al. (1964); Miles, Barrabee, and Finesinger (1951); Rioch and Lubin (1959); Rosenberg (1954); Zigler and Phillips (1961). Harris and Christiansen (1946) and Rosenbaum et al. (1956) show a nonsignificant relationship.

Three out of four more diverse estimates of intellectual skills are in the same direction (Barry & Fulkerson, 1966; McNair, Lorr, Young, Roth, & Boyd, 1964; Sullivan, Miller, & Smelser, 1958). One obvious way of understanding these findings is that psychotherapy requires learning, and those who learn most readily do better.

Affect

We found nine studies of psychotherapy in which initial anxiety level was assessed. In five, a significant relationship was obtained between high initial anxiety and a criterion of change (Gallagher, 1954; Gottschalk et al., 1967; Hamburg et al., 1967; Kirtner & Cartwright, 1958a; Luborsky, 1962). Nonsignificant studies were Bergin and Jasper (1969); Distler, May, and Tuma (1964); Katz et al. (1958); Roth, Rhudick, Shaskan, Slobin, Wilkinson, and Young (1964). In one "nonsignificant" study (Distler et al., 1964), a positive significant relationship was found for women and a nonsignificant one for men. In sum, five and "one-half" studies confirm that *patients with high anxiety at the initial evaluation or at beginning of treatment are the ones likely to benefit from psychotherapy*. High initial anxiety probably indicates a readiness, or at least an openness, for change.

Under the heading of Other Affects we have listed five other studies suggesting that it is not only initial anxiety which is a good prognostic sign, but the presence of any strong affect, such as depression (Astrup & Noreik, 1966; Conrad, 1952; Gallagher, 1954; Gottschalk et al., 1967; Uhlenhuth & Duncan, 1968). Patients with flattening of affect have a poor prognosis (Astrup & Noreik, 1966). These findings are not unique for psychotherapy; they appear to be a good prognostic sign for a variety of other treatments; for example, treatment by drugs (Beecher, 1959) or, possibly, no formal treatment at all, as in the case of acute depression. The overall conclusion about affects is that *almost any affect is better than no affect, and that anxiety and depression are probably the two "best" initial affects*. The presence of these strong affects may indicate the patient is in pain and asking for help. The absence of affect very likely goes along with a state in which the patient is not reaching out for help, or has given up.

In two studies the number of complaints on the Symptom Check List was found to be a positive sign (Stone, Frank, Nash, & Imber, 1961; Truax, Wargo, Frank, Imber, Battle, Hoehn-Saric, Nash, & Stone, 1966)—the implication may be the same, that the patient is in pain and asking for help. The Symptom Check List score is probably not primarily a "severity of illness" measure; it is best classified here along with anxiety and other affects.

Ethnocentrism

Ethnocentrism is a significantly negative predictor in two out of three studies (Barron, 1953a; Tougas, 1954; it is insignificant in Rosen, 1954).

Human relations interest

Four studies show this to be a promising characteristic of patients in psychotherapy (Gottschalk et al., 1967; Isaacs & Haggard, 1966; Rayner & Hahn, 1964; Rosenbaum et al., 1956).

Coping or defensive style

Defensiveness was shown in two out of three studies to be negatively related to improvement in psychotherapy (Strupp et al., 1963; Zolik & Hollon, 1960; with one nonsignificant—Raskin, 1949).

Somatic concern

Somatic and health concerns were shown to be negative indicators in two studies (Rosenberg, 1954; Stone et al., 1961).

Self-awareness, insight, and sensitivity

Three out of five studies showed these qualities were positively related to outcome (Conrad, 1952; Rosenberg, 1954; Zolik & Hollon, 1960—nonsignificant were the studies of Raskin, 1949; Rosenbaum et al., 1956).

Age

Older patients tend to have a slightly poorer prognosis. Of 11 studies, 4 show that younger patients profited more from psychotherapy (Casner, 1950; Hamburg et al., 1967; Stone et al., 1961; Zigler & Phillips, 1961). Nonsignificant results were obtained by Bloom (1956), D. S. Cartwright (1955), Gaylin (1966), Gottschalk et al. (1967), Seeman (1954). The two negative studies that found older patients did better were in the context of a limited age range (Conrad, 1952; Knapp, Levin, McCarter, Wermer, & Zetzel, 1960).

Sex

In five studies men and women have about the same chances of benefiting from psychotherapy (D. S. Cartwright, 1955; Gaylin, 1966; Hamburg et al., 1967; Knapp et al., 1960; May, 1968). In two studies, however, the women did better (Mintz, Luborsky, & Auerbach, 1971; Seeman, 1954).

Social achievements

In general, *patients with higher social achievements are better suited for psychotherapy*. This would be expected, because people who can achieve in spheres requiring social skills should also do so in psychotherapy. Various social achievements have been examined: socioeconomic (social class), occupational, educational, and marital. Of these, educational achievement has most supporting studies (Bloom, 1956; Casner, 1950; Hamburg et al., 1967; McNair et al., 1964; Sullivan et al., 1958). Of the two nonsignificant studies (Knapp et al., 1960; Rosenbaum et al., 1956), the study by Knapp et al. was based on uniformly well-educated psychoanalytic patients.

Combinations of these achievements into comprehensive measures of social competence have been successful predictors of improvement with psychotherapy (Stone et al., 1961) and with hospitalization (Zigler & Phillips, 1961).

Student status

Three studies (D. S. Cartwright, 1955; Casner, 1950; Rogers & Dymond, 1954) found that student status is associated with improvement; one found that it makes no difference (Gaylin, 1966). The facilitation provided by student status is probably a function of the similarity felt between the patient and therapist and/or the fact that being a student *implies* social competence. The same reasoning may partly explain the finding that professional people, including patients who are analytic candidates or psychiatrists, are more likely to complete treatment than the general population patients (Hamburg et al., 1967).

Previous psychotherapy

Findings in three studies (Hamburg et al., 1967; Klein, 1960; McNair et al., 1964) agree that previous psychotherapy makes no significant difference in predicting the outcome of a patient's current psychotherapy! It is hard to explain; it would seem natural to expect that previous response would predict future response.

Patient factors (judged from the sessions)

This obviously is a profitable area. Most of the studies involving judgments of the early phases of the treatment turned out to be predictive of the final outcome. There is a higher percentage of successful prediction on this basis—a sample of the patient's actual behavior in treatment—than on the basis of the patient's state *before* he begins treatment.

Likability has been rated from segments of tape recordings and is significantly related to the outcome of treatment (Stoler, 1963, 1966). Under the heading Patient Factors Before Treatment, another study is positive (Strupp et al., 1963), and one is nonsignificant (Gottschalk et al., 1967). Patient "attractiveness for psychotherapy" described earlier may well be a similar concept, and was significantly related to outcome. In general, liking a patient may tend to be associated with the inclination to believe the patient is attractive as a patient for psychotherapy, and these judgments *may* actually provide favorable conditions for growth, as Rosenthal and Jacobson (1968) found for school children.

Much successful prediction has come from Rogers' process scale composed of seven strands which, in his first paper on the topic (Rogers, 1959), he called relationship to feeling, degree of incongruence, manner of experiencing, communication of self, construing of experiencing, relationship to problems, and manner of relating to others. They have been altered slightly in later studies by Rogers and his students. One of the most repeatedly successful is manner of experiencing (a term first suggested by Gendlin). It implies that the patient is capable of experiencing deeply and immediately, *and* of being reflectively aware about this feeling. A low score indicated the patient was remote from his experiencing and unable to understand its implicit meanings. Scales have been developed by Gendlin, Beebe, Cassens, and Oberlander (1968) and others which show fairly good interjudge reliability; the scales are based upon very brief segments—4 minutes of the treatment session. Of the six studies involved with the Experiencing scale, all are positively and significantly related to the patient's improvement (Gendlin, Jenney, & Shlien, 1960; Gendlin et al., 1968; Kirtner, Cartwright, Robertson, & Fiske, 1961; Tomlinson, 1967; Tomlinson & Hart, 1962; Walker, Rablen, & Rogers,

1960). The findings by Gendlin et al. (1968) that patients do better who *start* treatment with a higher level of "process" is consistent with the major trend for greater assets before treatment to be a positive portent—"the rich get richer."

A long series of studies involving the discomfort-relief quotient (Dollard & Mowrer, 1953) was based on objective word counts of patients' statements. Some of the studies showed that decrease in the discomfort-relief quotient (increased comfort) indicates successful outcome of psychotherapy, and some were nonsignificant (Mowrer, Hunt, & Kogan, 1953).

II. Therapist Factors

Therapist factors (assessed apart from the session)

Only three topics among the variety of explored therapist factors have noteworthy relationships to outcome: the therapist's level of experience, his skill, and his interest pattern.

Thirteen studies were found dealing with level of experience. Eight of these showed a significant positive relationship to the patient's improvement (Barrett-Lennard, 1962; Cartwright & Lerner, 1963; Cartwright & Vogel, 1960; Katz et al., 1958; Knapp et al., 1960; Miles et al., 1951; Myers & Auld, 1955; Rice, 1965). The four studies with nonsignificant findings were Fiske et al., 1964; Grigg, 1961; Mindess, 1953; Sullivan et al., 1958. One study was difficult to classify because it showed that inexperienced therapists performed well, but only under limited circumstances (R. Cartwright & Lerner, 1963).

In three of five studies, therapist's skill was shown to positively influence recovery (Klein, 1965; Nash, Hoehn-Saric, Battle, Stone, Imber, & Frank, 1965; Nichols & Beck, 1960; insignificant were Imber, Frank, Nash, Stone, & Gliedman, 1957; Muench, 1965).

Several studies on therapists' interest patterns, mainly using the Strong Vocational Interest Blank with a key developed by Betz (1963) for Type A therapists (problem-solving approach) versus Type B therapists (mechanical interests) showed significant relationships to patient improvement for schizophrenic patients. Most of the reports seem based upon the same or successive samples of Phipps Psychiatric Clinic patients and therapists (e.g., Betz & Whitehorn, 1956; Whitehorn & Betz, 1954, 1957), except for the study by Lichtenberg (1958; also described by Betz, 1963) which was based upon a sample from Sheppard and Enoch Pratt Hospital. However, McNair, Callahan, and Lorr (1962) found a reverse effect: Neurotic patients of Type B therapists improved significantly more than neurotic patients of Type A therapists. However, a more careful evaluation needs to be made of the Type A versus Type B therapist distinction. The replication by Stephens and Astrup (1963, 1965), using the same Phipps Clinic patient sample but controlling for form of schizophrenia, revealed no relationship between Type A or B therapists and discharge status. Also, multivariate taxonomic studies suggest more than two value types (cf. Welkowitz, Cohen, & Ortmeyer, 1967).

Aside from predicting the outcome of psychotherapy, the A–B dichotomy has some substance, as shown by its correlations with other dimensions (see reviews by Carson, 1967 and Silverman, 1967). A-type therapists, for example, are more field dependent than B-type therapists on the Witkin Rod and Frame test (Pollock & Kiev, 1963).

Therapist factors (judged from the sessions)

Empathy may be a promising therapist variable, as judged from psychotherapy sessions (either by judges from the tape and transcript, or by patient or therapist from their experiences with each other in the therapy session). It is significant in three out of six studies when rated from brief tape samples of the session (Rogers, Gendlin, Kiesler, & Truax, 1967; Truax, 1963; Truax et al., 1966), but the same or other measures of empathy are nonsignificant in studies by Bergin and Jasper (1969), Rogers et al. (1967), Mintz et al. (1971). In four out of six findings based on ratings by the patient and the therapist, empathy is significant (Barrett-Lennard, 1962; Cartwright & Lerner, 1963; Feitel, 1968; Lesser, 1961) and nonsignificant for other measures (in Cartwright & Lerner, 1963; Lesser, 1961). When combined with Warmth and Genuineness, the predictive power of empathy is increased (Truax et al., 1966), and similarly with other variables in the "Relationship Inventory" (Barrett-Lennard, 1962).

The implication seems clear: *The therapist's empathy (and other related qualities) facilitates the patient's gains from psychotherapy.* But what seems like a clear implication, on closer inspection may prove to be more complicated. The causal direction of the relationship may not be one-way: Patients who are improving, or who reveal to the therapist their capacity to improve, may elicit from him more empathy, or may attribute to him more empathy!

III. The Match Between Patient and Therapist (Assessed Apart from the Sessions)

Fourteen studies deal with some form of similarity between therapist and patient. Nine show a positive relationship: greater similarity is associated with better outcome (Graham, 1960; Hollingshead & Redlich, 1958; Landfield & Nawas, 1964; Lesser, 1961; Sapolsky, 1965; Schonfield, Stone, Hoehn-Saric, Imber, & Pande, 1969; Sheehan, 1953; Tuma & Gustad, 1957; Welkowitz et al., 1967). Some measures were not significant: similarity of profile shape on the MMPI (Carson & Llewellyn, 1966; Lichtenstein, 1966) and *Q*-sort similarity of patient's and therapist's ideal selves (Hunt, Ewing, LaForge, & Gilbert, 1959). One report also contained a significant negative relationship between similarity of patient's and therapist's self-perceptions and progress in treatment (Lesser, 1961), and one a curvilinear relationship for MMPI profile shapes (Carson &

Heine, 1962). The variety of forms of positive similarity includes social class, interests, values, and compatibility of orientation to interpersonal relations. A feeling of similarity seems to provide a more significant relationship between the therapist and patient and, therefore, a better outcome to treatment.

IV. Treatment Factors

Different types of treatment probably have differential effects, but it is hard to know what type of treatment has what effect. The large array of quantitative studies contains only a few of each treatment type, and therefore offers only a few tentative trends:

1. Three studies compared individual versus group psychotherapy. Baehr (1954) found individual psychotherapy to be slightly superior to group psychotherapy, but Imber et al. (1957) found no differences at the end of 6 months of treatment; Stone et al. (1961) found none 5 years later; Pearl (1955) found group treatment superior. No generalization is therefore possible.

2. Three studies found the *combination* of individual and group psychotherapy was better than either individual or group psychotherapy alone (Baehr, 1954; Conrad, 1952; Peck, 1949).

3. Surprisingly few reports in the literature compare the effectiveness of psychotherapy and pharmacotherapy. The three studies we found of schizophrenic patients (Fairweather, Simon, Gebhard, Weingarten, Holland, Sanders, Stone, & Reahl, 1960; Grinspoon, Ewalt, & Shader, 1968; May, 1968) suggest that psychotherapy combined with pharmacotherapy is more effective than psychotherapy alone, but in most ways not more effective than pharmacotherapy alone. Similar trends emerged from studies of *neurotic* patients (Daneman, 1961; Gibbs, Wilkins, & Lauterbach, 1957; Lorr, McNair, Weinstein, Michaux, & Raskin, 1961; Lorr, McNair, & Weinstein, 1963; Rickels, Cattell, Weise, Gray, Yee, Mallin, & Aaronson, 1966; Roth et al., 1964), but this latter group is less well-controlled and the role of psychotherapy as a treatment method was limited. In all of these latter studies the treatment, generally on a once-a-week basis, did not exceed 8 weeks.

School of treatment usually made no measurable difference, according to a handful of studies where the most frequent comparisons involved client-centered, psychoanalytic, and Adlerian therapy (R. Cartwright, 1966; Heine, 1953; Shlien, Mosak, & Driekers, 1962; Tougas, 1954).

It has been thought—at least since Otto Rank—that treatments which are structured from the outset as time-limited, might perform as well as time-unlimited treatment. Most of the research so far has shown no significant difference between the two time conditions (Frank, Gliedman, Imber, Stone, & Nash, 1959; Henry & Shlien, 1958; Pascal & Zax, 1956; Shlien, 1957; Shlien et al., 1962).

In 20 of 22 studies of essentially time-unlimited treatment, *the length of treatment was positively related to outcome; the longer the duration of treatment or the more sessions, the better the outcome!* It is a temptation to conclude—

and it may be an accurate conclusion—that if psychotherapy is a good thing, then the more the better. Other interpretations, however, may also fit: (*a*) Patients who are getting what they need, stay in treatment longer; those who are not, drop out sooner. (*b*) Therapists may overestimate positive change in patients who have been in treatment longer. A complimentary trend may also operate—therapists often assume some minimum number of sessions are needed before real change can occur, so that early dropouts tend to get poor outcome ratings.

In three out of three studies, a long and mandatory wait between the time of applying for psychotherapy and beginning it is negatively related to outcome (Gordon & Cartwright, 1954; Roth et al., 1964; Uhlenhuth & Duncan, 1968). Two main implications may be drawn from these results: First, the practice of using the patient as his own control by having him wait for psychotherapy and retesting him during the waiting period has in itself a negative impact on his future psychotherapy. The waiting experience may be a negative one and therefore cannot be accepted as a neutral, no-therapy period. Second, clinics with long waiting lists should be aware of these studies, and should try to provide service close to the time the patient applies for it.

Comparison of results with those of "drop-out versus stay-in psychotherapy"

Studies in which the criterion for outcome is "dropping out versus staying in treatment" have been excluded from the review, since there is no *explicit* evidence that this variable is consistently related to the amount of gain a patient makes. There is, however, some indirect evidence from studies showing that *length of treatment* is positively related to gain from psychotherapy.

Fulkerson and Barry (1961) have reviewed this area, but the only extensive survey is by Brandt (1965) of factors influencing patients to drop out. It provides some interesting comparisons with the present review. Brandt concluded there is little uniformity in the data presented, the variables controlled, the variables investigated, the base lines, the definitions, and the findings reported in 25 studies dealing with premature terminators among adult patients in long-term individual outpatient psychotherapy. Of the 29 variables investigated by 18 researchers and research teams (in Brandt's review), only sex, age, and marital status consistently did not differentiate between dropouts and remainers. The only variables which consistently differentiated between the two groups were personality characteristics. The personality characteristics and methods for determining them differed widely from one study to another.

Brandt made no attempt to compare his findings with those for predicting outcome of psychotherapy in general; nor did he explain the consistencies in the data he presented. In his table summarizing the dropout studies which do or do not differentiate between remainers and terminators for 18 studies and 29 predictors, he did not note that for education, five of the seven studies showed that higher education goes along with staying in treatment—as is noted in our review. For occupation, four of the seven studies which mentioned occupational status showed a positive relationship to remaining—almost the same as in our review. Marital status appears in six studies; in all six there is no differentiation between the two groups; this is also similar to our review in which four of the five studies showed no significant difference in marital status. For personality characteristics, seven out of seven differentiate. (Brandt does not indicate which personality characteristics were mentioned most frequently.) For the Rorschach, four out of six studies differentiate; this is similar to our review. Seven out of seven studies in which age is mentioned showed no differentiation between remainers and terminators—this is not similar to our review, which often indicates age to be inversely related to amount of gain from treatment. There was no difference between the sexes in two out of two studies; this is somewhat the same as in our review.

Lorr, Katz, and Rubenstein (1958) reported the cross-validation of a test battery (Terminator-Remainer Battery) designed to predict early termination of psychotherapy. The Terminator-Remainer battery consists of subtests taken from the Manifest Anxiety Scale, the Behavior Disturbance Scale, and the *F* Scale, as well as sociability, ideal-actual self, education, vocabularly, and motivation (therapist's rating). Remainers have a history of being less impulsive—with less antisocial behavior and more anxiety, more self-criticality, and less inclination to endorse rigid irrational beliefs. They are also more retiring in interpersonal relationships, better educated, have better vocabularies, and are considered by therapists to be more highly motivated for psychotherapy. Three studies of Terminator-Remainer battery have had useful predictive power for a veteran population. However, few of the ratings or tests (as compared with background factors) added significantly to the Terminator-Remainer battery. The one that added most was the therapist's rating of patient's motivation for psychotherapy. Remainers and terminators seemed to be two separate patient populations who reacted differently in psychotherapy. The Terminator-Remainer battery and other measures can identify many in these two groups. Therapists have some influence, but not a large one, on the proportions of both populations they can hold in treatment.

In conclusion, many of these characteristics of remainers versus dropouts seem similar to those from our review of factors influencing outcome of psychotherapy.

Overall Conclusions About the Main Factors Influencing Outcome of Psychotherapy

Main findings from the survey

It is easy to become overimpressed with the limits of the group of quantitative studies by the limits of the individual studies. Most of the single studies are weak reeds because of their small sample size, small number, unreliability of measures, and brevity of treatment. Although we may sometimes be steered the wrong way because all the studies on certain predictors may be subject to the same error, in taking them together and trying to discern agreements and disagreements, some consistencies emerge which probably will stand up to further testing. *It adds fiber to a finding when it is resilient enough to appear in different groups and by different assessment methods.* When there have been divergent results on the same qualities, it has sometimes—though less often than anticipated—been possible to review the studies and locate the probable responsible agent in the nature of the patient groups or criterion measures. Much more of this type of reviewing remains to be done.

The list in Table 1 contains the essence of the quantitative research on the predictors of benefiting from psychotherapy. It may have value as a guide in the selection of patients and therapists, as well as for elucidating the process of psychotherapy. A brief formulation of the necessary ingredients for psychotherapy, based on Table 1, follows:

1. Most research conclusions have been about the patient, especially of the patient as he was *before* treatment: the more adequate his general personality functioning, the better his future course in psychotherapy. Similarly, the higher his intelligence and other intellectual skills, the better his future in psychotherapy. Patients most likely to succeed in treatment come highly motivated for it and expect it to help. The treatment is best begun at a time when the patient is upset and shows it by high levels of anxiety and distress and the presence of other affects such as depression. Younger patients often are more pliable and make more changes. Higher educational attainment and other social achievements probably are in part an expression of adequate general personality functioning, intelligence, and motivation. During treatment patients do better who are likable and capable of deeply experiencing and reflecting on their experiencing.

2. Much less has been established about the therapist: his experience level and skill, as well as his ability to show empathy during the session, seem important.

3. The match between the patient and therapist is facilitated by similarities in values, attitudes, interests, and social class. The patient's intellectual and social attainments may increase his sense of having more in common with the therapist.

4. The comparative studies of type, methods, and schools of treatment are insufficient; those that exist are inconsistent. Treatment factors, therefore, have had little established about them (possibly such treatment factors are less potent than patient and therapist factors), except that those patients do better who start treatment when they apply for it (and presumably are more ready for it) and persist in it longer. Some studies indicate that time-limited therapy does not do worse than time-unlimited, and that group therapy added to individual therapy does better than either one separately. Psychotherapy with pharmacotherapy tends to be slightly more effective than psychotherapy alone, but in most ways not more effective than pharmacotherapy alone—especially for schizophrenic patients.

Some promising predictive combinations

It seems a safe, overall conclusion that factors in the patient and therapist, and in the patient-therapist interaction, *combine* in some way to eventuate in the gains of psychotherapy. Such interactions have been shown very neatly for pharmacology studies where the giver of the drug, the expectations of the patient, and the patient's qualities are as important as the nature of the drug itself in determining the effects of the drug (Rickels, 1968). Nevertheless, only a small part of the psychotherapy research has tried combinations of predictors:

1. The section Patient Factors Before Treatment points to the same conclusion suggested by Luborsky (1962): *High affect (anxiety and other forms of distress) with high integration or ego strength form a good combination of prognostic conditions for change through psychotherapy.*

2. A combination of high patient motivation with high therapist empathy was found to be especially advantageous by Cartwright and Lerner (1963).

3. Gottschalk et al. (1967) constructed a successful regression equation for predicting the outcome of short-term treatment. It is composed of a combination of severity of illness, level of anxiety, and capacity for object relations.

4. Truax et al. (1966) found increased success in predicting improvement by combining empathy, warmth, and genuineness.

5. A multidimensional prognostic index of 32 items was developed both on clinical grounds and on the basis of this review and is being tested in several populations (Auerbach & Luborsky). It should be useful for clinicians who wish to try this combination of promising variables as part of their evaluations of patients for psychotherapy. No such index has ever been constructed for nonpsychotic patients. It will be informative to compare its predictive power with indexes for psychotic patients (Lorr, Wittman, & Schanberger, 1951; Thorne, 1952), and with indexes for predicting susceptibility and recovery from physical illness (Thurlow, 1967).

6. In no studies of nonpsychotic patients has there been adequate representation of both the therapist and patient variables; therefore no estimates can be made of the relative contribution of the patient versus therapist to the variance of outcome. Probably the sicker the patient, the less impact a therapist can have—assuming the generalization that openness to constructive change varies with severity of illness. However, it seems unlikely that the study by Astrup and Noreik (1966) on psychotic patients applies equally to nonpsychotic ones—that it is almost entirely the patient's initial state which determines his future course either with or without psychotherapy!

Comparison of the quantitative survey with clinical wisdom

Clinical knowledge has assembled much more wisdom than the quantitative has managed to garner. Although clinical lore has a higher percentage of error, it addresses itself to the array of issues which the clinician must confront now. What follows are a few of the outstanding discrepancies in the two literatures:

1. Quantitative studies, in their stress upon the qualities of the patient and the relationship with the therapist, give far less weight to the technique of treatment than do clinical writings. Accuracy of interpretation has had relatively little quantitative work done on it, except for the work on empathy (which may or may not be the same)—and here the accuracy of the empathy has not been adequately explored. It is damaging to some of the research on empathy that estimates of therapist's empathy can be reliably rated on the basis of the therapist's statements alone, independent of whether the judge has read what the patient has said (Truax, 1966).

2. The tremendous emphasis in the clinical literature on the importance of providing insight to the patient has had no quantitative investigation in relation to outcome variables, except for two studies of initial insight which gave divergent results: Raskin (1949), Zolik and Hollon (1960).

3. Nothing exists in the quantitative literature on qualities of the patient which make him amenable to various forms of treatment. The clinical literature is full of such discussions, which are neatly summarized by Wallerstein et al. (1956). A frequent reason for conducting a diagnostic evaluation is to decide on the patient's suitability for psychoanalysis versus other forms of treatment. There are dozens of clinical articles on how to make this judgment, but no quantitative ones. At the present time the best conclusion from the quantitative literature is that those patients who are most suitable for psychotherapy are also the ones most suitable for psychoanalysis.

4. A large part of the clinical literature is based on long-term treatment; almost all the quantitative research is on short-term treatment.

Methodological Evaluation of the Studies

Evaluation of criterion

1. The most frequent criterion measure, and usually the only one, is the therapist's gross improvement rating. The fact that only one criterion measure is used is a significant limitation; the fact that it is an improvement rating rather than a raw difference score is psychometrically advantageous. On the other hand, the fact that it is provided by the therapist, a committed participant in the therapeutic exchange, is a distinct disadvantage. At too many points where a relationship is found (e.g., for empathy or length of treatment), the causal relationship may be the reverse of what is supposed, or due to other factors. Although both the therapist and patient may be biased judges, their estimates have some face validity and should be used along with the estimates of outside judges.

It seems unlikely that *improvement* ratings (whether by therapist, patient, or outside observer) should be given up (in favor of the "residual gain scores" or "target symptom approach" to be described). At first glance, improvement ratings seem poor because the judge can hardly be expected to recall the exact level at which the patient started as a base for estimating the improvement.

A difference score corrected for initial level might seem to be the only answer. On soberer reflection, however, one should look more kindly upon the improvement score because the judge can give his own weight to the *quality* of the improvement (and he can be reminded of the initial level) while any difference score *might* be more arbitrary.

2. Where several criterion measures are available, correlations among them are usually low and often not statistically significant. The only criterion measure which tends to have consistent significant correlations with other criterion measures is the therapist's ratings of success or improvement (e.g., Fiske et al., 1964). The fact that it is the *therapist's* rating of improvement which is most used is advantageous from this point of view, but see paragraph 1 of this section.

3. Since many different kinds of changes occur in psychotherapy and measures of these are often not highly correlated, we cannot speak of *the* predictors of change in psychotherapy. According to Fiske et al. (1964), four main change factors are identifiable: favorable self-evaluation, adequacy as measured by TAT, therapist's perception of change, and patient's reported symptoms. A predictor of one kind of change may not and probably will not predict another kind of change. We have not taken this into account in the summary of the number of significant studies, but have tried to consider this in the discussion. (Humor about psychiatry has long recognized this: There was the man who had just paid $50 to a psychiatrist to cure his inferiority complex—that is, unfavorable self-evaluation criterion—who left the session and on his way home got fined $50 for talking back to a policeman—that is, social-conformity criterion.)

4. Dropping out *versus* staying in psychotherapy probably has some similarity to other outcome criteria such as therapist's rating of improvement, because: (*a*) The initial-state correlates of drop-out versus stay-in appear to be similar to those for improvement ratings, as shown in a preceding section, Comparison of Results of Drop-Out versus Stay-In Psychotherapy. (*b*) Drop-out versus stay-in is probably related to the number of sessions; the latter is highly correlated with the usual criteria of outcome. (*c*) Patients who drop out early are often viewed as not improving.

5. Few studies use as a criterion of change a "residual gain score," that is, scores from which the correlation of "pre" and "post" has been removed, and none allow for the effects of error components of scores on correlations. Instead, they use as a criterion an *improvement* or *success* rating, or sometimes raw difference scores. Those studies which use difference scores tend to obtain zero or negative correlations with predictors (Cartwright & Roth, 1957; Fiske et al., 1964; Luborsky, 1962).

The use of raw difference scores $D = Y - X$ ("post" minus "pre") is dubious on two grounds: First, the intent in D is to have a measure free of differences in "pre," that is, for r_{XD} to equal zero. Yet it is an algebraic necessity that r_{XD} not, in general, equal zero. Thus, D does not accomplish the purpose for which it is intended. Further, the "finding" that r_{XD} is negative is virtually mandated by the algebra, and moreover, this correlation is spurious in that both X and $D = Y - X$ share the same measurement error in X, resulting in the irony that the larger the error in X (the lower X's reliability), the larger (negative) is r_{XD}.

Second, the reliability of D scores is generally poor, thus attenuating all correlations or group differences which involve it. The use of residual difference scores, $Y \cdot X$, that is, Y from which X has been removed by linear regression (or, equivalently, the use of $D \cdot X$ "residual gain scores"), results in a score which correlates zero with X. Although this is an improvement over D scores, it removes the *observed* X out of *observed* Y (or D), whereas what is wanted, as Tucker, Damarin, and Messick (1966) argued, is *true* X out of *true* Y (or D). Their "base-free measure of change" $\hat{G}$ replaces observed scores with true scores in the residualization. Their very useful article gives formulas for the reliability of $\hat{G}$ scores, and the correlation of $\hat{G}$ with other single variables as well as other $\hat{G}$ scores. These formulas all require reliability coefficients for X, which is a most desirable bit of information, however the scores are to be used. On psychometric grounds, if any function of pre- and postscores is to be used as criterion methods, we would recommend $\hat{G}$.

6. Almost all of these studies are geared to predict the *amount* of change. However, Brenman (1952) observed that a small change in a crucial area may make a huge difference for a patient. If the criterion measure was a more tangible and reasonable one—for example, *the type of change the patient needs or desires*, the predictability of the criterion might be increased. Only a few studies have taken this direction of trying to predict changes in certain areas. The Johns Hopkins group is one of the few who tried to predict changes in "target symptoms" (Battle, Imber, Hoehn-Saric, Stone, Nash, & Frank, 1966).

7. Prediction might be more successful and more useful to the therapist when it is geared toward the prediction of the *types of problems that will occur in the course of the treatment*. The majority of the predictions made in the Menninger Foundation Psychotherapy Research Project were aimed toward prediction of behavior during treatment (Sargent, Horowitz, Wallerstein, & Appelbaum, 1968.) Unfortunately, final analyses of data are not yet complete.

8. Very few of the studies have follow-up assessment, that is, an assessment beyond the end of the psychotherapy. This is a deficiency because some patients do continue to change in the year or two following the termination of their psychotherapy. However, it is not a major deficit because correlations between end-of-treatment assessments and follow-up assessments tend to be high.

Predictor problems

1. Many studies make predictions from single predictors to a single criterion. Yet in making predictions clinically, we never rely on one predictor. A more desirable approach would be to use multiple predictors, moreover, to use them in multivariate form and in ways which facilitate the discovery of nonlinear and configurational relationships (Cohen, 1968). Of the 166 studies, only a few are moderately comprehensive in the *number* of predictive (and

criterion) variables; hardly any used multivariate data-analytic forms. In the comprehensive category are the University of Chicago Counseling Center Study by Rogers and Dymond (1954); Fiske et al. (1964); the series at Johns Hopkins Phipps Clinic, for instance, Frank et al. (1959); Gottschalk et al. (1967); Rogers et al. (1967); and the Menninger Study (Wallerstein et al., 1956).

2. Most of the studies, if they do have more than one predictor variable, do not include variables from *both* the patient and the therapist at the same time.

3. Much of what is considered to be prediction seems really to be an evaluation of the patient as he is now, with the expectation that he will be somewhat the same later as he is now. (It is like the story of the man who asked of his Rabbi, "How will life be for me if I move across the river?" The Rabbi asked, "Well, tell me; how is life for you now?" The man replied, "It is bitter." The Rabbi then forecast, "It will be bitter across the river.") There seems to be good reason for this; for example, McNair et al. (1964) found that initial score on seven measures is the best predictor of later score on the same measures. The experience of prediction in the Menninger Study (Luborsky, 1962) also suggests that the best estimate of where the patient will be at the end of therapy is to be made from a proper evaluation of where the patient is now, then adding to that level some moderate but not too large increase. (There is a tendency for the judges to expect that patients who are very sick will not gain as much as they do, and a tendency across all patients to expect more change to take place than actually does.)

4. The predictors and the setting of treatment often interact. This has been investigated systematically only in terms of predictors related to early release from mental hospitals (Cohen, 1968). Cohen found that a prognostic variable or set of variables depended on which other variables or sets were partialled out or controlled. Some variables (education, church attendance) are related to early release in opposite ways, from one hospital to another. Marital and hospitalization history variables are important predictors and are consistent across hospitals, as are some psychologist-rated admission symptom factors.

5. A successful prediction of change has to take into account the type of change that the patient and therapist are aiming for. Not taking this into account can lead to markedly different estimates of improvement or success of the treatment. One patient, for example, presented as his main target problem at the beginning of treatment a hopelessness, futility, and a suicidal inclination, all starting 6 months earlier with the loss of a friend. The same patient had become an overt homosexual during the preceding 3 to 4 years. If a change from homosexuality to heterosexuality were taken by the therapist or patient as the target goal, the treatment would legitimately have been considered a failure. As it was, the patient ended up the treatment still with homosexual tendencies, but feeling less hopeless and futile, and both the patient and therapist independently agreed upon the treatment's success.

6. What is the best way to evaluate these predictive variables? Are tests adequate, or can most of what is needed be evaluated through nontest

indicators? Most predictive variables can be evaluated by interviewing the patient, or through a sample of the early sessions of psychotherapy. A few can be evaluated through tests such as those for intelligence and for general personality functioning (e.g., Rorschach).

Other problems of method

1. Almost all of these studies are based on groups of patients who are diverse in type and in initial severity of illness. Predictions within more homogeneous subgroups should produce better results for some variables. On the other hand, other variables (e.g., age) might "wash out" in homogeneous subgroups. Luborsky (1962) and Luborsky and Schimek (1964) found that for the neurotic patients (rated above 50 on the Health–Sickness Rating Scale), anxiety seemed to serve as an impetus to improve, but for the borderline or psychotic patients (50 or below on the Health–Sickness Rating Scale), anxiety did not or could not serve this useful purpose. In the present review we have noted the predictors which apply to neurotic versus psychotic groups. Future prediction studies might succeed better by attempting to predict in even more homogeneous groups or, equivalently, by the use of Group × Predictor interaction variables. These are variables which account for criterion variance due to predictors correlating to different degrees in different groups (Cohen, 1968).

2. Almost all of these studies are based on relatively short-term treatment. Most of the treatment lengths are less than 30 to not more than 40 sessions. The only exceptions are psychoanalytic treatments (Klein, 1960; Knapp et al., 1960); a psychoanalytic practice survey (Hamburg et al., 1967); and the Menninger project (Wallerstein et al., 1956) which is still not complete partly because the research project itself becomes long-term when long-term treatment is being investigated. Essentially, then, the results of this review apply to short-term treatment. The factors influencing change might well be similar for long-term treatment, but we can find little evidence from the quantitative literature. One slight evidence for similarity of some results for short- and long-term treatment comes from Cartwright, Kirtner, and Fiske (1963). When they selected a group of patients who had 37 or more sessions and intercorrelated the criteria of change, the results were comparable to the entire sample—the change variables were no more highly intercorrelated for this subgroup.

3. *In virtually every study, there is no control over or systematic knowledge of the obtaining of counsel through other than psychotherapy.* In only a few studies is an effort made to find out about the use of other resources; for instance, the "situational variables" interview in the Menninger study (Sargent, Modlin, Faris, & Voth, 1959), or a questionnaire on seeking or receiving guidance from a variety of sources (Paul, 1967). In terms of drug research, it would be like testing responsiveness to a drug when allied substances are freely available and no record is kept of what else has been ingested by the subject.

4. In most studies no effort has been made to determine the *quality*

of the psychotherapy offered to each patient; it must vary widely. The earliest remedy for this was begun by Rogers' (1959) methods of scoring process.

5. If there is an inclination to publish significant results and not to publish insignificant ones, it would influence what we have available to survey (Cohen, 1962)! We have no evidence that this happens more frequently in this area than in others. The percentage of nonsignificant studies reported may be of interest—it is approximately 24%. From this we see that investigators *do* seem to report, and editors accept, nonsignificant results fairly frequently; how often they refrain is not known. But bias against nonsignificant results is known to exist. Also, the larger percentage of significant results might be expected—it is our faith that if an investigator has a hunch that a certain variable is significant, he is more apt to be right than wrong.

6. Individuals must differ in their readiness to change, either with or *without* treatment, or regardless of what type of treatment is offered. We have placed this point near the end of our review to emphasize it: Our survey is limited to the factors which influence change as a result of psychotherapy *only for those who have started psychotherapy. For most of the studies surveyed, therefore, it cannot be determined whether the type of individual who profits most would also have profited from another form of treatment, or from change-inducing experiences which usually are not designated as psychotherapy—or indeed from nothing more than the mysterious changes attributed to the passage of time.* The patient who presents himself with many assets for psychotherapy may be especially capable of achieving his ends by a variety of means—by a variety of psychotherapies, by medications, or by other resources such as talking with the bartender, with friends, with his minister, or by "keeping his own counsel." By applying the Prognostic Index for Psychotherapy or other prognostic instruments to groups treated by a variety of methods, we might learn more about the issue of general readiness to change.

The need for a new cross-validation study

The present review should lead directly to cross-validation studies of the predictors listed in Table 1. One of these is now in progress. It incorporates the essence of the promising predictors and some of the above methodological suggestions such as the use of long-term treatment, tape recordings of the treatment to permit intensive process scoring, and multivariate analysis of the predictors with various criteria of outcome.

Summary

An exhaustive survey has been made of quantitative studies of factors influencing the outcome of psychotherapy. The content conclusions are listed under the heading Overall Conclusions About the Main Factors Influencing Outcome of Psychotherapy; the methodological conclusions are listed under the heading Methodological Evaluation of the Studies—both in preceding sections of this review.

References

APFELBAUM, B. (1958). *Dimensions of Transference in Psychotherapy.* Berkeley and Los Angeles: University of California Press.

ASTRUP, C., & KOREIK, K. (1966). *Functional Psychoses, Diagnostic and Prognostic Models.* Springfield, Ill.: Charles C. Thomas.

BAEHR, G. O. (1954). The comparative effectiveness of individual psychotherapy, group psychotherapy, and a combination of these methods. *Journal of Consulting Psychology*, **18**, 179–183.

BARRETT-LENNARD, G. T. (1962). Dimensions of therapist response as causal factors in therapeutic change. *Psychological Monographs*, 76 (43, Whole No. 562).

BARRON, F. (1953). Some test correlates of response to psychotherapy. *Journal of Consulting Psychology*, **17**, 235–241.

BARRY, J., & FULKERSON, S. (1966). Chronicity and the prediction of duration and outcome of hospitalization from capacity measures. *Psychiatric Quarterly*, **40**, 104–121.

BATTLE, C., IMBER, S., HOEHN-SARIC, R., STONE, A., NASH, E., & FRANK, J. (1966). Target complaints as criteria of improvement. *American Journal of Psychotherapy*, **20**, 184–192.

BEECHER, H. K. (1959). *Measurement of Subjective Responses: Quantitative Effects of Drugs.* New York: Oxford University Press.

BERGIN, A., & GARFIELD, S. (eds.), (1970). *Handbook of Psychotherapy and Behavior Change.* New York: Wiley.

BERGIN, A. E., & JASPER, L. G. (1969). Correlates of empathy in psychotherapy: A replication. *Journal of Abnormal Psychology*, **74**, 477–481.

BETZ, B. J. (1963). Bases of therapeutic leadership in psychotherapy with the schizophrenic patient. *American Journal of Psychotherapy*, **17**, 196–212.

BETZ, B. J., & WHITEHORN, J. C. (1956). The relationship of the therapist to the outcome of therapy in schizophrenia. *American Psychiatric Association Psychiatric Research Reports*, **5**, 89–105.

BLOOM, B. L. (1956). Prognostic significance of the underproductive Rorschach. *Journal of Projective Techniques*, **20**, 336–371.

BRADY, J. P., ZELLER, W. W., & REZNIKOFF, M. (1959). Attitudinal factors influencing outcome of treatment of hospitalized psychiatric patients. *Journal of Clinical and Experimental Psychopathology*, **20**, 326–334.

BRANDT, L. W. (1965). Studies of "dropout" patients in psychotherapy: A review of findings. *Psychotherapy: Theory, Research and Practice*, **2**, 2–13.

BRENMAN, M. (1952). *On Teasing and Being Teased and the Problem of "Moral Masochism." Psychoanalytic Study of the Child.* New York: International Universities Press.

CARSON, R. C. (1967). *A* and *B* therapist "types"; A possible critical variable in psychotherapy. *The Journal of Nervous and Mental Disease*, **144**, 47–54.

CARSON, R. C., & HEINE, R. W. (1962). Similarity and success in therapeutic dyads. *Journal of Consulting Psychology*, **26**, 38–43.

CARSON, R. C., & LLEWELLYN, C. E. (1966). Similarity in therapeutic dyads. *Journal of Consulting Psychology*, **30**, 458.

CARTWRIGHT, D. S., (1955). Success in psychotherapy as a function of certain actuarial variables. *Journal of Consulting Psychology*, **19**, 357–363.

CARTWRIGHT, D. S., KIRTNER, W. L., & FISKE, D. W. (1963). Method factors in changes associated with psychotherapy. *Journal of Abnormal and Social Psychology*, **66**, 164–175.

CARTWRIGHT, D. S., ROBERTSON, R. J., FISKE, D. W., & KIRTNER, W. L. (1961). Length of therapy in relation to outcome and change in personal integration. *Journal of Consulting Psychology*, **25**, 84–88.

CARTWRIGHT, D. S., & ROTH, I. (1957). Success and satisfaction in psychotherapy. *Journal of Clinical Psychology*, **13**, 20–26.

CARTWRIGHT, R. D. (1966). A comparison of the response to psychoanalytic and client-centered psychotherapy. In L. Gottschalk & A. Auerbach (eds.), *Methods of Research in Psychotherapy.* New York: Appleton-Century-Crofts.

CARTWRIGHT, R. D., & LERNER, B. (1963). Empathy, need to change, and improvement and psychotherapy. *Journal of Consulting Psychology*, **27**, 138–144.

CARTWRIGHT, R. D., & VOGEL, J. L. (1960). A comparison of changes in psychoneurotic patients during matched periods of therapy and no therapy. *Journal of Consulting Psychology*, **24**, 121–127.

CASNER, D. (1950). Certain factors associated with success and failure in personal-adjustment counseling. *American Psychologist*, 5, 348.

COHEN, J. (1962). The statistical power of abnormal-social psychological research: A review. *Journal of Abnormal and Social Psychology*, **65**, 145–153.

COHEN, J. (1965). Some statistical issues in psychological research. In B. Wolman (ed.), *Handbook of Clinical Psychology*. New York: McGraw-Hill.

COHEN, J. (1968). Prognostic factors in functional psychosis: A study in multivariate methodology. *Transactions of the New York Academy of Sciences*, **30**, 833–840.

COHEN, J. (1968). Multiple regression as a general data-analytic system. *Psychological Bulletin*, **70**, 426–443.

CONRAD, D. C. (1952). An empirical study of the concept of psychotherapeutic success. *Journal of Consulting Psychology*, **16**, 92–97.

DANEMAN, E. A. (1961). Imipramine in office management of depressive reactions (a double blind clinical study). *Diseases of the Nervous System*, **22**, 213–217.

DISTLER, L. S., MAY, P. R., & TUMA, A. H. (1964). Anxiety and ego strength as predictors of response to treament in schizophrenic patients. *Journal of Consulting Psychology*, **28**, 170–177.

DOLLARD, J., & MOWRER, O. (1953). A method of measuring tension in written documents. In O. Mowrer (ed.), *Psychotherapy: Theory and Research*. New York: Ronald Press.

FAIRWEATHER, G., SIMON, R., GEBHARD, M., WEINGARTEN, E., HOLLAND, J., SANDERS, R., STONE, G., & REAHL, J. (1960). Relative effectiveness of psychotherapeutic programs: A multicriteria comparison of four programs for three different patient groups. *Psychological Monographs*, 74 (5, Whole No. 492), 26.

FISKE, D. W., CARTWRIGHT, D. S., KIRTNER, W. L. (1964). Are psychotherapeutic changes predictable? *Journal of Abnormal and Social Psychology*, 69, 418–426.

FRANK, J., GLIEDMAN, L., IMBER, S., STONE, A., & NASH, E. (1959). Patients' expectancies and relearning as factors determining improvement in psychotherapy. *American Journal of Psychiatry*, **115**, 961–968.

FREUD, S. (1913). On beginning the treatment. In James Strachey (ed.), *The Standard Edition of Complete Psychological Works of Sigmund Freud*. Vol. 12. London: Hogarth Press and Institute of Psychoanalysis, 1964.

FREUD, S. (1937). Analysis terminable and interminable. In James Strachey (ed.), *The Standard Edition of Complete Psychological Works of Sigmund Freud*. Vol. 23. London: Hogarth Press and Institute for Psychoanalysis, 1964.

FULKERSON, S. C., & BARRY, J. R. (1961). Methodology and research on the prognostic use of psychological tests. *Psychological Bulletin*, **58**, 177–204.

GALLAGHER, J. J. (1954). Test indicators for therapy prognosis. *Journal of Consulting Psychology*, **18**, 409–413.

GAYLIN, N. (1966). Psychotherapy and psychological health: A Rorschach function and structure analysis. *Journal of Consulting Psychology*, **30**, 494–500.

GENDLIN, E. T., BEEBE, J., CASSENS, J., & OBERLANDER, M. (1968). Focusing ability in psychotherapy, personality, and creativity. In J. M. Shlien, H. F. Hunt, J. D. Matarazzo, & C. Savage (eds.), *Research in Psychotherapy*. Vol. 3. Washington, D.C.: American Psychological Association.

GENDLIN, E. T., JENNEY, R., & SHLIEN, J. (1960). Counselor ratings of process and outcome in clinet-centered therapy. *Journal of Clinical Psychology*, **16**, 210–213.

GIBBS, J. J., WILKINS, B., & LAUTERBACH, C. G. (1957). A controlled clinical psychiatric study of chlorpromazine. *Journal of Clinical and Experimental Psychopathology: Quarterly Review of Psychiatry and Neurology*, **18**, 269–283.

Section III: Psychotherapy

GLIEDMAN, L., STONE, A., FRANK, J., NASH, E., & IMBER, S. (1957). Incentives for treatment related to remaining or improving in psychotherapy. *American Journal of Psychotherapy*, **11**, 589–598.

GOLDSTEIN, A. P. (1960). Therapist and client expectation of personality change in psychotherapy. *Journal of Counseling Psychology*, **7**, 180–184.

GOLDSTEIN, A. P., & SHIPMAN, W. G. (1961). Patient expectancies, symptom reduction, and aspects of the initial psychotherapeutic interview. *Journal of Clinical Psychology*, **14**, 129–133.

GOODMAN, N. (1960). Are there differences between fee and non-fee cases? *Social Work*, **5**, 46–52.

GORDON, T., & CARTWRIGHT, D. S. (1954). The effect of psychotherapy on certain attitudes towards others. In C. Rogers & R. F. Dymond (eds.), *Psychotherapy and Personality Change*. Chicago: University of Chicago Press.

GOTTSCHALK, L. A., MAYERSON, P., & GOTTLIEB, A. A. (1967). Prediction and evaluation of outcome in an emergency brief psychotherapy clinic. *Journal of Nervous and Mental Disease*, **144**, 77–96.

GRAHAM, S. R. (1960). The influence of therapist character structure upon Rorschach changes in the course of psychotherapy. *American Psychologist*, **15**, 415. (Abstract)

GRIGG, A. E. (1961). Client response to counselors at different levels of experience. *Journal of Counseling Psychology*, **8**, 217–225.

GRINSPOON, L., EWALT, J. R., & SHADER, R. (1968). Psychotherapy and pharmachotherapy in chronic schizophrenia. *American Journal of Psychiatry*, **124**, 1645–1652.

HAMBURG, D. A., BIBRING, G. L., FISHER, C., STANTON, A. H., WALLERSTEIN, R. S., WEINSTOCK, H. I., & HAGGARD, E. (1967). Report of Ad Hoc Committee on central fact-gathering data of the American Psychoanalytic Association. *Journal of the American Psychoanalytic Association*, **15**, 841–861.

HARRIS, R. E., & CHRISTIANSEN, C. (1946). Prediction of response to brief psychotherapy. *Journal of Psychology*, **21**, 269–284.

HEINE, A. M. (1953). A comparison of patients' reports on psychotherapeutic experience with psychoanalytic, nondirective and Adlerian therapists. *American Journal of Psychotherapy*, **7**, 16–25.

HENRY, W. E., & SHLIEN, J. (1958). Affective complexity and psychotherapy: some comparisons of time-limited and unlimited treatment. *Journal of Projective Techniques*, **22**, 153–162.

HOLLINGSHEAD, A. B., & REDLICH, F. C. (1958). *Social Class and Mental Illness*. New York: Wiley.

HOLT, R., & LUBORSKY, L. (1958). *Personality Patterns of Psychiatrists*. Vol. 2. Topeka: The Menninger Foundation.

HUNT, J. MCV., EWING, T., LAFORGE, R., & GILBERT, W. (1959). An integrated approach to research on therapeutic counseling with samples of results. *Journal of Counseling Psychology*, **6**, 46–54.

IMBER, S., FRANK, J., NASH, E., STONE, A., & GLIEDMAN, L. (1957). Improvement and amount of the therapeutic contact: An alternative to the use of no-treatment controls in psychotherapy. *Journal of Consulting Psychology*, **21**, 309–315.

ISAACS, K. S., & HAGGARD, E. A. (1966). Some methods used in the study of affect in psychotherapy. In L. A. Gottschalk & A. H. Auerbach (eds.), *Methods of Research in Psychotherapy*. New York: Appleton-Century-Crofts.

KARUSH, A., DANIELS, G., O'CONNOR, J., & STERN, L. (1968). The response to psychotherapy in chronic ulcerative colitis: I. Pretreatment factors. *Psychosomatic Medicine*, 30 (3), 255–276.

KATZ, M. M., LORR, M., & RUBINSTEIN, E. A. (1958). Remainer patients' attributes and their relation to subsequent improvement in psychotherapy. *Journal of Consulting Psychology*, **22**, 411–413.

KIRTNER, W. L., & CARTWRIGHT, D. S. (1958). Success and failure in client-centered therapy as a function of client personality variables. *Journal of Consulting Psychology*, **22**, 259–264. (a)

KIRTNER, W. L., CARTWRIGHT, D. S., ROBERTSON, R. J., & FISKE, D. W. (1961). Length of therapy in relation to outcome and change in personal integration. *Journal of Consulting Psychology*, **25**, 84–88.

KLEIN, H. (1960). A study of changes occurring in patients during and after psychoanalytic treatment. In P. Hoch & J. Zubin (eds.), *Current Approaches to Psychoanalysis.* New York: Grune & Stratton.

KLEIN, H. (1965). *Psychoanalysts in Training: Selection and Evaluation.* New York: Columbia University Psychoanalytic Clinic for Training and Research.

KLOPFER, B., KIRKNER, F., WISHAM, W., & BAKER, G. (1951). Rorschach prognostic rating scale. *Journal of Projective Techniques*, **15**, 425–428.

KNAPP, P. H., LEVIN, S., MCCARTER, R. H., WERMER, H., & ZETZEL, E. (1960). Suitability for psychoanalysis: a review of 100 supervised analytic cases. *Psychoanalytic Quarterly*, **29**, 459–477.

LANDFIELD, A. W., & NAWAS, M. M. (1964). Psychotherapeutic improvement as a function of communication and adoption of therapist's values. *Journal of Counseling Psychology*, **11**, 336–341.

LESSER, W. M. (1961). The relationship between conseling progress and empathic understanding. *Journal of Counseling Psychology*, **8**, 330–336.

LICHTENBERG, J. (1958). A statistical analysis of patient care at the Sheppard and Enoch Pratt Hospital. *Psychiatric Quarterly*, **32**, 13–40.

LICHTENSTEIN, E. (1966). Personality similarity and therapeutic success: a failure to replicate. *Journal of Consulting Psychology*, **30**, 282.

LIPKIN, S. (1954). Clients' feelings and attitudes in relation to the outcome of client-centered therapy. *Psychological Monographs*, 68, (1, Whole No. 372).

LORR, M., KATZ, M. M., & RUBINSTEIN, E. (1958). The prediction of length of stay in psychotherapy. *Journal of Consulting Psychology*, **22**, 321–327.

LORR, M., MCNAIR, D. M., & WEINSTEIN, G. J. (1963). Early effects of chlordiazepoxide (Librium) used with psychotherapy. *Journal of Psychiatric Research*, **2**, 257–270.

LORR, M., MCNAIR, D. M., WEINSTEIN, G. J., MICHAUX, W. W., & RASKIN, A. (1961). Meprobamate and chlorpormazine in psychotherapy: some effects on anxiety and hostility of outpatients. *Archives of General Psychiatry*, **4**, 381–389.

LORR, M., WITTMAN, P., & SCHANBERGER, W. (1951). An analysis of the Elgin Prognostic Scale. *Journal of Clinical Psychology*, **7**, 260–262.

LUBORSKY, L. (1962). The patient's personality and psychotherapeutic change. In H. H. Strupp & L. Luborsky (eds.), *Research in Psychotherapy.* Vol. 2. Washington, D.C.: American Psychological Association.

LUBORSKY, L. (1969). Research cannot yet influence clinical practice. (An evaluation of Strupp and Bergin's study, "Some empirical and conceptual bases for coordinated research in psychotherapy; a critical review of issues, trends, and evidence.") *International Journal of Psychiatry*, 7, (3) 135–146.

LUBORSKY, L., & SCHIMEK, J. (1964). Psychoanalytic theories of therapeutic and developmental change: implications for assessment. In P. Worchel & D. Byrne (eds.), *Personality Change.* New York: Wiley.

MAY, R. (1968). *Treatment of Schizophrenia.* New York: Science House.

MCNAIR, D. M., CALLAHAN, D. M., & LORR, M. (1962). Therapist "type" and patient response to psychotherapy. *Journal of Consulting Psychology*, **26**, 425–429.

MCNAIR, D. M., LORR, M., YOUNG, H. H., ROTH, I., & BOYD, R. W. (1964). A three-year follow-up of psychotherapy patients. *Journal of Clinical Psychology*, **20**, 258–264.

MILES, H. W., BARRABEE, E. L., & FINESINGER, J. E. (1951). Evaluation of psychotherapy, with a follow-up of 62 cases of anxiety neuroses. *Psychosomatic Medicine*, **13**, 83–105.

MINDESS, M. (1953). Predicting patient's response to psychotherapy: a preliminary study designed to investigate the validity of the Rorschach Prognostic Rating Scale. *Journal of Projective Techniques*, **17**, 327–334.

MINTZ, J., LUBORSKY, L., & AUERBACH, A. (1971). Dimensions of psychotherapy: a factor-analytic study of ratings of psychotherapy sessions. *Journal of Consulting and Clinical Psychology*, **36**, 106–120.

Section III: Psychotherapy

MOWRER, O. H., HUNT, J. MCV., & KOGAN, L. (1953). Further studies utilizing the discomfort-relief quotient. In O. H. Mowrer (ed.), *Psychotherapy: Theory and Research.* New York: Ronald Press.

MUENCH, G. A. (1965). An investigation of the efficacy of time-limited psychotherapy. *Journal of Counseling Psychology*, **12**, 294–298.

MYERS, J. K., & AULD, F. (1955). Some variables related to outcome of psychotherapy. *Journal of Clinical Psychology*, **11**, 51–54.

NASH, E., HOEHN-SARIC, R., BATTLE, C., STONE, A., IMBER, S., & FRANK, J. (1965). Systematic preparation of patients for short-term psychotherapy. II. Relation of characteristics of patient, therapist, and the psychotherapeutic process. *Journal of Nervous and Mental Disease*, **140**, 374–383.

NICHOLS, R. C., & BECK, K. W. (1960). Factors in psychotherapy change. *Journal of Consulting Psychology*, **24**, 388–399.

PASCAL, G. R., & ZAX, M. (1956). Psychotherapeutics: success or failure? *Journal of Consulting Psychology*, **20**, 325–331.

PAUL, G. L. (1967). Insight vs. desensitization in psychotherapy two years after termination. *Journal of Consulting Psychology*, **31**, 333–348.

PEARL, D. (1955). Psychotherapy and ethnocentrism. *Journal of Abnormal and Social Psychology*, 50, 227–229.

PECK, R. E. (1949). Comparison of adjunct group therapy with individual psychotherapy. *Archives of Neurology and Psychiatry*, **62**, 173–177.

POLLACK, I. W., & KIEV, A. (1963). Spatial orientation and psychotherapy: An experimental study of perception. *Journal of Nervous and Mental Disease*, **137**, 93–97.

RASKIN, N. J. (1949). An analysis of six parallel studies of the therapeutic process. *Journal of Consulting Psychology*, **13**, 206–221.

RAYNER, E. H., & HAHN, H. (1964). Assessment for psychotherapy: A pilot study of psychological test indications of success and failure in treatment. *British Journal of Medical Psychology*, **37**, 331–342.

RICE, L. N. (1965). Therapist's style of participation and case outcome. *Journal of Consulting Psychology*, **29**, 155–160.

RICKELS, K., CATTELL, R. B., WEISE, C., GRAY, B., YEE, R., MALLIN, A., & AARONSON, H. G. (1966). Controlled psychopharmacological research in private psychiatric practice. *Psychopharmacologia*, **9**, 288–306.

RIOCH, M. J., & LUBIN, A. (1959). Prognosis of social adjustment for mental hospital patients under psychotherapy. *Journal of Consulting Psychology*, **23**, 313–318.

ROGERS, C. (1957). The necessary and sufficient conditions of therapeutic personality change. *Journal of Consulting Psychology*, **21**, 95–103.

ROGERS, C. R. (1959). A tentative scale for measurement of process in psychotherapy. In E. A. Rubinstein & M. B. Parloff (eds.), *Research in Psychotherapy*. Vol. 1. Washington, D.C.: American Psychological Association.

ROGERS, C. R., & DYMOND, R. F. (eds.), (1954). *Psychotherapy and Personality Change.* Chicago: University of Chicago Press.

ROGERS, C. R., GENDLIN, E., KIESLER, D., & TRUAX, C. (eds.), (1967). *The Therapeutic Relationship and Its Impact: A Study of Psychotherapy with Schizophrenics.* Madison: University of Wisconsin Press.

ROSEN, E. (1954). Ethnocentric attitude changes and rated improvement in hospitalized psychiatric patients. *Journal of Clinical Psychology*, **10**, 345–350.

ROSENBAUM, M., FRIEDLANDER, J., & KAPLAN, S. (1956). Evaluation of results of psychotherapy. *Psychosomatic Medicine*, **18**, 113–132.

ROSENBERG, S. (1954). The relationship of certain personality factors to prognosis in psychotherapy. *Journal of Clinical Psychology*, **10**, 341–345.

ROSENTHAL, R. I., & JACOBSON, L. (1968). *Pygmalion in the Classroom: Teacher Expectation and Pupil's Intellectual Development*. New York: Holt, Rinehart & Winston.

ROSENZWEIG, S. (1936). Some implicit common factors in diverse methods of psychotherapy. *American Journal of Orthopsychiatry*, **6**, 412–415.

ROTH, I., RHUDICK, P. J., SHASKAN, D. A., SLOBIN, M. S., WILKINSON, A. E., & YOUNG, H. (1964). Long-term effects on psychotherapy of initial treatment conditions. *Journal of Psychiatric Research*, **2**, 283–297.

SANFORD, N. (1962). Discussion of papers on measuring personality change. In H. Strupp & L. Luborsky (eds.), *Research in Psychotherapy*. Vol. 2. Washington, D.C.: American Psychological Association.

SAPOLSKY, A. (1965). Relationship between patient-doctor compatibility, mutual perception, and outcome of treatment. *Journal of Abnormal Psychology*, **70**, 70–76.

SARGENT, H., HOROWITZ, L., WALLERSTEIN, R., & APPLEBAUM, A. (1968). Prediction in psychotherapy research: A method of transferring clinical judgments into testable hypotheses. *Psychological Issues*, **6**, No. 21.

SARGENT, H., MODLIN, H., FARIS, M., & VOTH, H. (1959). Situational variables. *Bulletin of the Menninger Clinic*, **22**, 148–166.

SCHONFIELD, J., STONE, A., HOEHN-SARIC, R., IMBER, S., & PANDE, S. (1969). Patient-therapist convergence and measures of improvement in short-term psychotherapy. *Psychotherapy: Theory, Research, and Practice*, **6**, 267–271.

SCHROEDER, P. (1960). Client acceptance of responsibility and difficulty of therapy. *Journal of Consulting Psychology*, **24**, 467–471.

SEEMAN, J. (1954). Counselor judgments of therapeutic process and outcome. In C. Rogers & R. F. Dymond (eds.), *Psychotherapy and Personality Change*. Chicago: University of Chicago Press.

SHEEHAN, J. G. (1953). Rorschach changes during psychotherapy in relation to the personality of the therapist. *American Psychologist*, **8**, 434. (Abstract)

SHLIEN, J. M. (1957). Time-limited psychotherapy: an experimental investigation of practical values and theoretical implications. *Journal of Counseling Psychology*, **4**, 318–322.

SHLIEN, J. M., MOSAK, H., & DRIEKERS, R. (1962). Effects of time limits: a comparison of two psychotherapies. *Journal of Counseling Psychology*, **9**, 31–34.

SIEGEL, N., & FINK, M. (1962). Motivation for psychotherapy. *Comprehensive Psychiatry*, **3**, 170–173.

SILVERMAN, J. (1967). Personality trait and "perceptual style" studies of the psychotherapists of schizophrenic patients. *Journal of Nervous and Mental Disease*, **145**, 5–17.

SNYDER, W. (1947). The present status of psychotherapeutic counseling. *Psychological Bulletin*, **44**, 297–386.

STEPHENS, J. H., & ASTRUP, C. (1963). Prognosis in "process" and "non-process" schizophrenia. *American Journal of Psychiatry*, **119**, 945–953.

STEPHENS, J. H., & ASTRUP, C. (1965). Treatment outcome in "process" and "non-process" schizophrenics treated by "A" and "B" types of therapists. *Journal of Nervous and Mental Disease*, **140**, 449–456.

STOLER, N. (1963). Client likability: A variable in the study of psychotherapy. *Journal of Consulting Psychology*, **27**, 175–178.

STOLER, N. (1966). The relationship of patient-likability and the A-B psychiatric resident types. (Doctoral dissertation, University of Michigan) Ann Arbor, Mich.: University Microfilms.

STONE, A., FRANK, J. D., NASH, E., & IMBER, F. (1961). An intensive five-year follow-up study of treated psychiatric outpatients. *Journal of Nervous and Mental Disease*, **133**, 410–422.

STRUPP, H. H., & BERGIN, A. (1969). Some empirical and conceptual bases for coordinated research in psychotherapy: a critical review of issues, trends, and evidence. *International Journal of Psychiatry*, **7**, 18–90. (a)

STRUPP, H. H., & BERGIN, A. E. (1969). Research in Individual Psychotherapy: A Bibliography. (USPHS Publication No. 1944 (OC-7M-07) Washington, D.C.: National Institutes of Mental Health.

STRUPP, H. H., WALLACH, M. S., JENKINS, J. W., & WOGAN, M. (1963). Psychotherapists' assessments of former patients. *Journal of Nervous and Mental Disease*, **137**, 222–230.

SULLIVAN, P. L., MILLER, C., & SMELSER, W. (1958). Factors in length of stay and progress in psychotherapy. *Journal of Consulting Psychology*, **22**.

THORNE, F. C. (1952). The prognostic index. *Journal of Clinical Psychology*, **8**, 42–45.

THURLOW, J. (1967). General susceptibility to illness: A selective review. *Canadian Medical Association Journal*, **97**, 1397–1404.

TOLMAN, R. S., & MAYER, M. M. (1957). Who returns to the clinic for more therapy? *Mental Hygiene*, **41**, 497–506.

TOMLINSON, T. M. (1967). The therapeutic process as related to outcome. In C. R. Rogers (ed.), *The Therapeutic Relationship and Its Impact*. Madison: University of Wisconsin Press.

TOMLINSON, T. M., & HART, J. T. (1962). A validation of the process scale. *Journal of Consulting Psychology*, **26**, 74–78.

TOUGAS, R. R. (1954). Ethnocentrism as a limiting factor in verbal therapy. In C. Rogers & R. Dymond (eds.), *Psychotherapy and Personality Change*. Chicago: University of Chicago Press.

TRUAX, C. B. (1963). Effective ingredients in psychotherapy: An approach to unraveling the patient-therapist interaction. *Journal of Counseling Psychology*, **10**, 256–263.

TRUAX, C. B. (1966). Influence of patient statements on judgments of therapist statements during psychotherapy. *Journal of Clinical Psychology*, **22**, 335–337.

TRUAX, C. B., WARGO, D. G., FRANK, J. D., IMBER, S. D., BATTLE, C. C., HOEHN-SARIC, R., NASH, E., & STONE, A. (1966). Therapist empathy, genuineness, and warmth and patient therapeutic outcome. *Journal of Consulting Psychology*, **30**, 395–401.

TUCKER, L. R., DAMARIN, F., & MESSICK, S. (1966). A base-free measure of change. *Psychometrika*, **31**, 457–473.

TUMA, A. H., & GUSTAD, J. W. (1957). The effects of client and counselor personality characteristics on client learning in counseling. *Journal of Counseling Psychology*, **4**, 136–141.

UHLENHUTH, E., & DUNCAN, D. (1968). Subjective change in psychoneurotic outpatients with medical student therapists. II. Some determinants of change. *Archives of General Psychiatry*, **18**, 532–540.

WALKER, A., RABLEN, R. A., & ROBERS, C. R. (1960). Development of a scale to measure process change in psychotherapy. *Journal of Clinical Psychology*, **16**, 79–85.

WALLERSTEIN, R., ROBBINS, L., SARGENT, H., & LUBORSKY, L. (1956). The psychotherapy research project of the Menninger Foundation. Rationale, method, and sample use. *Bulletin of the Menninger Clinic*, **20**, 221–280.

WELKOWITZ, J., COHEN, J., & ORTMEYER, D. (1967). Value system similarity: Investigation of patient-therapist dyads. *Journal of Consulting Psychology*, **31**, 48–55.

WHITEHORN, J., & BETZ, B. (1957). A comparison of psychotherapeutic relationships between physicians and schizophrenic patients when insulin is combined with psychotherapy and when psychotherapy is used alone. *American Journal of Psychiatry*, **113**, 907–910.

WINDLE, C. (1952). Psychological tests in psychopathological prognosis. *Psychological Bulletin*, **49**, 451–482.

WOLBERG, L. R. (1967). *The Technique of Psychotherapy*. New York: Brune & Stratton.

ZAX, M., & KLEIN, A. (1960). Measurement of personality and behavior changes following psychotherapy. *Psychological Bulletin*, **57**, 435–448.

ZIGLER, E., & PHILLIPS, L. (1961). Social competence and outcome in psychiatric disorders. *Journal of Abnormal and Social Psychology*, **63**, 264–271.

ZOLIK, E. S., & HOLLON, T. N. (1960). Factors characteristic of patients responsive to brief psychotherapy. *American Psychologist*, **15**, 287. (Abstract)

DAVID L. GEISINGER

Controlling Sexual and Interpersonal Anxieties

In this article, Dr. Geisinger presents a case history of a woman who was treated by means of behavior therapy. It is particularly instructive because of the wide variety of techniques that were employed. This not only illustrates the use of these techniques, but also shows behavior therapy to be a multifaceted approach that can incorporate a multitude of clinical techniques. The inclusion of three separate hierarchies in the Appendix should help make the technique of systematic desensitization more clear. The Editor's Notes, which are distributed throughout the article, were contributed by Drs. Krumboltz and Thoresen, the editors of the book in which this paper originally appeared.

The following case is not a typical one. No case is really typical in that each hinges upon a variety of factors which, when considered in their entirety, tend to be unique to a particular client and problem. A case presentation, however, can provide examples or elements which are common to other settings with other clients. One central issue is that of generalizability: what can be learned from this one case that will be applicable to other cases?

Learning the Principles

Principles of interaction, intervention and modification, not specific and unvarying techniques, are the elements which are most important to extract from any case study. Each technique is capable of undergoing an almost infinite variety of alterations depending upon the circumstances surrounding its application and the individuals involved.[1] Such alterations, moreover, *should* be made, since counseling must be flexible and individualized if it is to be maximally effective. The flexibility, however, must not be dictated by mere

[1] Editors' Note: The counselor actually needs both. Mastery of a given set of techniques coupled with an understanding of the principles underlying them provides the necessary foundation from which the counselor can build.

Reprinted from "Controlling Sexual and Interpersonal Anxieties" by David L. Geisinger, in *Behavioral Counseling: Cases and Techniques* edited by John D. Krumboltz and Carl E. Thoresen. Copyright © 1969 by Holt, Rinehart and Winston, Inc. Reprinted by permission of Holt, Rinehart and Winston, Inc. and Dr. Geisinger.

whim, but by a solid familiarity with the principles of human behavior. The case presented here employed techniques based primarily on principles of classical and operant conditioning.

All clients do not progress as smoothly or so positively as this one. Counseling was greatly enhanced in the present instance by the client's high motivation, her diligence in doing the assignments given her, and the splendid co-operation and support of her husband.

In addition, what may be termed "relationship factors" played an influential part in the outcome of this case. The type of relationship involved here was a relaxed one of deep trust, mutual respect, and warmth. In many respects the relationship was more like that of student and teacher than that of client and counselor in the more traditional sense.[2]

The Case of Naomi

Naomi was a 23-year-old married woman who came from a lower middle-class background. As a child she lived with her grandparents after her parents divorced, returning to live with her mother at the age of 18. Her mother, stepfather, and grandparents were alcoholics, and she was a frequent witness to the vociferous arguments which often occurred when they had been drinking. She noted that she was often spanked with a strap or slapped for minor infractions. Her mother and her grandparents had had a puritanical attitude toward sex, and she noted that her parents as well as her grandparents always slept in separate bedrooms. She recalled her mother informing her that her grandfather used to force her grandmother into bed every night. The subject of sex was avoided or, on occasion, talked about in a very pejorative way. As a consequence of her exposure to these and other negative attitudes and experiences she avoided any sexual or romantic involvements during her high school years. After she left high school she found that she was able to interact with members of the opposite sex only when her anxiety was reduced by drinking large amounts of alcoholic beverages. Drinking had not, however, become a problem in later life.

She married at the age of 21. Her husband was a graduate student in the behavioral sciences and was described as a sensitive, thoughtful person who was quite devoted to her. She stated that, in general, she and her husband got along very well.

Sensitivity, shyness, and sex

At the time she began counseling there were several areas of concern to her which, because of their pervasiveness, caused her considerable

[2] Editors' Note: What is termed "relationship factors" indeed may be crucial to what happens. However, this "relationship" actually involves a host of complex present and past behaviors, for example, verbal and nonverbal responses by counselor and client coupled with covert activities such as thoughts, attitudes, and sets. When a counselor acts in a manner producing this "good relationship," he becomes a much more powerful model and reinforcing agent for his client.

anxiety during much of her waking day. These concerns were (1) an exaggerated sensitivity to criticism from anyone in her environment particularly from her husband and people in the office where she was a secretary; (2) a marked lack of assertiveness, a shyness, and a tendency to withdraw from social and interpersonal interactions; (3) numerous and persistent feelings of jealousy about her husband which she was aware had no factual basis; (4) painful feelings of discomfort and anxiety about sex, accompanied by a desire to avoid all conversations or situations in which there was even a remote sexual reference.

Her mood was almost always rather gloomy and her facial expression tended to be pained and cheerless. Her physical appearance seemed to mirror this mood: her clothes were drab, unattractive, and ill-fitting, her hair was rarely combed. She was about 40 pounds overweight. In general she conveyed the impression of a person who did not care about her physical appearance, yet in discussion she revealed a definite concern and displeasure with the way she looked. She indicated that she would have liked to take better care of herself, but that most of the time her feelings of self-disgust and her ensuing depressions seemed to rob her of all desire or motivation to work at changing any of these aspects of her appearance.

Concerning her sexual anxiety, she felt that although she loved her husband very much, and although he was a good, attentive, and thoughtful lover, she experienced little pleasure during sex. Most often, intercourse proved to be somewhat painful, although the pain was not especially severe. She was able to experience orgasm sporadically, but most of the time it was accompanied by considerable feelings of guilt. This guilt was related to her inability to put a stop to what she thought might be a "homosexual" fantasy which would drift into her imagination during lovemaking: a nude, faceless woman sexually provoking a faceless man. She felt more stimulated by the image of the woman than by the image of the man. She stated that she had never actually had a homosexual encounter and did not know the origin or reason for this fantasy.

I decided to see her in counseling on a once-a-week basis with the understanding that when the need arose we would see her husband as well. She was told that certain of her problems could most effectively be dealt with by enlisting her husband's support and co-operation. She reported that her husband would be eager to participate in any way he could.

Variety of techniques

A broad-spectrum approach to counseling was decided upon to deal with the problems of excessive sensitivity to criticism, lack of social assertiveness, and undue sexual anxiety. The following techniques were selected: (1) assertive training, (2) behavior rehearsal, (3) group verbal interaction, (4) thought-stopping, (5) flooding techniques, and (6) systematic desensitization. With regard to desensitization, three separate anxiety hierarchies were constructed in the areas of personal criticism, general sexual stimuli, and jealousy concerning her husband.

The first hour and much of the second were spent in history-taking and in the detailed examination of the circumstances surrounding her various anxieties and depressions. The ongoing behavioral analysis focused on the contingencies of her uncomfortable feelings and maladaptive behavior patterns: when and where did they become manifest, who was present at these times, what was she thinking and doing when they appeared, and what did she do to gain some measure of relief from her discomfort.[3]

"THOUGHT-STOPPING" AND COUNTERCONDITIONING. During the second session, in discussing sexual anxiety, I told her in the future to open her eyes during lovemaking and at the final stages of orgasm to look directly at her husband. The point was made that orgasm could, and often did, operate as a powerful positive reinforcement for the stimuli associated with it. Since she had had many orgasms while imagining the homosexual fantasy, this image had become predominant during intercourse. I informed her that in no way did this persistent image mean that she was a homosexual. Opening her eyes during orgasm and looking directly at her husband would interfere with the guilt-producing scene and she would gradually begin to associate her attention and imagination to thoughts of her husband making love to her.[4]

At this point her husband was brought in and both of them were given instructions to engage in as much foreplay as possible prior to intercourse without extending it so far that the situation would begin to become tense and uncomfortable. The relationship between foreplay, vaginal lubrication, relaxation of the muscles in the vaginal walls, and easier, painless intercourse was discussed. Questions that either of them had about sexual technique were solicited and answered in a calm, factual manner.

The following week she reported that she had kept her eyes open during lovemaking and had looked at her husband at the moment of orgasm. She found that she was able to exclude all the former thoughts about her guilt-producing fantasy. She felt a sense of relief about this and also about the fact that the extension of time spent in foreplay had resulted for the first time in the complete absence of pain during intercourse. Orgasm had occurred on both occasions of sexual intercourse during the week.

BEGINNING SYSTEMATIC DESENSITIZATION. The third hour was spent in having her refine and elaborate some of the particular settings in which her anxiety became manifest. A description of the process of desensitization and its rationale was given along with a manual on constructing a hierarchy. She

[3] Editors' Note: Initial attention to such specifics is very important, and often neglected, in helping the counselor discover what antecedents may be causing the behavior and what consequences may be maintaining the behavior.

[4] Editors' Note: Stated differently, the physical act of lovemaking, especially orgasm, would be associated by contiguity with positive visual stimuli, that is, her husband's face rather than with her anxiety producing fantasy.

was asked to begin thinking about specific situations in the areas of criticism, jealousy, and sex. Examples of relevant items within each of these topics were given such as, "Driving home from work with Aaron (her husband), you notice him staring at a very attractive woman standing on a corner," and, "You are walking to the store alone and two men drive by slowly and whistle at you."

BEHAVIOR REHEARSAL AND ASSERTIVE TRAINING. During the fourth and fifth sessions behavior rehearsal and assertive training were started. The client reported that her boss had given her an excess amount of work, often resulting in her having to work overtime without compensation in order to finish. She felt angry and resentful about this and was considering leaving her job. I pointed out that she often seemed to take flight from other situations when she felt pressured and abused. It would be helpful for her to learn how to cope more directly with these situations in the future as an alternative to escaping from them.

Using role-playing, I played the part of her employer and she played herself in a typical office interaction. At first her responses were faltering and inadequate and she seemed very ill-at-ease. A tape recording of this behavior rehearsal was played back to her with my suggestions as to how she might improve her communication and be more assertive.[6] She tried again to role-play the same scene. This time she was hostile in a very exaggerated way. Again the tape was played back to her and she laughed when she heard how angrily she had expressed herself. I reversed roles and played her part in the office setting while she played the part of her employer. This modeling technique enabled her to learn in an explicit manner a new way of behaving with her boss. After a few more rehearsals she was able to handle the situation smoothly and comfortably. She was told to practice what she had learned whenever the opportunity arose, both at work and in other settings.

The following week I received a letter from the client which contained the following passages:

> Something that made me feel badly last week was what I interpreted as apathy from you in regard to the notes that I had compiled during the week prior to our last session. (The client often brought in extensive and detailed notes about what had gone on during the week and would read them to me instead of telling me spontaneously what had gone on.) I had spent quite a bit of time writing down everything I considered important, and when I left your office, I felt that my notes had been a worthless waste of time. In addition, I felt like a guinea pig while reading the notes to you ... I was very uneasy at the end of the last session concerning your not getting up at the end. I didn't know when the session was over and didn't know when to leave. I felt like I was being put to some kind of test or game.

[6] Editors' Note: Good use of a modeling technique, in this case having the client observe her own behavior.

Lastly, she asked if I would reduce her fee since she was finding it difficult to pay for counseling because her husband was a student and she herself earned only a modest salary. At the bottom of the page, in a postscript, she stated: "I feel guilty for having written this letter."

During the next session I complimented her for having had the courage to write the letter, stating that I knew how difficult it must have been for her to do so. I used the letter as a cogent example of her growing ability to assert herself. I stated that the letter represented an important start in a series of "successive approximations" toward the goal of being able to assert herself in any situation. I then requested that she tell me in person the information she had conveyed in the letter. When she had done this, I complimented her again and told her that I would be happy to reduce the fee as she had requested.[7] I informed her that my not getting up at the end of the last session was not a test or a game but merely an oversight, adding that if she had not had the courage to bring it to my attention, she would have continued to be puzzled by it. Other instances where she failed to ask for clarification of certain matters at her job were called to her attention in order to emphasize the proper time for, and kinds of, assertive behaviors. Further behavior rehearsals concerning this area were practiced near the end of the session.

Continuing desensitization

Several sessions were then spent in teaching her the technique of progressive relaxation (Jacobson, 1938). She was told to practice this technique at home for two 15-minute periods daily. At about this time she stated that she had always felt particularly anxious at the time of her menstrual periods. She had claimed that she would like to be able to have the convenience of using an internal device such as a tampon but found that her anxiety made the insertion of such devices painful. We agreed to include the insertion of such devices as an item on her "general sexual anxiety" hierarchy.

By the twelfth session considerable progress on the desensitization of the hierarchy had been made. Her mood in the office had undergone a perceptible change—she smiled a good deal more and stated that she was feeling more comfortable at work. She reported an instance in which she was able to be more assertive with her boss with no associated anxiety. Work was begun in the desensitization of her sensitivity to innocuous personal criticism and in the area of jealousy about her husband, Aaron.

During the fourteenth session she said, "Yesterday I was actually joking with Mr. Tomkins (office manager) at the office—I can't believe it!"

Desensitization in the three areas mentioned previously continued during the latter half of each subsequent counseling session. For the most part, several items on each of the three hierarchies were presented to the patient during

[7] Editors' Note: This probably was an immediately reinforcing consequence for her being assertive!

a given session. The first half of each session was devoted to a review of her progress and a general discussion of other issues that had arisen during the week. When matters of particular significance arose which required longer discussion, the amount of time spent on desensitization proper was reduced.[8]

During the fifteenth session once again Naomi was asked to move to another chair in the office—a large, comfortable recliner chair. The room was darkened a bit by drawing the window blinds. She was then instructed to shut her eyes and recline in the chair while beginning to give herself instructions to relax. Since she had frequently practiced relaxation at home as well as having gone through many relaxation sessions in the office while receiving explicit verbal instructions from me, it was no longer necessary to give her these specific instructions in order to get her to relax. She was now able to reach a deeply relaxed state by herself in only five minutes.

She was told to signal by raising her left index finger when she felt very relaxed. After she had done this I told her that if during the course of any of the imagination sequences she became at all anxious or tense, she was to indicate this to me by raising her right index finger.

Items 23 and 24 from the "general sexual anxiety" hierarchy were presented to her along with item 14 on the "criticism" hierarchy and item 12 on the "jealousy" hierarchy. Each item was repeated until the criterion of three presentations with no reporting of anxiety was met.[9]

The items were presented for the first time for 5 seconds, the second time for 10 seconds, the third time for 20 seconds. From time to time "perception checks" were made by asking the client to signal if she was able to imagine vividly the item being described to her. These perception checks are a useful adjunct to the desensitization procedure in that they give the counselor feedback as to whether the client has not been signaling because, perhaps, she has not been able to imagine the scenes being described rather than because she didn't experience anxiety. In addition, this technique also permits the counselor to know if, as happens on rare occasions, the client has gradually lapsed into sleep.

The last item presented during the hour was, as always, an item describing an experience in which the client felt particularly calm and peaceful. In Naomi's case this was a description of herself being served breakfast in bed by Aaron during a particular Sunday morning. Having the last scene in the desensitization sequence be a pleasant one tends to

[8] Editors' Note: This brings up an important question. Would counseling prove just as effective or even more so without these discussions during the first half of each session? The answer may lie in some optimal combination of certain amounts and kinds of discussion with certain types of clients having particular problems.

[9] Editors' Note: An interesting question is raised here, in terms of efficiency and effectiveness, about working on several specific problems. In Naomi's case she was explicitly dealing with her problems of sexual anxiety, criticism, and jealousy. Is it more effective to complete desensitization on one problem before going on to another? Or do concurrent efforts such as working on three hierarchies, as in this case, actually interact to foster more rapid change?

ensure that the procedure itself does not become associated with an anxiety-producing experience, since the last item in a chain of events is usually the one which is most clearly remembered.

Evidence of progress

During the seventeenth session she reported the following progress: (1) she had used a tampon during the second day of her menstrual cycle, after trying unsuccessfully during the first day, and was able to do so quite easily with no pain; (2) while at a new friend's house she played the piano in front of several people though formerly she had been too self-conscious and frightened of making mistakes to do this; (3) she called up a prospective employer who had delayed making a definite commitment to her and told him diplomatically but assertively that she expected to hear from him one way or the other about a particular job.

She entered the next hour stating, "A number of people have told me I've completely changed, that I'm a new person." Though she continued to wear drab, ill-fitting clothing and no make-up, her mood continued to be optimistic and, in contrast to her former appearance, her facial expressions were more animated. In view of the fact that she had no pressing problems that she wanted to discuss, the hour was devoted in its entirety to the desensitization procedure, as were the next two sessions.

Jealousy and appearance

During the twenty-second session, she indicated that she was still excessively jealous of Aaron's attention. She expressed her discouragement about the fact that the desensitization did not seem to be working in this area. "I still get upset whenever Aaron's concern, time or interest is spent on other people, even other men. I get especially upset whenever Aaron looks at any woman. It seems like a setback." I assured her that it was not a setback but that perhaps it was an indication that we were not working on the most basic dimension relating to her feelings of jealousy. I was unable, however, to arrive at any alternatives at the time and, to some extent, secretly shared her discouragement. I told her, however, that we would continue to explore this subject in future sessions until we could discover the basis for her difficulty.

After thinking about the matter during the intervening week I began to suspect that the patient's jealousy of her husband's attention might be related to her feelings about her own appearance. She had, after all, occasionally hinted about her dissatisfaction with the way she looked, and it was apparent that her self-concept had been a poor one for many years. Aaron, however, prided himself on what he felt was his well-balanced sense of values. He often derogated what he called the "superficial aspects of life," among which was a concern with "mere appearance" such as attractive, stylish clothing and make-up, while laying strong emphasis on matters of intellect. This message was an irritating paradox to the patient because Aaron would often notice other women who were obviously not of shining intellect while commenting enthusiastically about their attractive appearances. Naomi had grown quite reluctant to spend any money on improving her own appearance though it seemed that she would welcome the opportunity to do so if she were not criticized for it.

With this in mind, I began the next session by commenting on how much better she looked since she had been on her diet. I brought up the fact that she would soon have to buy new clothes to accommodate her new figure. She picked up this topic with great enthusiasm and began to elaborate upon it, essentially supporting the hypothesis I had made earlier. She indicated that she was particularly upset by Aaron's criticism and as a result had gone without any make-up for over a year. She added that she was also in great need of a new coat since the one she now wore was practically falling apart.

We discussed Aaron's inconsistency: that he talked one way but behaved in another in that he was actually very responsive to women who were physically attractive. She decided gradually to improve her physical appearance the following week. In addition, we went through several behavior rehearsals in which I played the part of Aaron and she played herself bringing up the matter of buying new clothes.

Naomi entered the twenty-fourth session wearing a new coat. She noted that Aaron had been "a pushover" and had made no protest whatsoever when she brought up the subject of purchasing new clothing. She had begun to wear eye-liner and some mascara, and even though Aaron did not remark about it one way or the other, she said, "I'm feeling much better about myself." She added that she did not have any feelings of jealousy during the week.

"*Flooding*" *sex talk*

During the next session, she expressed concern that "sex-talk" in conversation continued to make her quite anxious. "Certain words trigger my anxiety, it seems, especially when Aaron is around." I asked her what these words were and she mentioned among others the following terms: chick, babe, broad, lay, fuck, cunt, whore, prostitute, screw, bubble-dance, tits, knockers, boobs, seduce, make, breasts, figure, shape, nude, shack-up, sexy, voluptuous, orgy, harem, bigamy, knocked-up, piece of ass.

The procedure of "flooding" was described to her and in accord with this she was instructed to read the list of words to herself at least 15 times a day for the next two weeks. She was also told to make up sentences that incorporated these words and to read these sentences aloud to Aaron several times each day, after which Aaron was to read them back to her.

It was further suggested that they try to inject some humor into this homework assignment in order to speed up the process of desensitization, since humor is, in most instances, strongly incompatible with anxiety.[10]

Two weeks later she and her husband returned to the office. They had done the exercises diligently and with good results. Her anxiety about the "sex-talk" had diminished markedly, and she was much more comfortable participating in social conversation.

Some Changes

At this time Aaron was graduating from the university and had accepted a job in another city. It was generally agreed that this move fortunately coincided with what seemed to be an appropriate stopping point in counseling. Naomi had changed considerably. She had eliminated several phobias, had become more assertive, was more relaxed in her social interactions, her sex life had improved as did her relationship with her husband in general, and perhaps most importantly, her thoughts and feelings about herself had undergone decided improvement.

An interesting sidelight to this case occurred ten months later. The author and his colleague, who was familiar with the case, were attending a professional meeting and noticed Aaron sitting in the audience on the other side of the room. During the coffee break we approached him to say hello and I naturally asked how his wife was getting along. He smiled broadly and without saying anything he tapped a young woman on the shoulder who was standing near him chatting with another group of people and said, "You can ask her yourself." When she turned around and greeted us, we found it hard to believe our eyes. It was Naomi. Her hair had been cut and set in an attractive new style, her figure was lithe, she was wearing a bright new dress, tastefully applied make-up, and had even changed her eye-glass frames, from the large, unflattering ones she formerly wore. She seemed poised, outgoing and obviously at ease as she told us how well things had been going for her.[11]

[10] Editors' Note: In this example a type of "graduated flooding" is used since Naomi was not asked to say these words in normal social situations. "Flooding" and other techniques based in part on operant extinction such as implosive therapy may seem quite different from systematic desensitization based on the principle of counterconditioning. Both procedures, however, are quite similar, focusing on the repetitive exposure to stress producing stimuli without aversive consequences. Gradual exposure to stressful stimuli may in the long run prove more effective since excessive anxiety is not aroused and the opportunity for adaptive responses to occur is increased.

[11] Editors' Note: Some "stories" still do have happy endings!

Appendix

General Sexual Anxiety Hierarchy

1. Patricia (a married woman who works in my office) is flirting with some men in the office; she is calling them "honey," "sweetie," and occasionally holds their hands.
2. I am walking downtown during my lunch hour. There is a man standing up against a building who is staring at a woman as she walks by him. The woman doesn't notice him.
3. I am walking downtown during my lunch hour. There are two men standing on a corner who scrutinize a woman as she walks by them. She doesn't notice them, but after she walks by the men look at each other and grin.
4. I am sitting at my desk at the office. Three men are waiting for the elevator. I look up and notice that they are all looking at me.
5. I am driving to the store alone and see a carload of men trying to pick up two girls. The girls seem slightly self-conscious, but it is obvious that they are enjoying it.
6. I am walking to the store alone and two men drive by and whistle at me.
7. My husband and I go to a new friend's house. In the living room is a profile drawing of a nude (from the waist up).
8. I am with my husband at a friend's house. On a coffee table there is a copy of "Playboy" magazine casually opened to a page containing a color photograph of a voluptuous nude woman.
9. I'm in my office and the door to Mr. Tomkins' (office manager) office is open. I hear him telling a dirty joke on the telephone in a low voice. After telling the joke he laughs heartily and says, "Isn't that awful?"
10. I am in the office with Bob (a junior executive) and Mr. Gordon (my boss). Mr. Gordon says to Bob, "I'd like to do nothing but chase women."
11. I am sitting on the toilet at home. I am beginning to give myself a douche by inserting the nozzle into my vagina.
12. I'm sitting at my desk in the office. As a workman walks by my office, he quickly sticks his head in the door and says, "Hi, beautiful."
13. I'm walking to the store and two men across the street make kissing noises at me.
14. I'm at the office and Bob is explaining procedures to me. While he is talking, he is looking at my breasts.
15. I'm in a small store and it is rather crowded. As a strange man steps past me he casually puts his hands on my waist.

16. Downtown I see a woman wearing heavy makeup who is standing on a corner as though she wants to be picked up.
17. At my parents' home, my father says, "A woman's duty is to her husband; he is the master and she'll do as he desires."
18. At my parents' home, my mother and father have just come home from seeing a burlesque show, and they are discussing the shapes of the women performers.
19. I'm at a movie. A woman who is partially clothed is shown on the screen and men in the audience whistle and shout.
20. I'm at a movie. Partially clothed women are shown dancing on the screen. The men in the audience whistle, shout and laugh.
21. Ralph (a friend) is at our house. He's telling of a movie he saw in which a very long line of beautiful girls are waiting to enter the bedroom of the male star.
22. I'm walking down the hall in the office building. Some workmen are doing electrical work and as I walk by they look at my breasts, hips, and thighs.
23. I'm at the office and Mr. Gordon is giving directions to another girl as to how to get to the camera store. He says, "It's right next door to where the topless girls are."
24. I am at home sitting on the toilet putting a tampon in my vagina.
25. I'm walking with another girl downtown. A drunk man staggers out of a bar and says, "Care to spread your legs, honey?"
26. I'm at the doctor's office and he is spreading the opening of my vagina in order to give me a pelvic examination.
27. My husband, our friend Don, and I are driving downtown. Don points to a woman and says, "Boy, that woman has big breasts."
28. While waiting for the bus I see a sign carved into the wooden bus shelter saying, "All waves throw a good fuck."
29. Bob, Mr. Gordon, and I are in the office. Mr. Gordon stands in front of me, looks at my breasts and says, "Never let a challenge go by."

Criticism Hierarchy

1. At the office building Cathy, another secretary, says, "Why don't you wear your hair down?"
2. Mr. Tomkins, the boss, asks, "Have you registered to vote?" I reply, "No," and he says jokingly, "You stinker!"
3. At the office one of my letters is returned to me by Dorothy the district manager's secretary. She has put red marks all over the letter with the statement added, "Please check spelling of names, and counties."
4. At home while playing darts with Aaron I shoot a dart which comes close to the target and Aaron says, "Just a little higher, Hon."

5. At class the teacher says, "Naomi, how can this statement be proven?" I shrug my shoulders and he frowns.
6. Alice, one of the clerks at the office, tells me, "You have a tiny rip in the back of your dress."
7. While doing poorly at darts, Aaron suggests, "Why don't you try holding the dart differently?"
8. At the office, the boss brings back a letter I've composed and says, "Next time it might be better not to be so blunt in telling the customer that he's made an error."
9. Aaron is looking at some math problems I've done at home and says, "These two are right, but in this one you have cancelled the numerators by mistake."
10. At home I receive a letter from my grandmother stating, "You had better start settling down and staying at one job."
11. At home I am telling Aaron of a new route to the bridge. He replies, "That freeway doesn't go to the bridge; it ends up downtown."
12. While shooting darts poorly at home, Ken suggests, "Maybe leaning forward would help."
13. At the office building I go to the mail room to make Xerox copies. As I am leaving the mail room, the clerk sarcastically says, "Don't go out of here without picking up your mail."
14. At the office the mail room clerk brings me the mail and notes that I'm not doing anything. He says, "Here's something for you to do while you're resting."
15. At the office building a man says to me when I'm buying a candy bar, "That's fattening, you know."
16. At the office while taking shorthand, I misunderstand a word and send the letter out with the wrong word in it. The boss's attention is called to the error and he tells me, "You should have caught that."
17. At home I receive a letter from mother after I've told her that I'm drawing unemployment, and she implies I'm a thief by the statement: "People like Dad work hard all their lives putting money into that fund, and then small-time crooks come along and drag it out."
18. At the office I'm talking to an irate man on the phone who says, "What have you people been doing? I've been waiting for my travel orders for a week!"
19. I am crossing the street and am half way to the other side when the light changes to "Don't Walk." A man drives by me and says, "Read the signs!"
20. I am walking out of a post office downtown at the same time a man is entering the building and he says to me, "You're using the wrong door."
21. At home I receive a letter from my grandmother in which she states, "Dad is disgusted with you."
22. At home I am trying to awaken Aaron and am rubbing the bottom of his foot. He irritably says, "That doesn't go over."

23. I start eating a bowl of ice cream at home and Aaron disgustedly looks on and says, "It's not the ice cream so much—it's the amount. I don't know how you can eat so much without getting sick."
24. At home Aaron said, "Your thighs used to be so big that I could see no distinction where your butt ended and your thighs began."

Jealousy Hierarchy

1. Aaron and I are at Ron and Dora's house. Aaron and Ron are talking to each other and laughing.
2. At home I am reading a letter from Aaron's mother and in it she mentions various female relatives of his.
3. At home Aaron tells me that Jack helped him look for apartments all afternoon.
4. Aaron and I are in the supermarket. Aaron bumps into a woman and cordially says, "Pardon me."
5. At home Aaron says he saw the movie "Sound of Music" while I was gone, and he enjoyed it very much.
6. In front of the office building I introduce Aaron to Helen (another secretary), and he is very charming and cordial.
7. At school a girl asks a question in physics class and Aaron looks at her.
8. Aaron and I are at the roller skating rink and he asks a woman of about 50 years of age to skate with him.
9. Ron, Dora, Aaron, and I are at the Xanadu Ballroom and Aaron is waltzing with Dora.
10. I introduce Aaron to Cathy outside the office building and he is very charming.
11. At home Aaron is telling me about his course and says of his female teacher, "She's pretty sharp in some ways."
12. Aaron and I are at Norton's restaurant and Aaron is courteous and pleasant to the attractive waitress.
13. Aaron and I are at a restaurant, and an attractive woman sitting near us keeps staring at him.
14. Aaron and I are at the roller rink. It is the girls' turn to have the floor to themselves for doing tricks, and Aaron watches them intently.
15. Aaron and I are downtown during lunch hour and there are numerous well-dressed, attractive women all around us.
16. Aaron and I are at a dancing studio and the good-looking female dancing instructor is dancing with him.
17. Aaron looks at a billboard in town which shows a sexy-looking woman with a low-cut dress on.
18. Driving home from work, Aaron stares at a woman with a good figure who is standing on the corner.
19. Aaron and I are at Norton's restaurant. A waitress with a good figure swings her hips when she walks by and Aaron looks her up and down.

20. Aaron and I are at Steve's house. We are sitting opposite to Steve and his wife, Lois. Lois is wearing a skirt and has her legs pulled up to her chest so that Aaron can see her crotch area.
21. Aaron and I are at a friend's house. We are about to leave and a woman who boards there comes out to the doorway of her bedroom in her panties and bra. She looks at us and says, "You aren't leaving so early, are you?"

ROBERT J. SMITH

A Closer Look at Encounter Therapies

In this paper, Dr. Smith examines encounter groups as a potential therapeutic vehicle, pointing out differences between those groups and more traditional approaches to group therapy. He sees the encounter movement in the context of current cultural phenomena, with the purported emphasis on individuality and feeling being consistent with social developments among the youth culture. The emphasis on feeling is in contrast with the emphasis on thought in more traditional therapies, which have incorporated some encounter techniques in an attempt to integrate new developments. Dr. Smith ends with a call for definitive research, which is the most sensible way to settle sharp differences in opinion about the efficacy of therapeutic approaches.

It is now recognized as a historical truism that the climate of the times exerts important pressure in shaping artifacts of any given era. This would seem especially true of theories as artifacts, shaped as they are by the persons who have propounded them. It is again a truism that theories do not come "full-blown from the head of Zeus." Yet, they are liable to become especially visible or exciting or generate particular support when the social climate is of a nurturant character.

It is this writer's thesis that the sociocultural climate of contemporary America is peculiarly suited to the theory and technique which underlie what I choose to label, "encounter therapies," and has resulted in their remarkable fruition and dissemination in the culture to levels rarely touched by other psychotherapeutic efforts.

Reprinted from the *International Journal of Group Psychotherapy*, **20** (1970), 192–209, with the permission of International Universities Press and Dr. Smith.

The present writer joins with Jacques Barzun (1959) in believing that intellect is in a state of serious decline. Barzun has somewhat loosely defined intellect as:

> . . . the capitalized and command form of live intelligence; it is intelligence stored up and made into habits of discipline, signs and symbols of meaning, chains of reasoning and spurs to emotion—a shorthand and a wireless by which the mind can skip connections, recognize ability and communicate truth [1959, p. 4].

Present-day observers are wont to point to the aridity of a society built along rational, "scientific" lines, e.g., technologic and positivistic, particularly as regards the "crisis in values" that Western culture is said to be facing. However, in eschewing "rational technologies," intellect may be an unfortunate victim of the distaste with which elements of the culture regard some of the admittedly sterile products of an overly ordered society; it is the baby going out with the bath water problem. The emphasis on feeling and doing may be at the expense of the critical function of intellect, a function which traditionally has served to leaven emotional excess. I would contend that the current decline and distrust of intellect has contributed markedly to the rise of an "encounter group" philosophy.

After a brief consideration of some contemporary areas in which intellect seems to be suffering obvious inroads, I would like to examine in some detail the method and theory of encounter therapies as these function both within the general climate of psychology and, more specifically, among psychotherapies.

In education, Barzun (1959) reminds us that we have seen the subversion of Dewey's "teaching by doing" and even more formal "content-centered" approaches into "doing without comprehension," the "child-centered curriculum" that Sputnik I and warnings by such as Admiral Rickover have only partially allayed, and then because of essentially non-intellective motives (Rickover, 1963). Emphasis has been transduced to "life adjustment" with consequent devaluation of the intellectural command of subject matter.

In higher education, student activism in the civil rights movement and "stop the (Vietnam) war" campaigns have served as impetus for a powerful swing to the opinion that education must serve a demonstrable public (social) purpose. Ivory tower, uninvolved, dispassionate intellect, viewing social encounters from a far, lofty perch, while perhaps never more than an ideal in America, has been seriously castigated. Solving problems in the abstract, leaving it to others to translate them into social action, has been pooh-poohed by activists both in and out of academia; the academies are challenged to become "committed."

In popular music we have seen the emergence of "rhythm and blues" and "rock" as the dominant style, a far cry from the (socially) sophisticated lyrics and traditional melodies of Rodgers and Hart, or Kern, or Coward, of thirty and forty years ago. The current emphasis is to "do your own dance" (make it up!) to the tune, letting the "big beat" carry you away from your inhibitions. The dancers "... are linked only by their common need for the relaxation of tensions and the emotional sensations that briefly provide them with an aroused sense of self. As an expression of the lack of self-identity, the Twist is a symptom of the social pathology of this culture" (Levine, 1966, p. 210).

Now "sensory saturation" is in vogue, and crazy-quilt lighting patterns and "psychedelic" wall paintings add their sensory assault on gyrating dancers.

Recent "message" songs are likely to be couched in simple language decrying traditional values, hypocrisy, the adult world, etc. Black "soul," the seemingly indefinable, has captured youthful fancies, and attempted definitions—of the music as illustrative of a style of life—abound.

Contemporary drama, too, seen in films and theatre, has more and more moved toward the physical, the emotive, the expression of feeling. And this is not simply the fruit of the Freudian revolution, for the theatre of Ibsen and O'Neill was replete with Freudian symbols and situations. Today, however, with Albee, Ionesco, Beckett, Genet, and others, there is a concentration on feeling tone and confrontation of a clearly existential, "gut-level" type. The plays of an earlier day traditionally had some sort of rational structure: a beginning, middle, and end, with action flowing along some sort of linear time sequence. Today's aptly termed "theater of the absurd" (Esslin, 1961) knows no such bounds. Performers frequently mingle with the audience, and the latter is sometimes pulled up on the stage and into the action in such a way that one may experience trouble delineating the cast from the audience. Traditional dramatic forms are eschewed for the more dreamlike, manifestly "absurd" sequences now routinely performed (Tolpin, 1968).

Finally, contemporary "hippiedom" as a manifestation of distrust in the rational ordering of society and the championing of sensual experience as a good per se is yet another cultural force running counter to intellect. Adler (1968) has used the term "antinomian" to describe the contemporary "hippie." Historically this term "designated those values and behaviors that challenged ecclesiastical authority and questioned the moral law—hence its appropriateness for current unconventional behavior" (p. 336).

Within psychology, too, a challenge to intellect appears to have manifested itself.

General Psychology

One hears talk in this decade of a "third stream" in psychology. Such a movement avows a form of "enlightened humanism" aiming to chart a course between cold, laboratory emphasis on psychological science as represented by apparatus and animal research and speculative psychoanalytic formulations and other "arty" approaches which may be long on theory but short on empirical research (cf. Maslow, 1962). Leaders of the American current of this stream, often taking their cue from European existential thinkers, generally decry the positivistic philosophy upon which laboratory psychology has built its station (Koch, 1964; American Psychological Association, 1967) and place a re-emphasis on man the experiencer, his phenomenology, on self theory, etc. A quote from Maslow (1962) imparts the flavor of this approach:

> The existentialists along with many other groups are helping to teach us about the limits of verbal, analytic, conceptual rationality. They are part of the current call back to raw experience as prior to any concepts or abstractions. This amounts to what I believe to be a justified critique of the whole way of thinking of the western world in the twentieth century, including orthodox positivistic science and philosophy, both of which badly need reexamination [pp. 13–14].

Psychotherapy

The psychotherapeutic endeavor has been the aspect of psychology which has most epitomized the trend away from intellect. The "thirdstream" leaders come essentially from a clinical therapeutic background. In Burton's words:

> Since psychotherapy can in the long run only reflect the decadent social scene that the patient brings to the consulting room—and so, too, the psychotherapist himself as a part of that same culture—it is understandable that libido conflict as a wide explanatory principle for the neuroses, and the "couch" as the principal technique of encounter, began to fade in efficacy decades ago. Indeed, the patient no longer could or would stand for this form of lonely psychiatric encounter and insisted on more care, love and intimacy than was given. In his indigenous perspicacity as a human being, the patient became less and less impressed with the intellectual juggling we called psychodynamics [1967, pp. xii–xiii].

This trend may be seen specifically in gestalt therapy's emphasis on physical and emotional action. Emphasizing this is Polster's (1966) judgment of gestalt therapy's three primary emphases: (1) encounter (of therapist and patient in here and now relation), (2) the heightening of (total) awareness and, (3) experiment (action, see examples below).

Gestalt therapists, expanding the holistic analyses of perception attributed to the gestalt theoreticians of academic psychology, e.g., Wertheimer, Koffka, and Kohler, and incorporating the action-oriented approach of Kurt Lewin, have emphasized the unitary nature of the human organism as regards "physical and mental holism" (Perls et al., 1951). Thus, their therapeutic endeavor concentrates on having the client experience, in as many "contact spheres" as possible (contact of organism and environment), rapport with the world about. Perhaps it is the traditional Western tendency to adduce verbal solutions to "problems in living" that has contributed to the major emphasis given physical "exercises" by the gestalt therapists.

Expanded self-awareness is also encouraged through such procedures as the following:

> Concentrate on your "body" sensation as a whole. Let your attention wander through every part of your body. How much of yourself can you feel? To what degree and with what accuracy does your body—and thus you—exist [Perls et al., 1951, p. 86]?

While the thinking or cognitive function is not gainsaid, the importance of body states are emphasized, as seen in the following "experiment" suggested to a client:

> Attempt to mobilize some particular pattern of body-action. For instance, tighten and loosen the jaw, clench the fists, begin to gasp. You may find that this tends to arouse a dim emotion—in this case frustrated anger. Now, if to this experience you are able to add the further experience—a fantasy, perhaps—of some person or thing in the environment which frustrates you, the emotion will flare up in full force and clarity [Perls et al., 1951, p. 98].

This emphasis very closely parallels the methodology of encounter therapists.

Encounter groups

There is a growing, nay, leaping, movement in psychotherapy which, at least on American shores, has already attained major proportions. These are the therapeutic endeavors which emphasize direct physical, emotive confrontations and are called variously sensitivity, T-, encounter and marathon group therapies. They have spread massively, if haphazardly, to a host of domains, many of which are clearly outside traditional psychotherapeutic pathways. There are groups sponsored by such diverse organizations as clerical, nursing, and business, as well as marital and seemingly just plain "fun" groups! The present discussion will be confined to those which have surfaced in the psychological literature.

Therapies emphasizing the emotive are neither unique nor previously unknown. The present writer has elsewhere (1964) discussed the relatively strong emphasis on emotion in Freudian psychotherapy as it might compare with, say Adlerian or Rational-Emotive psychotherapy. However, even within the Freudian paradigm, intellect has its day when (intellective) insight follows on emotional catharsis. Moreover, physical activity has not been emphasized in the psychoanalytic movement.

Within encounter or sensitivity or T-groups (following Schutz [1967], I use these more or less interchangeably) the client (group member) is encouraged to become physically and emotionally involved at the outset. Numerous techniques are utilized to this end. Schutz (1967) describes several. Persons who are "locked up" in themselves may be "unlocked" by being stretched back-to-back with another person. Persons who have had difficulty making "contact" with others may be asked in a group to close their eyes, stretch out their hands, and explore space around them, ultimately touching and exploring the bodies of other group members. "Wordless" sessions are sometimes utilized to stymie verbal transactions which are felt to have a shielding effect. To develop a sense of trust one person is bade to relax and group members pass him gently from one to another.

It is thus clear that the body, as an active agent, assumes overriding importance in the strategy of the encounter therapies. "The manner in which a person holds his body indicates his mood, his background, and his present accessibility to human interchange" (Schutz, 1967, p. 36).

Schutz discusses and illustrates how physical acting out, e.g., beating one's fist repeatedly against a pillow, can serve to change one's ideation, for example, as regards an imagined victim of such a beating. The emphasis is on the muscle system and the body action is used as the prime element for influencing attitudes and feelings.

With the advent of groups meeting in intensive interaction for full weekends or longer, i.e., marathon groups, we come to the extreme of the encounter method. Such extended sessions are well calculated to break down the inhibitions of those who might, in typical one-hour sessions, successfully dodge or thwart involvement in the physicalism and emotionalism of the group. Stoller (1968) has noted that the effort here is to break down conventional reserves as seen in role-playing, mask-wearing, and "distancing" techniques.

A recently popular subtype of marathon is the nude encounter (Bindrim, 1968) where clothes, seen by some therapy practitioners as the last barrier to emotional meeting, are eliminated. The groups, varying between being led by a skilled, i.e., psychotherapeutically sophisticated, leader, a lay person, or being leaderless, are paced through a variety of experiences calculated to produce a state of "joy." In Schutz's (197) words:

> A man must be willing to let himself be known to himself and to others. He must express and explore his feelings and open up areas long dormant and possibly painful, with the faith that in the long run the pain will give way to a release of vast potential for creativity and joy [pp. 16–17].

Participants in such groups are encouraged to experience strong, varied sensory input. They may touch a congenial partner; they may smell pleasurable objects and taste pleasant stimuli. "This process of sensory saturation led to a mild drugless 'turn-on' or peak state of experiencing" (Bindrim, 1968, p. 182).

Critique—Methodological

A recent review of T-group training for management personnel (Campbell and Dunnette, 1968) is relevant to an examination of the encounter therapies (the former, to the extent that they differ from the latter, do so in that they are commonly composed of businessmen seeking training for better organizational functioning). These authors indicated a list of eight assumptions underlying T-group theory, and five are borrowed (and paraphrased) here as pertinent to the methodology of psychotherapeutic group encounters. It is assumed:

1. That group members can articulate constructive feedback.
2. That group members can achieve at least rudimentary agreement on the important aspects of the situation.
3. That psychological safety (to let down barriers) can be achieved within hours, even among strangers.
4. That anxiety, normally created at the outset, facilitates learning.
5. That transfer of training occurs between the "cultural island" represented by the group and "back home."

Let us examine these in light of what is known or represents a credible (until proven otherwise) hypothesis about groups.

Encounter group members do seem to articulate some sort of consensus (Bach, 1968; Schutz, 1967; Stoller, 1968). Thus, they begin focusing on specific behaviors by certain group members. Why did John get angry when Sue pushed Bill down? The group is likely quickly to fasten on John and force him to an examination of his feelings, and he may be encouraged (even psychologically manipulated) into acting out. Groups in the typical literature have been high level as regards education and experience, so it comes as no surprise that they are able quickly to adopt a psychologizing stance.

As regards safety to reveal personality quirks, encounter groups do appear to emphasize the freedom of their atmosphere. While this may be expected to enhance the letting down of defensive barriers, it poses a greater problem as concerns transfer to a real-life situation. Still, in their research review, Campbell and Dunnette (1968) summarized that the T-group training did seem to induce "back home" behavioral changes, as seen by associates of T-group members compared with nontreated control subjects. These authors noted, however, that because of the inadequacy of experimental controls, it could not be said whether self-perception changes were greater or lesser following T-group experience when compared with other types of group experience, the simple passage of time, or the mere act of filling out a self-description questionnaire. The authors reported an interesting study by Underwood (1965) which, with a limited number of subjects, suggested that T-group participants made more changes than did controls, but the changes were viewed by reporting colleagues as unfavorable in regard to their jobs! Might it be because the job situation poses a reality vastly different from the T-group experience? More research here is clearly required.

The purpose of creating anxiety within the group setting, according to Campbell and Dunnette (1968), is for "... shaking up or jarring loose the participant from his preconceived notions and habitual forms of interacting so that feedback may have its maximum effect" (p. 76). But they noted that the research on learning is equivocal on this point, and they reported that there is some suggestion that learning is more effective under states low in anxiety. The resolution of this issue must also await future findings.

The literature on groups and aspects of groups is vast and growing rapidly, but little of it seems to have been incorporated into encounter group discussions or strategies. That much "happens" in such groups is undeniable. To sort out the operative forces so that systematic control and understanding will result seems of paramount importance. The Campbell and Dunnette review pleads for more concentration on the effects of sensitivity training on markedly differing individuals. They note that laboratory (T-group) training to date seems to proceed as if it had the same effects on everyone: "Given a particular kind of outcome, certain kinds of people may benefit from T-group training while others may actually be harmed" (1968, p. 76).

How does a variational trainer role—active, passive, or whatever—affect group process? It is Garwood's (1967) contention that the trainer is the major force in what transpires in sensitivity training. In the words of Campbell and Dunnette:

> It is surprising indeed that essentially no research has been done on the differential effects of change in the trainer role, in spite of frequent allusions in the literature to the crucial role played in the T-group by the trainer's behavior. Questions concerning the optimal procedures for giving feedback, for enhancing feelings of psychological safety, and for stimulating individuals to try new behaviors should also be investigated [1968, p. 100].

We know by now a good deal about the dynamics of persons and groups. We know that task-oriented groups evolve a different structure and dynamic from that seen in maintenance-oriented groups. We know that variational leader-follower relations affect group structure and that sex of members and physical placement of participants are factors, etc. Yet, encounter group practitioners seem blithely unaware or unconcerned with such material. It is as if, catching a glimpse of the nirvana that such joy-inspiring group experiences appear to be stretching toward, it is enough simply to count the personal testimonials of participants as they depart for "back home."

In essence, this is what the research reported by Bach (1967, 1968) consists of. His research has concerned the postencounter attitudes of "marathonians." While they overwhelmingly report positive as opposed to negative experiences (and Bach has made an analysis of what dimensions of experience seem most valuable to his respondents; e.g., aggression-confrontation is prized), there is no evaluation, from this research series, of the marathon group as a technique judged against other techniques, or of marathon clients compared to others, etc. Counter to this criticism is a recent study by Uhlemann and Weigel. They found that "significant others" in the lives of 12 marathon group participants viewed the latter as showing significantly more movement toward (self-) desired behavioral goals following marathon experience than did a control group of nonparticipants. While such research is difficult to carry out, particularly with any amount of experimental rigor, it is a crucial consideration, since elementary social psychology suggests that respondents from a group experience will traditionally report positive experiences. Campbell and Dunnette (1968) noted:

> ... it may be argued that the crucial factor in T-group training is how each *individual* feels at the end of the training program and that investigating hypotheses concerning human behavior or assessing performance change is of little consequence. This view is quite legitimate so long as the T-group assumes a status similar to that enjoyed by other purely individual events such as aesthetic appreciation or recreational enjoyment—events from which each individual takes what he chooses [p. 101].

Yet, if this technique is put forth as a serious change agent, as would seem to be implicit in the expectancies of those who pay a fee as well as in the hopes of the practitioners, then the importance of assessing lasting elements of "joy" seems obvious. Many a technique or idea is gratifying initially, only to produce ennui and disillusion when it becomes "fad for fad's sake." Dunnette warned in an earlier publication (1966):

> In industrial psychology, a most widespread current fashion is the extensive use by firms of group process or sensitivity-training programs; the effectiveness of such programs is still proclaimed solely on the basis of testimonials, and a primary rationale for their inadequate evaluation is that they are a form of therapy and must, therefore, be good and worthwhile [pp. 346-347].

Spotnitz (1968), discussing Stoller's exposition of "accelerated interaction," i.e., marathon groups, observed:

> ... To feel exhilarated and renewed is not invariably therapeutic. The dropping of masks and "learning that the masks are not so necessary" disregards the fact that some masks are vitally needed ego defenses. Some patients are unable to build bridges until they have outgrown their need for barriers. In short, the primary shortcoming of this paper [of Stoller's] is that it argues for the exposure of patients to an experience that may be desirable for some and undesirable for others without establishing any objective criteria for participation. A selection of candidates for accelerated interaction based primarily on "the feelings of the group leader" seems to be a rather hit-or-miss policy [pp. 236–237].

It is interesting to have one of our medical brethren remind us of the importance of objective methodology! House (1967) too has made a strong recommendation for the screening of participants in T-groups. He calls for "careful preselection of participating individuals by means of adequate psychometric instruments to screen out as effectively as is possible any persons for whom this method might prove potentially overwhelming" (p. 29).

What about the demands placed on the individual group members? Let us assume a volunteer who, having heard about marathon groups, being curious but knowing little, elects to join one for an extended weekend. He pays a fee, perhaps makes a considerable journey, and finds himself among a small group of strangers all of whom expect something valuable to happen to them. There are powerful demands operative in such a setting. As an example, it might be extremely difficult to partake of such a group and not be "internally convinced" (and consequently play the part) that one was undergoing significant positive experiences in the group. There are pressures to be socially appropriate (this may mean behaving very unsocially!) in the group, to enter the spirit of the leader's cues and physical exercises, even pressure from wanting to "get one's money's worth."

A cornerstone of the encounter program seems to be perseverance, demanded of the patient by the therapist in the therapeutic milieu. An example is that two persons who may dislike one another have been required to meet regularly for a specified period regardless of whether or not they would like to continue doing so. Schutz (1967) has remarked that they commonly work out a satisfactory relationship. One wonders whether a demand of this strength, no matter what its nature, might produce much the same result. I am suggesting that the powerful leader demand here may create the attitude, e.g., stemming from acquiescence, rather than any intrinsic organismic change having occurred.

Critique—Theoretical

One could say that the arc from traditional moral suasion techniques of a bygone era, with their emphasis on "telling the patient what he must do," to nude marathon groups and "doing your own thing," is no less than 180 degrees. Of course, in the latter instance, one's "own thing" is regularly subject to group demands and expectancies so it is not completely "free form." Still, the differences are many and fundamental. The view of the nature of man and such attendant things as his happiness, goals, optimal modes of functioning, etc., appears vastly different when one chooses to emphasize the physical-emotional aspect, on one hand, or intellect, on the other. Stoller (1968a) has contended:

> It is easy to see how I would appear to stand for a kind of frenzied mindlessness, a kind of psychic orgy. As I have indicated, people require a frame of reference and their need for understanding what is happening to them is extremely important. What I have found is that people come to this very readily following an intense experience and do not have to have the elements of a system fed into them. Under such an arrangement, the ideations emerge as though they were their own discoveries rather than bits of teaching given them [p. 257].

How do group members "come to this frame of reference"? This writer would again hazard that the dynamic of group and leader demand and expectancy serve as powerful conditioners. We need look no further than Mesmer (Zilboorg and Henry, 1941) to witness the power of suggestion in therapy. In spite of Stoller's (sort of) disclaimer, the subordination of intellect is clear both from the techniques and the premises cited. Parloff (1968), responding to Stoller, countered:

> The debate between those who would place primary emphasis on cognitive processes and those who would stress affect in explaining the therapeutic process is not new. Moreover, it has long been conceded that thinking without feeling does not appear to produce enduring therapeutic effects. Nor has it been found that expression of feeling in the absence of thinking has enjoyed any great therapeutic success [p. 242].

In similar vein, Anthony (1968) noted:

> The emphasis on experience rather than insight also savors of adolescence. For these therapists, to paraphrase Socrates, the unexperienced life is not worth living and the examined life is a hindrance rather than a help. "Self-knowledge is irrelevant" [p. 250].

We have seen that encounter therapies lay heavy stress on the role of the body as a conditioner of emotionality. This view calls to mind the James-Lange theory. In this theory, body changes directly follow the perception of an exciting event, and these body changes are then said to constitute the sum and substance of the emotion. Perls, Hefferline, and Goodman have specifically marked the affinity of gestalt therapy with James-Lange:

> The celebrated James-Lange theory of emotion as a reaction to bodily movements—for instance, running away gives rise to fear or weeping gives rise to sorrow—is half right. What needs to be added is that the bodily actions or condition are also a relevant *orientation to*, and a potential *manipulation of*, the environment; for example, it is not just running, but running *away*, running away from *something*, running away from something *dangerous*, that constitutes the situation of fear" [Perls et al., 1951, p. 98, italics in original].

However, James was aware that the *content* of the fear or attraction was a necessary part of the emotional sequence; he simply wanted to deny that the emotion was a "mental affection," as other theories had maintained. In subsequent discussion, Perls, Hefferline, and Goodman (1951) placed increasing emphasis on cognition (p. 99)—considerably greater than would seem fit under James' rubric. They went on to suggest that the presumed division of body and mind may be common to us because we have, in effect, not become "whole," i.e., are incipient neurotics. Still, it will hardly serve the logic of their metatheory to argue that only the healthy experience wholeness.

In any event, at the operating level, encounter group strategies give primacy to body changes over ideation in much the way that James-Lange stressed (Schutz, 1967). How adequate is the James-Lange theory?

Cannon (1927) severed the viscera of experimental animals yet obtained typical rage and other emotional response patterns under appropriate stimulation. Furthermore, the same visceral changes occurred in varying emotional states. Cannon and Sherrington's research indicated that it was the region of the thalamus which mediated emotional responsiveness, not peripheral mechanisms.

James (see Golightly, 1953), in defending his position, insisted that statements about overt behavior were not equivalent to those concerning subjective experience. Goldstein (1968) has made a similar statement, arguing that emotional behavior and emotional experience must be distinguished. This returns an implicit dualism re the mind-body issue, and is especially interesting when one considers that Goldstein speaks from a behavioristic orientation. At this stage of the game, the James theory (Lange had been almost exclusively concerned with physiology) remains, as Lindsley (1951) characterized it, an irrefutable hypothesis and not especially influential. Certainly the evidence for it is less demonstrable (measurable) than that used to buttress the centralist positions of Cannon, Sherrington, and other physiologists. This does not mean that encounter therapeutics are building on a false foundation. However, the desire to emphasize physical elements may result in distortion of the importance that imagery and intellection may have on emotion—and this even disregarding the possible intercession of suggestion as an emotional conditioner, as noted above.

A theoretical assumption that Campbell and Dunnette (1968) attributed to T-groups but that is equally applicable to encounter groups is that virtually everyone lacks interpersonal competence; that is, they tend to have distorted self-images, faulty perceptions, etc. While such an assumption is likely, by its very nature, to remain an open question, its importance may turn on the method by which prospective group members are recruited. If voluntary clients enter the group and are free to leave at will with no stigma, then in a sense they are defining themselves as in some need of treatment. But in the writer's experience this is not always the case. College courses have been run in sensitivity group fashion, and enrollment has been quasi-voluntary, i.e., a "required course." It has been used with captive audiences who were not adequately apprised of what the purpose of the technique was. It has been advertised as a sort of gay experience, a "happening." And these groups were conducted by leaders of considerable formal psychological training. The old question from social psychology, "When is a volunteer a volunteer?" remains with us and is very pertinent here.

Perhaps the central issues posed by encounter and marathon methodology play on the massive popularity they have achieved in record time. If they were esoteric techniques undertaken by a few practitioners in the sanctity of their offices, they would be of interest, but less stringently so. However, we meet them increasingly at every turn, and they appear rapidly to be passing out of the hands of experienced professionals. This same problem has already come to issue in the sensitive area of the ethics of psychological testing (American Psychological Association, 1965). Since our discipline was lax in policing testing, some has been imposed from the outside. It is not surprising if one feels prone to do some soul-searching as regards ethics at this juncture.

Is there a compelling necessity to the encounter therapy premise that the healthiest or most desirable relationships are invariably those in which one's inmost feelings, emotions, etc., are laid bare? That many persons are "bottled up" to others in these areas is demonstrably true, and some sort of confrontation with their own emotions may be eminently desirable, but this position, in the limiting case, seems to assume that conventional, even intellectual, rapprochement between, let us say, very superior individuals, is cultural, dishonest, and suspect, and this writer would vote such a theoretical bias debatable. Spotnitz (1968) has commented (perhaps unduly harshly):

> Current interest in the so-called marathon groups suggest that we are now encountering in the field of psychological medicine a phenomenon paralleling the search, in biological medicine, for one panacea for all known disease processes. That search has been abandoned; it demonstrated the necessity of devising and refining specific procedures for the treatment of different conditions [p. 238].

Anthony (1968) has written:

> *In the arena of acceleration therapy, acting out becomes the rule rather than the resistance* ... Ideally, as I see it, affect and cognition should go hand in hand, sensitively balanced to fit the needs of the passing therapeutic situation ... *There is a need to know as well as to feel, and both should find a place in the balanced therapeutic process* [p. 253, italics in original].

This observer would close by noting that new approaches deserve trial and encouragement in the art-science field of psychotherapy where dogma has often overridden reality. There is room and need for innovation, and those who press for change can be forgiven a certain pioneering zeal. Perhaps it is the popularization and consequent distortion of this strategy which has winged the conscience of this observer. As is usual when science meets the public, the former are alert to limitations which frequently have not filtered down to an eager public (Schutz, 1967, pp. 11–12). It is to be hoped that the present article may balance what seems a premature, overdetermined acceptance of an interesting and challenging therapeutic technique. Careful, long-term evaluation will alone tell if the value of the method will make it a stock in trade of the practicing psychotherapist.

References

Adler, N. (1968). The antinomian personality: The hippie character type. *Psychiatry*, **31**, 325–338.

American Psychological Association (1965). Special issue: Testing and public policy. *Amer. Psychologist*, **20**, 857–993.

AMERICAN PSYCHOLOGICAL ASSOCIATION (1967). Committee on the Scientific and Professional Aims of Psychology (1967). The scientific and professional aims of psychology. *Amer. Psychol.*, **22**, 49–76.

ANTHONY, E. J. (1968). Discussion. *This Journal*, **18**, 249–255.

BACH, G. R. (1967). Marathon group dynamics: II. dimensions of helpfulness: Therapeutic aggression. *Psychol. Rep.*, **20**, 1147–1158.

BACH, G. R. (1968). Marathon group dynamics: III. disjunctive contacts. *Psychol. Rep.*, **20**, 1163–1172.

BARZUN, J. (1959). *The House of Intellect*. New York: Harper Bros.

BINDRIM, P. (1968). A report on a nude marathon. *Psychotherapy: Theory, Research & Practice*, **5**, 180–188.

BURTON, A. (1967). *Modern Humanistic Psychotherapy*. San Francisco: Josey-Bass.

CAMPBELL, J. P., and DUNNETTE, M. D. (1968). Effectiveness of T-group experiences in managerial training and development. *Psychol. Bull.*, **70**, 73–104.

CANNON, W. B. (1927). The James-Lange theory of emotions: A critical examination and an alternative theory. *Amer. J. Psychol.*, **39**, 106–124.

DUNNETTE, M. D. (1966). Fads, fashions, and folderol in psychology. *Amer. Psychol.*, **21**, 343–352.

ESSLIN, M. (1961). *The Theatre of the Absurd*. Garden City, N.Y.: Doubleday & Co.

GARWOOD, D. S. (1967). The significance and dynamics of sensitivity training programs. *This Journal*, **17**, 457–472.

GOLDSTEIN, M. L. (1968). Physiological theories of emotion: A critical historical review from the standpoint of behavior theory. *Psychol. Bull.*, **69**, 23–40.

GOLIGHTLY, C. L. (1953). The James-Lange theory: A logical post-mortem. *Philos. of Sci.*, **20**, 286–299.

HOUSE, R. J. (1967). T-group education and leadership effectiveness: A review of empirical literature and a critical evaluation. *Personnel Psychol.*, **20**, 1–32.

JAMES, W., and LANGE, C. G. (1922). *The Emotions*. Baltimore: Williams & Wilkins Co.

KOCH, S. (1964). Psychology and emerging conceptions of knowledge as unitary. In, *Behaviorism and Phenomenology*, T. W. Wann (ed.). Chicago: University of Chicago Press.

LEVINE, E. M. (1966). The twist: A symptom of identity problems as social pathology. *Israel Ann. Psychiat. & Related Disciplines*, **4**, 198–210.

LINDSLEY, D. B. (1951), Emotion. In, *Handbook of Experimental Psychology*, S. S. Stevens (ed.). New York: Wiley.

MASLOW, A. H. (1962). *Toward a Psychology of Being*. New York: Nostrand.

PARLOFF, M. B. (1968). Discussion. *This Journal*, **18**, 239–249.

PERLS, F., HEFFERLINE, R. F., and GOODMAN, P. (1951). *Gestalt Therapy*. New York: Dell.

POLSTER, E. (1966). A contemporary psychotherapy. *Psychotherapy: Theory, Research & Practice*, **3**, 1–6.

RICKOVER, H. G. (1963). *American Education, A National Failure*. New York: Dutton.

SCHUTZ, W. C. (1967). *Joy: Expanding Human Awareness*. New York: Grove Press.

SMITH, R. J. (1964). A note on rational-emotive psychotherapy: Some problems. *Psychotherapy: Theory, Research & Practice*, **1**, 151–153.

SPOTNITZ, H. (1968). Discussion. *This Journal*, **28**, 236–239.

STOLLER, F. H. (1968). Accelerated interaction: A time limited approach based on the brief, intensive group. *This Journal*, **18**, 220–235.

STOLLER, F. H. (1968a). Discussion. *This Journal*, **18**, 255–258.

TOLPIN, M. (1968). Eugene Ionesco's "The Chairs" and the theatre of the absurd. *Amer. Imago*, **25**, 119–139.

UHLEMANN, M. R., and WEIGEL, R. G. Behavioral Change Outcomes of Marathon Group Counseling. Unpublished manuscript.

UNDERWOOD, W. J. (1965). Evaluation of laboratory method training. *Training Director's Journal*, **19**, 34–40. Cited in Campbell, J. P., and Dunnette, M. D. (1968).

ZILBOORG, G., and HENRY, G. W. (1941). *A History of Medical Psychology*. New York: Norton.

CHARLES SEASHORE

What Is Sensitivity Training?

Sensitivity training is an area of enormous current interest, and probably much misunderstanding. The term has been used to embrace a variety of types of growth groups, such as encounter groups, T-groups, marathons, and so on. Before its current vogue, sensitivity training referred to a procedure that occurred in a T- (for training) group. Dr. Seashore describes the methods and goals of these groups in a manner that may help to clarify some of the mystery that surrounds them. However, in general these groups take on different forms depending upon the training and predilections of the leader. While participation in such a group, which has been referred to as therapy for normal people, may provide an interesting and possibly helpful experience, it is important to know the qualifications of the leader before joining such a group.

Sensitivity training is one type of experience-based learning. Participants work together in a small group over an extended period of time, learning through analysis of their own experiences, including feelings, reactions, perceptions, and behavior. The duration varies according to the specific design, but most groups meet for a total of 10–40 hours. This may be in a solid block, as in a marathon weekend program or two to six hours a day in a one- or two-week residential program or spread out over several weekends, a semester, or a year.

The sensitivity training group may stand by itself or be a part of a larger laboratory training design which might include role playing, case studies, theory presentations, and intergroup exercises. This paper focuses mainly on the T Group (the *T* stands for *training*) as the primary setting for sensitivity training. However, many of the comments here also apply to other components of laboratory training.

A Typical T-Group Starter

The staff member in a typical T Group, usually referred to as the trainer, might open the group in a variety of ways. The following statement is an example:

Reprinted from the *NTL Institute News and Reports*, **2** (1968), with the permission of the NTL Institute and Dr. Seashore.

> This group will meet for many hours and will serve as a kind of laboratory where each individual can increase his understanding of the forces which influence individual behavior and the performance of groups and organizations. The data for learning will be our own behavior, feelings, and reactions. We begin with no definite structure or organization, no agreed-upon procedures, and no specific agenda. It will be up to us to fill the vacuum created by the lack of these familiar elements and to study our group as we evolve. My role will be to help the group to learn from its own experience, but not to act as a traditional chairman nor to suggest how we should organize, what our procedure should be, or exactly what our agenda will include. With these few comments, I think we are ready to begin in whatever way you feel will be most helpful.

Into this ambiguous situation members then proceed to inject themselves. Some may try to organize the group by promoting an election of a chairman or the selection of a topic for discussion. Others may withdraw and wait in silence until they get a clearer sense of the direction the group may take. It is not unusual for an individual to try to get the trainer to play a more directive role, like that of the typical chairman.

Whatever role a person chooses to play, he also is observing and reacting to the behavior of other members and in turn is having an impact on them. It is these perceptions and reactions that are the data for learning.

Underlying Assumptions of T-Group Training

Underlying T-Group training are the following assumptions about the nature of the learning process which distinguish T-Group training from other more traditional models of learning:

1. *Learning responsibility.* Each participant is responsible for his own learning. What a person learns depends upon his own style, readiness, and the relationships he develops with other members of thc group.
2. *Staff role.* The staff person's role is to facilitate the examination and understanding of the experiences in the group. He helps participants to focus on the way the group is working, the style of an individual's participation, or the issues that are facing the group.
3. *Experience and conceptualization.* Most learning is a combination of experience and conceptualization. A major T-Group aim is to provide a setting in which individuals are encouraged to examine their experiences together in enough detail so that valid generalizations can be drawn.
4. *Authentic relationships and learning.* A person is most free to learn when he establishes authentic relationships with other people and thereby increases his sense of self-esteem and decreases his defensiveness. In authentic relationships persons can be open, honest, and direct with one another so that they are communicating what they are actually feeling rather than masking their feelings.

5. *Skill acquisition and values.* The development of new skills in working with people is maximized as a person examines the basic values underlying his behavior as he acquires appropriate concepts and theory and as he is able to practice new behavior and obtain feedback on the degree to which his behavior produces the intended impact.

The Goals and Outcomes of Sensitivity Training

Goals and outcomes of sensitivity training can be classified in terms of potential learning concerning individuals, groups, and organizations.

1. *The individual point of view.* Most T-Group participants gain a picture of the impact that they make on other group members. A participant can assess the degree to which that impact corresponds with or deviates from his conscious intentions. He can also get a picture of the *range of perceptions* of any given act. It is as important to understand that different people may see the same piece of behavior differently—for example, as supportive or antagonistic, relevant or irrelevant, clear or ambiguous—as it is to understand the impact on any given individual. In fact, very rarely do all members of a group have even the same general perceptions of a given individual or a specific event.

   Some people report that they try out behavior in the T Group that they have never tried before. This experimentation can enlarge their view of their own potential and competence and provide the basis for continuing experimentation.
2. *The group point of view.* The T Group can focus on forces which affect the characteristics of the group such as the level of commitment and follow-through resulting from different methods of making decisions, the norms controlling the amount of conflict and disagreement that is permitted, and the kinds of data that are gathered. Concepts such as cohesion, power, group maturity, climate, and structure can be examined using the experiences in the group to better understand how these same forces operate in the back-home situation.
3. *The organization point of view.* Status, influence, division of labor, and styles of managing conflict are among organizational concepts that may be highlighted by analyzing the events in the small group. Subgroups that form can be viewed as analogous to units within an organization. It is then possible to look at the relationships between groups, examining such factors as competitiveness, communications, stereotyping, and understanding.

   One of the more important possibilities for a participant is that of examining the kinds of assumptions and values which underlie the behavior of people as they attempt to manage the work of the group. The opportunity to link up a philosophy of management with specific behaviors that are congruent with or antithetical to that philosophy makes the T Group particularly relevant to understanding the large organization.

Research on Sensitivity Training

Research evidence on the effectiveness of sensitivity training is rather scarce and often subject to serious methodological problems. The following generalizations do seem to be supported by the available data:

1. People who attend sensitivity training programs are more likely to improve their managerial skills than those who do not (as reported by their peers, superiors, and subordinates).
2. Everyone does not benefit equally. Roughly two-thirds of the participants are seen as increasing their skills after attendance at laboratories. This figure represents an average across a number of studies.
3. Many individuals report extremely significant changes and impact on their lives as workers, family members, and citizens. This kind of anecdotal report should be viewed cautiously in terms of direct application to job settings, but it is consistent enough that it is clear that T-Group experiences can have a powerful and positive impact on individuals.
4. The incidence of serious stress and mental disturbance during training is difficult to measure, but it is estimated to be less than one per cent of participants and in almost all cases occurs in persons with a history of prior disturbances.

Section IV

Recent Issues and Trends

This is a time in the development of the field of abnormal psychology when some rather major innovative movements are under way. These represent much more than a simple case of a new way of looking at old problems, although there is certainly some of that taking place. The more innovative programs that are emerging are really addressing themselves to a problem that is different from the one that typically engaged the mental health professional up to recent years. Where the traditional worker adopted the stance of waiting for a person to come to him with a complaint that could be classified and worked on in some time-honored way, many who are concerned about helping psychology make an even greater impact on society's problems are redefining the object of their concern. For such people criminal behavior, doing poorly at school and dropping out, alcoholism, even failure to approach living up to one's potential are all problems that must be dealt with. In addition, the idea of attempting to prevent the development of problems that must be dealt with in the clinic or hospital is also prominent.

By redefining the problem in such a way, the mental health worker is called upon to reexamine many of the assumptions that had been fundamental to the way he worked traditionally. He must also begin to understand the problem he is grappling with in different terms and his own role must be redefined. Finally, he must develop entirely new vehicles through which services can be delivered to his target group. Most of the following papers deal with various aspects of these problems.

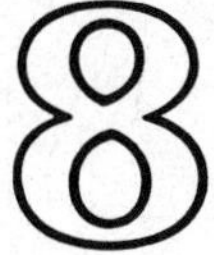

Issues and Emergent Programs

The papers in this chapter deal with the soil from which the community psychology approach grew, and some of the basic issues that must be grappled with in its development. In addition, examples are offered of specific programs that have been applied in different settings.

GERALD CAPLAN

Community Psychiatry—Introduction and Overview

The paper that introduces this section on community psychology is actually an introduction to community psychiatry written by one of that field's pioneers, Dr. Gerald Caplan. What Caplan says about the forces stimulating the development of community psychiatry, and the phases through which community psychiatry has passed in its development is equally valid for community psychology. Particularly noteworthy is Caplan's depiction of the need for community approaches, the internal conflict suffered by traditionally trained professionals attempting to develop such approaches, and the new professional role that the community mental health worker is attempting to define.

The material that has been omitted in the editing of this paper focuses on the development of new theoretical models for the community area, and issues in training professionals for work in the community. Readers interested in this material should consult the original reference.

Abridged from Chapter 1, Community Psychiatry—Introduction and Overview by G. Caplan in S. E. Goldston (ed.), *Concepts of Community Psychiatry*. Bethesda, Md.: National Institute of Mental Health, Public Health Service Publication No. 1319, 1965, pp. 3–18, with the permission of Dr. Caplan and the National Institute of Mental Health.

Over the past few years, community leaders have become increasingly interested in people suffering from mental disorders. This interest has arisen partly because of the need to conserve manpower—especially skilled manpower—in a period of rapid technological development; and partly because of the increasing assumption of responsibility by Government for the personal welfare of citizens. In the United States this interest was strikingly manifested by President Kennedy's message to Congress on February 5, 1963. This was a sequel to the Mental Health Study Act of 1955, which established the Joint Commission on Mental Illness and Mental Health, and it followed the publication of the report of that Commission in 1961.

The special significance of the President's message was that it called upon Congress to take the lead and to shoulder responsibility for the prevention and treatment of mental subnormality and mental disorder throughout the country. This is to be accomplished by providing Federal support for community programs which are planned to combat these ills on a wide scale by means of locally coordinated services. The message expresses dissatisfaction with our past ineffectual attack on mental illness through the treatment of individual patients in mental hospitals. It brushes aside some of the major recommendations of the Joint Commission to improve the mental hospital system as the core of a new program, and replaces these by a proposal to establish a series of interlocking community services and facilities. This emphasized the President's demand for a completely new approach. He advocated a focus on the total population of mentally disordered, and the development of services to identify and satisfy the whole range of their needs, rather than the provision, as in the past, of institutions to which certain of them will be admitted in order to remedy particular aspects of their problems.

The President's call to action must evoke a response not only among legislators but also among psychiatrists. In the past we have operated within the framework of our professional mandate to treat sick individuals. We have looked to the community to provide us with the institutions and other practical resources to allow us to deploy our psychiatric methods and techniques in order to fulfill our mission. Most of us have not been satisfied with these resources, and some of us have also not been satisfied with the restriction of our professional mandate to the treatment of individual patients. We have felt that unless psychiatrists are entrusted with the task of dealing with all the manifestations of mental ill health wherever they exist in the population, and unless we are provided with the necessary sanction and resources to fulfill this task, our efforts to treat those individual casualties, who are referred to us, must always be relatively ineffective in significantly reducing the total load of mental suffering and disability among community members.

The President's message offers us just such an opportunity. It calls for the establishment of coordinated programs of community psychiatry in place of facilities for the treatment of sick individuals.

Community Psychiatry is based upon the acceptance by psychiatrists of responsibility for dealing with all the mentally disordered within the confines of a community. This responsibility focuses upon current cases, but also spreads to potential cases through programs of primary prevention.

The psychiatrist in traditional clinical practice accepts responsibility only for his own patients. He restricts his interest to those individuals who come to his office, clinic, or hospital, and who are involved in a personal professional relationship with him. He usually exercises some selection over those whom he accepts for diagnosis, treatment, or management, and he legitimately narrows his practice to particular diagnostic, age, or socio-economic categories. In contrast, the community psychiatrist accepts responsibility for helping those of all ages and classes, who are suffering from disorders of all types, wherever they occur in the community. Some will be defined by themselves or others to be suffering from psychiatric disorders and will have been sent or will have come to a psychiatric facility. Others will be under general medical care because their presenting symptoms were defined as physical illness. Others will be defined as maladjusted in the educational, social, occupational, or religious fields and may be struggling on their own, or they may be receiving help from family and friends, or from the professional or administrative workers in those fields. The extent of the population for which the community psychiatrist feels responsible is difficult to determine accurately because mental disorder is arbitrarily differentiated from other forms of deviance and shades off into variations of acceptable patterns of adjustment behavior. Let us not embark on a lengthy debate about the difficult borderline cases. We can define the mentally unhealthy population for practical purposes as all those who manifest abnormalities of behavior or thinking which most psychiatrists would diagnose as being due to mental subnormality, psychosis, neurosis, psychosomatic disorder, personality disorder, and the other illnesses listed in the *A.P.A. Manual of Mental Disorders*, whether or not the individuals concerned, or others, have already defined these people as mentally disordered.

This emphasizes a fundamental problem which confronts the community psychiatrist. He differs from his traditional colleagues in having to provide services for a large number of people with whom he has had no personal contact, and of whose identity and location he has no initial knowledge. He cannot wait for patients to come to him, because he carries equal responsibility for all those who do not come. A significant part of his job consists of finding out who the mentally disordered are and where they are located in his community, and he must deploy his diagnostic and treatment resources in relation to the total group of sufferers rather than restrict them to the select few who ask or are referred for help.

These difficulties are compounded in those programs which also encompass primary prevention. These programs seek to lower the rate of new cases of mental disorder in a community by reducing harmful influences and by increasing the capacity of individuals to adjust and adapt in a reality based way to their life difficulties. Here the community psychiatrist is dealing with those who are not yet sick. He can concentrate his efforts to some extent by giving highest priority to populations at special risk, either because they are the focus of particular harmful forces or because they are especially vulnerable; but despite this, he clearly must deal with numbers of people of a magnitude which far surpasses anything in the experience of the traditional psychiatrist.

The only legitimate limitation of the population focus of the community psychiatrist is the boundary of his community. This may be geographic or functional, i.e., his community may be located within the local limits of a city, region, or State, or it may be a functional community such as an industrial firm, an army unit, a trade union, or the Peace Corps, whose members are bound together by organizational ties and not necessarily by living in one place. Certain types of community have both a geographic and a functional boundary, like colleges, hospitals, or factories. The population of such communities, although sometimes large, is usually relatively easy to investigate and define—as contrasted with the complex situation in a city or county community—because it has been developed by design in relation to stated missions and goals. It seems plausible that lessons learned by psychiatrists in these simpler communities might apply to the more complex ones. Before we proceed to our discussion of the major problems which confront the psychiatrist who accepts responsibility for the community psychiatric program of a city, county, or State, it may be helpful to review briefly some of the experience of psychiatrists working in institutions such as colleges or factories.

The history[1] of college and industrial psychiatric programs is often characterized by a succession of phases. In the beginning it is usual for the psychiatrist to be asked to diagnose and either to treat, or to refer for treatment, individual students or workers whose disordered behavior has aroused attention. The psychiatrist makes use of his traditional methods and skills, and his practice has few special characteristics apart from the more formal structuring of the referral and dispositional channels. Soon, however, the psychiatrist begins to focus more than usual on the social forces and environmental pressures impinging on his patients, because in the relatively closed system of the institution these are more easily visible to him than in the open community. He begins to learn about the conditions of work in different departments, and he finds it easier than in outside practice to identify etiological factors in the patient's current environment. This has more than diagnostic significance. The psychiatrist begins to include in his treatment plan the active manipulation of the organizational aspect of his patient's life. This is aided by his building up collaborative relationships with key figures in the administrative hierarchy of the organization.

[1] This section has been influenced by recent discussions with Harold Bridger of the Tavistock Institute of Human Relations in London and with Dr. J. J. O'Dwyer, Principal Medical Adviser of Unilever, Ltd.

The next phase is characterized by the psychiatrist becoming interested in common elements, whether etiological or clinical, among patients coming from certain departments. He becomes sensitive to variations in the numbers of cases referred at different times, and he begins to search for changes in the social and physical milieu of the units of the organization, to which he ascribes pathogenic significance, and which he tries to modify in the interests of groups of his patients.

From this, it is a short step to starting a continuing survey of the flow of patients of varying categories from different units in the organization. He then develops an interest in finding some way of extending the validity of these records by identifying those other disturbed people who do not come to his clinic because of their own low motivation or because their administrators do not refer them. In an organization, such as a factory, which keeps such records of individual performance as quantitative and qualitative productivity figures, punctuality, absenteeism, sick leave, and the like, the psychiatrist soon finds that many criteria are available to him, in addition to the clinical manifestations of referred patients, if he wishes to chart variations in individual performance which are probably related to mental disorder.

By now, it will be seen that the psychiatrist has extended his focus beyond the population of his current patient load. He has begun to investigate the environment of his organization not only as it influences his present patients but also as it may affect now and in the future those disordered people whom he is not seeing.

This widening of focus will probably by now also have been influenced by requests from the administrators of the organization for his help in handling problems of selection and personnel placement and promotion. If he accedes to these requests, he will find that he is using his clinical skills and his knowledge of personality and human relations and needs not only to deal with persons suspected of mental disorder, but also to predict the fitness of healthy persons to deal effectively with particular situations without endangering their mental health. He will also be exercising some influence upon the nature of the population in the organization, and hopefully he will be reducing the risk of mental disorder by excluding vulnerable candidates and by preventing the fitting of round pegs into square holes.

At this stage, if not before, the psychiatrist will be facing the fundamental problem of how best to deploy his own resources, and those of the assistants who have probably been added to his unit as the demands for his services have increased. Although the range of his interests has broadened, his basic concern still remains the reduction of suffering and disability among the mentally disordered in the organization. His awareness of their numbers and condition has increased, as has also his understanding of the environmental forces inimical or conducive to their welfare.

One conclusion should be clear to him by this time. The problem is too big to handle on the traditional basis of the diagnosis and treatment of individuals. No organization can afford to maintain a psychiatric staff big enough to diagnose and treat adequately each of its members who is mentally disturbed. Even with the most effective selection system to screen out disturbed or potentially disturbed candidates for admission, the expectable environmental stresses of any organization, added to the spontaneous incidence of unpredictable disturbances of endogenous or extra-organization origin, will result in too many patients for such an approach.

If the problem is dealt with by reducing referrals or building waiting lists for intake or treatment, suffering will continue and the productivity of disordered individuals will deteriorate, and also of those other members of the organization who are dependent upon them for support or for the flow of materials and services. Referral to outside treatment resources is no way out, because most private and community agencies are already full, or soon would be if the organization radically increased its volume of referrals. Apart from humanitarian and administrative considerations, the problem cannot be dealt with by discharging a major portion of the sufferers from the organization, because many of them in industry are likely to be skilled employees who are in scarce supply, or in college they are talented students who, apart from their mental difficulties, are of great promise.

This apparent impasse in planning the deployment of psychiatric resources is the turning point in the development of the program. Some psychiatrists are so wedded to their traditional individual-patient diagnosis and treatment approach that they see no way out. Their machine gets clogged up with increasing numbers of patients who are referred from all sides by administrators who have become alerted to problems of mental disorder and who have got to know the psychiatrists and to respect them. At the same time the psychiatrists are exposed to increasing demands for nonclinical help in selection, in personnel management, and in counseling administrators. Lengthening the waiting lists, and interrupting intake—those easy defense mechanisms of psychiatrists in the open community—may be tried, but they lead to the rapid build-up of frustration and resentment in the relatively closed community of an organization. In this setting the visibility of the psychiatrist is greater, as is also the amount of control over him. He may be able to extricate himself by retracing his steps and progressively walling himself off, cutting down his contacts, and narrowing his focus. The alternative is to abandon ship!

The history of psychiatric programs in colleges and industries brings to our attention some psychiatrists who did not reach this sorry state because they interrupted their development at an earlier stage, but also many who have resolved this crisis, or even circumvented it earlier, by a radical shift in orientation which has carried them onto a different plane of professional functioning. These psychiatrists no longer base their programs on the traditional assumption that mental disorder, like any illness, should if at all possible be diagnosed and treated by a medical specialist and on the corollary assumption that a mentally disordered individual who is not personally treated by a pyschiatrist is likely to suffer more intensely and for a longer period than if he were. Instead, they begin to operate on the assumption that mental disorder is often caused or aggravated by unhealthy forms of life adjustment, and that when it occurs there are many possibilities available to the sufferer, and the social network of which he is part, to modify their mutual relationships so that a healthier equilibrium will be obtained, which in turn will have a beneficial effect on the disorder.

In a community, a variety of regularly occurring mechanisms exist which may stimulate all concerned in such instances to change the pattern of their relationships. These include social pressures brought into play by alterations in the smooth functioning of the work or social situation. They include the actions of administrators who try to modify the organizational life to produce a better fit between the sufferer and others in order to improve output. They include informal patterns of support by peers, and the operations of a variety of caregiving professionals—personnel and health workers inside the organization, and clergymen, social workers, and counselors in the outside community. Among all these influences the psychiatrist occupies an important position. He has a special contribution to make, which can often be helpful. But he is one among many, and often one or more of the other possibilities might produce as good or better results than if his aid were involved.

The traditional assumptions drive the psychiatrist to see all sufferers personally because he feels that any alternative is second best or even harmful. The second assumption leads to a more leisurely survey of the possibilities. The psychiatrist realizes that as one of the many helpful forces in the community he should evaluate the others and then decide in accordance with each set of circumstances the amount of profit to be gained by his intervention, and whether this should take the form of personal interaction with the sufferer or of supporting the helpful influence of other elements in the system, or of some combination of these. The predicted profit can then be related to the outlay of effort. Since this approach does not necessarily involve a contractual arrangement with the sufferer, whose case may be considered on the basis of information supplied by others, the psychiatrist is free to deploy his efforts in such a way as to benefit the largest number of sufferers in the organization, rather than being forced to deal in a preordained way with each successive case.

From this derives the paradox that the psychiatrist who takes the traditional individual-patient point of view affects less patients than the other and yet is always pressed for time. He is at the mercy of the chance nature of his patient flow. He feels that what he has to do is determined by the number and type of the patients he happens to see. In contrast, the second psychiatrist controls his own operations in the light of explicit judgments of the whole field of forces. He is therefore able to operate at maximum efficiency by choosing the most favorable and opportune moments for his interventions and by utilizing available leverage points so that other helpers in the field of forces multiply his own efforts. This psychiatrist does not feel pressed for time because in his planning he is constantly taking into account the amount of his available resources of time and energy, and the proportions to be deployed in relation to the priority of alternative goals.

His methods include individual diagnostic and treatment contact with certain types of case, and in addition, a whole range of indirect methods which foster the supportive or remedial contributions of the other caregiving persons and services of the institution. The indirect methods consist mainly in offering individual and group consultation to administrators and caregivers on how best to deal with a person currently in crisis or showing signs of disorder. If successful, such consultation has a carryover which will enable similar cases to be handled in the future without having to invoke the aid of the psychiatrist. The effect of this is that gradually more and more cases are handled within the social system of the organization without referral and even without consultation.

The final step for the industrial and college psychiatrist is that he becomes interested in what Dr. O'Dwyer the Principal Medical Adviser of Unilever has called "the health of the firm." By this he means the quality of its organization which affects the well-being of its component parts and ultimately the morale and the health of its workers. The psychiatrist is called in by the administrators for consultation not only in respect to the management of the malfunctioning of an individual or a group of workers, but also in regard to any policy issue which may significantly affect the interrelationships of groups and individuals. Eventually, those who established the policies which govern the entire structure and functioning of the organization delay major decisions until he has given his views on the probable repercussions of their actions on the mental health of their workers. The administrators may or may not accept his advice, but in any case they take into account the mental health implications of different courses of action before deciding. If their plan involves a hazard for certain individuals and groups they may build into it some additional provisions to counteract the emotional burden or to compensate for it.

ERNEST G. POSER

The Effect of Therapists' Training on Group Therapeutic Outcome

One of the most critical problems in the mental health field is in the area of manpower shortage. The number of well-trained psychotherapists does not nearly satisfy the need for such people. One reaction to this problem has been the development of a number of treatment paradigms that do not rely on the trained professional. Such novices as housewives, college students, and parents of disturbed children have been enlisted in an attempt to cope with manpower problems. This raises the question of whether these less well-trained people are competent to deal with the complex issues of treatment of the mentally ill. In this paper, Dr. Poser examines the efficacy of a group of untrained college students, as compared to professionals, in group therapy with schizophrenic patients, and finds the two groups to be similarly effective, with the advantage, although slight, resting with the nonprofessionals. Dr. Poser quite correctly indicates that it is impossible to draw conclusions from this research that go beyond the specific method of treatment and type of patient studied, but it is of interest that a good deal of other evidence supports the generality of the finding that nonprofessionals can be highly effective therapeutic agents.

The present manpower shortage in the mental health professions has given new impetus to investigations concerned with therapist variables in studies of therapeutic outcome. Hence, it is not surprising that recent work in this field, notably by Anker and Walsh (1961), Beck, Kantor, and Gelineau (1963), Rioch, Elkes, Flint, Usdansky, Newman, & Silber (1963), and Schofield (1964) should have focused attention on what appear to be the active therapeutic ingredients of the patient-therapist interaction. All of these authors suggest that effective therapy can be carried out by personnel without professional training, and most of them provide objective evidence in support of this view.

Truax (1963) and his associates also drew attention to nonacademic qualifications of therapists by their ingenious demonstration that those rated

---

Reprinted from the *Journal of Consulting Psychology*, **30** (1966), 283–289, with the permission of the American Psychological Association and Dr. Poser.

high with respect to certain human qualities, such as "accurate empathy," tend to improve the psychological functioning of schizophrenics, while therapists rated low in empathy actually impair the clinical status of their patients. The therapist's personality attributes with which Truax is concerned are essentially those previously elaborated by Rogers (1957), who does not feel that special intellectual professional knowledge—psychological, psychiatric, medical, or religious—is required of the therapist. In this context he observes that "intellectual training and the acquiring of information has, I believe, many valuable results—but becoming a therapist is not one of those results [p. 101]." This view is consistent with the speculation that nonprofessional workers, possibly selected in accordance with Truax's criteria, could do effective therapy, at least with certain types of patients.

There is urgent need for studies seeking to define those aspects of the treatment process which crucially affect therapeutic outcome. Without such information, it is difficult to distinguish between the necessary and the superfluous conditions of therapeutic personality change. But it may be misleading to think of the variance accounting for therapeutic outcome only in terms of active versus inactive ingredients, if the term "active" is meant to imply the deliberate application of some theory or procedure to the conduct of psychotherapy. There may be a third source of therapeutic change related to the familiar placebo effect operative in most other forms of medical and psychiatric treatment. Because, strictly speaking, there is no such thing as "inert" psychotherapy in the sense that placebos are pharmacologically inert, the term "placeboid" might serve to describe this effect in psychotherapy.

Rosenthal and Frank (1956) have dealt with the placebo phenomenon in some detail and conclude that

> . . . improvement under a special form of psychotherapy cannot be taken as evidence for: (*a*) correctness of the theory on which it is based; or (*b*) efficacy of the specific technique used, unless improvement can be shown to be greater than, or qualitatively different from that produced by the patients' faith in the efficacy of the therapist and his technique—"the placebo effect" [p. 300].

More recently, Frank, Nash, Stone, and Imber (1963) have shown that some psychiatric patients recover simply as a result of attending a clinic or receiving placebo, without psychotherapy or other treatment being given.

Such studies, however, do not bear on the crucial problem of placeboid effects in the psychotherapeutic interaction itself. They do not tell us whether some of the supposedly active ingredients of therapy, such as the theoretical training or experience of the therapist, for instance, are or are not relevant to therapeutic outcome. Could it be that such behavior change as does occur posttherapeutically is due to other factors not hitherto considered to be necessary antecedents of therapeutic change? Fiedler (1950) and others have already shown that adherents of widely disparate theoretical persuasions achieve much the same results in psychotherapy, and more recently similar findings have been reported by Gelder, Marks, Sakinofsky, and Wolff (1964) with respect to the comparative outcome of psychotherapy and behavior therapy. Though rich in implication, none of these studies were specifically designed to test for placeboid effects in therapeutic outcome. To do so, according to Rosenthal and Frank (1956), requires, in addition to the therapy under study, the application of

> another form of therapy in which patients had equal faith, so that the placebo effect operated equally in both, but which would not be expected by the theory of therapy being studied to produce the same effects [p. 300].

The present study constitutes an attempt to provide a controlled experiment in line with the above suggestion.

The therapeutic technique under study was group therapy with chronic schizophrenics. The fact that such therapy is most often carried out by psychiatrists, social workers, occupational therapists, and psychologists (Poser, 1965) suggests that training in one of these professions is commonly regarded as an appropriate, if not essential, prerequisite for the successful group therapist. To test the validity of this assumption three treatment conditions were compared in this investigation.

In the first, group therapy was conducted by highly trained psychiatrists, social workers, and occupational therapists. In the second condition all therapists were undergraduate students without previous training or experience relevant to the care of mental patients. Because a comparison of two treatments in terms of their effectiveness would be meaningless without first demonstrating the validity of the outcome criterion to be applied, a control group of untreated patients was also included.

In terms of Rosenthal and Frank's statement cited above, the untrained therapists in the present investigation were thought to provide a form of treatment which, by virtue of their lacking professional sophistication, would prove to be less effective than that offered by trained personnel. This, at least, would be the prediction if it is true that training and experience are relevant to therapeutic outcome. At the same time, there was no reason to believe that the patients had more faith in the trained than the untrained therapists, since they were in the main unaware of this distinction. Hence placeboid effects, if any, could operate equally in both therapeutic situations. In fact, the untrained therapists are here conceptualized as contributing nothing but placeboid effect, much as the pharmacologically inert substance does in a placebo-controlled drug study. By corollary, the theoretical sophistication and past experience of a trained therapist is, for the purpose of this study, viewed as the active ingredient in the therapeutic process. In other words, it is proposed that such therapeutic effectiveness as untrained therapists do attain is attributable to nonspecific aspects of the helping relationship, such as activation, sympathy, opportunity for verbal ventilation, regularity of attendance, and the like. These would appear to be formally comparable to the nonspecific factors thought to underlie placebo responses as, for instance, attention giving, expectation inducing, pill ingestion, and many other situational variables familiar to the drug therapist. Many of these variables are highly effective in the treatment of certain physical disabilities, as placebo studies of patients with headaches (Jellinek, 1946) or the common cold (Diehl, Baker, and Cowan, 1940) have abundantly shown. A similar phenomenon may operate in psychotherapy, which would account for the near-ubiquitous two-thirds improvement rate consequent upon most forms of psychotherapy.

Method

Subjects. A total of 343 male chronic schizophrenics was studied. They represent almost the entire male schizophrenic population of a 1,500-bed hospital, only assaultive patients and those suffering from known organic brain damage having been excluded. Their median age was 47 years (range 20–73). All of them had been hospitalized uninterruptedly for at least 3 years. Their median length of hospitalization was 14 years, with a range from 3 to 44 years.

The vast majority of these patients were receiving phenothiazine medication at the time of the study. This was continued throughout, and only in emergencies was medication changed during the course of the project.

Therapists. The untrained therapists consisted of 11 young women between the ages of 18 and 25. All were undergraduate students in one of Montreal's universities, and most had never had a course in psychology. None intended to enter a mental health profession, nor had any of them ever visited a mental hospital. No attempt was made to select a particular type of applicant. Anyone who expressed interest in the project and accepted the terms of employment was enrolled. They were paid at the standard rate for summer employment at that time and were asked to consent to the taking of numerous psychological tests which were to be used for subsequent investigation. As an additional control, two inpatients—one an alcoholic and the other suffering from hysteria—were asked to act as untrained therapists.

The professional therapists were seven psychiatrists, six psychiatric social workers, and two occupational therapists. In addition to their formal professional qualifications, that is, certification in psychiatry, all the psychiatrists had had from 5 to 17 years of professional experience. All but one had previously done group psychotherapy, and three were specialized in this area. Their ages ranged from 35 to 50, and all were male.

All social workers had had postgraduate professional training leading to a degree and at least 5 years' professional experience. Two were specialized in group work, and all but two had had previous experience doing case or group work with psychotic patients. Their ages ranged from 36 to 43, and two out of the six were male.

The two occupational therapists had professional experience of 5 and 7 years' duration, respectively, and this included some mental hospital work. Both were female, one aged 27 and the other 30.

None of the therapists taking part in this project was on the staff of the hospital where this work was done, nor were any of the patients known to the therapists prior to the start of the project. All were paid at the rate appropriate to their profession.

Tests. Selection of these was guided by three considerations. First, the performance required had to be within the behavioral repertoire of chronic schizophrenic patients. Second, preference was given to tests which had previously been demonstrated to differentiate normals from psychotics. Since a large number of patients were involved, the third criterion was purely practical—those tests were chosen which could be administered in a relatively short space of time.

The final test battery consisted of two psychomotor, two perceptual, and two verbal tests, in addition to the Palo Alto Hospital Adjustment Scale (McReynolds & Ferguson, 1946), intended to provide a quantitative estimate of the patients' adjustment in the hospital. The tests were:

1. Speed of tapping (TAP). (The number of taps on a reaction key in 10 seconds.)
2. A test of visual reaction-time (RT) involving choice.
3. The Digit-Symbol test (DS) of the Wechsler-Bellevue Scale I.
4. A color-word conflict test (Stroop), in which the score reflects the time taken by the patient to read 100 color names under three conditions of increasing difficulty (Thurstone & Mellinger, 1953).
5. Verbal fluency (VF). (The number of different animals named in 1 minute.)
6. The Verdun Association List (VAL), a 20-item word-association test devised by Sigal (1956) to discriminate between working and nonworking mental hospital patients.

All of these tests were individually administered immediately before or after therapy. Occasionally a patient was found untestable before or after therapy. Such patients were seen by another examiner, so that no patient was given a zero score on any test unless he had been given two opportunities to take it from a different examiner on each occasion.

Procedure. The 343 patients were selected for this project by the psychiatric staff of the hospital. Each patient was assigned to a group in such a way that every unit of 10 patients would be matched as closely as possible with every other unit in terms of the patients' age, severity of illness, and length of hospitalization. Following this, the groups were compared with respect to their mean test performance prior to therapy. Where major disparities between groups were noted, individual patients were exchanged, so that all groups were roughly comparable with respect to age, clinical status, length of hospitalization, and test performance prior to therapy.

At this stage six groups (one of them composed of 13 patients) were picked at random to serve as untreated controls. Patients in these groups received the usual hospital care, but were excluded from all forms of group treatment other than routine occupational therapy. The remaining 28 groups were each assigned to a therapist picked at random from among the project staff available at the time. The project extended over three periods of 5 months. In the first of these, 11 untrained therapists took part; in the second, seven professional and one untrained therapist; and in the final period, eight professional and one untrained therapist.

Each therapist met his or her group during 1 hour daily 5 days a week for a period of 5 months. A special attendant saw to it that patients would join their groups at the appropriate time and place. Even so, one or two patients in almost every group refused to attend regularly. Their absences were recorded, and only those patients who attended at least two-thirds of all available sessions were re-evaluated at the end of the 5-month period. This reduced the total number of patients included in the study from 343 to 295. At the time of the post-therapy retest no group had less than six members who met the attendance criterion.

Both the trained and untrained therapists were quite free to conduct their therapy sessions in any way they wished. Wherever possible, the materials or facilities they required were provided by the hospital, but at no time did the project director offer suggestions for procedure or in any way facilitate communication among therapists while the project was under way. To get some idea of each therapist's approach, a few sessions of every group were attended by an observer. Also, each therapist was asked to keep a daily record of his group's activities. Some therapists used only verbal communication during therapy; others arranged activities ranging from party games and dancing to "communal" painting and public speaking. All stressed interaction among members of their group.

Results

The pre- and post-therapy test scores of all patients were subjected to covariance analysis. The covariance adjusted posttherapy scores of the untreated control group were then compared to those of the patients treated by lay therapists (Table 1) and those of the professional therapists (Table 2), respectively. This was done for each of the six tests separately. On all tests, with the exception of the Stroop, a high score indicates better performance than a low score.[2]

Similar comparisons were made between the posttherapy scores of patients receiving lay therapy and those treated by professionals (Table 3). Finally, in Table 4, interprofessional comparisons are made between the posttherapy test behavior of patients treated by social workers and psychiatrists.

It appears from these tables that the largest number of significant differences in test behavior occur between the untreated group and those groups treated by lay therapists. Four out of the six tests reflect significantly better performance by the patients of lay therapists. The VAL approaches significance in the expected direction.

On comparing the test behavior of the untreated with that of patients treated by professionals, only two out of the six tests show significant superiority of the latter group (Table 2).

[2] The reversal of direction in the Stroop test scores arises from the raw score's being expressed as a ratio.

TABLE 1 *Covariance adjusted posttherapy scores of untreated patients and those treated by lay therapists*

Treatment		TAP	VF	VAL	DS	RT	Stroop
Untreated controls	Mean	45.763	11.699	26.218	20.428	.169	2.508
($N = 63$)	*SD*	9.772	4.449	6.580	7.204	.054	.768
Treated by lay therapists	Mean	49.735	12.600	28.786	24.135	.197	1.025
($N = 87$)	*SD*	10.222	4.370	8.264	6.812	.063	.698
	t	2.308†	1.295	1.801*	2.922**	2.613	2.336‡

* $p < .10$.
† $p < .05$.
‡ $p < .02$.
** $p < .01$.

TABLE 2 *Covariance adjusted posttherapy scores of untreated patients and those treated by professional therapists*

Treatment		TAP	VF	VAL	DS	RT	Stroop
Untreated controls	Mean	45.763	11.699	26.218	20.428	.169	2.508
($N = 63$)	*SD*	9.772	4.449	6.580	7.204	.054	.768
Treated by professional therapists	Mean	46.372	10.948	28.104	23.187	.154	.835
($N = 145$)	*SD*	9.894	3.061	6.950	5.612	.049	.579
	t	.387	1.148	1.427	2.313‡	1.688	2.903**

‡ $p < .02$.
** $p < .01$.

A direct comparison of patients treated by lay and professional therapists reveals a significantly better performance on the part of those treated by the former on three of the six tests (Table 3). It is of interest to note that the standard deviation on every test is smaller for the group of patients treated by professional therapists.

Table 4 suggests that there is no significant difference between post-therapeutic test performance of patients treated by social workers and the performance of those treated by psychiatrists.

Because the study began with patients treated by lay therapists, it was possible before the end of the project to retest some of the patients and most

TABLE 3 *Covariance adjusted posttherapy scores of patients treated by lay and professional therapists*

Treatment		TAP	VF	VAL	DS	RT	Stroop
Treated by lay therapists	Mean	49.735	12.600	28.786	24.135	.197	1.025
($N = 87$)	*SD*	10.222	4.370	8.264	6.812	.063	.698
Treated by professional therapists	Mean	46.372	10.948	28.104	23.187	.154	.835
($N = 145$)	*SD*	9.894	3.061	6.950	5.612	.049	.579
	t	2.331†	2.899**	.588	.930	4.998§	.356

† $p < .05$.
** $p < .01$.
§ $p < .001$.

TABLE 4 *Covariance adjusted posttherapy scores for patients treated by social workers and psychiatrists*

Treatment		TAP	VF	VAL	DS	RT	Stroop
Treated by social workers	Mean	47.332	10.613	27.687	22.324	.154	1.025
($N = 53$)	*SD*	10.222	3.05	6.618	6.603	.063	.656
Treated by psychiatrists	Mean	46.252	11.212	28.011	23.307	.151	.755
($N = 60$)	*SD*	8.978	3.162	7.899	5.459	.040	.561
	t	.564	.743	.203	.688	.249	.321

of the untreated controls who took part in the first phase of the investigation. These scores, obtainable from 61 patients, constitute a 3-year follow-up and are presented in Table 5. To save time, only four of the original six tests were given in this part of the study, and a *t* test for correlated means was used to evaluate the difference between the two test sessions, separated by 3 years. Table 5 shows that test performance after 3 years was still significantly better than it was before treatment on all of the tests used. That this result was not a function of greater familiarity with the tests at follow-up—by which time each patient had taken them twice before—is indicated by the result of retesting 23 untreated controls after 3 years. Only on the tapping test did they show significantly better performance on follow-up, much as they had done on the first retest after 5 months.

In an effort to get some measure of change in the patients' ward behavior,

TABLE 5 *Three-year follow-up of schizophrenics treated by lay therapists* ($N = 61$)

Stage		TAP	VF	RT	VAL
Before treatment	Mean	38.84	9.02	326.24	19.08
	SD	19.63	5.50	405.09	14.07
Three years later	Mean	48.15	10.52	183.07	24.20
	SD	17.50	6.43	320.04	14.53
	t	4.22§	2.58‡	3.61§	3.32**

‡ $p < .02$.
** $p < .01$.
§ $p < .001$.

the Hospital Adjustment Scale was administered to 80 patients, all of whom had been treated by lay therapists. The scale was administered before treatment, and again after 5 months. On each occasion it was completed both by the nursing supervisor and an attendant familiar with the patients. The supervisor's ratings showed significant improvement between test and retest, but the attendants' ratings did not. It was felt that this equivocal result reflected little more than the greater ego-involvement of the supervisors, whose wish to see the project succeed might well have influenced their ratings.

Unfortunately it was not possible to have the scale completed by personnel sufficiently familiar with the patients to assess their behavior and yet unaware of their participation in the project. For this reason and also because of the ward staff's strong resistance to the time consuming task of filling out the scale it was not administered to subsequent therapy groups.

Discussion

The objection may be made that changes in psychological test performance, as employed in this study, do not constitute a relevant criterion of therapeutic outcome. The usual alternatives are rating scales, questionnaires, or the comparison of discharge rates before and after therapy. None of these seemed appropriate for the present patient population, consisting as it did of schizophrenics with many years of hospitalization. The behavioral repertoire of such patients is so limited that rating scales are difficult to complete, as our own attempt at using the Hospital Adjustment Scale clearly showed. For the same reason, questionnaires completed by the patients would be hard to interpret. Discharge rates during and after therapy were compared, but showed no significant difference between treated and untreated groups. Nor would this be expected in the light of previous findings, such as those of Beck et al. (1963). Their study showed that in a sample of 120 psychotics, those who were discharged during the Harvard undergraduate volunteer program had, on the average, been hospitalized for 4.7 years, whereas the undischarged patients had been hospitalized for 12.4 years. This is consistent with earlier studies, suggesting that after 4 years of hospitalization only 3% of patients are likely to be discharged.

With one exception (Stroop) the verbal and performance tests employed in the present investigation were known from earlier work to discriminate effectively between psychotics and normals. It therefore seems justified to interpret significant incremental change in the treated groups' test behavior as reflecting therapeutic gain. This conclusion is validated by the absence of such change in the untreated control group on five out of the six tests. That the TAP did show significant improvement on retest of the control group may reflect the greater emphasis placed on activity programs for mental patients in recent years. On the other hand, since tapping was the first test to be administered to each patient, initial performance on it may have been impaired by apparatus stress or the novelty effect of the test situation.

Why lay therapists should have done somewhat better than professional therapists in facilitating the test behavior of their patients remains a matter of conjecture. It seems likely that the naïve enthusiasm they brought to the therapeutic enterprise, as well as their lack of "professional stance" permitted them to respond more freely to their patients' mood swings from day to day. Certainly, the activities in which they engaged their patients had a less stereotyped character than that offered by their professional counterparts. On the other hand, the greater standard deviation in the test behavior of those treated by lay therapists suggests that they may have helped some of their patients at the expense of others. Professional therapy, by contrast, seems to have had a more even effect on all participants.

The 3-year follow-up data for the untrained group are highly encouraging and support the conclusion that the therapy given achieved more than transient activation. It is planned to carry out similar follow-up studies on the patients treated by professional therapists.

The groups treated by fellow patients were too small to make quantitative assessment very meaningful. Their results were, however, treated separately in the covariance analysis and showed no significant difference from patients treated by lay or professional therapists. They received excellent cooperation from their fellows, as evidenced by their group attendance record, which showed full attendance in one group and 8 out of 10 in the other. Those who knew the patient-therapists clinically agreed that participation in the project had enhanced their mental health. Both are now discharged after prolonged hospitalization.

To extend the conclusions from this study beyond its present context, that is, the outcome of group therapy with chronic schizophrenics, would clearly be premature. When viewed in relation to the literature reviewed at the outset of this paper, the present findings do, however, support the conclusion that traditional training in the mental health professions may be neither optimal nor even necessary for the promotion of therapeutic behavior change in mental hospital patients.

References

ANKER, J. M., & WALSH, R. P. (1961). Group psychotherapy, a special activity program, and group structure in the treatment of chronic schizophrenics. *Journal of Consulting Psychology*, **25**, 476–481.

BECK, J. C., KANTOR, D., & GELINEAU, V. A. (1963). Follow-up study of chronic psychotic patients "treated" by college case-aide volunteers. *American Journal of Psychiatry*, **120**, 269–271.

DIEHL, H. S., BAKER, A. B., & COWAN, D. W. (1940). Cold vaccines, further evaluation. *Journal of the American Medical Association*, **115**, 593–594.

FIEDLER, F. E. (1950). A comparison of therapeutic relationships in psychoanalytic, non-directive and Adlerian therapy, *Journal of Consulting Psychology*, **14**, 436–445.

FRANK, J. D., NASH, E. H., STONE, A. R., & IMBER, S. D. (1963). Immediate and long-term symptomatic course of psychiatric out-patients. *American Journal of Psychiatry*, **120**, 429–439.

GELDER, M. G., MARKS, I. M., SAKINOFSKY, I., & WOLFF, H. H. (1964). Behavior therapy and psychotherapy for phobic disorders: Alternative or complementary procedures? Paper presented at the 6th International Congress of Psychotherapy, London.

JELLINEK, E. M. (1946). Clinical tests on comparative effectiveness of analgesic drugs. *Biometrics Bulletin*, **2**, 87.

MCREYNOLDS, P., & FERGUSON, J. T. (1946). *Clinical Manual for the Hospital Adjustment Scale*. Palo Alto: Consulting Psychologists Press.

POSER, E. G. (1966). Group therapy in Canada: A national survey. *Canadian Psychiatric Association Journal*, **11**, 20–25.

RIOCH, M. J., ELKES, C., FLINT, A. A., USDANSKY, B. S., NEWMAN, R. G., & SILBER, E. (1963). National Institute of Mental Health pilot study in training mental health counselors. *American Journal of Orthopsychiatry*, **33**, 678–689.

ROGERS, C. R. (1957). The necessary and sufficient conditions of therapeutic personality change. *Journal of Consulting Psychology*, **21**, 95–103.

ROSENTHAL, D., & FRANK, J. D. (1956). Psychotherapy and the placebo effect. *Psychological Bulletin*, **53**, 294–302.

SCHOFIELD, W. (1964). *Psychotherapy: The Purchase of Friendship*. Englewood Cliffs, N.J.: Prentice-Hall.

SIGAL, J. (1956). The Verdun Association List. Unpublished doctoral dissertation, University of Montreal.

THURSTONE, L. L., & MELLINGER, J. J. (1953). *The Stroop Test*. University of North Carolina, The Psychometric Laboratory.

TRUAX, C. B. (1963). Effective ingredients in psychotherapy: An approach to unraveling the patient-therapist interactions. *Journal of Counseling Psychology*, **10**, 256–263.

M. BREWSTER SMITH[1] and NICHOLAS HOBBS[2]

The Community and the Community Mental Health Center[3]

One of the most significant material impetuses to the development of community approaches to treating mental disorder has been the federal support program for establishing community mental health centers. The purpose of these centers was to bring treatment services closer to the community and making such services more readily available than was characteristically true under the traditional state hospital system. The hope was that community mental health centers would alleviate the need for large, isolated institutions that serve as a last resort for those with very serious problems. In actual fact, the mental health centers that have been developed have sprung up in a variety of locations and under the auspices of many different groups. As a result, there tends to be relatively little similarity between any two centers, and many are not vastly different from traditional mental hospitals and clinics.

In their paper Smith and Hobbs attempt to describe the spirit that was intended to guide the establishment of mental health centers. In the process they set forth important guidelines for what should be the ideal approach in the establishment of such service agencies.

Throughout the country, states and communities are readying themselves to try the "bold new approach" called for by President John F. Kennedy to help the mentally ill and, hopefully, to reduce the frequency of mental

[1] M. Brewster Smith is Professor of Psychology and Director of the Institute of Human Development at the University of California, Berkeley. He was Vice President of the Joint Commission on Mental Illness and Health and was formerly President of the Society for the Psychological Study of Social Issues and Editor of the *Journal of Abnormal and Social Psychology*.

[2] Nicholas Hobbs is Provost of Vanderbilt University and Director of the John F. Kennedy Center for Research on Education and Human Development at Peabody College. He was Vice-Chairman of the Board of Trustees of the Joint Commission on Mental Illness and Health and is currently President of the American Psychological Association and Vice President of the Joint Commission on Mental Health of Children.

[3] This statement was adopted on March 12, 1966, by the Council of Representatives as an official position paper of the American Psychological Association.

Reprinted from *American Psychologist*, **21** (1966), 499–509, with the permission of the American Psychological Association and M. B. Smith.

disorders. The core of the plan is this: to move the care and treatment of the mentally ill back into the community so as to avoid the needless disruption of normal patterns of living, and the estrangement from these patterns, that often come from distant and prolonged hospitalization; to make the full range of help that the community has to offer readily available to the person in trouble; to increase the likelihood that trouble can be spotted and help provided early when it can do the most good; and to strengthen the resources of the community for the prevention of mental disorder.

The community-based approach to mental illness and health attracted national attention as a result of the findings of the Joint Commission on Mental Illness and Health that was established by Congress under the Mental Health Study Act of 1955. After 5 years of careful study of the nation's problems of mental illness, the Commission recommended that an end be put to the construction of large mental hospitals, and that a flexible array of services be provided for the mentally ill in settings that disrupt as little as possible the patient's social relations in his community. The idea of the comprehensive community mental health center was a logical sequel.

In 1962, Congress appropriated funds to assist states in studying their needs and resources as a basis for developing comprehensive plans for mental health programs. Subsequently, in 1963, it authorized a substantial Federal contribution toward the cost of constructing community mental health centers proposed within the framework of state mental health plans. It appropriated $35,000,000 for use during fiscal year 1965. The authorization for 1966 is $50,000,000 and for 1967 $65,000,000. Recently, in 1965, it passed legislation to pay part of the cost of staffing the centers for an initial period of 5 years. In the meantime, 50 states and 3 territories have been drafting programs to meet the challenge of this imaginative sequence of Federal legislation.

In all the states and territories, psychologists have joined with other professionals, and with non-professional people concerned with mental health, to work out plans that hold promise of mitigating the serious national problems in the area of human well-being and effectiveness. In their participation in this planning, psychologists have contributed to the medley of ideas and proposals for translating the concept of comprehensive community mental health centers into specific programs. Some of the proposals seem likely to repeat past mistakes. Others are fresh, creative, stimulating innovations that exemplify the "bold new approach" that is needed.

Since the meaning of a "comprehensive community mental health center" is far from self-evident, the responsible citizen needs some guidelines or principles to help him assess the adequacy of the planning that may be underway in his own community, and in which he may perhaps participate. The guidelines and discussion that are offered here are addressed to community leaders who face the problem of deciding how their communities should respond to the opportunities that are opened by the new Federal and state programs. In drafting what follows, many sources have been drawn upon: the monographs and final report of the Joint Commission, testimony presented to Congress during the consideration of relevant legislation, official brochures of the National Institute of Mental Health, publications of the American Psychiatric Association, and recommendations from members of the American Psychological Association who have been involved in planning at local, state, and national levels.

The community mental health center, 1966 model, cannot be looked to for a unique or final solution to mental health problems: Varied patterns will need to be tried, plans revised in the light of evaluated experience, fossilized rigidity avoided. Even as plans are being drawn for the first comprehensive centers under the present Federal legislation, still other bold approaches to the fostering of human effectiveness are being promulgated under the egis of education and of economic opportunity programs. A single blueprint is bound to be inadequate and out of date at the moment it is sketched. The general approach underlying these guidelines may, it is hoped, have somewhat more enduring relevance.

Throughout, the comprehensive community mental health center is considered from the point of view of members of a community who are seeking good programs and are ultimately responsible for the kind of programs they get. The mental health professions are not to be regarded as guardians of mental health, but as agents of the community—among others—in developing and conserving its human resources and in restoring to more effective functioning people whose performance has been impaired. Professional people are valuable allies in the community's quest for the health and well-being of its members, but the responsibility for setting goals and major policies cannot be wisely delegated.

Community Involvement and Community Control

For the comprehensive community mental health center to become an effective agency of the community, community control of center policy is essential.

The comprehensive community mental health center represents a fundamental shift in strategy in handling mental disorders. Historically, and still too much today, the preferred solution has been to separate the mentally ill person from society, to put him out of sight and mind, until, if he is lucky, he is restored to normal functioning. According to the old way, the community abandoned its responsibility for the "mental patient" to the distant mental hospital. According to the new way, the community accepts responsibility to come to the aid of the citizen who is in trouble. In the proposed new pattern, the person would remain in his own community, often not even leaving his home, close to family, to friends, and to the array of professional people he needs to help him. Nor would the center wait for serious psychological problems to develop and be referred. Its program of prevention, detection, and early intervention would involve it in many aspects of community life and in many institutions not normally considered as mental health agencies: the schools, churches, playgrounds, welfare agencies, the police, industry, the courts, and community councils.

This spread of professional commitment reflects in part a new conception of what constitutes mental illness. The new concept questions the appropriateness of the term "illness" in this context, in spite of recognition that much was gained from a humanitarian viewpoint in adopting the term. Mental disorders are in significant ways different from physical illnesses. Certainly mental disorder is not the private misery of an individual; it often grows out of and usually contributes to the breakdown of normal sources of social support and understanding, especially the family. It is not just an individual who has faltered; the social systems in which he is embedded through family, school, or job, through religious affiliation or through friendship, have failed to sustain him as an effective participant.

From this view of mental disorder as rooted in the social systems in which the troubled person participates, it follows that the objective of the center staff should be to help the various social systems of which the community is composed to function in ways that develop and sustain the effectiveness of the individuals who take part in them, and to help these community systems regroup their forces to support the person who runs into trouble. The community is not just a "catchment area" from which patients are drawn; the task of a community mental health center goes far beyond that of purveying professional services to disordered people on a local basis.

The more closely the proposed centers become integrated with the life and institutions of their communities, the less the community can afford to turn over to mental health professionals its responsibility for guiding the center's policies. Professional standards need to be established for the centers by Federal and state authorities, but goals and basic policies are a matter for local control. A broadly based responsible board of informed leaders should help to ensure that the center serves in deed, not just in name, as a focus of the community's varied efforts on behalf of the greater effectiveness and fulfillment of all its residents.

Range of Services

The community mental health center is "comprehensive" in the sense that it offers, probably not under one roof, a wide range of services, including both direct care of troubled people and consultative, educational, and preventive services to the community.

According to the administrative regulations issued by the Public Health Service, a center must offer five "essential" services to qualify for Federal funds under the Community Mental Health Centers Act of 1963: (*a*) *inpatient care* for people who need intensive care or treatment around the clock; (*b*) *outpatient care* for adults, children, and families; (*c*) *partial hospitalization*, at least day care and treatment for patients able to return home evenings and weekends, perhaps also night care for patients able to work but needing limited support or lacking suitable home arrangements; (*d*) *emergency care* on a 24-hour basis by one of the three services just listed; and (*e*) *consultation and education* to community agencies and professional personnel. The regulations also specify five additional services which, together with the five "essential" ones, "complete" the comprehensive community mental health program: (*f*) *diagnostic service*; (*g*) *rehabilitative service* including both social and vocational rehabilitation; (*h*) *precare and aftercare*, including screening of patients prior to hospital admission and home visiting or halfway houses after hospitalization; (*i*) *training* for all types of mental health personnel; and (*j*) *research and evaluation* concerning the effectiveness of programs and the problems of mental illness and its treatment.

That the five essential services revolve around the medically traditional inpatient-outpatient core may emphasize the more traditional component of the comprehensive center idea somewhat at the expense of full justice to the new conceptions of what is crucial in community mental health. Partial hospitalization and emergency care represent highly desirable, indeed essential, extensions of the traditional clinical services in the direction of greater flexibility and less disruption in patterns of living. Yet the newer approach to community mental health through the social systems in which people are embedded (family, school, neighborhood, factory, etc.) has further implications. For the disturbed person, the goal of community mental health programs should be to help him and the social systems of which he is a member to function together as harmoniously and productively as possible. Such a goal is more practical, and more readily specified, than the elusive concept of "cure," which misses the point that for much mental disorder the trouble lies not within the skin of the individual but in the interpersonal systems through which he is related to others. The emphasis in the regulations upon consultation and public education goes beyond the extension of direct patient services to open wide vistas for imaginative experimentation.

The vanguard of the community approach to mental health seeks ways in which aspects of people's social environment can be changed in order to improve mental health significantly through impact on large groups. Just as a modern police or fire department tries to prevent the problems it must cure, so a good mental health center would look for ways of reducing the strains and troubles out of which much disorder arises. The center might conduct surveys and studies to locate the sources of these strains; it might conduct training programs for managers, for teachers, for ministers to help them deal with the problems that come to light. By providing consultation on mental health to the governing agencies of the community, to schools, courts, churches, to business and industry, the staff of the center can bring their special knowledge to bear in improving the quality of community and family life for all citizens. Consultation can also be provided to the state mental hospitals to which the community sends patients, to assist these relics of the older dispensation in finding a constructive place in the new approach to mental health. Preferably, revitalized state hospitals will become integral parts of the comprehensive service to nearby communities.

In performing this important and difficult consultative role, the mental health professionals of the center staff do not make the presumptuous and foolish claim that they "know best" how the institutions of a community should operate. Rather, they contribute a special perspective and special competencies that can help the agencies and institutions of community life—the agencies and institutions through which people normally sustain and realize themselves—find ways in which to perform their functions more adequately. In this endeavor, the center staff needs to work in close cooperation with other key agencies that share a concern with community betterment but from different vantage points: councils of social agencies, poverty program councils, labor groups, business organizations, and the like. To promote coordination, representatives of such groups should normally be included in the board responsible for the center's policies.

Communities may find that they want and need to provide for a variety of services not specifically listed among the "additional services" in the regulations issued by the Public Health Service: for example, a special service for the aged, or a camping program, or, unfortunately, residences for people who do not respond to the best we can do for them. The regulations are permissive with respect to additional services, and communities will have to give close and realistic attention to their own needs and priorities. For many rural areas, on the other hand, and for communities in which existing mental health services are so grossly inadequate that the components of a comprehensive program must be assembled from scratch, the present regulations in regard to essential services may prove unduly restrictive. Communities without traditions of strong mental health services may need to start with something short of the full prescribed package. So long as their plan provides for both direct and indirect services, goes beyond the traditional inpatient-outpatient facility, and involves commitment to movement in the direction of greater comprehensiveness, the intent of the legislation might be regarded as fulfilled.

Many of the services that are relevant to mental health will naturally be developed under auspices other than the comprehensive center. That is desirable. Even the most comprehensive center will have a program that is more narrowly circumscribed than the community's full effort to promote human effectiveness. What is important is that the staff of the center be in good communication with related community efforts, and plan the center's own undertakings so as to strengthen the totality of the community's investment in the human effectiveness of its members.

Facilities

Facilities should be planned to fit a program and not vice versa.

The comprehensive community mental health center should not be thought of as a place, building, or collection of buildings—an easy misconception—but as a people-serving organization. New physical facilities will necessarily be required, but the mistake of constructing large, congregate institutions should not be repeated. The danger here is that new treatment facilities established in medical centers may only shift the old mental hospital from country to town, its architecture changed from stone and brick to glass and steel. New conceptions are needed even more than new facilities.

Small units of diverse design reflecting specific functions and located near users or near other services (such as a school or community center) might be indicated, and can often be constructed at a lesser cost than a centralized unit linked to a hospital. For example, most emotionally disturbed children who require residential treatment can be effectively served in small residential units in a neighborhood setting removed from the hospital center. Indeed, there is the possibility that the hospital with its tense and antiseptic atmosphere may confirm the child's worst fears about himself and set his deviant behavior.

Each community should work out the pattern of services and related facilities that reflects its own problems, resources, and solutions. The needs and resources of rural areas will differ radically from those of urban ones. Every state in the nation has its huge mental hospitals, grim monuments to what was once the latest word in treatment of the mentally ill, and a major force in shaping treatment programs ever since. It should not be necessary to build new monuments.

Continuity of Concern

Effective community action for mental health requires continuity of concern for the troubled individual in his involvements with society, regardless of awkward jurisdictional boundaries of agencies, institutions, and professions.

A major barrier to effective mental health programing is the historical precedent of separating mental health services from other people-serving agencies—schools, courts, welfare agencies, recreational programs, etc. This is partly a product of the way of thinking that follows from defining the problem as one of illness and thus establishing the place of treatment and the professional qualifications required to "treat" it. There are thus immense gaps in responsibility for giving help to people in trouble. Agencies tend to work in ignorance of each other's programs, or at cross purposes. For example, hospital programs for emotionally disturbed children often are operated with little contact with the child's school; a destitute alcoholic who would be hospitalized by one community agency is jailed by another.

Current recommendations that a person in trouble be admitted to the total mental health system and not to one component of it only fall short of coming to grips with the problem. The laudable aim of these recommendations is to facilitate movement of a person from one component to another—from hospital to outpatient clinic, for example, with minimum red tape and maximum communication among the professional people involved.

Such freedom of movement and of communication within the mental health system is much to be desired. But freedom of movement and of communication between systems is quite as important as it is within a system.

No one system can comprise the range of mental health concerns to which we are committed in America, extending from serious neurological disorders to include the whole fabric of human experience from which serious —and not so serious—disorders of living may spring. Mental health is everyone's business, and no profession or family of professions has sufficient competence to deal with it whole. Nor can a mental health center, however comprehensive, encompass it. The center staff can and should engage in joint programing with the various other systems with whom "patients" and people on the verge of trouble are significantly involved—school, welfare, industry, justice, and the rest. For such joint programing to reflect the continuity of concern for the individual that is needed, information must flow freely among all agencies and "systems." The staff of the center can play a crucial role in monitoring this flow to see to it that the walls that typically restrict communication between social agencies are broken down.

Reaching Those Who Most Need Help

Programs must be designed to reach the people who are hardly touched by our best current efforts, for it is actually those who present the major problems of mental health in America.

The programs of comprehensive community mental health centers must be deliberately designed to reach all of the people who need them. Yet the forces generated by professional orthodoxies and by the balance of public initiative or apathy in different segments of the community—forces that have shaped current "model" community mental health programs—will tend unless strenuously counteracted to restrict services to a favored few in the community. The poor, the dispossessed, the uneducated, the "poor treatment risk," will get less service—and less appropriate service—than their representation in the community warrants, and much, much less service than their disproportionate contribution to the bedrock problem of serious mental illness would demand.

The more advanced mental health services have tended to be a middle-class luxury; chronic mental hospital custody a lower-class horror. The relationship between the mental health helper and the helped has been governed by an affinity of the clean for the clean, the educated for the educated, the affluent for the affluent. Most of our therapeutic talent, often trained at public expense, has been invested not in solving our hard-core mental health problem—the psychotic of marginal competence and social status—but in treating the relatively well-to-do educated neurotic, usually in an urban center. Research has shown that if a person is poor, he is given some form of brief, mechanical, or chemical treatment; if his social, economic, and educational position is more favored, he is given long-term conversational psychotherapy. This disturbing state of affairs exists whether the patient is treated privately or in a community facility, or by a psychiatrist, psychologist, or other professional person. If the community representatives who take responsibility for policy in the new community mental health centers are indignant at this inequity, their indignation would seem to be justified on the reasonable assumption that mental health services provided at public expense ought to reach the people who most need help. Although regulations stipulate that people will not be barred from service because of inability to pay, the greatest threat to the integrity and usefulness of the proposed comprehensive centers is that they will nonetheless neglect the poor and disadvantaged, and that they will simply provide at public expense services that are now privately available to people of means.

Yet indignation and good will backed with power to set policy will not in themselves suffice to bring about a just apportionment of mental health services. Inventiveness and research will also be indispensable. Even when special efforts are made to bring psychotherapy to the disturbed poor, it appears that they tend not to understand it, to want it, or to benefit from it. They tend not to conceive of their difficulties in psychological terms or to realize that talk can be a "treatment" that can help. Vigorous experimentation is needed to discover ways of reaching the people whose mental health problems are most serious. Present indications suggest that methods hold most promise which emphasize actions rather than words, deal directly with the problems of living rather than with fantasies, and meet emergencies when they arise without interposing a waiting list. Much more attention should also be given to the development of nonprofessional roles for selected "indigenous" persons, who in numerous ways could help to bridge the gulf between the world of the mental health professional and that of the poor and uneducated where help is particularly needed.

Innovation

Since current patterns of mental health service are intrinsically and logistically inadequate to the task, responsible programing for the comprehensive community mental health center must emphasize and reward innovation.

What can the mental health specialist do to help people who are in trouble? A recent survey of 11 most advanced mental health centers, chosen to suggest what centers-in-planning might become, reveals that the treatment of choice remains individual psychotherapy, the 50-minute hour on a one-to-one basis. Yet 3 minutes with a sharp pencil will show that this cannot conceivably provide a realistic basis for a national mental health program. There simply are not enough therapists—nor will there ever be—to go around, nor are there enough hours, nor is the method suited to the people who constitute the bulk of the problem—the uneducated, the inarticulate. Given the bias of existing facilities toward serving a middle-class clientele, stubborn adherence to individual psychotherapy when a community can find and afford the staff to do it would still be understandable if there were clear-cut evidence of the superior effectiveness of the method with those who find it attractive or acceptable. But such evidence does not exist. The habits and traditions of the mental health professions are not a good enough reason for the prominence of one-to-one psychotherapy, whether by psychiatrists, psychologists, or social workers, in current practice and programing.

Innovations are clearly required. One possibility with which there has been considerable experience is group therapy; here the therapist multiplies his talents by a factor of six or eight. Another is crisis consultation: a few hours spent in active intervention when a person reaches the end of his own resources and the normal sources of support run out. A particularly imaginative instance of crisis consultation in which psychologists have pioneered is the suicide-prevention facility. Another very promising innovation is the use under professional direction of people without professional training to provide needed interpersonal contact and communication. Still other innovations, more radical in departure from the individual clinical approach, will be required if the major institutional settings of youth and adult life—school and job—are to be modified in ways that promote the constructive handling of life stresses on the part of large numbers of people.

Innovation will flourish when we accept the character of our national mental health problem and when lay and professional people recognize and reward creative attempts to solve it. Responsible encouragement of innovation, of course, implies commitment to and investment in evaluation and research to appraise the merit of new practices.

Children

In contrast with current practice, major emphasis in the new comprehensive centers should go to services for children.

Mental health programs tend to neglect children, and the first plans submitted by states were conspicuous in their failure to provide a range of services to children. The 11 present community programs described as models were largely adult oriented. A recent (1965) conference to review progress in planning touched occasionally and lightly on problems of children. The Joint Commission on Mental Illness and Health bypassed the issue; currently a new Joint Commission on Mental Health of Children is about to embark upon its studies under Congressional auspices.

Most psychiatric and psychological training programs concentrate on adults. Individual psychotherapy through talk, the favored method in most mental health programs, is best suited to adults. What to do with an enraged child on a playground is not normally included in curricula for training mental health specialists. It would seem that our plans and programs are shaped more by our methods and predilections than by the problems to be solved.

Yet an analysis of the age profile of most communities—in conjunction with this relative neglect—would call for a radically different allocation of money, facilities, and mental health professionals. We do not know that early intervention with childhood problems can reduce later mental disorder, but it is a reasonable hypothesis, and we do know that the problems of children are receiving scant attention. Sound strategy would concentrate our innovative efforts upon the young, in programs for children and youth, for parents, and for teachers and others who work directly with children.

The less than encouraging experience of the child guidance clinic movement a generation and more ago should be a stimulus to new effort, not an occasion for turning away from services to children. The old clinics were small ventures, middle-class oriented, suffering from most of the deficiencies of therapeutic approach and outreach that have been touched upon above. A fresh approach to the problems of children is urgently needed.

We feel that fully half of our mental health resources—money, facilities, people—should be invested in programs for children and youth, for parents of young children, and for teachers and others who work directly with children. This would be the preferable course even if the remaining 50% were to permit only a holding action with respect to problems of adults. But our resources are such that if we care enough we can move forward on both fronts simultaneously.

The proposal to place the major investment of our mental health resources in programs for children will be resisted, however much sense it may make, for it will require a thoroughgoing reorientation of the mental health establishment. New facilities, new skills, new kinds of professional people, new patterns for the development of manpower will be required. And new and more effective ways must be found to reach and help children where they are—in families and schools—and to assist these critically important social systems in fostering the good development of children and in coming to the child's support when the developmental course goes astray. This is one reason why community leaders and other nonprofessionals concerned with the welfare and development of people should be centrally involved in establishing the goals of community mental health centers. They can and should demand that the character of the new centers be determined not by the present habits and skills of professional people but by the nature of the problem to be solved and the full range of resources available for its solution.

Planning for Problem Groups That Nobody Wants

As a focus for community planning for mental health, the comprehensive center should assure that provision is made to deal with the mental health component in the problems of various difficult groups that are likely to "fall between the stools" of current programs.

Just as good community programing for mental health requires continuity of concern for the troubled individual, across the many agencies and services that are involved with him, so good programing also requires that no problem groups be excluded from attention just because their problems do not fit neatly into prevalent categories of professional interest, or because they are hard to treat.

There are a number of such groups of people, among whom problems of human ineffectiveness are obvious, yet whose difficulties cannot accurately or helpfully be described as mainly psychological: for example, addicts, alcoholics, the aging, delinquents, the mentally retarded. It would be presumptuous folly for mental health professionals to claim responsibility for solving the difficult social and biological problems that are implicated in these types of ineffectiveness. But it would also be irresponsible on the part of persons who are planning community mental health programs not to give explicit attention to the adequacy of services being provided to these difficult groups and to the adequacy of the attack that the community is making on those aspects of their problems that are accessible to community action.

Recently, and belatedly, national attention has been focused on the mentally retarded. This substantial handicapped group is likely to be provided for outside the framework of the mental health program as such, but a good community mental health plan should assure that adequate provision is in fact made for them, and the comprehensive center should accept responsibility for serving the mental health needs of the retarded and their families.

Some of the other problem groups just mentioned—e.g., the addicts and alcoholics—tend to get left out partly because treatment by psychiatric or psychological methods has been relatively unproductive. Naturally, the comprehensive center cannot be expected to achieve magical solutions where other agencies have failed. But if it takes the approach advocated here—that of focusing on the social systems in which problem behavior is embedded—it has an opportunity to contribute toward a rational attack on these problems. The skills that are required may be more those of the social scientist and community change agent than those of the clinician or therapist.

In planning its role with respect to such difficult groups, the staff of the center might bear two considerations in mind: In the network of community agencies, is humanly decent care being provided under one or another set of auspices? And does the system-focused approach of the center have a distinctive contribution to make toward collaborative community action on the underlying problems?

Manpower

The present and future shortage of trained mental health professionals requires experimentation with new approaches to mental health services and with new divisions of labor in providing these services.

The national effort to improve the quality of life for every individual—to alleviate poverty, to improve educational opportunities, to combat mental disorders—will tax our resources of professional manpower to the limit. In spite of expanded training efforts, mental health programs will face growing shortages of social workers, nurses, psychiatrists, psychologists, and other specialists. The new legislation to provide Federal assistance for the staffing of community mental health centers will not increase the supply of manpower but perhaps may result in some minor redistribution of personnel. If adequate pay and opportunities for part-time participation are provided, it is possible that some psychiatrists and psychologists now in private practice may join the public effort, adding to the services available to people without reference to their economic resources.

The manpower shortage must be faced realistically and with readiness for invention, for creative solutions. Officially recommended staffing patterns for community mental health centers (which projected nationally would require far more professionals than are being trained) should not be taken as setting rigid limitations. Pediatricians, general medical practitioners, social workers other than psychiatric ones, psychological and other technicians at nondoctoral levels should be drawn into the work of the center. Specific tasks sometimes assigned to highly trained professionals (such as administrative duties, follow-up contacts, or tutoring for a disturbed child) may be assigned to carefully selected adults with little or no technical training. Effective communication across barriers of education, social class, and race can be aided by the creation of new roles for specially talented members of deprived groups. New and important roles must be found for teachers, recreation workers, lawyers, clergymen. Consultation, in-service training, staff conferences, and supervision are all devices that can be used to extend resources without sacrificing the quality of service.

Mental health centers should find ways of using responsible, paid volunteers, with limited or extended periods of service. There is a great reservoir of human talent among educated Americans who want to contribute their time and efforts to a significant enterprise. The Peace Corps, the Vista program, Project Head-Start have demonstrated to a previously skeptical public that high-level, dependable service can be rendered by this new-style volunteer. The contributions of unpaid volunteers—students, housewives, the retired—can be put to effective use as well.

Professional Responsibility

Responsibility in the comprehensive community mental health center should depend upon competence in the jobs to be done.

The issue of who is to be responsible for mental health programs is complex, and not to be solved in the context of professional rivalries. The broad conception of mental health to which we have committed ourselves in America requires that responsibility for mental health programs be broadly shared. With good will, intelligence, and a willingness to minimize presumed prerogatives, professional people and lay board members can find ways of distributing responsibility that will substantially increase the effectiveness of a center's program. The tradition, of course, is that the director of a mental health center must be a psychiatrist. This is often the best solution, but other solutions may often be equally sensible or more so. A social worker, a psychologist, a pediatrician, a nurse, a public health administrator might be a more competent director for a particular center.

The issue of "clinical responsibility" is more complex but the principle is the same: Competence rather than professional identification should be the governing concern. The administration of drugs is clearly a competence-linked responsibility of a physician. Diagnostic testing is normally a competence-linked responsibility of a psychologist; however, there may be situations in which a psychiatrist or a social worker may have the competence to get the job done well. Responsibility for psychotherapy may be assumed by a social worker, psychiatrist, psychologist, or other trained person. The director of training or of research could reasonably come from one of a number of disciplines. The responsible community member, to whom these guidelines are addressed, should assure himself that there is a functional relationship in each instance between individual competence and the job to be done.

This issue has been given explicit and responsible attention by the Congress of the United States in its debates and hearings on the bill that authorizes funds for staffing community mental health centers. The intent of Congress is clear. As the Senate Committee on Labor and Public Welfare states in its report on the bill (Report No. 366, to accompany H.R. 2985, submitted June 24, 1965):

> There is no intent in any way in this bill to discriminate against any mental health professional group from carrying out its full potential within the realm of its recognized competence. Even further it is hoped that new and innovative tasks and roles will evolve from the broadly based concept of the community mental health services. Specifically, overall leadership of a community mental health center program may be carried out by any one of the major mental health professions. Many professions have vital roles to play in the prevention, treatment and rehabilitation of patients with mental illnesses.

Similar legislative intent was established in the debate on the measure in the House of Representatives.

Community members responsible for mental health centers should not countenance absentee directorships by which the fiction of responsibility is sustained while actual responsibility and initiative are dissipated. This is a deviee for the serving of professions, not of people.

Training

The comprehensive community mental health center should provide a formal training program.

The need for centers to innovate in the development or reallocation of professional and subprofessional roles, which has been stressed above in line with Congressional intent, requires in every center an active and imaginative training program in which staff members can gain competence in their new roles. The larger centers will also have the self-interested obligation to participate in the training of other professionals. Well-supervised professional trainees not only contribute to the services of a center; their presence and the center's training responsibilities to them promote a desirable atmosphere of self-examination and openness to new ideas.

There should be a director of training who would be responsible for: (*a*) in-service training of the staff of the center, in the minimum case; and, in the larger centers, (*b*) center-sponsored training programs for a range of professional groups and including internships, field placements, postdoctoral fellowships, and partial or complete residency programs; and (*c*) university-sponsored training programs that require the facilities of the center to give their students practical experience. Between 5% and 10% of the center's budget should be explicitly allocated to training.

Program Evaluation and Research

The comprehensive community mental health center should devote an explicit portion of its budget to program evaluation. All centers should inculcate in their staff attention to and respect for research findings; the large centers have an obligation to set a high priority on basic research and to give formal recognition to research as a legitimate part of the duties of staff members.

In the 11 "model" community programs that have been cited previously, both program evaluation and basic research are rarities; staff members are commonly overburdened by their service obligations. That their mental health services continue to emphasize one-to-one psychotherapy with middle-class adults may partly result from the small attention that their programs give to the evaluative study of program effectiveness. The programs of social agencies are seldom evaluated systematically and tend to continue in operation simply because they exist and no one has data to demonstrate whether they are useful or not. In this respect the "model" programs seem to be no better.

The whole burden of the preceding recommendations, with their emphasis on innovation and experimentation, cries out for substantial investment in program evaluation. Only through explicit appraisal of program effects can worthy approaches be retained and refined, ineffective ones dropped. Evaluative monitoring of program achievements may vary, of course, from the relatively informal to the systematic and quantitative, depending on the importance of the issue, the availability of resources, and the willingness of those responsible to take the risks of substituting informed judgment for evidence.

One approach to program evaluation that has been much neglected is hard-headed cost analysis. Alternative programs should be compared not only in terms of their effects, but of what they cost. Since almost any approach to service is likely to produce some good effects, mental health professionals may be too prone to use methods that they find most satisfying rather than those that yield the greatest return per dollar.

All community mental health centers need to plan for program evaluation;

the larger ones should also engage in basic research on the nature and causes of mental disorder and on the processes of diagnosis, treatment, and prevention. The center that is fully integrated with its community setting will have unique opportunities to study aspects of these problems that elude investigation in traditional clinic and hospital settings. That a major investment be made in basic research on mental health problems was the recommendation to which the Joint Commission on Mental Illness and Health gave topmost priority.

The demands of service and of research are bound to be competitive. Because research skills, too, are scarce, it is not realistic to expect every community mental health center to have a staff equipped to undertake basic research. At the very least, however, the leadership in each center should inculcate in its training program an attitude of attentiveness to research findings and of readiness to use them to innovate and change the center's practices.

The larger centers, especially those that can establish affiliation with universities, have an obligation to contribute to fundamental knowledge in the area of their program operations. Such centers will normally have a director of research, and a substantial budget allocation in support of research, to be supplemented by grants from foundations and governmental agencies. By encouraging their staff members to engage in basic studies (and they must be sedulously protected from encroaching service obligations if they are to do so), these centers can make an appropriate return to the common fund of scientific and professional knowledge upon which they draw; they also serve their own more immediate interests in attracting and retaining top quality staff and in maintaining an atmosphere in which creativeness can thrive. As a rough yardstick, every center should devote between 5% and 10% of its budget to program evaluation and research.

Variety, Flexibility, and Realism

Since the plan for a comprehensive community mental health center must allocate scarce resources according to carefully considered priorities tailored to the unique situation of the particular community, wide variation among plans is to be expected and is desirable. Since decisions are fallible and community needs and opportunities change, provision should be made for flexibility and change in programs, including periodic review of policies and operations.

In spite of the stress in these guidelines on ideal requirements as touchstones against which particular plans can be appraised, no single comprehensive center can be all things to all men. Planning must be done in a realistic context of limited resources and imperfect human talent as well as of carefully evaluated community needs, and many hard decisions will have to be made in setting priorities. In rural areas, especially, major alterations in the current blueprint would seem to be called for if needed services are to be provided. As a result, the comprehensive community mental health centers that emerge should be as unique as the communities to whose needs and opportunities they are responsive. This is all to the good, for as it has been repeatedly emphasized, there is no well-tested and prefabricated model to be put into automatic operation. Variety among centers is required for suitability to local situations; it is desirable also for the richer experience that it should yield for the guidance of future programing.

The need for innovation has been stressed; the other side of the same coin is the need for adaptability to the lessons of experience and to changing requirements of the community. Flexibility and adaptiveness as a characteristic of social agencies does not "just happen"; it must be planned for. The natural course of events is for organizations to maintain themselves with as little change as possible, and there is no one more conservative than the proponent of an established, once-radical departure. Plans for the new centers should therefore provide for the periodic self-review of policies and operations, with participation by staff at all levels, and by outside consultants if possible. To the extent that active program evaluation is built intrinsically into the functioning of the center, the review process should be facilitated, and intelligent flexibility of policy promoted. Self-review by the center staff should feed into general review by the responsible board of community leaders, in which the board satisfies itself concerning the adequacy with which the policies that it has set have been carried out.

This final recommendation returns once more to the theme, introduced at the outset, that has been implicit in the entire discussion: the responsibility of the community for the quality and adequacy of the mental health service that it gets. The opportunities are now open for communities to employ the mechanism of the comprehensive mental health center to take major strides toward more intelligent, humane, and effective provision for their people. If communities rise to this opportunity, the implications for the national problem of mental health and for the quality of American life are immense.

FRANK RIESSMAN

The "Helper" Therapy Principle

A significant development in community psychology has been the introduction of a variety of nonprofessional groups recruited and trained to provide many types of mental health services. One obvious reason for recruiting nonprofessionals is that professional manpower is in drastically short supply.

Reprinted from *Social Work*, **10** (1965), 27–32, with the permission of the National Association of Social Workers and F. Riessman.

Another reason is that many new community programs are attempting to reach target populations that have characteristically not been well understood or dealt with effectively by middle class mental health workers. The indigenous nonprofessional is, therefore, a necessary bridge to the lower class community.

In the paper that follows, Riessman makes a very important point concerning the nonprofessional movement. He asserts that there is considerable reason to believe that nonprofessionals who serve as helpers in mental health programs can derive important personal benefits from such a role. This, then, is an additional dividend of the community program that utilizes nonprofessionals. Making a "helper" of a person who has a serious problem himself may alleviate that problem as well as provide significant benefit for a number of other community members who need help.

An age-old therapeutic approach is the use of people with a problem to help other people who have the same problem in more severe form (e.g., Alcoholics Anonymous). But in the use of this approach—and there is a marked current increase in this tendency—it may be that emphasis is being placed on the wrong person in centering attention on the individual receiving help. More attention might well be given the individual who needs the help less, that is, the person who is providing the assistance, because frequently it is he who improves!

While it may be uncertain that people *receiving* help are always benefited, it seems more likely that the people *giving* help are profiting from their role. This appears to be the case in a wide variety of self-help "therapies," including Synanon (for drug addicts), Recovery Incorporated (for psychologically disturbed people), and Alcoholics Anonymous. Mowrer notes that there are over 265 groups of this kind listed in a directory, *Their Brother's Keepers.*[1] The American Conference of Therapeutic Self-Help Clubs publishes an official magazine, *Action,* describing some of the functions of these groups.

While there is still a need for firm research evidence that these programs are effective, various reports (many of them admittedly impressionistic) point to improvement in the givers of help rather than the recipients. Careful research evaluating these programs is needed, because there are numerous contaminating factors that may be contributing to their success, such as the leadership of the therapist, selection of subjects, and the newness or novelty of the program.

Although much of the evidence for the helper principle is observational and uncontrolled, there is one experimental investigation that provides at

[1] O. Hobart Mowrer, *The New Group Therapy* (Princeton, N.J.: D. Van Nostrand Co., 1964), p. iv.

least indirect verification or support of the principle. In a study by King and Janis in which role-playing was used, it was found that subjects who had to improvise a speech supporting a specific point of view tended to change their opinions in the direction of this view more than subjects who merely read the speech for an equivalent amount of time.[2] They describe this effect in terms of "self-persuasion through persuading others."

Volkman and Cressey formulate this principle as one of their five social-psychological principles for the rehabilitation of criminals:

> The most effective mechanism for exerting group pressure on members will be found in groups so organized that criminals are induced to join with non-criminals for the purpose of changing other criminals. A group in which criminal "A" joins with some non-criminals to change criminal "B" is probably most effective in changing criminal "A", not "B". . . .[3]

Perhaps, then, social work's strategy ought to be to devise ways of creating more helpers! Or, to be more exact, to find ways to transform *recipients* of help into *dispensers* of help, thus reversing their roles, and to structure the situation so that recipients of help will be placed in roles requiring the giving of assistance.

In most of the programs mentioned thus far the helpers and the helped have had essentially the same problem or symptom. The approach is carried one step further in Recovery Incorporated, in which emotionally disturbed people help each other even though their symptoms may differ.

A somewhat more indirect expression of the principle is found in the sociotherapeutic approach reported by Wittenberg some years ago.[4] Wittenberg found that participation in a neighborhood block committee formed to help other people in the neighborhood led to marked personality development and growth in a woman who had been receiving public assistance and who also had considerable personality difficulty.

Work of Nonprofessionals

Another variant of this principle is found in the work of indigenous nonprofessionals employed as homemakers, community organizers, youth workers, recreation aides, and the like. Some of these people have had serious problems in the recent past. Some are former delinquents. It has been observed, however, that in the course of their work, their own problems

[2] B. T. King and I. L. Janis, "Comparison of the Effectiveness of Improvised Versus Non-Improvised Role Playing in Producing Opinion Changes," *Human Relations*, Vol. 1 (1965), pp. 177–186.

[3] Rita Volkman and Donald R. Cressey, "Differential Association and the Rehabilitation of Drug Addicts," *American Journal of Sociology*, Vol. 69, No. 2 (February 1963), p. 139'

[4] Rudolph M. Wittenberg, "Personality Adjustment Through Social Action," *American Journal of Orthopsychiatry*, Vol. 18, No. 2 (March 1958), pp. 207–221.

diminished greatly.[5] One of the important premises of the HARYOU program is that "indigenous personnel will solve their own problems while attempting to help others."[6]

The helper therapy principle has at least two important implications for the nonprofessional of lower socioeconomic background: (1) Since many of the nonprofessionals to be recruited are former delinquents, addicts, AFDC mothers, and the like, it seems quite likely that placing them in a helping role can be rehabilitative for them. (2) As the nonprofessionals benefit from their new helping roles, they may actually become more effective workers and thus provide more help to others at a new level.

Thus, what is presented here may be a positive upward spiral in contrast to the better-known downward trend. That is, the initial helping role may be furnishing minimal help to the recipient, but may be highly beneficial to the helper, who in turn becomes more efficient, better motivated, and reaches a new stage in helping skill.

Therapy for the Poor

The helper principle probably has universal therapeutic application, but may be especially useful in low-income treatment projects for these two reasons:

1. It may circumvent the special interclass role distance difficulties that arise from the middle-class-oriented therapy (and therapist) being at odds with the low-income clients' expectations and style; the alienation that many low-income clients feel toward professional treatment agents and the concomitant rapport difficulties may be greatly reduced by utilizing the low-income person himself as the helper-therapist.

For the same reason much wider employment of neighborhood-based nonprofessionals in hospitals and social agencies as aides or social service technicians is recommended. Like the helper-therapist, they are likely to have considerably less role distance from the low-income client than does the professional.

2. It may be a principle that is especially attuned to the co-operative trends in lower socioeconomic groups and cultures. In this sense it may be beneficial to both the helper (the model) and the helped.

Students as Helpers

In Flint, Michigan, a group of fourth-grade pupils with reading problems was assigned to the tutelage of sixth-grade pupils who were also experiencing reading difficulties. It is interesting to note that while the fourth graders made

[5] *See* Gertrude Goldberg, "The Use of Untrained Neighborhood Workers in a Homemaker Program," an unpublished report of Mobilization For Youth, New York, N.Y., 1963; and *Experiment in Culture Expansion* (Sacramento, Calif.: State of California Department of Corrections, 1963).

[6] *Youth in the Ghetto* (New York: Harlem Youth Opportunities Unlimited, 1964), p. 609.

significant progress, the sixth graders also learned from the experience.[7] Mobilization For Youth has used homework helpers with a fair amount of success, in that the recipients of the help showed some measurable academic improvement.[8] It may be that even more significant changes are taking place in the high school youngsters who are being used as tutors. Not only is it possible that their school performance is improving, but as a result of their new role these youngsters may begin to perceive the possibility of embarking on a teaching career.

Schneider reports on a small study in which youngsters with varying levels of reading ability were asked to read an "easy" book as practice for reading to younger children. She observes:

> For the child who could read well, this was a good experience. For the child who could not read well it was an even better experience. He was reading material on a level within his competence and he could read it with pleasure. Ordinary books on his level of interest were too difficult for him to read easily and so he did not read books for pleasure. Reading for him was hard, hard work; often it left him feeling stupid and helpless. This time it was different ... he would be a giver; he would share his gift with little children just as a parent or teacher does.[9]

In a sense these children were role-playing the helper role in this experience, as they were reading aloud to adults in anticipation of later reading to small children.

The classroom situation illustrates an interesting offshoot of the helper principle. Some children, when removed from a class in which they are below average and placed in a new group in which they are in the upper half of the class, manifest many new qualities and are in turn responded to more positively by the teacher. This can occur independently of whether or not they play a helper role. But some of the same underlying mechanisms are operative as in the direct helper situations: the pupil in the new group is responded to more, he stands out more, more is expected of him, and generally he responds in turn and demands more of himself. Even though he may not be in the helper role as such, similar forces are at work in both cases, stimulating more active responses. (Unfortunately, this principle may be counteracted if the teacher treats the entire group as a "lower" or poorer group and this image is absorbed in an undifferentiated manner by all the members of the class.)

A connected issue worthy of mention is that in the new situations in the schools, where (hopefully) integration will be taking place, youngsters coming from segregated backgrounds will need help in catching up, in terms of reading

[7] Frank B. W. Hawkinshire, "Training Needs for Offenders Working in Community Treatment Programs," *Experiment in Culture Expansion* (Sacramento, Calif.: State of California Department of Corrections, 1963), pp. 27–36.

[8] "Progress Report" (New York: Mobilization For Youth, July 1964).

[9] Gussie Albert Schneider, "Reading of the Children, by the Children, for the Children." Unpublished manuscript, 1964. (Mimeographed.)

skills and the like. It is generally argued that the white middle-class children who do not need this extra assistance will suffer. Their parents want these youngsters to be in a class with advanced pupils and not to be "held back" by youngsters who are behind.

However, in terms of the helper principle, it may very well be that the more advanced youngsters can benefit in new ways from playing a teaching role. Not all fast, bright youngsters like to be in a class with similar children. We have been led to believe that if one is fast and bright he will want to be with others who are fast and bright and this will act as a stimulus to his growth. It does for some people, but for others it most certainly does not. Some people find they do better in a group in which there is a great range of ability, in which they can stand out more, and, finally—and this is the point of the helper principle—in situations in which they can help other youngsters in the classroom. In other words, some children develop intellectually not by being challenged by someone ahead of them, but by helping somebody behind them, by being put into the tutor-helper role.

As any teacher can report, there is nothing like learning through teaching. By having to explain something to someone else one's attention is focused more sharply. This premise seems to have tremendous potentiality that social workers have left unused.

Leadership Development

Carried one step further, the helper principle allows for the development of leadership in community organizations and the like. It has been found, for example, in tenant groups, that an individual might be relatively inactive at meetings in his own building, but display quite different characteristics when helping to organize another building. In the new situation, forced to play the helper role, leadership begins to emerge. The character of the new group, in which the individual is in a more advanced position vis-à-vis the remainder of the group, contributes toward the emergence of new leadership behavior. This is simply another way of saying that leadership develops through the act of leading. The art of leadership training may lie in providing just the right roles to stimulate the emergence of more and more leadership.

While some individuals fall more naturally into the helper or leader role (in certain groups), this role can be distributed more widely by careful planning with regard to the sociometry and composition of the group. When the group is fluid, the introduction of new members often encourages older members who were formerly in the follower role to assume a more active helping role.

Following King and Janis' lead, role-playing can be utilized to have a person who formerly was the recipient of help in the group now play a helper role, thus aiding him to persuade himself through persuading others.[10] Many similar group dynamic approaches can be used in order to utilize most fully the potentialities of the helper principle. Seating arrangements can be altered, individuals can be placed in key positions—for example, chairing small committees—and temporary classroom groupings can be formed in which pupils previously submerged by more advanced classmates are now allowed to become helpers or models for less advanced youngsters. The essential idea in all of this is to structure and restructure the groups so that different group members play the helper role at different times.

Helper Therapy Mechanisms

It may be of value to speculate briefly regarding the various possible mechanisms whereby the helper benefits from his helping role. Brager notes the improved self-image that probably results from the fact that a person is doing something worthwhile in helping someone in need.[11]

The King-Janis study suggests that becoming committed to a position through advocating it ("self-persuasion through persuading others") may be an important dimension associated with the helper role. Pearl notes that many helpers (such as the homework helpers) are "given a stake or concern in a system" and this contributes to their becoming "committed to the task in a way that brings about especially meaningful development of their own abilities."[12]

There is undoubtedly a great variety of other mechanisms that will be clarified by further research. Probably also the mechanisms vary depending on the setting and task of the helper. Thus helpers, functioning in a therapeutic context, whether as professional therapeutic agents or as nonprofessional "peer therapists," may benefit from the importance and status associated with this role. They also receive support from the implicit thesis "I must be well if I help others." People who themselves have problems (e.g., alcoholics, drug addicts, unwed mothers) should derive benefit from this formulation. Moreover, their new helper roles as such may function as a major (distracting) source of involvement, thus diverting them from their problem and general self-concern. There is no question also that individual differences are important so that some people receive much greater satisfaction from "giving," "helping," "leading," "controlling," "co-operating," "persuading," and "mothering."

Helpers operating in a teaching context, again both as professionals and nonprofessionals, may profit more from the cognitive mechanisms associated with learning through teaching. They need to learn the material better in order to teach it and more generalized academic sets may emerge from the

[10] Op. cit.

[11] George Brager, "The Indigenous Worker: A New Approach to the Social Work Technician," pp. 33–40, this issue.

[12] Arthur Pearl, "Youth in Lower Class Settings," p. 6. Paper presented at the fifth Symposium on Social Psychology, Norman, Okla., 1964.

teacher role. Finally, the status and prestige dimensions attached to the teacher role may accrue unforeseen benefits to them.

The helper in the leader role may benefit from some of the same factors related to the teacher and therapist roles as well as the "self-persuasion through persuading others" mechanism and their "stake in the system." In essence, then, it would seem that the gains are related to the actual demands of the specific helper role (whether it is teacher, leader, or therapist), plus the new feelings associated with the meaning and prestige of the role and the way the helper is treated because of the new role.

Cautions and Conditions

In a sense, the helper principle seems counter to the widely accepted psychological dictum that warns against therapist projection. The well-known danger, called to our attention by all of psychoanalytic theory and practice, indicates that a therapist with a specific problem may, unless he has understanding and control of this problem, project it to the person he is treating. Of course, in many of the cases cited this situation does not arise because both the treater and the treated suffer from the same malady. But in other cases when rehabilitated nonprofessional workers are hired to work with people who either have no specific problem or do not have the problems of the helper, the possibility of projection as well as psychological contagion has to be considered.

Two controlling devices are suggested to guard against the potential risk: (1) the helper should not be involved in any intensive treatment function unless he has considerable awareness of his problem and the projection issue, and (2) professional supervision is absolutely necessary; perhaps one of the difficulties of the amateur therapeutic self-help programs is the anti-professionalism that frequently characterizes them.

There is another potential danger residing in the helper therapy principle, especially if it is to be applied on a large scale. Much of the intrinsic value of the technique may depend on it operating in a relatively subconscious fashion. Once people know they are being placed in certain helping roles in order to be helped themselves, some of the power of the principle deriving from feelings of self-importance and the like may be reduced. That this is not entirely true is evident from role-playing situations in which the subjects know the object of the game but still are affected. Nevertheless, the question of large-scale manipulation of the principle, with the increased likelihood of mechanical and arbitrary application, does hold some danger that only careful observation and research can accurately evaluate.

Implications

The helper principle may have wide application in hospital groups (both in- and outpatient), prisons, correctional institutions, and so forth. Scheidlinger suggests that the principle may have powerful implications for social work's understanding of the therapeutic process in all group therapy. Not only are individual group members aided through helping other members in the group, but the group as a whole may be greatly strengthened in manifold ways as it continually offers assistance to individual group members.[13]

Levine suggests that in a variety of types of habit change, such as efforts to curtail cigarette smoking, the helper principle may have considerable validity. Smokers who are cast in the role of persuading other smokers to stop smoking have themselves been found to benefit from their commitment to the new antismoking prescription.[14]

The helper principle does not really require that only the helper profit or even that he benefit more than the person receiving help. Thus it is seen in the Flint, Michigan, study that the fourth graders receiving help benefited at least as much as the givers of help.[15] The helper principle only calls attention to the aid the helper receives from being in the helper role.

The helper principle has been utilized with varying degrees of awareness in many group situations. What we are calling for is more explicit use of this principle in an organized manner. Conscious planning directed toward the structuring of groups for the widest possible distribution of the helper role may be a decisive therapeutic intervention, a significant leadership training principle, and an important teaching device. It is probably no accident that it is often said that one of the best ways to learn is to teach. Perhaps also psychiatrists, social workers, and others in the helping professions are helping themselves more than is generally recognized!

[13] Conversation with Saul Scheidlinger, Community Service Society, New York, N.Y., January 18, 1964.

[14] Conversation with Sol Levine, Harvard University School of Public Health, Cambridge, Mass., January 12, 1964.

[15] Hawkinshire, op. cit.

GERALD CAPLAN

Problems of Training in Mental Health Consultation

One of the fundamental ways in which the mental health professional can extend his expertise is through consultation with others in the community whose work, though not directly concerned with mental health, brings them into contact with people who have mental health needs. Thus, the school teacher, clergyman, general practitioner, public health nurse, and the like can, with adequate preparation and support, serve important mental health needs of their clients. Caplan has been one of the mental health field's outstanding spokesmen with respect to this approach. Although the paper that follows is directed primarily toward training professionals for consultative functions, Caplan also says a good deal about his particular approach to this activity and provides some insight into how it developed.

My interest in mental health consultation was aroused in 1949, when as Director of the Lasker Mental Hygiene and Child Guidance Center of Hadassah in Jerusalem I accepted responsibility for supervising the mental health of about 16,000 children in the Youth Aliyah Immigrant Children's Organization in Israel. My budget allowed me a staff of five or six psychologists and social workers. I quickly found that at any point in time about 1,000 children were felt by their counselors and teachers or by the house mothers of the residential institutions in which they lived, to be in need of specialist mental health attention. I eventually convinced myself and my sponsors that the investigation and treatment of individual children was not an effective contribution to this problem. Instead, I developed a method of consultation with the teachers and child care workers in the institutions to help them handle the psychological problems of most of these children themselves within the framework of the organization's normal educational environment.[1]

[1] Rosenfeld, Jona M. and Gerald Caplan. "Techniques of Staff Consultation in an Immigrant Children's Organization in Israel." *The American Journal of Orthopsychiatry*, vol. XXIV, No. 1, January, 1954.

Abridged from Chapter 8, "Problems in Mental Health Consultation" by G. Caplan in S. E. Goldston (ed.), *Concepts of Community Psychiatry.* Bethesda, Md.: National Institute of Mental Health, Public Health Service Publication No. 1319, 1965, pp. 91–108, with the permission of Dr. Caplan.

In 1952, when I came to Harvard, I found that Erich Lindemann and his colleagues had been working along similar lines in offering consultation to the teachers of the Wellesley school system as an alternative to the traditional diagnosis and treatment of referred cases.[2]

During the following years I studied this method at the Wellesley Human Relations Service, and in 1954 I also began to use a consultation approach with public health nurses at one of the health centers of the city of Boston Health Department. At the same time I started a weekly seminar for psychiatrists, psychologists, and social workers working in the community clinics of the State Department of Mental Health. In this seminar we discussed the early experience of the participants in offering consultation to a variety of professionals in the community—schoolteachers, kindergarten teachers, probation officers, clergymen, policemen, public health nurses, welfare workers, and the like. On the basis of my studies at Harvard and Wellesley I began to develop a conceptual framework and to define a system of techniques of consultation, and this I fed into the seminar and modified in the light of discussions of the experience of the other workers in their different settings.

In 1959 I felt that my definition of the consultation method had sufficiently progressed so that it would lend itself to a formal evaluation study. By that time our early efforts in the health center had sufficiently impressed the Commissioner of Public Health of Boston that he had invited us to offer consultation on a citywide basis to all the public health nurses of his department. We accordingly set up a research project at Harvard School of Public Health financed by the NIMH,[3] to evaluate the results of a 3-year period of our type of consultation to the public health nurses of Boston, using as a control group nurses in adjoining towns which had no such program. The analysis of the data from this study is currently nearing completion.[4]

Meanwhile, we had begun to use our experience and facilities for the training of our community mental health students at Harvard School of Public Health. These are mainly experienced psychiatrists, psychologists, and psychiatric social workers who come to us for 1 academic year to study for a master's degree in public health, with community mental health as their field of special interest.[5] They spend about half their time studying traditional public health subjects, such as epidemiology, biostatistics, and public health administration; and the remainder of their time is devoted to the theory

[2] Caplan, Gerald, "Mental Health Consultation in Schools." *The Elements of a Community Mental Health Program*, proceedings of a round table at the 1955 Annual Conference. Milbank Memorial Fund, 40 Wall St., New York, N.Y.

[3] NIMH Research and Development Grant No. M-3442.

[4] Caplan, Gerald, Louise Howe, and Lenin Baler, *Exploratory Studies of Mental Health Consultation.* Transcript of Faculty Research Conference, Harvard School of Public Health, Dec. 13, 1961. Mimeographed document.

[5] This training program was transferred on July 1, 1964, to the newly established Laboratory of Community Psychiatry in the Department of Psychiatry of Harvard Medical School.

and practice of community psychiatry.[6] In recent years the latter has included learning the skills of mental health consultation.

In the beginning, the Harvard students attended the seminars I gave for the State workers, but eventually I began a special weekly seminar for them and I arranged for them to spend some time each week working in one of the State community mental health centers, where they were given an opportunity to practice consultation under the supervision of the senior clinic workers who had attended my seminars in the past.

Because of the design of our research in the Boston Health Department we could not use that setting in the field training of our students. The practical experience and the supervision they were getting in the State centers turned out to be uneven in quality. We were therefore pleased when the Boston Visiting Nurse Association asked us to provide a citywide consultation service to them similar to our program in the city health department. Three years ago we began arranging for our students to have their practicum experience within the framework of this service, and we began using the experienced consultants on our Harvard research staff as supervisors. When the data collection of our evaluation study was completed in 1961, we were asked to continue our program in the city health department on a service basis, and this together with the Visiting Nurse Association program currently provides us with about 200 potential consultees among public health nurses operating out of 20 nursing units. Each of our students now spends a weekly session thoughout the year offering consultation to these public health nurses, and is given an hour a week of individual supervision by one of our senior consultants. My seminar continues as in the past. During the first semester I discuss the theory of preventive psychiatry, the place of mental health consultation within this framework, and our systematic formulations on technique. During the second semester I clarify these concepts by case centered discussions focused on examples of the students' practical experience in consulting with the public health nurses.

Against this background I will now discuss some of the major issues we have encountered in the development of our training program, which I imagine may have relevance in other settings.

(1) *The development of techniques.* In a new field it may be necessary for teachers to provide opportunities for students to acquire knowledge about subjects in which the teachers have no special competence. It is probably an advantage however for the teachers to guide the students' explorations on the basis of some degree of technical expertness. The acquisition of the latter was in our case a slow process. It depended on being exposed to situations and accepting responsibilities, which forced us to acknowledge the inadequacy of our previous skills, and to break new ground. Already in Israel we had discovered that although many consultees were having difficulties in their work because of the intrusion of personal problems, we could not use our traditional

[6] Caplan, Gerald. "An Approach to the Education of Community Mental Health Specialists." *Mental Hygiene*, vol. 43, No. 2, April 1959, pp. 268–280.

psychotherapeutic methods in uncovering these subjective links and in helping them overcome their private emotional difficulties. Such an approach usually led to the arousal of anger and resistance, because the consultees resented being forced or seduced into the role of patients. We had to find ways of handling such a situation of personal emotional involvement, while at the same time respecting the boundaries of privacy in our consultees.

This involved us in various exploratory trial and error efforts, and in the necessity for a continuing clinical evaluation of the results of different technical maneuvers. In this work we found it particularly advantageous to have an ongoing study group of our staff, in which we could pool information about our field experiences, and derive a measure of objectivity from the reactions of others to our subjective descriptions and our appraisals of our own efforts. Such a staff study group, which I started in Israel and continued for several years at Wellesley and Harvard, forced us to record the process of interaction between ourselves and our consultees, and promoted the self-awareness which is an essential aspect in developing a professional method. Some practitioners may become highly skilled without consciously disciplining themselves in this way. Their learning takes place at a preconscious level, and although their competence increases with experience, they are often unable to explain what they have done in particular consultation situations. Their records are also not too clear. In the study group the other participants often succeeded in drawing out of them an account of what they had done, from which we were able to learn more than they themselves were aware of.

(2) *Conceptualization and definition.* Intuitive practitioners are valuable allies in developing a method such as consultation, but as teachers their value is largely restricted to offering themselves as role models in apprenticeship situations. In developing a body of knowledge which can be communicated to students of different personalities, so that despite variations in detail which are related to the idiosyncratic personal interplay between consultant and consultee, some professional consistency can be maintained, it is necessary to derive a set of general principles which describe and classify the regularly occurring problem situations and evaluate the range of effective ways of dealing with them.

In our case we faced the initial difficulty that the topic itself had previously not been defined. Many mental health specialists had talked to other professionals about the latter's work, and had collaborated with them in handling mentally disturbed people. Many psychiatrists had used the term consultation for such operations. They had also used the term in other connections, such as talking with parents about their children, talking with college students about their problems, and short-term therapeutic contacts with patients.

We felt that an essential step in building a body of knowledge was to define what we included in the term consultation and to differentiate this from similar operations. We thought we might be helped by seeing how consultants in other fields had defined their topic. We searched the literature in adult education, social work, nursing, social science, business management, and agricultural extension, but got little help. Many have written about consultation, but few satisfactory definitions are to be found.

We eventually decided on a definition which fitted our own framework of preventive psychiatry, and appeared to apply to a particular segment of the various operations being conducted by our workers. This definition was crystallized in 1954 and we have used it without major modification since then. We define mental health consultation as a process of interaction between a mental health specialist and a member of another profession in regard to the mental health aspects of the latter's work with a client or program, in which the consultant helps the consultee improve his effectiveness in handling the current problem and at the same time helps him increase his understanding of the issues involved so that he may be able to deal more adequately on his own with similar problems in the future.

In the early years of our program we were mainly interested in primary prevention, and we saw consultation as being a major instrument for helping people cope adequately with life crises through our offering consultation to community caregiving professionals who were in contact with them at crisis times. As our awareness of the range of problems encompassed by community psychiatry broadened, we emphasized the use of consultation to support caregiving professionals and administrators also in their management of the mentally disordered and retarded in programs of secondary and tertiary prevention.

Our delimitation of the method within our general framework of theory allowed us to specify its goals, and to differentiate it from similar methods which have been developed to achieve contiguous goals—such as psychotherapy, counseling, casework, supervision, and education. We had to specify the boundaries between these methods so that our students could learn the sets of techniques appropriate for each, and so that they could use each method consistently in their eventual community practice, when they would be called upon to handle complicated situations in which they would be faced by a tangle of goals and a bundle of overlapping and potentially conflicting role demands.

The essential characteristics of mental health consultation appeared to include the following: (*a*) The consultant focuses not only on the client's problem but also on the work situation of the consultee—the main question for the consultant is "Why is this consultee having difficulty with this client and asking me for help at this time?" The consultant must therefore pay attention to the total field of forces of the consultee institution in which he is involved together with the consultee and the client. (*b*) The consultant has no administrative authority over the consultee and accepts no responsibility for the latter's implementation of consultation recommendations. The consultee is thus free to accept or reject anything the consultant says. This freedom avoids the tensions of an authoritarian relationship and permits the consultee quickly to take over, as his own, any of the consultant's ideas which appeal to him. (*c*) Consultation continually fosters the professional autonomy of the consultee. It is based on an egalitarian relationship of two colleagues, each of whom has special competence in his own subject. (*d*) Although the consultant is sensitive to the feelings of the consultee and to the psychosocial forces of his institutional setting, the content of the consultation discussions is restricted by the consultant to the problems of the client. Personal problems of the consultee are never discussed directly, although they are sometimes handled vicariously in their displacement onto the client. (*e*) Consultation operates in general on an ad hoc basis in short series of one to four sessions invoked by the consultee or his supervisors because of a current work problem. The consultant has no systematic body of knowledge to impart in a circumscribed course. He expects to be called in from time to time over an indefinite period. Between consultation units the channels of communication are maintained, but there is no necessity for personal contact. The method is economical in time because it operates only in response to current need.

Having defined the limits of our method, we then attempted to subdivide into meaningful categories the regularly occurring sets of operations which our workers experienced in practice. We developed a fourfold classification of mental health consultation according to (*a*) whether it was invoked by the consultee for help with a particular client or else with an administrative problem, and (*b*) whether the consultant focused his efforts primarily on the client or administrative problem or primarily on the consultee. The four types were (1) Client centered case consultation, in which the consultant's primary goal is change in the client through diagnosing his case and prescribing remedial action to the consultee, (2) Program centered administrative consultation, which is the analog of this in relation to an administrative problem, (3) Consultee centered case consultation, in which the consultant's primary goal is to help the consultee improve his understanding and competence on the basis of handling the current client, and (4) Consultee centered administrative consultation, the analog of the latter is dealing with an administrative problem.[7]

As the work progressed, each of these types was further subdivided, its regularly occurring problems specified and categorized, and alternative ways of solving them described. For instance, the process of consultee centered case consultation was found to involve five overlapping phases: (*a*) *Preparing the Ground for Consultation*, which involves building up relationships between the consultant's agency and the consultee institution and working out a mutually agreed upon plan of operation which is eventually expressed in the form of a contract. (*b*) *Building and Maintaining the Individual Consultation Relationship*, which involves promoting reality-based perceptions in the consultee of the consultant as a helpful and understanding

[7] Ch. 8. "Types of Mental Health Consultation" in *Principles of Preventive Psychiatry*, by Gerald Caplan. Basic Books, New York, January 1964.

colleague who offers his specialized assistance with due respect for the consultee's own professional competence. (*c*) *Assessing the Consultation Problem*, which involves methods for exploring the consultee's account of his work difficulties in order to determine whether these are caused by lack of knowledge, skill, or self-confidence, or by distortions of functioning due to subjective interference. In the latter case, the consultant must explore further in order to pinpoint the specific difficulty which is being displaced onto the client. (*d*) *Delivering the Consultation Message* relates to the techniques to be used in helping the consultee overcome the distortions in his perceptions or expectations of the case. These techniques support him in achieving a reality-based view of the work situation while carefully avoiding the explicit uncovering of the personal factors which have contributed to the subjective interference with his professional functioning. (*e*) *Ending and Follow-Up* deals with the final phase of this consultation method. The consultant steps back and allows the consultee to return to the case enriched by the added understanding and emotional freedom he has obtained from the consultation. The consultee's increased effectiveness, in a situation in which he previously was at an impass, is the major factor in driving home the consultation message, so that he integrates his new wisdom and so that this may have a carryover in future cases. The consultant later evaluates the effectiveness of the consultation by finding out how this and similar problems have been subsequently dealt with by the consultee.

Over the years a body of theory began to emerge from such work, and this was used to guide the efforts of the staff consultants, whose practical experience in turn led to the evaluation and modification of the theoretical constructs. The latter began as classificatory concepts. They progressed to descriptions of expectable sequences, and eventually to postulates on causal relationships between technical interventions and goals. For instance, one commonly occurring type of consultee centered case consultation was found to involve a link between an unsolved psychological problem of the consultee and a disorder in his perception of the client. This was explicated theoretically as being caused by a disorder of professional objectivity due to the interference of a conceptual block in the consultee by the displacement of his personal problem onto the client. We formulated this block as a preconscious syllogistic theme of the consultee, which led him to expect as inevitable a particular bad outcome, whenever he encountered a certain category of case. We then developed a technique, which we called, "theme interference reduction," for investigating the nature of such a conceptual block and for interrupting its final common path, using the current work situation as a test case. This depends on accepting the consultee's formulation that the client fits the initial category, and then using the leverage of the consultation relationship to help him realize that the bad outcome he expects is not inevitable.[8]

[8] Ch. 9. "Methodology of Mental Health Consultation" in *Principles of Preventive Psychiatry*, by Gerald Caplan. Basic Books, New York, January 1964.

This technique strictly avoids discussing the personal link between the consultee and the client, and instead focuses on the client's situation as perceived by the consultee. The consultant helps the consultee invalidate his fantasy-distored preconceptions by enlarging his view of the realistic possibilities of the situation. If successful, this not only reduces his distortion of perception in the current case, but also the tension associated with the underlying theme so that he is freed to handle such cases in the future with less difficulty.

The development of concepts such as these has largely been based upon the detailed analysis of consultation records kept by the Harvard staff. It has been modified and kept close to reality by the continuing interchange with the workers in the state community mental health centers at their weekly seminars. This has prevented the growth of an ivory tower system, which is a constant hazard in a field such as ours.

EMORY L. COWEN

Emergent Directions in School Mental Health

A relatively common focus for preventive programs in the mental health field is the public school system. This is true for a number of reasons: pupils in the system are relatively young; they can be reached at a time in life when serious mental health problems have not yet become entrenched; the system gathers in virtually all of the youngsters in a given community; and parental cooperation is often easy to enlist because most parents would like to see their children succeed in school and respond promptly to signs that this is not happening. Perhaps the best known study devoted to the identification and prevention of emotional disorders in school children has been conducted by Cowen and his colleagues in Rochester, New York. The paper that follows provides an excellent summary of the development of that project and the many stages through which it has passed during the years of its existence.

Reprinted from *American Scientist*, **59** (1971), 723–733, with the permission of the *American Scientist* and Dr. Cowen.

More so than ever before, society today is appalled by precipitous awarenesses of serious social and human-adaptive problems such as explosive inner-city riots, antisocial behaviors in high school dropouts, the rampant, destructive problems of addiction, the shocking conditions of many of our institutions (e.g. mental hospitals, detention settings, and prisons), and the bombing of public buildings. Nowadays such events and circumstances are all too evident because of the immediacy and drama of reports in the public media. Profound social eruptions polarize reactions from the entirely repressive, at one extreme, to well-meaning, humanitarian surges to develop crash programs to overpower these social blights, at the other. However well conceived these programs may be, they are subject to the dangers of being crisis-motivated, palliative counter-measures rather than planned, reasoned, long-term approaches.

The obvious and vexing presence of social eyesores also generates political pressure for immediate solutions. Proposals that grow out of such an atmosphere often lead to heavily invested crash programs, characteristically directed to manifest current symptoms and designed to solve these problems by "overwhelming" them. There are, however, hidden assumptions behind even the best designed and executed of such programs. They start, for example, with at least two strikes against them by being directed to conditions that are already florid, entrenched, and basic to the individual's life economy.

Even if that were not so, programs targeted specifically to advanced, well-developed, adverse "end states" (e.g. addiction) rest on the tenuous assumption that such conditions have specific determinants and can be treated effectively by specific interventions. They overlook the strong possibility that many personally or socially unfortunate outcomes—the psychoses, alcoholism, addiction, crime and delinquency, the neuroses—merely reflect alternative, adverse "end solutions" to earlier life problems. Otherwise stated, it is more than admissible that effective generalized programs in early detection and prevention could cut down the flow of *many* different types of maladaptive end states—indeed most of those that fall under the umbrella of human disordered behavior.

If this argument has merit, it is not only appropriate but essential that society allocate a far greater share of its mental health resources to before-the-fact prevention rather than to costly, ineffective attempts at after-the-fact repair (which, in the last analysis, can be viewed analogically as applying undersized, frayed Band-Aids to profusely bleeding psyches). This point of view is well reflected in the recent report of the President's Task Force on the Mentally Handicapped (1970) which states on page 18: "By proverbial wisdom and common sense, prevention of disability is greatly to be preferred to treatment and rehabilitation." Schools, as social institutions that significantly shape the development of all human beings in modern society, are potentially ideal settings for preventive interventions.

Since the beginning of the current century, mental health professionals have been performing a variety of clinical services in American schools, reflecting two basic assumptions: (1) that schools have both the responsibility, and the potential, for promoting the child's psychological as well as his educational well-being and (2) that these two spheres of development are intimately intertwined—i.e. psychological maladaptation encourages educational failure and *vice versa.*

The day-to-day activities of school mental health professionals have long been guided by prevailing conceptions of pathological behavior and by a *reactive* orientation to deficit. Psychologists and social workers in the schools have been cast in the role of "experts" or "trouble-shooters," called on to do their magic in the face of significant educational or interpersonal failure. Striking and understandable parallels exist between the specific problems of school mental health today and the broader ones confronting society in this area: Professionals are in woefully short supply. Demand for assistance, and certainly latent need, far exceeds resources. Established helping techniques are limited in value and their distribution across social strata is inequitable. Thus, the meager firepower generated from scarce mental health resources is directed to a relatively small percent of florid, rooted dysfunctions, which, unfortunately, are precisely the ones with the poorest prognoses.

Recent surveys (Glidewell and Swallow 1969) indicate that roughly 30 percent of all children have school maladaptation problems ranging from mild to severe. In some quarters, that figure is as high as 70 percent. The absolute numbers thus implicated are staggering, and our present resource system cannot provide effective help for them. The magnitude of the mismatch between school-failure data and resource data dictates consideration of alternative conceptualizations and stratagems to guide future school mental health approaches. Greater attention must be directed to engineering school environments that potentiate adaptation, developing delivery systems that feature widespread early identification of ineffective school function, and creating interventions designed to short-circuit maladaptation. Such efforts must pay heed to the realities of current manpower shortages if they are to be successful. They must meet the twin challenges of identifying effective new manpower deployments and more socially utilitarian uses of scarce professional time.

We shall describe here the development and evaluation of a long-range program for early detection and prevention of school maladaptation which offers a logically attractive alternative to past after-the-fact, crisis-oriented school mental health delivery systems. Although the foregoing views were present in germinal form when our program started more than a decade ago, they were far less clearly articulated. At that time we were more impressed by several earthy, "battleline" observations hinting at weaknesses in the school mental health delivery system. The first, a point frequently made by teachers, was that 40 to 60 percent of class time was preempted by three or four children who were unable, for any of several reasons, to meet the challenge of school. This condition was unhealthy for the affected few, seriously undermined the educational environment of the many, and threatened the teacher's equanimity and well-being.

A second perturbing problem was the rash of referrals, some complicated and serious, in children about to move from elementary to high school. Typically, resources for dealing with such problems were not available. Study of these children's cumulative dossiers often indicated that prodromal signs had been present in fifth, or third, grade or even at the very start of the child's school career. Either appropriate services for the child had not been available earlier or people had hoped that, if they closed their eyes long enough, the difficulties would go away. Far from vanishing, in most cases they "picked up steam" over time, became rooted, and assumed even more serious proportions during the later elementary period.

Faced with many such serious chronic problems, we decided to allocate existing mental health resources to early detection and prevention at the primary level, even at the risk of losing traditional clinical services at the upper levels. Our hope was that this emphasis might sharply reduce the incidence of chronic school maladaptation and, with it, heavy later service demands. In a world of finite resources, such as the world of mental health today, critical decisions have less to do with whether a given objective (i.e. program) is "good" absolutely and more with which of many "goods" have the *greatest* prospective social value. Merely to perpetuate known programs without considering other possible allocations of the scarce resources restricts innovation by default. The value clearly reflected in our decision is that prevention is preferable to repair—indeed it is essential if truly effective school mental health programs are to develop.

The Early Years, 1958–1969

Our work on the Primary Mental Health Project (PMHP), spanning 13 years, falls into three periods. In the first, 1958 to 1963, new techniques for early identification of school maladaptation and a primitive program in early secondary prevention were developed. A school psychologist and a school social worker were assigned, full-time, to promote these ends in the primary grades of a single elementary school in Rochester, N.Y. Children in this school were largely from the upper-lower and lower-middle socio-economic strata and were ethnically representative of the city of Rochester at large, except for an underweighting of Negro and Jewish children.

Estimates of actual, or incipient, school maladaptation were formulated for first-grade children based on an amalgam of four sources: group psychological screening of intellectual and personality status, social work interviews with mothers, direct classroom observation, and teachers' reports of the child's behavior and educational status. Based on these data a dichotomous clinical judgment—red-tag vs non-red-tag—was rendered for each child. This was a private research diagnosis, to avoid labeling

Fig. 1 (*opposite*). *Comparison of third grade status of red-tag and non-red-tag children shows superior adjustment or academic achievement on all measures for the non-red-tag group.* Nurses ref., 3rd: *Mean, number of referrals to nurse.* Nurses ref., cum.: *Mean, number of referrals to nurse, 1st–3rd grades.* G.P.A.: *Mean, sum of end-of-year report card grades.* Rdg. comp., pctle.: *Mean, percentile score, SRA reading comprehension.* Reasoning, pctle.: *Mean, percentile score, SRA reasoning.* Arith. comput., pctle.: *Mean, percentile score, SRA arithmetic computation.* Ach.-apt. disc.: *Mean, discrepancy between achievement and aptitude.* MHCS rating: *Mean, maladjustment rating by mental-health professionals.* TBRS, total: *Mean, sum of teachers' behavior ratings for maladjustment.* TBRS, overall: *Mean, teachers' overall behavior rating for maladjustment.* Neg. choices, peers: *Mean, number of negative peer sociometric nominations.* % neg. choices, peers: *Mean, percent negative peer sociometric nominations.* Neg. choices, self: *Mean, number of negative role, self-nominations.* % neg. choices, self: *Mean, percent negative role, self-nominations.*

---

the child or promoting self-fulfilling prophecies. Red-taggers were those who had already manifested dysfunction or in whom such dysfunction seemed imminent; the non-red-taggers were children who had adapted adequately to school. Later research clarified the basis for this initially dichtomous clinical judgment, particularly the contribution of the social worker's interview, and established a framework for rendering continuous judgments of school adaptation (Beach et al. 1968). The red-tag judgment has been shown to relate to other salient facets of the child's behavior and performance, including school record and achievement data, and teacher and parent judgments (Zax et al. 1964; Liem et al. 1969; Cowen et al. 1970b).

About a third of the primary graders were classified red-tag, a figure that compares closely to Glidewell and Swallow's 30 percent school maladjustment datum (Cowen et al. 1963; Cowen et al. 1966a). These children were found to be functioning significantly more poorly than non-red-taggers on a variety of measures taken at the end of the third school year: school record indices, such as attendance and nurse-referrals; performance criteria, including report-card grades, standard, system-wide achievement tests, and achievement-aptitude discrepancy scores; behavioral and adjustive indices, including behavior ratings made by teachers and mental health professionals: and peer ratings of sociometric status.

Figure 1 graphically depicts significant differences between red-tag and non-red-tag groups on 14 criterion measures, at the end of third grade. In all instances the observed differences favor the non-red-tag group. Follow-up evaluation at seventh grade level (Zax et al. 1968) indicated that, without special intervention during the elementary period, the red-tag child's dysfunction and inability to achieve continued. Thus in seventh grade, red-taggers were less well accepted by peers, were judged as more maladjusted by teachers, and had poorer health records, lower grades, and lower scores on standard achievement tests than non-red-tagers.

Initial secondary preventive efforts, over a three-year period, were built around recasting the professional's role away from traditional one-to-one

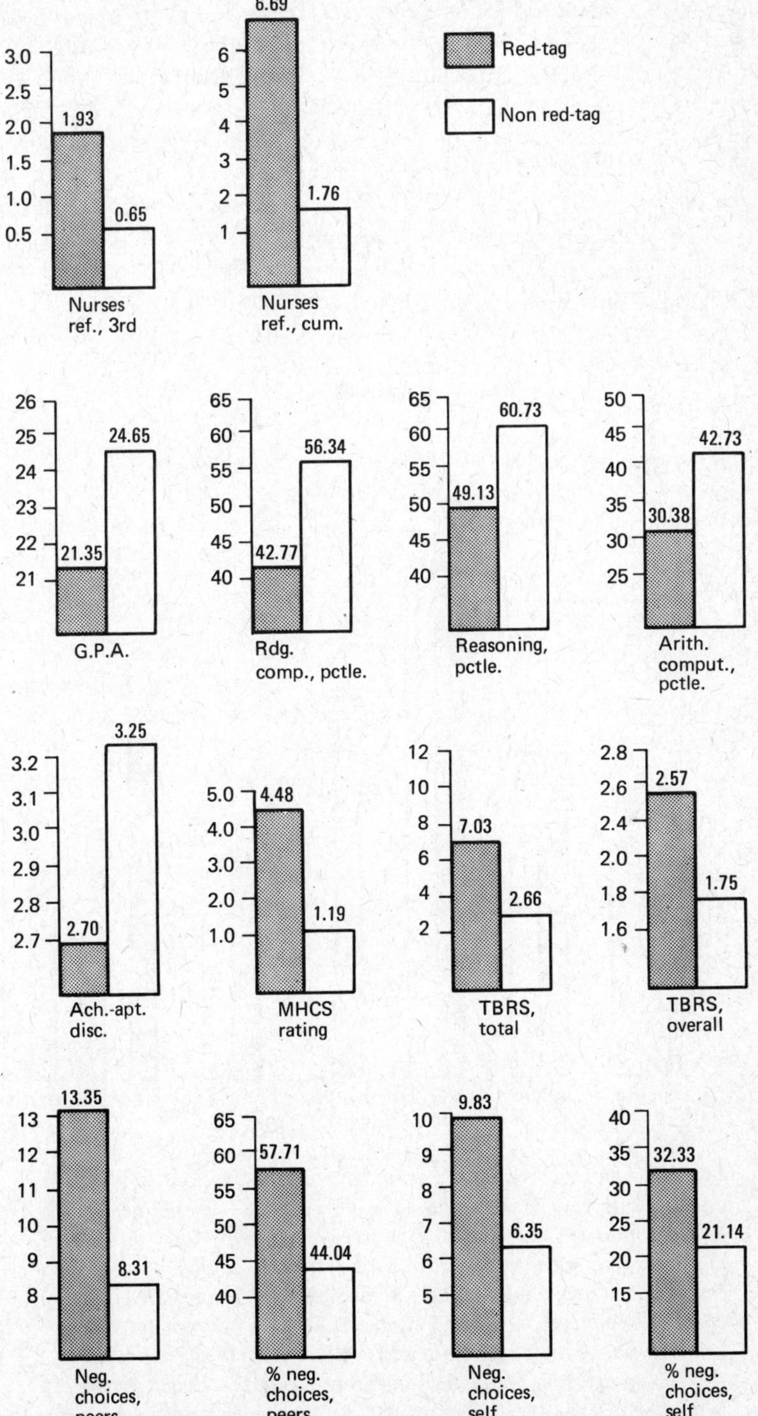
Red-tag
Non red-tag
3.0
2.5
2.0
1.5
1.0
0.5
1.93
0.65
Nurses
ref., 3rd
6
5
4
3
2
1
6.69
1.76
Nurses
ref., cum.
26
25
24
23
22
21
24.65
21.35
G.P.A.
65
60
55
50
45
40
56.34
42.77
Rdg.
comp., pctle.
65
60
55
50
45
40
60.73
49.13
Reasoning,
pctle.
50
45
40
35
30
25
42.73
30.38
Arith.
comput.,
pctle.
3.2
3.1
3.0
2.9
2.8
2.7
3.25
2.70
Ach.-apt.
disc.
5.0
4.0
3.0
2.0
1.0
4.48
1.19
MHCS
rating
12
10
8
6
4
2
7.03
2.66
TBRS,
total
2.8
2.6
2.4
2.0
1.8
1.6
2.57
1.75
TBRS,
overall
13
12
11
10
9
8
13.35
8.31
Neg.
choices,
peers
65
60
55
50
45
40
57.71
44.04
% neg.
choices,
peers
10
9
8
7
6
5
9.83
6.35
Neg.
choices,
self
40
35
30
25
20
15
32.33
21.14
% neg.
choices,
self

clinical services for acute flare-ups or crises, toward educative, resource, and consultative functions (Cowen et al. 1966a; Zax and Cowen 1969). At the end of the third school year, children in the prevention program (E's) were compared with peers from demographically similar, geographically contiguous control schools (C's) with traditional school mental health services. The E's significantly exceeded C's on seven measures, including fewer nurse referrals, higher grades and achievement test scores, superior achievement relative to aptitude, lower self-rated anxiety, and teacher behavior ratings indicating superior adjustment (Cowen et al. 1966a). Figure 2 depicts significant differences between experimental and control children.

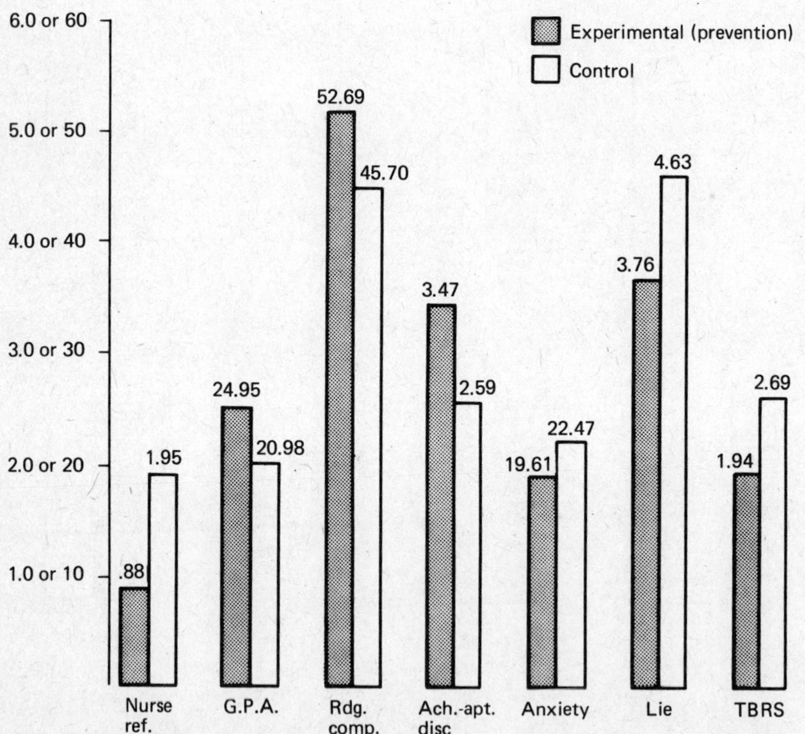

Fig. 2. *Comparison of third grade status of experimental (prevention) and control groups on seven criterion measures shows superior adjustment or academic achievement on each for prevention group.* Nurse ref.: *Mean, number of referrals to nurse, 3rd grade.* G.P.A.: *Mean, sum of end-of-year report card grades.* Rdg. comp.: *Mean, percentile score, SRA reading comprehension.* Ach.-apt. disc.: *Mean, discrepancy between aptitude and achievement.* Anxiety: *Mean, anxiety scale score (Childrens Manifest Anxiety Scale).* Lie: *Mean, lie scale score (Childrens Manifest Anxiety Scale).* TBRS: *Mean, teachers' overall behavior rating for maladjustment.*

The two key conclusions emerging from the initial work were that (1) ineffective function can be accurately identified early in the child's school career and, without intervention, it has serious later consequences, and (2) there are significant positive effects, along several important dimensions, of an early secondary prevention program. These findings established a base for pursuing related objectives within a common conceptual net.

Nonprofessional Aides

However accurate and efficient programs for early detection may be, their social value to date has been limited by an inability to follow through with appropriate remediation. This failing has been due both to the way society's interpersonal helping resources have been defined and to current acute shortages in professional mental health manpower. At the time we had to face this dilemma, important new explorations of the use of nonprofessionals in human service were getting under way. A central issue underlying such usage is whether the attributes required to help another person are those of I.Q., advanced specialty education, and professional degrees, or whether they are found in the spheres of personality, life experience, and stylistic variables. Given the shortage of resources, however, the choice we faced was either to repress identified problems or to develop new nonprofessional helping-services "checked and balanced" by alternative new professional roles.

Accordingly, we recruited a small group of six housewives, judged to be warm, natural, interpersonally adept, themselves effective mothers, with a strong interest in working with children, to serve as child-aides with maladapting primary-graders (Zax and Cowen 1967). These women came from middle-class backgrounds, had a median high school education, and were on the average in their early forties. Since we counted heavily on the aides' styles and reflexes, rather than on mastery of the content of a Ph.D. curriculum, training was focused and brief (6 weeks). Its two major purposes were to develop an understanding and way of thinking about school adjustment problems and to minimize the anxiety some aides felt about prospective human service contacts with maladapting children—a heretofore sacrosanct professional function. The didactic-discussion portion of training touched on aspects of early childhood development, behavior problems in children, parent-child relations, and, briefly, on teaching methods and techniques. Its clinical component included case-history materials, films about maladapting children, and direct classroom observation, each followed by discussion of the observed behavior. Frequency of child-observations increased as the start of actual service activities neared, facilitating a natural transition between training and on-the-job activities.

Aides were hired as half-time employees to permit regular, planful interactions with children experiencing difficulties. Teachers referred youngsters to the aide program for a variety of reasons: aggressive, disruptive behaviors; shyness, timidity, and undersocialization; and more classic learning disorders. After background information about the child, from various sources, was shared and objectives established, the aide began to meet regularly with him. At the core of the aide's contacts with the child is a committed human relation. Her specific activities vary depending on the child's problem and, thus, the goals established for him, as well as the personalities, interests, and styles of the two parties. Joint activities range from conversation to direct educational assistance, to recreational and play functions, to use of expressive media, etc. Evaluations of aide-seen vs comparable control children (see below), based on a series of rating scales tapping the child's behavioral and educational progress, indicated that the program is seen as effective by teachers, aides, and parents alike (Cowen 1968; Cowen, Dorr, Trost, and Izzo, in press).

The housewife-aide program gave impetus to development of several other, conceptually related, service programs for young school children using different helping personnel such as college students (Cowen et al. 1966b; Zax and Cowen 1967; Cowen et al. 1969), retired people (Cowen et al. 1968), indigenous neighborhood teenagers, inner-city mothers, and even fourth-graders (Cowen 1970; Cowen et al. 1970a; Cowen 1971a). Although these programs have a common conceptual base, they differ in details such as the nature and extent of the prior training of helpers, the loci and types of contacts between helper and child, and methods of supervision. They share common denominators, however, which, additively, point to an alternative approach to school dysfunction. All the programs focus on *young*, maladapting school children. They pivot around the strong commitment of the helping person to a child who needs assistance. They implicate key role-shifts by the school mental health professional in which traditional one-to-one clinical services are, in good measure, supplanted by educative, liaison, supervisory, consultative, and resource functions.

This redefined approach seems to have potential for expanding the reach of mental health helping activities in sorely needed geometric ways. To illustrate, a group of five half-time child-aides can see about 50 youngsters during the school year, for an average of thirty-five 40-minute sessions each. Not only are 50 children far more than the professional can see this intensively but they also represent a substantial proportion of the maladapting primary graders in any given school. While using nonprofessionals started as an expedient to meet professional manpower and fiscal problems, Sobey (1970) recently presented data suggesting that this development now stands on its own merits. Her survey of several hundred human service programs using nonprofessionals indicates that 85 percent report faster service, 89 percent, more extensive service, 84 percent, the ability to add new services, 76 percent, freeing up professional time, and 84 percent, gaining new viewpoints as a result of using nonprofessionals. In our program, ingredients such as the aides' strong motivation, their intrinsic "common sense," and the exciting challenge offered by the work combined to make this group a prospectively valuable asset in human service for maladapting children.

Recent Developments

The project's first decade developed methods for early detection of ineffective school function, studied its incidence, and assessed the efficacy of early secondary interventions. Research indicated that the model was workable and merited expansion from its initial experimental-demonstration base to one of broader system impact. Accordingly, in the late stages of the second project-period, after establishing a support base with responsible mental health planning groups in the community, discussions of how it might be extended were undertaken with Rochester City School District and several nearby county school districts. This period was marked by countless meetings, with school boards, superintendents, principals, and pupil personnel co-ordinators, around issues of feasibility and cost.

Ultimately a plan evolved to extend the project to six Rochester and five county schools in three adjacent districts. These eleven settings represented a wide range, including large (N = 1,100) and small (N = 140) schools; exclusively primary (kgn–3rd grade) and traditional elementary (kgn–7th grade) schools; locales ranging from the inner-city ghetto (97 percent nonwhite enrollment) to relatively affluent suburbia. While there were structural communalities in *how* participating schools were staffed (i.e. portions of the time of a social worker and psychologist plus *x* child-aides for each pair of schools), specifics varied as a function of resources. Thus, whereas one full-time psychologist, one full-time social worker, and 10 aides staffed each two Rochester city schools, county schools averaged one-quarter to two-fifths of a psychologist and social worker and fewer (e.g. 6–8) aides per pair of schools. Most aides work half-time except in inner-city schools, where need and job realities dictated full-time employment.

While different saturations, particularly in professional time, in the several settings detract from program uniformity, they accurately mirror the reality of the current resource scene. The challenge they present is: "Given fixed and less than ideal resources in a setting, what programs and personnel deployments are most promising?" The project as it now exists is hardly a series of eleven identical models from a Sears Roebuck catalogue; it is far more a federation of philosophically linked, like-minded, but highly individualistic programs. Its specific implementation and detail necessarily vary across schools because needs, problems, and, particularly, resources vary. The linking orientations that bring programs together under a single umbrella are: their shared emphasis on early detection and prevention of school maladaptation; their use of professionals as consultants and resource people, and building direct child-helping services around nonprofessional child-aides. Whatever its resource limits are, each setting thus seeks, realistically, to extend its individual and social impact.

The Program in Action

For the 1969–70 school year, the expanded PMHP had a six-month "build-up" period in the eleven participating schools during which professionals, many newly assigned, became known to school personnel, oriented them to project workings, made necessary space arrangements, and established referral systems. Training professionals and recruiting and training child-aides, each described more fully elsewhere (Cowen in press), also took place during the build-up period.

The program's actual child-serving operations began in March 1970. By then schools had generated ample slates of child-referrals. Roughly 330 children were seen during the three month "debugging" period in the spring of 1970. During the 1970–71 academic year, 531 children were referred to the program, including about 150 carry-overs from the preceding spring. PMHP has thus seen about 700 youngsters in its first year. This total, roughly 17 percent of the primary grade enrollment of participating schools, includes most youngsters with serious maladaptive problems who otherwise would have gone without help.

Most often, aides see children two times a week for relatively brief (30–40 minute) sessions. At peak, the aide group renders about 800 child-serving contracts weekly, suggesting by extrapolation that a program of this magnitude can generate at least 20,000 child-contracts anually. To cite two hypothetical extremes in resource allocation, one could choose to see 4,000 children five times each or 200 children 100 times each. Neither extreme makes sense as a uniform prescription. Interventions with children must necessarily reflect their individual needs and problems. Some children can profit from a brief contact every other week; others will need to be seen three times a week. Since specific empirical relations among types of maladaptation, frequency of contact, and outcome are not yet established, diverse allocations of aide resources are being explored.

For example, aides during the 1970–71 school year were trained in group approaches, for children who might particularly be helped by a sheltered group socialization experience. This development has two potential values: expanding the number of children who can be seen, and as an intervention-modality of choice for children with specific types of school maladaptation (e.g. the timid and the withdrawn). In inner-city settings, which are frequently characterized by sharp communication barriers between home and school that subvert the child's educational growth, aides have been used effectively as home visitors to open doors between families and a school establishment often seen as alien. The aides, themselves neighborhood people, offer "know-how" and a "style match" (Reiff and Riessman 1965) that help to gain entrance into heretofore impenetrable homes—a crucial first step in opening lines of communication.

How children get referred to PMHP and what, concretely, happens to them in their project experience bear further consideration. In their day-today contacts with children, teachers frame standards for behavior and educational development. They differ considerably in their reactions to departures from these expectancies. Children who show minor deviations are often effectively handled within the teacher's well-established repertoire of classroom-management techniques. However, when a problem defies "normal" handling or assumes "serious" proportions in her eyes, the teacher solicits help. PMHP stands as a potential resource in such instances. The principal difficulties that elicit the call for help are learning disabilities (e.g. the child who does not read), problems of withdrawal and undersocialization, and those of hyperactivity, aggressiveness, and distractibility. When the teacher determines that a more serious failing is present, or well along in process, she submits a referral to the mental health professionals indicating briefly the nature of the difficulty. Occasionally referrals come from other school personnel or from parents; in each case, however, formal recognition of a serious school adaptation problem energizes the helping process.

Available sources of information about the child are pooled at the time of referral. These include the referral statement itself; prior screening information (e.g. group intellectual, personality, and behavior measures) obtained routinely for all children early in the school year; and data from the social worker's contact with the mother. A staff conference is held, including mental health professionals serving as consultants, the teacher, prospective aide, and involved "others" (e.g. principal, nurse, lunchroom monitor) who interact with the child, to piece together available information, arrive at a preliminary understanding of his difficulties, and establish a set of working goals. Though on occasion another approach is recommended (e.g. social work contact with mother or a set of procedures for more effective classroom management), most often the child is assigned to meet regularly with an aide, with a particular set of objectives in mind.

Case History

A résumé of a composite case may give a clearer picture of the modus operandi.

> Bobby, a second-grader, was brought to the team's attention by his teacher. He was extremely disruptive in the classroom and aggressive to peers in the school corridors, gymnasium, and lunchroom. "Unless given complete attention and constant priase," said his teacher, "he strikes out at anyone near him and has tantrums." Although evidencing above-average potential in earlier intellectual screening, Bobby had already been left back once and now was identified as the *bête noire* of the primary grades. He was on the threshold of suspension from school.
>
> Social work contact with his mother indicated an unstable family history. The oldest of four children, Bobby was the product of a stormy marriage that ended in divorce when he was four. His mother remarried and came to Rochester where, in the next four years, the family moved six times, and Bobby attended four schools with assignment to seven different classrooms.

At an initial staff conference, the boy's teacher, the mental health professionals, school principal, lunchroom monitor, and prospective aide pieced together a view of Bobby as a child who has spent his first years in an uncertain, ever-changing, menacing psychological world, who had learned to expect misfortune, and whose behavior was designed to prove and confirm his belief that his environment was hostile and people untrustworthy. On the positive side, Bobby had established interests in arts and model-making, his family situation was now more stable, and his mother showed genuine concern for his wellbeing.

Objectives and guidelines were established for those who would have frequent contact with Bobby. Most important were: trying to stabilize a positive, trusting view of his world; shoring up his battered self-concept; offering praise and support only for real achievement; and setting realistic limits firmly. He was assigned to see an aide twice weekly.

Thereafter, when Bobby challenged his teacher with his overt provocations, she unswervingly dealt with each transgression in a way that clearly labeled the action—but not the child—as unacceptable. After some time, this damped his need to act out; in fact, one day he said to his mother that his teacher "was really fair and I deserved to be punished!"

Bobby's initial approach to his aide was marked more by aloofness and disinterest than by the heralded pattern of aggressive provocation. The aide accepted his style and pacing without pushing him. When, after this early fencing, Bobby ventured several half-hearted, almost transparent attempts at provocation, the aide's response was again firm but accepting. His relation with the aide became more enthusiastic, and he became involved in high-level artistic and creative activities that won him deserved approval and support.

The teacher, aide, and mental health consultants conferred several times during the year to compare notes. It was clear within six weeks that the boy had "turned the corner." The frequency and intensity of his environmental testing had diminished sharply, and his formerly deficient academic work had improved markedly. Apparently, two relations of trust and security had been established, with a resultant change in Bobby's view of the world. This was helped along by further stabilization in his home situation, by his mother's clearer understanding, with the help of the social worker, of Bobby's perceptions, and by his mother's development of more effective ways to interact with him in critical choice-point situations.

The boy met with his aide 57 times during the eight-month school year. Two years later, he was showing above-average academic progress and was well accepted by his classmates. Virtually all signs of his prior Dennis-the-Menace behavior had disappeared.

Further Training and New Roles

Training for all project personnel is seen as on-going and open-ended. Professionals continue to have regular biweekly training sessions, as a "committee of the whole," to consider current problems of project conduct and management. They provide on-the-job supervision and case-review sessions for aides. Supervision, though regularized, varies in format across schools and includes both individual and group contacts. Teacher involvement is facilitated through extensive use of substitute teachers, which allows regular teachers to participate with professionals and aides, in conferences concerning the children during school hours. Several principals regard the teachers' continuing growth in understanding and sensitivity, gained through participation in discussions of problem instances with teams and consultants and then translated to more effective, direct battle-line handling of classroom situations, as the principal project benefit. If the teacher learns to cope with budding dysfunction more effectively in the classroom, an important step toward primary prevention has been achieved.

Project staff provide extensive consultation to participating schools, with a broad range of objectives. Among the most basic is to strengthen the hand of program participants so that they can come to function more independently. "Modeling" the consultant's role for school professionals and professionals-in-training furthers this end. Another consulting objective is to clarify project aims and roles continually so that they can be carried out most effectively. When difficulties come up (e.g. misuse of project resources, inadequate supervision, disagreements between team members), the consultant fulfills important information-finding and trouble-shooting roles. The format of consultation varies. There are individual meetings with school personnel, group conferences with child-aides and/or with teachers, and frequent case-centered consultations on specific problem children, with teachers, aides, and professionals.

Currently, to extend the projects' consulting arm, four senior aides have assumed consultative responsibilities. These women, each with six years of prior supervised experience with children, serve as resource-persons for new aides. The decision to use senior aides as consultants was not a manpower expedient; rather, it grew out of our experience in training nonprofessionals, where we discovered that contact with seasoned aides was among the most useful, informative, and reassuring of all possible experiences for aides-in-training. While use of senior aides as consultants is new and still in the process of "finding its own level," initial reactions to it have been positive. The consulting aide brings experience and perspective to the beginner re specific problems that develop in contacts with children, "models" the aide role, and participates in individual and group supervision by professionals, representing another vantage point and set of experiences. Project staff supervise these senior aide activities.

The delivery system described, aiming as it does for geometric expansion of helping services, requires, in addition to new manpower uses, changing professional roles. The professional abandons a substantial portion of traditional, direct clinical service functions in favor of activities elsewhere described as mental health "quarter-backing" (Cowen 1967; Cowen 1971a; Zax and Cowen, 1972). The cadre of nonprofessionals brought into line-contact roles extends the mental health helping arm significantly by bringing service to a substantial segment of maladapting school children who might otherwise become casualties of the system. The ultimate proof of the model rests in the empirical, rather than philosophical, arena. Way-station empirical indicants have been encouraging (see Fig. 2).

Reality, logic, and cost economics favor this new approach. For example, five half-time aides, at a total cost of about 50 percent of one full-time mental health professional, bring service to perhaps ten times as many children. If the initial relatively minor cost-increment of hiring aides averts personally disastrous and socially costly outcomes, such as institutional placement for mental disability, addiction, delinquent and criminal behavior, or less drastic ones, such as foster-home or special-class placement, then the model holds promise for important long-term financial as well as human gain. The professional in this new program in no sense becomes obsolescent; rather he assumes new, more socially utilitarian roles that significantly extend the reach of needed services.

Research Components

From the start, the project has heavily emphasized research. Some of its early findings were described in the preceding text. Current project research is extensive; however, anchored as it is in a real, sometimes volatile world, the research is often hampered by extraneous external "noise" that detracts from a theoretical ideal of antiseptically pure laboratory work. Our research net touches, directly or indirectly, roughly 20,000 people, including children, teachers, parents, school personnel, and mental health professionals and nonprofessionals. Thus, sheer problems of numbers are overwhelming. Moreover, many of our "responders" understandably feel distant, or removed, from the research operation. They do not clearly perceive how marks on a piece of paper today can have much to do with effective education tomorrow. Consequently we expect, and get, a certain amount of careless responding, overt noncooperation, and passive aggression. The entire research operation is far less clean than the tightly controlled laboratory investigation. Impure data, weakened experimental designs, and absence of ideal controls are, for us, chronic hazards.

Another order of research problem stems from the rapid flux of the current urban educational scene. New programs are continually being introduced. School structures and compositions are changing. In Rochester, for example, there has been much interest in, and at times acrimonious debate about, redistricting schools to achieve racial balance. The Rochester School Board voted in the spring of 1970 to establish two such racially balanced zones, including, as it happened, two project schools. An immediate consequence of this decision was that these schools became kgn-3 structures rather than kgn-6. Because of the considerable investment in the redistricting plan, the shift in structure was understandably accompanied by other, hopefully salutary, changes (e.g. smaller classes, introduction of teacher-aide personnel, special reading programs, "voluntary" teachers).

While such drastic change can, in part, be neutralized experimentally by using comparably "zoned-but-non-project" control schools, rapid change in school structures breeds a host of additional problems for the researcher. Some schools—and it is their autonomous right to do so—have, for example, eliminated grading completely or have introduced prose reports as substitutes. Others have abandoned the one-teacher/one-class notion that has long pervaded primary education, and now rotate children to several class groupings and teachers, for different subject areas or pursuits. Without arguing the merits of these changes, the fact that grades and teacher judgments, heretofore bellwether evaluation criteria, are simply unavailable or no longer comparable across schools renders the already complex challenge of long-term project evaluation extraordinarily difficult. An incidental irony is added when educational change, which an experimenter may favor as a professional or as a citizen, undercuts long years of heavily invested program development and carefully evolved experimental design.

Nor are the foregoing problems static, "one-shot" concerns. To the contrary, today's social sands shift with ever-accelerating speed. In Rochester, for example, the school board, the city's basic education policy-making and planning body, is a partisan group. Each November thus holds a potential for change that can seriously affect programs and research evaluations. All this makes for very real, built-in research risk, since basic change in school organization or programs becomes experimental noise confounding the supposed "main effect" of concern—the project itself. We have little control over the powerful social forces underlying educational change. The project sits in a real and, at the moment, thoroughly mercurial urban world. Unquestionably its research findings will be affected and limited by this fact.

Such realistic limitations notwithstanding, research on all facets of the project proceeds energetically. Past studies and those underway include methodological and substantive investigations, outcome evaluations, process analyses, selection and prediction studies, and examination of the complex interrelations among these classes of variables.

We are, of course, centrally concerned with the effectiveness of the program and its components (i.e. outcome). In the immediate sense, this calls for specific evaluation of the aide program, based on comparison of the behavioral and educational development of youngsters exposed to it and otherwise comparable controls. Over longer periods our evaluation framework will be broadened to allow comparison of *all* children in project vs control schools on relevant measures of educational and personal development. Subtler aspects of the overall outcome question are also of concern, as for example: Do children with particular types of referral problems (e.g. undersocialization) profit more, or less, from the program than others (e.g. children referred for hyperactivity and aggression)? Are there relations between aide attributes and effectiveness with one or another type of child?

In a retrospective study of program outcomes (Cowen, Dorr, and Pokracki, in press), mothers of 36 children seen by child aides, an average of two years earlier, for an average of 55 sessions, were asked to judge the child's *current* status on a series of 7-point "change"-rating scales reflecting specific dimensions, such as getting along at home, getting along in school, peer relations, and attitude to school. Mothers and interviewers independently judged that significant growth had occurred in the child's subsequent educational and interpersonal development. Some of the findings of this study are depicted in Figure 3. Thus, relatively stable intermediate as well as short-term gain may be assumed to result from the aide program. The target children in question, almost without exception, had also made normal academic progress in the intervening period.

More microscopic study of the aide-child interaction is of interest to us both absolutely (i.e. descriptive accounts of what takes place during such contacts) and in terms of relations between process elements and many other variables, including outcome indices, aide characteristics, and structural aspects of program (professional and resource characteristics, nature of referrals, etc.). Accordingly, we have developed a comprehensive process-analysis form,

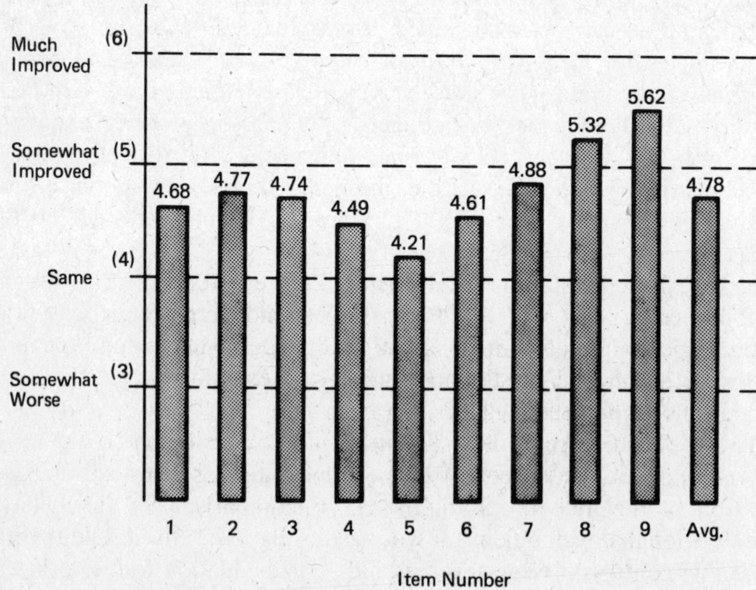

Fig. 3. *Mean pooled parent and interviewer follow-up ratings for children seen two years earlier by child aides. Each, except variable 5, indicates statistically significant improvement.* 1: *Actual educational performance.* 2: *Getting along with teachers.* 3: *Getting along with schoolmates.* 4: *Getting along with parents.* 5: *Getting along with siblings.* 6: *Getting along with neighborhood kids.* 7: *Degree of happiness.* 8: *Attitude toward school.* 9: *Extent of project's responsibility for observed changes (from complete to none).* Avg.: *Average improvement scores based on items 1–9.*

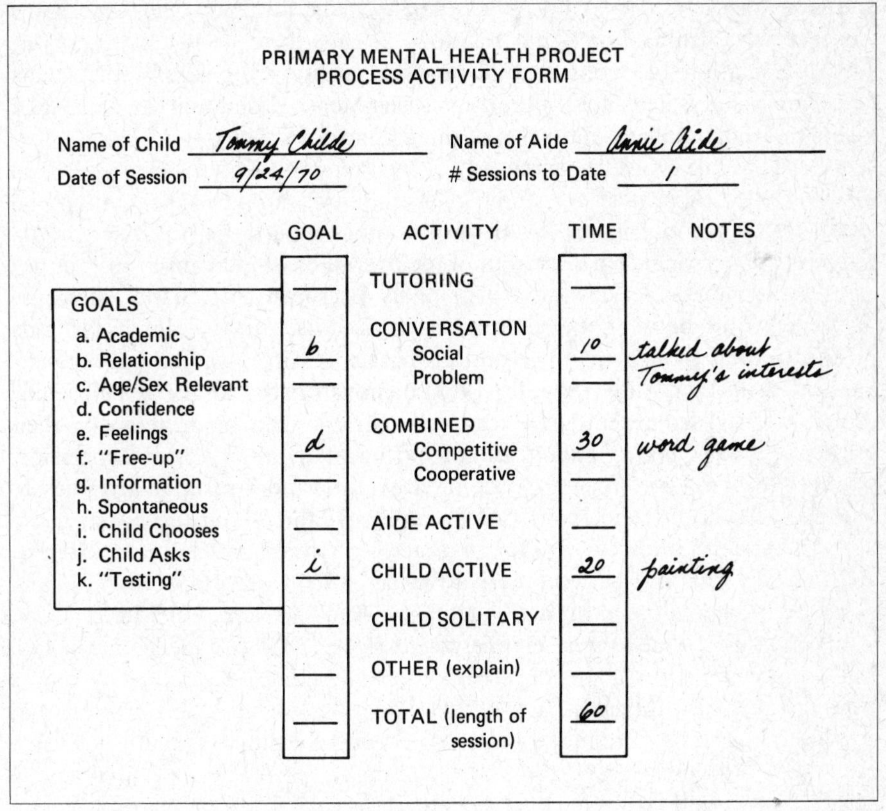

PRIMARY MENTAL HEALTH PROJECT
PROCESS ACTIVITY FORM

Name of Child Tommy Childe   Name of Aide Annie Aide
Date of Session 9/24/70   # Sessions to Date 1

GOALS
a. Academic
b. Relationship
c. Age/Sex Relevant
d. Confidence
e. Feelings
f. "Free-up"
g. Information
h. Spontaneous
i. Child Chooses
j. Child Asks
k. "Testing"

GOAL	ACTIVITY	TIME	NOTES
___	TUTORING	___	
	CONVERSATION		
b	Social	10	talked about
___	Problem	___	Tommy's interests
	COMBINED		
d	Competitive	30	word game
___	Cooperative	___	
___	AIDE ACTIVE	___	
i	CHILD ACTIVE	20	painting
___	CHILD SOLITARY	___	
___	OTHER (explain)	___	
___	TOTAL (length of session)	60	

Fig. 4. *Process-analysis form for aide goals and aide activities with children.*

including characterizations of both aide goals and actual aide activities with children (McWilliams 1971). This form (shown in Fig. 4) is completed biweekly by each aide for each child she is seeing, a procedure that yielded about 4,500 completed process forms for the 1970–71 school year.

Data such as these permit study of a number of significant questions, as for example: What is the overall nature of the aide-child interaction process and how does it change over time? Are these overall, or time-period, differences in process for different types of referrals (e.g. acting out vs withdrawn vs children with learning disabilities)? Do settings differ in emphases and contact procedures as evidenced by different process reports? Are there relations between specific goals established for a child and the use of particular process activity categories? What relations exist between goals and/or process activities and outcomes? Is there a relation between aide characteristics (e.g. personality factors, interest, attitudes, etc.) and how aides interact either with children in general or with specific groups?

Development of process information, particularly as it relates to outcome and aide-characteristics data, is essential. In addition to the theoretical value of establishing functional relations among these classes of variables, such information has considerable practical utility when fed back to participating schools (e.g. for optimizing assignment of children to aides and identifying maximally useful ways of interacting with them).

Considerable progress has already been made in identifying characteristics of child-aides. An interview study (Cowen, Dorr, and Pokracki, in press) showed that school mental health professionals agreed well in assessing 18 job-relevant personal characteristics of the overall child-aide applicant sample.

Furthermore, interviewing professionals discriminated reliably, along all 18 dimensions, between those accepted and those turned down for aide positions, even though the applicant group, as a whole, was homogeneously "select." A further study (Sandler 1970) demonstrated that the selected aide sample differed from demographically comparable controls in terms of their greater empathy, higher affiliative and nurturant qualities, lesser aggression, stronger teaching and social service interests, and more positive attitudes to schools and school-related concepts. The extensive three-hour test battery used to evaluate aides and controls is being factor-analyzed. We hope to examine more closely relations between derivative factor scores and both process and outcome measures based on aides' actual work with referred children.

As a project that heavily emphasizes early detection of ineffective school function, we are necessarily concerned with developing and refining screening procedures. Given the fact that our early identification programs now extend to many thousands of school children, we require techniques that are simple (i.e. easily responded to by the neophyte), brief, reliable, valid, and easy to score. To this end we have done a methodological study comparing several brief and lengthier teacher-screening measures for detecting early school maladaptation (Cowen et al. 1971a). A device shown by this research to be well-suited for mass screening of primary-graders is the AML Behavioral Rating Scale (Brownbridge and Van Vleet 1969), an 11-item scale reflecting the factors of aggressiveness (A), moodiness (M), and learning disability (L). Teachers complete this form for all children early in the school year. Forms are scored and the data summarized within 24 to 48 hours. Test norms have been prepared and distributed to school mental health professionals. When test data are returned, summaries are prepared for school use, identifying children whose A, M, or L or sum AML scores exceed given percentiles. Readministration of the AML at the end of the school year permits comparison of children seen by aides to otherwise comparable controls.

Further AML research is in progress, as for example more refined norming studies, factor-analytic studies, and validation studies (e.g. comparing AML scores of project-referred and nonreferred children, and relating referral statements about children to AML profiles). We are also experimenting with variations in the AML test format (e.g. in item-wording, rating-point descriptions, number of rating points). Other specific studies using this measure are also underway, as for example studies of sex and developmental differences and comparisons of AML profiles of promoted vs nonpromoted children.

While the project's research emphasis is on outcome, process, and aide-characteristics data and their interrelations, additional work is in progress that does not neatly fit these pigeonholes. For example, we are vitally concerned with developing information on utilization of project resources (Cowen et al. 1971b). Such work, while "unglamorous," provides two important classes of information: establishing the scope and "power" of the model used and developing concrete facts about specific utilization patterns for individual schools. The former information, combined with effectiveness data, makes possible cost/benefit analyses that facilitate comparison of the present approach both to traditional school mental health programs and other interventions (e.g. foster-home care, residential treatment, etc.) which stand as likely alternatives to this program. Preliminary cost/benefit analyses suggest that while the project involves a relatively small immediate cost increment, particularly for aide salaries, long-range savings accrued by averting more drastic and costly interventions are considerable. Providing concrete utilization data to individual schools allows each to see graphically how it has deployed its own (finite) resources, whether such use gives an optimal "needs/resources" match, and, if not, to correct course so as better to approach that balance.

School mental health consultation is central to the project's operation at two levels: consultation provided by project staff to schools; and that provided by school mental health professionals, within schools, to principals, teachers, aides, and other school personnel. The term consultation has had ever-increasing usage in the past decade and is defined in so many ways that it has assumed a catch-all quality. We hope, by using a largely naturalistic approach (i.e. recording consulting sessions and categorizing their component events), to identify more operationally the nature of consultation (i.e. what consultants actually *do* and how varied these interventions are) and its consequences (i.e. which consultative actions produce positive or negative outcomes and under what circumstances).

Project evaluation has heretofore been limited to relatively short-term effects. However, through the availability in this community of the comprehensive, cumulative Psychiatric Register of hospital, clinic, and private contacts with mental health practitioners, the temporal scope of follow-up evaluation is being extended. Together with the Register group we are conducting a follow-up study of the subsequent psychiatric history of 600 children who were seen through PMHP as firstgraders between 1958–1963 and screened (red-tag vs non-red-tag) for early school maladaptation. For this group—now ages 13–19—seven to twelve years have elapsed since the initial screening. The study thus seeks to establish whether children identified as maladapting at age six, and their families, have had different psychiatric histories than non-identified peers.

The preceding examples illustrate, without exhausting, the category "project-related" studies. The project's nature and scope are such that it offers broad opportunities to explore a variety of questions pertaining specifically to early detection and prevention of dysfunction; adaptation to school; selection, training, and use of nonprofessionals; new roles for mental health professionals; and, more generally, issues of child development.

Overview

The foregoing account indicates that the project rests on a particular set of assumptions from which new programming and manpower uses logically derive. Key assumptions include the following: (1) Much of our mental health effort must be directed to the very young and to the institutions that shape their developments. (2) There is need for greater emphasis on mental health programs that help the many to adapt effectively rather than on programs that react to marked adaptive failure in the few. Schools offer unique opportunities for the former type of programming. (3) Early detection and prevention of dysfunction are preferable to after-the-fact patchwork. The older, more entrenched the maladaptation, the more difficult and costly it is to cope with, and the greater the danger of irreparable personal consequences.

Given these assumptions, the following are our most important program emphases: (1) Introduction of widespread, early screening techniques for detection of school maladaptation. (2) Use of nonprofessional child-aides, selected for their warmth, facility in interpersonal relations, and interest in children, to bring immediate assistance to children identified as functioning ineffectively. (3) Development of preventive interventions designed to strengthen the hand of school personnel to deal with problems before they become negatively labeled, and to forestall the dire, cumulative consequences of educational failure. (4) Redefining the role of the school mental health professional as a consultant, trainer, and resource person for the many, rather than as a person largely restricted to one-to-one clinical services, on a crisis basis, for the severely malfunctioning few.

Whatever the satisfactions of the project experience, however much one may be persuaded that its delivery system is both logical and effective, there is a growing conviction on our part that it is insufficient. It has thus far been a program for early secondary prevention, and has not engaged the critical challenges of primary prevention. There are several reasons why this is so. First, primary prevention requires knowledge and skills that far transcend those of the mental health professional. Second, it has an ethereal quality because its pay-off criteria are abstract and futuristic. Schools by contrast, are heavily oriented to concrete, immediate problems that must be solved, if not instantly, then five minutes hence. In periods of fiscal austerity, school mental health priorities, like those in the emergency room of a hospital, are given to glaring here-and-now difficulties. That such an approach often guarantees future stultification rarely concerns those who must meet today's crises.

It is sure that no matter how a school is set up, it is an institution that profoundly influences child development. The choice we face is whether that influence is to be random or informed. Accordingly, the most important future role we can envision for the school mental health professional is as a social system analyst and social engineer. His challenge—and opportunity—must be measured in terms of how he can help to build health rather than how he can combat pathology. Optimally conceived, the school environment should potentiate adaptation for all children.

References

BEACH, D. R., E. L. COWEN, M. ZAX, J. D. LAIRD, M. A. TROST, and L. D. IZZO (1968). Objectification of a screening procedure for early detection of emotional disorder. *Child Development*, **39**, 1177–88.

BROWNBRIDGE, R., and P. VAN VLEET (1969). *Investments in Prevention: The Prevention of Learning and Behavior Problems in Children: Evaluation Report*. San Francisco, California: Pace I. D. Center.

COWEN, E. L. (1967). Emergent approaches to mental health problems: An overview and directions for future work. In E. L. Cowen, E. A. Gardner, and M. Zax (eds.), *Emergent Approaches to Mental Health Problems*. New York: Appleton-Century-Crofts, pp. 389–455.

COWEN, E. L. (1968). The effectiveness of secondary prevention programs using nonprofessionals in the school setting. *Proceedings, 76th Annual Convention, APA*, **2**, 705–06.

COWEN, E. L. (1970). Training clinical psychologists for community mental health functions: description of a practicum experience. In I. Iscoe & C. D. Spielberger (eds.), *Training and Research in Community Mental Health*. New York. Appleton-Century-Crofts, pp. 99–124.

COWEN, E. L. (1971a). On broadening community mental health practicum training for clinical psychologists. *Professional Psychology*, **3**, 159–168.

COWEN, E. L. (in press). A new approach to school mental health services. Chapter in NIMH–OED Manual for Community Mental Health Centers.

COWEN, E. L., R. L. CARLISLE, and G. KAUFMAN, (1969). Evaluation of a college student volunteer program with primary graders experiencing school adjustment problems. *Psychology in the Schools*, **6**, 371–75.

COWEN, E. L., J. M. CHINSKY, and J. RAPPAPORT (1970a). An undergraduate practicum in community mental health. *Community Mental Health Journal*, **6**, 91–100.

COWEN, E. L., D. A. DORR, and A. R. ORGEL (1971a). Interrelations among screening measures for early detection of school dysfunction, *Psychology in the Schools*, **8**, 135–39.

COWEN, E. L., D. A. DORR, and F. POKRACKI (in press). Selection of nonprofessional child-aides for a school mental health project. *Community Mental Health Journal*, **8**.

COWEN, E. L., D. A. DORR, I. N. SANDLER, and S. A. MCWILLIAMS (1971b). Utilization of a nonprofessional child-aide, school mental health program. *Journal of School Psychology*, **9**, 131–36.

COWEN, E. L., D. A. DORR, M. A. TROST, and L. D. IZZO (in press). A follow-up study of maladapting school children seen by nonprofessionals. *Journal of Consulting and Clinical Psychology*, **36**.

COWEN, E. L., J. HUSER, D. R. BEACH, and J. RAPPAPORT (1970b). Parental perceptions of young children and their relation to indices of adjustment. *Journal of Consulting and Clinical Psychology*, **34**, 97–103.

COWEN, E. L., L. D. IZZO, H. MILES, E. F. TELSCHOW, M. A. TROST, and M. ZAX (1963). A mental health program in the school setting: description and evaluation. *Journal of Psychology*, **56**, 307–56.

COWEN, E. L., E. LEIBOWITZ, and G. LEIBOWITZ (1968). The utilization of retired people as mental health aides in the schools. *American Journal of Orthopsychiatry*, **38**, 900–09.

COWEN, E. L., M. ZAX, L. D. IZZO, and M. A. TROST (1966a). The prevention of emotional disorders in the school setting: a further investigation. *Journal of Consulting Psychology*, **30**, 381–87.

COWEN, E. L., M. ZAX, and J. D. LAIRD (1966b). A college student volunteer program in the elementary school setting. *Community Mental Health Journal*, **2**, 319–28.

GLIDEWELL, J. C., and C. S. SWALLOW (1969). *The Prevalence of Maladjustment in Elementary Schools*. Report prepared for the Joint Commission on Mental Illness and Health of Children. Chicago: University of Chicago Press.

LIEM, G. R., A. W. YELLOTT, E. L. COWEN, M. A. TROST, and L. D. IZZO (1969). Some correlates of early detected emotional dysfunction in the schools. *American Journal of Orthopsychiatry*, **39**, 619–26.

MCWILLIAMS, S. A. (1971). Process analysis of a school-based mental health program. Unpublished Ph.D. dissertation, University of Rochester.

President's Task Force on the Mentally Handicapped (1970). *Action against mental disability*. Washington, D.C.: United States Government Printing Office.

REIFF, R., and F. RIESSMAN (1965). The indigenous nonprofessional: a strategy of change in community action and community mental health programs. *Community Mental Health Journal*. Monograph No. 1.

SANDLER, I. N. (1970). Characteristics of women working as child-aides in a school-based preventive mental health program. Unpublished Ph.D. dissertation, University of Rochester.

SOBEY, F. (1970). *The Nonprofessional Revolution in Mental Health*. New York: Columbia University Press.

ZAX, M., and E. L. COWEN (1967). Early identification and prevention of emotional disturbance in a public school. In E. L. Cowen, E. A. Gardner & M. Zax (eds.), *Emergent Approaches to Mental Health Problems*. New York: Appleton-Century-Crofts, pp. 331–51.

ZAX, M., and E. L. COWEN (1969). Research on early detection and prevention of emotional dysfunction in young school children. In C. D. Spielberger (ed.), *Current Topics in Clinical and Community Psychology*, Vol. I. New York: Academic Press, pp. 67–108.

ZAX, M., and E. L. COWEN (1972). *Abnormal Psychology: Changing Conceptions*. New York: Holt, Rinehart & Winston.

ZAX, M., E. L. COWEN, L. D. IZZO, and M. A. TROST (1964). Identifying emotional disturbance in the school setting. *American Journal of Orthopsychiatry*, **34**, 447–54.

ZAX, M., E. L. COWEN, J. RAPPAPORT, D. R. BEACH, and J. D. LAIRD (1968). Follow-up study of children identified early as emotionally disturbed. *Journal of Consulting and Clinical Psychology*, **32**, 369–74.

EMANUEL HALLOWITZ and FRANK RIESSMAN

The Role of the Indigenous Nonprofessional in a Community Mental Health Neighborhood Service Center Program

A major problem in developing programs that have a preventive impact on a community is developing a "handle" or entrée that permits the professional to bring his skills to bear on those who could benefit by them. Children can be readily engaged through schools, nurseries, recreational facilities, and the like, but adults are more difficult to contact. In the following paper, Hallowitz and Riessman describe a program that they have designed for bringing mental health-type service to relatively deprived neighborhoods. In this program, as in many others, considerable use is made of nonprofessionals, in this case people indigenous to the neighborhoods in which they work. The storefront service center offers its services in connection with a wide variety of problems, many of which can hardly be classified even broadly as being mental health problems. Nevertheless, although the role of the center in connection with many such problems is not vastly different from that of the old-time ward politician, efforts are made to render such services in a way that provides a model that the recipient of help can himself emulate. It is intended that this feature of the program will build skills that will contribute to the overall adequacy of functioning.

The Lincoln Hospital Mental Health Services represents an attempt to develop a comprehensive network of community mental health services in a highly disadvantaged urban area of New York City (4).

The Hospital district served is located in the Southeast Bronx. It is a congested, old section of the city suffering physically and socially from the classic ills of such areas: deteriorated housing; high mobility; high rates of juvenile delinquency, school dropouts, narcotic addiction, infant mortality,

Reprinted from the *American Journal of Orthopsychiatry*, **37** (1967), 766–778.

etc.[1] Most of its 350,000 inhabitants are Puerto Rican (55 per cent) or Negro (25 per cent).

In planning a strategy of intervention, it was important to keep in mind that throughout the city, services to low-income persons, particularly newcomers to urban centers, either have been inadequate or so organized and operated as to limit their full use by the poor. Because the public service agencies are fragmented, complex and bureaucratic, they constitute a frustrating, powerful and seemingly insurmountable network of barriers (2, 3). Also, the voluntary family and children's agencies have only one office each to serve the entire Bronx (former neighborhood offices and outposts have been consolidated in the interest of economy). Each is located (as are many of the public agencies) in middleclass neighborhoods at considerable distance from those who need the service most. Moreover, the traditional ways of operating waiting lists, weekly appointments, long-term service and emphasis on "talking through" are not consonant with the needs, the experience, or the life-style of low-income people (5, 8).

It was this view of our district—the people, their needs and the pattern of existing services—that impelled us to develop a network of Neighborhood Service Centers,[2] staffed by indigenous nonprofessionals under professional supervision.

The Neighborhood Service Center

In 1965 the Lincoln Hospital Mental Health Services established three Neighborhood Service Centers. The first opened on February 22, the second on June 29, the third on December 22. Two of these centers are located in a storefront at street level; the third is one flight up. Each Center serves a radius of five blocks (approximately 50,000 people) and each is staffed by five to ten nonprofessional mental health aides from the neighborhood and one or two professional mental health specialists who serve as Neighborhood Service Center director and assistant director.

[1] Compared to the Bronx, as a whole, most of the Lincoln area falls into the lowest quartile of median family income ($3,700–$5,400) and educational attainment (7.6–8.8 years) and the highest rate of male unemployment in this area is approximately twice that of the Bronx average. Similarly, the amount of overcrowded housing and school facilities are about twice that of the Bronx as a whole.

In addition, compared to the Bronx, as a whole: (1) Rates for juvenile delinquency offenses are 25 per cent higher. (2) Rates of venereal disease among youth under 21 are three times greater in some neighborhoods of the Lincoln area and $1\frac{1}{4}$ times as high as in other areas. (3) The rate of public assistance cases is approximately twice as high. (4) Admission rates to state mental hospitals are 40 per cent higher from this area. (5) Although reliable figures are not available, estimates of the percentage of deliveries of the Lincoln Hospital Obstetrical Service, in which there is no legal father, run as high as 70 per cent. (Comparable figures for the Bronx, as a whole, are not available.)

[2] The Neighborhood Service Center Program is supported by a grant from the United States Office of Economic Opportunity.

The core of the NSC program is its role as a "psychosocial first-aid station"; the Center is a place where people can bring any type of problem. This formula allows residents the possibility of receiving immediate help and comfort without having to define their problem in a way appropriate for the help-giving system (1). Moreover, the fact that the Center is located in the midst of the neighborhood it is to serve provides visibility and relatedness to the community that often is lacking in the more established agencies. In addition, the employment of indigenous nonprofessionals, their naturalness and the informal atmosphere of the setting confirm the "open door" policy and enable freer contact communication on the part of "clients" from the area.

The Neighborhood Service Center may be viewed as the first port of entry into the service system. The Center worker assumes the responsibility for helping the resident to define his problem and to determine the specific service that he and his family may require. He serves as a bridge between the resident and the service agency. The aide interprets to the resident the program and services of the agency. What might he realistically expect to receive? What are his rights and privileges? What can the agency expect of him? Similarly before making a referral, where indicated, the worker will contact the agency to interpret the specific needs of this client, his style of operation and behavior, his anxiety and fears, so that the agency may in turn gear its service to individualized needs.

In this *expediter* role, the Neighborhood Service Center worker may act as translator, negotiator, advocate, counselor, etc., and even as coordination link between a number of agencies offering services to the same family.

The problems that are brought to the Neighborhood Service Center run the *gamut of human misery* from helping a resident make application for project housing to requests for assistance in more complex and stressful situations. These situations include aiding a parent accept the need for service to a retarded child; helping a family recognize the need to apply for public assistance and helping them to establish their eligibility; helping a family which has just received an eviction notice; helping a family to obtain and use medical and health care: helping a family plan for an aged parent; helping a pregnant unmarried girl and her family to secure appropriate aid; and helping a resident to accept and obtain needed psychiatric services.

In some cases, on-the-spot advice and guidance is sufficient. In others, giving information as to where services can be obtained is sufficient. But usually the seeker of services must be helped to know how to make application, how to deal with the bottlenecks or red tape, and he particularly may need the encouragement and support of the nonprofessional worker to maintain motivation, dignity and self-esteem in the early stages of seeking and receiving services. In still other cases, the service required is not readily available (waiting list) and the Neighborhood Service Center worker is called upon to engage in a "holding action"—to use his knowledge and skill to keep a crisis situation from deteriorating further.

From February 22, when our first Center opened, to December 31, 7,119 different people were served by the two Neighborhood Centers.[3] (Statistics for the third Center have been excluded since it did not begin operations until the last week in December.)

Perhaps a clearer picture of the scope of the activities can be gained by limiting examinations to the six-month period (July–December) when both Centers were in full operation.

During this period 6,220 *new* cases came for services, an average of 1,037 *new* cases a month. Projecting this figure for a full year's operation would give us a total of 6,220 individuals a year per Center. Since the size of the average family coming to the Center is 3.9, it is not unreasonable to state that *indirectly each Center will touch the lives of some 25,000 people in the area it serves.*

The Mental Health Aide

Use of indigenous nonprofessionals as mental health aides in our Neighborhood Service Centers is dictated by two reasons: (1) the tremendous shortage of professional personnel requires that new sources of manpower be tapped and (2) our belief that the indigenous nonprofessional has special attributes that can be used to advance our program and service goals.

The mental health aides are a mixed group in terms of race, age, sex and language background.[4] All are Puerto Rican or Negro. Most are without much formal education. These are people who come from the neighborhood and have experienced poverty themselves. Although they are not sophisticated about mental health problems, they have "savvy," developed from their struggle to survive.

The mental health aide is not a junior social worker, psychologist or psychiatrist. He is more the good friend, good neighbor or perhaps the "friendly visitor" of the early days of social work. Although the mental health aide needs to maintain some objectivity and some detachment, it is of a different order than is required of the professional. The mental health aide intervenes directly in the lives of the clients on a peer level. He can attend funerals, weddings, baptisms and other social events. He is a "friend in need," potential counselor, a model and a sustainer of hope. In his attempts to influence behavior or to assist in problem solving, he relies most heavily on techniques of giving information, advice and counsel, persuasion and environmental manipulation. His manner, his language and his closeness to the life and style of the community enable the resident to develop a trust and confidence not so readily offered the professionals. It is this trust and

[3] These statistics are clearly underestimated since during the first five months no records were kept of contacts that required comparatively simple handling by the aides. It should also be kept in mind that these figures do not include contacts either in person or by phone with collateral sources such as teachers, ministers, social investigators, police, probation officers, housing managers and social workers.

[4] 14 men and 20 women; 18 Puerto Ricans, 16 Negroes; 16 between ages of 21–30, 13 between 31–40, four between 41–50 and one aged 72.

confidence which enables the aide to mediate successfully or bridge the gap between the resident and the professional. It is also this trust and confidence that facilitate the identification process with the aide and increase his power to influence attitudes and behavior.

Although the mental health aide works directly with the client from the moment the client enters the store, the aide always has available to him professional consultation and supervision from the center director and the back-up services of the Lincoln Hospital Mental Health Service Clinic.

To illustrate how the mental health aides can be helpful to people in trouble, let us look at some case examples.

Miss Martinez

Miss Martinez came to the Center reporting that she was eight months pregnant and that her common-law husband had deserted her last month. She worked until two weeks ago, but had been forced to stop working and had to move into a basement apartment with a brother and his family. The few dollars she had accumulated were now gone and she had applied to the Welfare Department for assistance. They had rejected her at intake because they contended that she must know the whereabouts of her common-law husband: they couldn't believe that she could live with a man for two years and not know more about him.

The aide, who spoke Spanish, explained to Miss Martinez why Welfare had to make an investigation and encouraged her to tell whatever she could about her husband. All she knew was that he worked for a cab company, but didn't know which company or where he had lived prior to their getting together. The aide suggested to her that they go together to the police station to see if it were possible to locate her husband. (The aides have had excellent relations with the Police Department—they have visited the police station on a number of occasions, and various policemen have dropped in at the Center to chat and keep warm). The captain of the station, upon hearing the details of the case, dispatched a member of his staff to the central taxicab bureau. There it was discovered that the woman's husband was in fact a cab driver, that he was wanted on charges, but could not be located and had disappeared. These facts were then reported to the Department of Welfare Intake Unit, who felt that they were sufficient to warrant opening the case for further investigation.

When the aide checked with the investigator assigned to the case shortly afterward, he was told that the field supervisor would not fully accept the evidence that was presented and still could not believe that the woman didn't know where her husband was.

Uncertain of what his role should be at this stage, the aide turned to his professional supervisor. The latter, in the presence of the aide phoned the investigator and subsequently the Department of Welfare supervisor. The aide was able to observe his supervisor moving from the stage of reasonable discussion to the point of righteous indignation, pointing up that the record was clear, that the woman had worked and was self-maintaining during eight months of pregnancy, that our aide had visited the home and had observed the living conditions and found they were as the woman had reported them, that it was not atypical for a woman in these circumstances not to know more about the husband than she did and the very fact that the Police Department couldn't locate the husband should be proof enough of her cooperativeness, her dependability and reliability.

That afternoon the investigator stopped by the Neighborhood Service Center to talk further with our aide. The aide indicated that we wanted to work cooperatively with Welfare, that we didn't want to serve as a pressure group and pointed up all of the things which the aide had done prior to raising this issue. The investigator agreed that the woman could receive Welfare assistance, arranged for an emergency allocation including back payment for carfares; the grant also included money for a layette and for future carfare which would enable her to take advantage of the prenatal service at Lincoln Hospital.

The aide then helped Miss Martinez find more adequate living quarters. On the day she moved, which happened to be a Saturday, the aide assisted her with the moving, helped her to wash down the walls, hang curtains, etc. (This is highly significant as the nonprofessional is now providing a model to the helpee, the client—a model which seems to say that helping people even outside the line of duty, not on a work day, is a good thing. The nonprofessional was functioning as one neighbor helping another and was implicitly suggesting a model whereby the helpee in the future might help another neighbor. He was persuading by example in line with our goal of *transforming clients into helpers and citizens.*)

Shortly after delivery of the baby, the woman stopped by the Center to see the mental health aide. She was relaxed and friendly and obviously enjoying the baby. She indicated to the aide that in a couple of months she would like to return to work. There was a neighbor who could care for the baby during the day at a modest stipend. She complained to the aide that her problem is that she has no marketable skills. She had taken some commercial course work when she was in high school, but these skills were very rusty. The aide was able to arrange a modified training program for her while she was at home with the baby. This was worked out in cooperation with the Department of Welfare. When she is ready to return to work, both the aide and the social investigator will attempt to find suitable employment for her.

Mrs. Garcia

When Mrs. Garcia swallowed a large number of aspirins and appeared as an emergency patient at Lincoln Hospital, the staff psychiatrist ascertained that she was not a psychotic woman. Apparently, she was reacting to a problem with her husband and her suicide attempt was the classic "cry for help," a way of getting attention and assistance from "the system." After talking with her at some length and after deciding that Mrs. Garcia was not likely to repeat her suicide attempt, the psychiatrist made an appointment for her to return to the hospital the following week. Since she was so distraught, he called the Neighborhood Service Center and asked to have one of the aides come over and pick up the lady, to work with her and obtain further information about her family problems.

This was arranged. An aide escorted Mrs. Garcia to the storefront, picking up her sister on the way, and all three sat down together. Mrs. Garcia's husband had been beating her for some time, she reported. When he went out and came home at 3 a.m. and she complained, he beat her. If she didn't complain, he accused her of not caring, and beat her.

Recently the situation had become worse; her husband had thrown her out of the house, put a new lock on the door, and told his wife that he wouldn't allow her to see the children anymore. In desperation she fled to her sister's apartment. But next day, a neighbor told her that her children had cried all night, and this sent her into the hysterical fit which culminated in her taking the pills.

The aide listened attentively. He then asked his supervisor, the center director, to join the conference. After talking for about half an hour—the aide, Mrs Garcia, her sister and the supervisor made a plan together. The aide would visit Mrs. Garcia's husband at home and have a long, informal talk with him.

As the plan was discussed, the supervisor grew a little anxious and said to the aide, "How do you feel about going there?" The aide, a short stout man, responded, "What do you mean?" The supervisor was a little embarassed, but said, "Well, Mr. Garcia sounds fairly tough." Whereupon, the aide said rather simply, "Well, I can protect myself, can't I?" and the supervisor responded, "Oh, yes, of course."

It was clear the next morning that the supervisor's alarm was misplaced. The two men had sat until late in the night, talking about the old days in Puerto Rico where both of them had been born, the problems they shared in New York, their views about women and the neighborhood. In the course of it all, the aide explained to Mr. Garcia that unless something was worked out amicably with his wife, the situation would grow more difficult. Now that the hospital had been involved in a suicide attempt, the police and the courts could easily step in and the aide was sure that Mr. Garcia didn't really want all that trouble. Mr. Garcia firmly agreed that the children could be given over at least temporarily to Mrs. Garcia, provided she returned to Puerto Rico.

"But she doesn't want to go back to Puerto Rico," the supervisor interjected upon hearing the story.

At this point the aide, with a very calm expression said, "One thing at a time."

A few days later, he was able to persuade Mr. Garcia to let his wife have their apartment and the children, at least for the time being, and he helped Mr. Garcia to find a room.

(The next step is to get women like Mrs. Garcia to come and help other people—to come to the monthly meetings, to join committees or just to help on a one-to-one basis when the aide calls her for something, because she is likely to become healthier and stronger if she's involved in the helping process.)

It should be kept in mind that as significant and meaningful as it may be, the provision of psychosocial first aid through the Neighborhood Service Centers is not seen as the sole aim; the aides are also a vehicle for intervention in community mental health issues. In facilitating services for residents from a whole variety of social agencies and institutions, the aides come in intimate contact with deliverers of service and, particularly, low echelon management. They have a twofold focus in working with these personnel: one, to insure that the resident receives adequate service and, two, to enlarge the perspective of the agents of the traditional institution and to increase their understanding of the unique needs, attitudes and values of the resident population. In this manner, although the policies of the institutions may not be directly or immediately changed, it is hoped that the manner in which the policies are implemented and the quality of the services rendered will be affected. While the aides are functioning in this direction, the professionals of the Neighborhood Service Center and the professionals of the Lincoln Hospital Mental Health Services are working with higher-echelon staff of these agencies and institutions, attempting to affect policies and practices at this level.

Because the Neighborhood Service Center has become the place in the community to which residents turn in time of crisis, the Center is able to keep abreast of the kinds of psychosocial problems with which the residents have to cope, the services needed and their availability. Likewise, the gaps, limitations and deficiences in the formal service structure and in the informal alternative arrangements currently employed by the community, are detected more readily. Thus, the Center is an important source of information on the nature of social changes needed, as well as a possible focus from which changes can arise.

Therefore, in addition to helping people meet their individual and family problems, the Neighborhood Service Center program is directed toward the development of community participation. (These activities are not reflected in the service statistics.) The objective is to engage the population receiving service at the Center in a graduated series of tasks of increasing complexity beginning with individual service and moving toward an involvement in large-scale community action.

Our target population is composed of those segments of the poor who are most in need of services; have been least active in their own behalf; and have limited experience with meetings, organized activities and formal leadership. One mechanism for this achievement is the community meeting where periodically all of the people who have visited the Center for service are invited. This community meeting is organized, planned and conducted by the mental health aides. At the meeting the aides assist the participants in identifying some of the major neighborhood problems and elicting their ideas about how they may work toward some amelioration or solution. Committees are formed to work on specific problems, and periodically they report back their activities to the large group. The aide who works with the committee must be careful that the task it sets for itself is comparatively simple and easily accomplished. As the group begins to succeed, the aide encourages it to take on tasks of increasing complexity and encourages collaboration with other community groups interested in the same neighborhood problems.

The many varied activities of the aides can be classified under the following headings:

Direct Services: specific assistance in finding employment and housing, giving advice and counsel, giving information, finding resources, expediting services and offering psychological support.

Community Action: organizing community meetings and socials, developing action committees (Hospital Committee, Tenants' Groups, Welfare Committee, Block Association, etc.).

Community Education: organizing and conducting campaigns (voter registration), disseminating information on job opportunities, planned parenthood, surplus foods, and publishing a newsletter.

Social Planning: convening meetings with agency representatives (welfare, police, schools, family agencies), participating in councils of social agencies (South Bronx Community Council, South East Bronx United).

Selection and Training of Mental Health Aides

There is no question that the effectiveness of the mental health aides depends on careful selection and subsequent training. It was fortunate that each time there were openings for a new group of aides, our recruiting efforts yielded many more applicants than the number of positions available. The ratio of applicants to positions available varied from 5 : 1 to 15 : 1.

It was immediately apparent that it would be of little use to rely on traditional methods of selecting employees; that is, to do an initial screening of application forms and to then conduct individual interviews with what appeared to be promising candidates. For one, the application forms were not designed to reveal those personal characteristics that might be related to adequate functioning as a mental health aide and secondly, individual interviews for such large numbers would be extremely time-consuming. We, therefore, devised a group selection process which was heavily influenced by the work of Margaret Rioch (6) and our colleagues, Melvin Roman and Seymour Kaplan.

Our first step was to convene a meeting of all applicants in which the nature of the position, salary, personnel practices and selection procedures were discussed. Opportunities for the applicant to comment and ask questions were provided. This initial procedure not only saved an enormous amount of time but it insured a uniform explanation of the job, work conditions, etc. On the basis of this initial presentation, a number of applicants decided not to proceed with their application. Similarly, we were able to spot some who by their manner and behavior seemed inappropriate choices and were thus screened out.

Following this initial meeting the remaining applicants were divided into small groups of no more than 10. Each small group was interviewed by the codirectors of the program or a codirector and a member of the training staff. The interviews were observed through a one-way mirror by four judges: a psychologist, a social worker, a psychiatrist and a nurse. In subsequent screening aides also were used as judges. Interestingly enough, there was a high correlation between their ratings and those of the professionals.

The group interview was directed toward ascertaining the candidates' attitudes toward the neighborhood—whether or not they rejected the people who lived in the area; attitudes toward people on welfare; feelings about discrimination, minority groups, disturbed people, etc. We used such open-ended questions as: "what kind of troubles do you think children have in this neighborhood"; "what do you think about welfare"; "what kind of troubles do you think parents have"; "what are the things you like or don't like about this neighborhood"; "what do you think about the police? the schools? etc." Invariably, differences of opinion led to a spontaneous interchange between group members. The leaders and the judges had an opportunity to observe how members of the group were able to present their viewpoints; with what tenacity they were held; to what extent members were open to other viewpoints; to what extent they played it safe; to what extent they were submissive, dominant, etc. Also typically, members of these groups were able to reveal personal experiences so that some judgment could be made as to degree of self-awareness, capacity for introspection, ability to cope with anxiety, frustration, hurt and disappointment.

Applicants were rated by the judges with regard to the following characteristics: empathy, attitude toward authority, comfort in the group, ability to communicate ideas and feelings, trainability and flexibility, capacity for self-awareness, reaction to stress, pathology, and relevant work and life experiences. The judges were particularly concerned that the people selected be "bridge" people; that is, they be able to communicate with ourselves, the professionals, and with people in the neighborhood. Though it was originally anticipated that after narrowing the applicant group to a reasonable number, we would use the individual employment interview as the final step of the selection process, both the judges and the leaders of the group interviews felt that it was not necessary and instead another group session was held of the more promising candidates for final selection. It seemed apparent that the group interview method provided a much clearer picture of ego functioning and ego capacity than could be obtained through the individual interview method.

The training program for the mental health aides is divided into three phases (7):

1. A prejob period of three weeks in which the training is based at Lincoln Hospital Mental Health Clinic. The emphasis in this phase is on operational tasks such as assisting the intake team at the Clinic, conducting door-to-door surveys in the community, escorting selected clients to clinic appointments and visits to various social agencies, for example, the Department of Welfare, the Police Department, schools, etc. Job simulation and role playing are central features of the training in this phase. Didactic presentations are kept to a minimum.

2. Following the three-week intensive training program, the aides are placed at the Neighborhood Service Center for a period of two weeks where one-half of their day is devoted to specific service to residents of the area and the other half is spent in further training based now on their on-the-job experiences.

3. On-going training takes place continuously at the Center. We estimate that approximately one-fifth of the work week is spent on further training. Some of this is accomplished through the individual supervisory conference with the director of the Neighborhood Service Center and through on-the-spot conferences that the aide requests as needed. Systematic training is provided through the regularly scheduled seminar with the training staff in which there is an attempt to refine interviewing skills, to teach new skills such as group interviewing and community organization and to deepen the aides' understanding of individual and family dynamics. Weekly staff meetings serve as another vehicle for deepening their knowledge and refining their skills.[5]

Evaluation

In addition to defining the role of the Neighborhood Service Center in a broad strategy of community mental health intervention, we are also particularly interested in assessing the contribution that the indigenous nonprofessional can make under professional supervision. Though our experience to date has been encouraging, it has not been without problems—problems that inhere in the nonprofessionals themselves, problems that inhere in the professionals, problems that inhere in our traditional modes of organizing and operating a service program.

The aides, coming as they do from a disadvantaged population, bring to the job many of the same strong feelings toward the power structure as is evident in the target population. On the one hand, there is fear, suspicion and distrust that they will be exploited, fired out of hand, discriminated against because of color, ethnic background or religion. On the other hand, supervisors and administrative personnel are invested with an omnipotence and omniscience and that somehow by association with us, they too, may become all powerful. The feeling that the professionals know everything and they know nothing is often balanced by counter feelings that it is only they who really care about the poor; that it is only they, the nonprofessionals, who really know what is going on; that they, the nonprofessionals, are down to earth while the professionals are on cloud nine. We also see operating simultaneously both the wish to learn from the professionals and an anti-intellectual attitude in which reading, education and knowledge are deprecated.

Not unrelated to the above, but also stemming from their life experiences, we find strong evidences of rivalry and competition between the aides, balanced at times by a cohesion and a cooperativeness in the face of the common enemy "the professional," or on those occasions when they have an

[5] We have experienced some of the usual conflict between the training and supervisory staffs. Initially, the supervisory staff felt that the preservice training and in-service training was not sufficiently attuned to on-the-job needs. The training staff, on the other hand, felt that the aides' skills were not being sufficiently developed. The development of regular channels for joint planning and communication has eased this. Continued clarification of respective roles and responsibilities should ease this further.

opportunity to demonstrate as a group their competency, such as in planning the opening of a Center, running of a Center Christmas party or community meeting, etc.

Insecure as individuals, they gain their feeling of security and strength as a group. Of interest is the fact that when one of their group is singled out by the professionals for special praise, feelings of rivalry are stirred and often it is perceived as the power structure's attempt to play favorites and in a sense, to divide and conquer.

Though the aides are delighted when they are initially "accepted into the system" and revel in their new status as mental health aides, they soon discover they are still low man on the totem pole. Struggle ensues to define their role more clearly and to attain a higher status than they are originally assigned.

As can readily be seen, all the above has a major impact on the learning process, their ability to engage in a supervisory process and in their response to administrative requirements and expectations.

In regard to problems inherent in the professional; the professional who engages in work with nonprofessionals is also subjected to conflicting emotions and attitudes. On the one hand, he enjoys the superior status and the omniscience and omnipotence invested in him by the nonprofessional. On the other hand, he feels anxious and resentful when he cannot live up to this expectation. Similarly, though he is eager to see the nonprofessional develop his skills and to take on more complex tasks, at the same time he is reluctant to give responsibility to the nonprofessional and to allow him much independence of action or judgment. The belief that a nonprofessional cannot do a quality job in relation to clients impels the professional to seek many ways of controlling and directing the nonprofessional's activity. The traditional difficulties that nonprofessionals have, for example, in recording and keeping records, increases the professional's anxiety that the nonprofessional will do damage. The professional's tendency to gather facts, to reflect, to plan a course of action and to be deliberative in his interventions, is threatened by the aide's more active and immediate response to client need. The professional's respect for traditional ways of operating, regard for channels of communication, lines of authority, etc., are threatened by the aide's more spontaneous and informal ways of functioning. Perhaps the sharpest conflict is seen in the professional's clinging to traditional ways of structuring programs and offering supervision to the aides, and the difficulty in adapting traditional methods to meet the needs and the style of the nonprofessional. For example, however well motivated we have been in offering a regular weekly conference to the aide for supervision, we failed to recognize initially that a supervisory conference meant one thing to the professional and another thing to the aide. Initially, the aide saw the supervisory conference as a schoolboy being called on the carpet in the principal's office to account for his poor school performance and his poor behavior.

Understandably, the professional who comes to work with the nonprofessional brings with him the frame of reference he has developed in his previous work experiences, which by and large, has been in professional settings. He therefore tends to view the nonprofessional's behavior, his attitudes and his work performance in line with his previously established frame of reference. In other words, he tends to measure or evaluate the aides in terms of traditional standards, in spite of an intellectual understanding that the old frame of reference no longer applies. To put it another way, the professional may be willing to start where the nonprofessional is at point A, but he indicates in his behavior and attitude that the nonprofessional had better move to point Z darn quick.

In regard to administrative practices and routines, we have discovered that much that the professional takes for granted as standard operating procedure is not quite so easy for the nonprofessional to accept. There is no doubt in our mind that part of the difficulty encountered in this area stems from the fact that the aides have not had the opportunity to fully develop work habits. Another problem is our tendency to continue blindly to impose organizational structures, routines and procedures that made sense in the traditional professional setting without examining their applicability to a new set of circumstances.

It is unfortunate that the above difficulties and complications sound overwhelming. There are many things on the positive side that far outweigh the difficulties enumerated; not the least of these is the aides' enthusiasm, dedication and conviction about the program and its goals. Another "plus" is the honesty and capacity for self-examination on the part of the professionals and their willingness to re-examine cherished beliefs and to experiment with new methods of operation and use of one's professional self.

The struggle between the nonprofessional and the professional has been kept, in our opinion, to a minimum for a number of reasons in addition to those noted above. From the beginning, we made a conscious effort to use the small group as a vehicle for cementing relationships between nonprofessionals and as a vehicle for airing of concerns on the part of the professional and the nonprofessional. We have provided many opportunities for the aides to participate as a group, and as a group to gain a sense of its own strength, power and competence. Similarly, we employed the small group to discuss differences among professional staff and to identify problems and issues and to consider alternative courses of actions. As each group of nonprofessionals (and professionals) developed its own sense of competence, there was less need on the part of individuals or on the part of groups to engage in power struggles.

Though our experience with nonprofessionals is limited, our findings are most encouraging. It seems fairly clear to us that nonprofessionals can provide and expedite service for large numbers of disadvantaged families. Extrapolating from the statistics presented, we can estimate that more than 6,000 families a year may be seen at each of the centers. Moreover, as indicated in the case illustrations, it is evident that nonprofessionals can intervene in critical situations, engage comparatively pathological people in meaningful relationships, stimulate them to take action in their own behalf, mobilize community resources, and serve as a bridge between the client-in-need and the professional service. We also are able to see that the nonprofessional is able to do quite a number of tasks that usually are carried out by the professional, but really do not require professional training and experience. In this manner, we are able to extend the outreach of the professional service to have an impact, at least to some degree, on considerably more people than would be possible by using professional personnel alone. The aides also have influenced the delivery of professional service, both within our organization and others. They have interpreted to the professionals the particular needs of the target population, their customs and their style of adaptation. This has increased the understanding of the professionals working with this population and has enabled many professionals to make appropriate adaptations in their helping techniques.

We also have seen our aides serve as effective role models for people in the community. Many of them have become active in their own buildings and neighborhoods; they assist neighbors and friends with personal problems and become active in organizations dedicated to improving neighborhood conditions. Both in their private life and in their job life, they have been able to provide some community leadership. They have organized delegations to appear at public hearings, have been spokesmen for these groups, and have helped others take leadership.

Pleased as we are with the growth and development of the aids and the quality of their work, we are not unmindful of some of their limitations. There is much yet for them to learn, and we hope to refine their skill in simple intervention techniques. We have every confidence that they will master these and move on to more complicated tasks which require deeper understanding of individual and group dynamics and a higher order of intervention techniques. We are committed to test to the limit the contribution that a nonprofessional can make in a community mental health program.

References

1. Caplan, Gerald (1964). *Principles of Preventive Psychiatry*. Basic Books, p. 102.
2. Cloward, Richard (1963). Social class and private social agencies. *Proceedings of the Annual Meeting of the Council on Social Work Education.*
3. Furman, Sylvan, et al. (1963). Social class factors in the flow of children to outpatient psychiatric facilities. Presented to American Public Health Association.
4. Peck, Harris B., Seymour Kaplan, & Melvin Roman (1966). Prevention, treatment and social action: A strategy of intervention in a disadvantaged urban area. *American Journal of Orthopsychiatry*, **36**, 57–68.
5. Riessman, Frank (1965). New approaches to treatment for low income people. *Social Work Practice*. National Conference on Social Welfare. 174–187.
6. Rioch, Margaret, et al. (1963). National Institute of Mental Health, pilot study in training mental health counselors. *American Journal of Orthopsychiatry*, **33**, 678–689.
7. Roman, Melvin & Sally Jacobson (1965). Progress Report: Training of mental health aides. Lincoln Hospital Mental Health Services. (mimeo)
8. Schneiderman, Leonard (1965). Social class, diagnosis & treatment. *American Journal of Orthopsychiatry*, **35**, 99–105.

A. PEARL and F. RIESSMAN

Poverty and New Careers for Nonprofessionals

Programs to prevent mental disorder in deprived, inner-city, adult populations are often difficult to implement. This is because the culturally impoverished, poorly educated, inner-city dweller has such limited prospects for leading a life satisfying even some of his most basic needs that the mental health worker has little to offer him that seems superior to the rewards of petty crime, drunkenness, and irresponsible living. The solution that Pearl and Riessman offer to this problem in the selection that follows involves providing jobs in the human services field for the undereducated and underprivileged. Many of the ideas set forth in this selection have formed the basis of "new career" programs that have been established throughout the country.

This chapter has been abridged to omit a section describing future prospects for the new careers movement and another that is critical of large scale emergency programs that hope, through large expenditures of funds, to solve complex social problems. The reader who is interested in this material should consult the original source.

This book deals with a current and unforgiveable shame of the United States of America, the name of which is poverty. For too many years widespread and pervasive poverty has existed in this country and the public has been either unaware or unconcerned about the problem. Today there is awareness and concern, frenzied activity and legislation, demonstration programs, and volunteers in the field—all functioning with but one stated ambition—to help the poor. The concern is laudable although the activity might not be.

There should be no confusion on one point. *Poverty will not be easy to eradicate.* Poverty is not a superficial blemish on an otherwise healthy structure. It is not a passing phase of a society in flux. The causes of poverty are deep-seated. Short term stop-gap measures will not bring about a permanent solution to the problem. The need to reorganize and revitalize many

---

of the structures and institutions central to society is the alternative to relegating large numbers of citizens to a spectator class—a permanent, stable "nonworking" class, whose children and grandchildren will also be unable to perform meaningful functions in our society. The prospect of many millions of Americans in such a nonproductive situation is not a science-fiction terror. The danger is real and upon us.

This presentation will include a description of the problem, an analysis of its causes and effects, an evaluation of suggested remedies, and a proposal for redress of the condition.

The complex of goals of the new career proposal includes the following:

1. A sufficient number of jobs for all persons without work.
2. The jobs to be so defined and distributed that placements exist for the unskilled and uneducated.
3. The jobs to be permanent and provide opportunity for life-long careers.
4. An opportunity for the motivated and talented poor to advance from low-skill entry jobs to any station available to the more favored members of society.
5. The work to contribute to the well-being of society.

To devise a program which will provide, in sufficient numbers, socially useful, compensated positions and which will also furnish equal chances for upward mobility, is no small task. If the poor and the currently unemployable are going to be brought into productive society there must be some determination of the capabilities of this group. What can the poor do? How can useful functions be developed that will meet the limitations of the population? What must be done to educate the uneducated in the labor force? What must be done to prevent future uneducated generations from developing? What responsibilities for providing the necessary jobs should be delegated to private industry? And, what is the public sector's responsibility? These are the basic questions confronting us.

It must be abundantly clear that in the solution of poverty every aspect of American life will undergo change. Organizational structures and institutions which have come to be accepted as basic and immutable must be transformed. Education in particular must be reappraised and adjustments must be made at every level. However, as will be stressed here, the modifications which take place must be keyed to the needs of the society. No good can come from a panic which demands change only for change's sake.

The methods of securing and changing employment in this country must also be overhauled. There is too much slippage between the referral office and the job. Too much of the job-securing mechanism concern is in satisfying the short-term needs of the employer. There is no articulated process for the job-seeker to obtain security. Too much of the risk in job preparation is absorbed by those least able to absorb risk—the poor. Civil service merit systems based primarily on an ability to perform written examinations may need to be updated to allow all persons, regardless of background, a more equal chance to obtain career placements.

The roles played by highly-skilled technicians and professionals need to be reviewed. Many functions currently performed exclusively by professionals must be delegated to persons with limited education, experience, and skill. Society insists that training take place prior to job placement. Such a system made sense (although it reinforced inequality) when only a small percentage of the population was engaged in highly skilled occupations, while most of the work force required little formal training. This condition no longer exists. Most of the needs of society can be satisfied only by the highly-skilled and the well-trained. In an era of rapid technological development even the skills of the professional rapidly become obsolete. Training cannot be considered a prerequisite for employment. While this is often understood for some functions it is not yet appreciated as a general proposition. There can be no end to poverty unless it is fully appreciated that, for the most part, training for the poor must take place *after* employment is secured. This may not be necessary in the future, when all of the population, rich and poor alike, are well-educated. But today, and certainly for the next decade, at least, many millions of persons will be seeking employment who have not had adequate education. This group, not only because of its plight, but also because it contains the parents of future generations, is the norm-setter. The poor job-seeker of the 1960's will develop and model the value systems, loyalties, and aspirations of those who are to benefit from new approaches to education. They must be permitted to play a useful, meaningful role in today's world. There can be no sacrifice of a population of today under the mantle of concern for tomorrow. Inability to deal with the poor of today will be transmitted to the poor of tomorrow.

Ours has been, and still is, a vigorous society. Growth has been rapid, and in the exciting, untrammeled course of that growth, much of the institutional structure has grown up unplanned. This lack of planning is often given accolades equal to those awarded the accomplishments. But the course of growth has necessitated interdependence and reliance upon government-sponsored activity. There is no denying the importance of the public sector, nor is there a path back from it. Education, welfare, recreation, and corrections are public responsibilities. A consequence of unimpeded and unplanned growth is lack of continuity and linkage between institutions, organizations, and agencies. This deficiency in connection is most strongly felt by the poor since they lack resources of their own. There is often no passageway for the poor from education to employment, from institutional commitment to living in free society, from economic calamity back to a sound economic footing. With limited resources, skill, and flexibility, the poor have little chance to recover from serious injury or prolonged illness. If there is to be a path from poverty, not only must there be change within structures, but there also must be integration between structures.

Changes of the nature outlined above can only come about when there is public consensus for their necessity. Therefore, many entrenched belief systems must be reconsidered and many myths exposed, with more adequate concepts offered in exchange.

One such fabrication places full responsibility on the poor. The details may vary, but there is a common theme; the poor are poor because of innate inferiority, a lack of desire—or the romantic variation—because they want to live the good, simple life. All of these are status-quo positions, implying that there is no cause for alarm and that the situation truly requires no change.

A variation of the theme is that the poor become poorer because they react violently, impulsively, and senselessly against middle-class values; or, conversely, the poor remain poor because the middle class can only maintain relative superiority by denying the poor equal access to opportunities.

This book will espouse an emphatic rejection of the desirability or inevitability of wholesale poverty. It is our thesis that no segment of our society stands to gain over the long run from the existence of a nonproductive class.

The poverty issue presents the United States with a totally new crisis, one that defies previously used solutions. It is a chronic crisis which does not lend itself to any partisan political position and would only worsen if atavistic procedures were employed as remedial measures. The crisis, on one hand involves the permanent poor, and on the other, involves an inability to provide, in sufficient numbers, persons to fill the most needed technological and professional roles. In over-simplified terms, there exists simultaneously large numbers of people without jobs and a great many jobs without people.

It is difficult to estimate accurately the number of jobs currently unfilled. There is a tendency for all operations to "make-do" with what is available. Administrations are often given credit for a "sound fiscal" operation when savings accrue from unfilled budgeted positions. However, there can be no doubt that were there thousands more fully accredited teachers, social workers, librarians, engineers, nurses, and doctors, the economy would absorb them.

The jobs which are needed are primarily in the public sector or are sustained by public financing. One reason that it is difficult to estimate job vacancies precisely is that definition of need is arbitrary. The public, through elected representatives, makes this determination. There are no established efficiency standards or guidelines to be applied to operations which are designed to provide helping services. Nor can there be any.

The value of an educated child, for example, cannot be reduced to a simple accounting of income obtained from tax investments. Adequate health, education, welfare, and recreation are available only to citizens of an affluent society. All societies need as much of these services as can be afforded.

The central thesis of this book is that in an affluent automated society the number of persons needed to perform such tasks equals the number of persons for whom there are no other jobs.[1]

[1] Impoverished nations with relatively few persons in helping services are not without need for these services. They are simply unable to afford them.

The persons without jobs are not difficult to identify. They are the unskilled, the uneducated. In disproportionate numbers they are young; they are Negro. They are likely to remain poor and so are their children. There is almost nothing that they can do about it. Lack of control over destiny is a unique feature of today's poverty. The poor of the past, because of differences in structure and organization of society, had a much better chance to change status than do the poor of today. (The Negro poor of the past—the slave—was an exception. He was denied opportunity to improve himself and the consequences of enforced poverty have an important bearing on the existing scene. In subsequent chapters, the particular problems of the Negro poor are discussed in detail).

The distinguishing feature of the modern economic scene is that unskilled labor is ceasing to be a necessary component of functioning society. Traditionally, the poor have possessed one marketable commodity—unskilled labor. By means of their labor the poor could gain a toehold on the economic ladder, and many of the children of these poor could advance to higher stations through education or entrepreneurial enterprise. Technological advancement was on the side of the poor (in the long run, at least). Technological advance stimulated the economy and provided work opportunity. The history of the United States can almost be charted by immigration of impoverished people linked to specific technological changes.

Railroading was but one technological development of the 19th century, which, on a mass scale provided entrance to viable society for the poor immigrant. Many members of the establishment proudly refer to antecedents who, as poor immigrants, worked the mines, laid the track, or manned the foundaries and mills. It was this profound influence of technological advance on the economy that encouraged immigration. If there had been nothing for the unskilled immigrant to do, the "dream" of America, the open society would not have been sustained. The promise of America continued because it was based on a hard core of truth.

The automotive industry further stimulated the economy and provided continued opportunity for the unskilled laborer. Technological advances in the 20's and 30's led to the assembly line which was specifically designed for the unskilled laborer. Complexity and variability of job performance was reduced to an absolute minimum. The essential feature of the assemly line was the reduction of job complexity to allow for interchangeability of workers regardless of skill. In a variety of settings increased affluence was accomplished at the expense of the skilled craftsman. Technological advance in shoemaking resulted in modern assembly line production, new jobs for the unskilled, and the elimination of the highly-skilled craftsman. Job evolution, however, has come full circle. The unskilled workers' functions, to a large extent created by the machine, are now being replaced by the machine.

Automation must be recognized for what it is, a permanent fixture in American life which will enable private industry to produce efficiently, increase the gross national product, *and*—eliminate jobs. John I. Snyder,

President and Chairman of U.S. Industries, Inc., estimates that two million jobs are eradicated each year by automation.[2]

A magnificent year for the general economy was 1963. There was a healthy increase in gross national product; a new high was set for median income. In this same year, however, rising unemployment widened an even greater economic gap between the poor and nonpoor, and the Negro and non-Negro. Between 1957 and 1962, 500,000 fewer workers produced significantly more goods and one million jobs were eliminated in agriculture, although farm surpluses continued to accumulate.[3]

The future augers for more of the same; the unskilled worker is to be replaced by automated devices and the labor force augmented by the trained technicians. It is projected that approximately the same number of persons will be employed as laborers in 1975 as was employed in 1960—a period in which it is expected that 20 million more workers will enter the labor market. There will be in excess of a million and a half fewer workers in agricultural pursuits in 1975 than there were in 1960. These workers and their families will steadily flow to urban centers where they will lack resources, skills, and education—possessing only the qualities necessary to become part of the permanent poor.

To expect the private sector to absorb these additional workers while being confronted with decreasing need of currently employed, meagerly skilled workers is unrealistic. Industry can engage in extensive job analyses and by redefinition create a considerable number of jobs which do not require extensive training or experience and industry should be encouraged along these lines by government subsidy. However, the greatest potential for new careers is in the public sector.

To offset the relative loss of employment in the private sector, there has been rapid growth in the public domain:

> Total government civilian employment rose from 5.5 million in 1947 to 9.2 million in 1962. . . . The addition of 3.7 million public employees accounted for one-third of the total increase in non-agricultural employment in the post war years.[4]

The bulk of the growth has been in education and health. In these areas the number of persons presently employed exceed by over 60 per cent the number employed 10 years ago.[5]

The New Career Concept

The new career concept has as a point of departure the creation of jobs normally allotted to highly-trained professionals or technicians, but which could be performed by the unskilled, inexperienced, and relatively untrained

[2] Snyder, John I., The Myths of Automation, *American Child*, 1964, Vol. 46, No. 1.

[3] United States Labor Department, *Manpower Report of the President and a Report on Manpower, Requirements, Resources, Utilization and Training*, U.S. Government Printing Office, Wash., 25, D.C., 1963.

[4] *Ibid.*, p. 16.

[5] *Ibid.*, p. 16.

workers; or, the development of activities not currently performed by anyone, but for which there is a readily acknowledged need and which can also be satisfactorily accomplished by the unskilled worker.

Detailed descriptions of both reconstituted job endeavors and creation of new activities are to be found in later chapters. In both instances there is a common need for careful scrutiny of the job function for the purpose of defining duties which are structured at the level of the jobless.

Providing jobs which the poor can perform is only a first step along the path to a new career. The job must be made permanent and must be incorporated into the matrix of the industry or agency. If the position, for example, is in government, there must be legitimation of the activity by civil service certification and incorporation of the function into the agency table of organization. In the private sector, created positions must, by similar procedures, become securely fused into the organic operation.

Persons filling entry positions must have latitude for limited advancement without being required to undergo extensive additional training. This type of opportunity is generally available to governmental and private agency personnel assigned to clerical or non-professional services. Advancement within the "same line" provides an inducement to "life career" for the least capable and gifted. For the many who aspire to more, and are capable of it, such a narrow range of possible achievement would hardly suffice.

The chance for truly substantial advancement in job station is crucial to the new career concept. If significant rise to higher stations is to be a genuine possibility for the entering unskilled worker, then jobs which will require knowledge, experience and skill, and present more challenge than the entry positions, must be created. These jobs would have to be intermediate between the unskilled beginning duty and the terminal professional status. To be eligible for an intermediate position a worker would be required to perform notably at the less advanced position and participate in a training program offered partially on the job and partially in a sequence of college courses (or receive training which could be allowed college credit).

Establishing a continuum ranging from nonskilled entry positions, extending through intermediate sub-professional functions, and terminating in full professional status, changes the nature of the upward mobility in our society. No longer would professional status be attained *only* by first completing between five and eight years of college. The requiring of this training *prior* to entrance into a field of endeavor effectively eliminates almost all of the poor from eligibility. A sequence beginning with the unskilled aide and proceeding through an assistant (two years of college equivalence plus experience); an associate (four years of college equivalence plus experience); and terminating in an accreditation as professional is manageable and opens areas to which the poor can now hardly hope to aspire.

If such a program were accepted in the field of medicine, it would be possible for a person to enter the field as a hospital aide (menial worker, only); graduate to a medical assistant (engage in slightly more responsible work); move upward to a medical associate (engage in a more demanding relationship with patients under direct supervision of doctor); continue up a sequence of increasing challenge and responsibility until ultimately the status of medical doctor was reached.

The unique quality of the new career proposal might be best emphasized by consideration of the present inability of a registered nurse to obtain credit for training and skill toward becoming a medical doctor. It is proposed that ultimately such a course would be available. The nurse-to-doctor sequence, while probably more fraught with difficulty than most, would indicate the nature of resistance to be encountered and overcome before the new career concept can be come a reality.

Probably only a small percentage of the persons who would enter a new career sequence as nonskilled aides would emerge as full-fledged professionals. Each advance based on merit would constitute a screening process which only the most sensitive, motivated, and capable would ford, but while all might not achieve the highest rung, the *opportunity* for attainment of a higher station would be available to all.

It is not recommended that there be only this arduous and circuitous route to professional status. The traditional path to the M.D., the Ph.D., the education or social work degree would be always an available alternative. However, there would be advantages to the aspiring professional in the development of a sequence of "landings" designed for subprofessionals. At the present time, if a student fails to attain full professional status there is no defined role for him. A person might invest almost a decade in education, only to be informed that he is not to be allowed to become a professional. There is no designated function for the "almost" doctor, lawyer, teacher, social worker, or psychologist. If a sequence of positions had been established, the person unable to attain full status might be eligible for an intermediate position.

Defining the Entry Jobs

For *full* implementation of the new career concept there must be large-scale study of the activities performed by professionals in the fields mentioned above (and others) to delineate specific duties and functions which the unskilled can perform. Such studies must define precisely the relative challenge, complexity, and time expended on each function. The number of jobs required at each level and the number of levels necessary for a complete sequence can be *initially* estimated from the results obtained from such a study. Continued study would be needed for revision of job needs and duties arising from changing situations and technological development.

Inauguration of the new career concept should not, however, await the conclusions of an extensive job study. There is need for immediate test of the concept by demonstration and experimentation in a diversity of settings, with a broad range of persons, and in the performance of a variety of tasks.

There is sufficient experience for initial experimentation. An educated reckoning of job activities which the unskilled can perform can be continually refined after experimentation. Research, while needed, cannot be an excuse for inactivity. It is only through activity that data can be obtained for use in evaluation and further development.

On the other hand, the exigencies of the moment cannot justify unthinking exuberance. *Any* activity is not necessarily good activity. The plight of the poor is tragic and action is needed, but the action which is needed is long-term commitment to an ultimate solution, not a transient concern with superficialities.

ALVIN TOFFLER

Coping with Tomorrow

The selection that follows is a chapter from a best selling book, *Future Shock*, by Alvin Toffler. The book documents the dizzyingly rapid series of changes that have taken place technologically and socially in recent years. The chapter of the book that is reprinted here is devoted to suggesting ways of coping with such change. It, therefore, represents an excellent example of steps that may be taken to prevent emotional and psychological disorganization to which all who live in such a changing milieu are vulnerable.

In the blue vastness of the South Pacific just north of New Guinea lies the island of Manus, where, as every first-year anthropology student knows, a stone age population emerged into the twentieth century within a single generation. Margaret Mead, in *New Lives for Old*, tells the story of this seeming miracle of cultural adaptation and argues that it is far more difficult for a primitive people to accept a few fragmentary crumbs of Western technological culture than it is for them to adopt a whole new way of life at once.

"Each human culture, like each language, is a whole," she writes, and if "individuals or groups of people have to change . . . it is most important that they should change from one whole pattern to another."

There is sense in this, for it is clear that tensions arise from incongruities between cultural elements. To introduce cities without sewage, anti-malarial

---

medicines without birth control, is to tear a culture apart, and to subject its members to excruciating, often insoluble problems.

Yet this is only part of the story, for there are definite limits to the amount of newness than any individual or group can absorb in a short span of time, regardless of how well integrated the whole may be. Nobody, Manus or Muscovite, can be pushed above his adaptive range without suffering disturbance and disorientation. Moreover, it is dangerous to generalize from the experience of this small South Sea population.

The success story of the Manus, told and retold like a modern folk tale, is often cited as evidence that we, in the high-technology countries, will also be able to leap to a new stage of development without undue hardship. Yet our situation, as we speed into the super-industrial era, is radically different from that of the islanders.

We are not in a position, as they were, to import wholesale an integrated, well-formed culture, matured and tested in another part of the world. We must invent super-industrialism, not import it. During the next thirty or forty years we must anticipate not a single wave of change, but a series of terrible heaves and shudders. The parts of the new society, rather than being carefully fitted, one to the other, will be strikingly incongruous filled with missing linkages and glaring contradictions. There is no "whole pattern" for us to adopt.

More important, the transience level has risen so high, the pace is now so forced, that a historically unprecedented situation has been thrust upon us. We are not asked, as the Manus were, to adapt to a new culture, but to a blinding succession of new temporary cultures. This is why we may be approaching the upper limits of the adaptive range. No previous generation has ever faced this test.

It is only now, therefore, in our lifetime, and only in the techno-societies as yet, that the potential for mass future shock has crystallized.

To say this, however, is to court grave misunderstanding. First, any author who calls attention to a social problem runs the risk of deepening the already profound pessimism that envelops the techno-societies. Self-indulgent despair is a highly salable literary commodity today. Yet despair is not merely a refuge for irresponsibility; it is unjustified. Most of the problems besieging us, including future shock, stem not from implacable natural forces but from man-made processes that are at least potentially subject to our control.

Second, there is danger that those who treasure the status quo may seize upon the concept of future shock as an excuse to argue for a moratorium on change. Not only would any such attempt to suppress change fail, triggering even bigger, bloodier and more unmanageable changes than any we have seen, it would be moral lunacy as well. By any set of human standards, certain radical social changes are already desperately overdue. The answer to future shock is not non-change, but a different kind of change.

The only way to maintain any semblance of equilibrium during the super-industrial revolution will be to meet invention with invention—to design new personal and social change-regulators. Thus we need neither blind acceptance nor blind resistance, but an array of creative strategies for shaping, deflecting, accelerating or decelerating change selectively. The individual needs new principles for pacing and planning his life along with a dramatically new kind of education. He may also need specific new technological aids to increase his adaptivity. The society, meanwhile, needs new institutions and organizational forms, new buffers and balance wheels.

All this implies still further change, to be sure—but of a type designed from the beginning to harness the accelerative thrust, to steer it and pace it. This will not be easy to do. Moving swiftly into uncharted social territory, we have no time-tried techniques, no blueprints. We must, therefore, experiment with a wide range of change-regulating measures, inventing and discarding them as we go along. It is in this tentative spirit that the following tactics and strategies are suggested—not as sure-fire panaceas, but as examples of new approaches that need to be tested and evaluated. Some are personal, others technological and social. For the struggle to channel change must take place at all these levels simultaneously.

Given a clearer grasp of the problems and more intelligent control of certain key processes, we can turn crisis into opportunity, helping people not merely to survive, but to crest the waves of change, to grow, and to gain a new sense of mastery over their own destinies.

Direct Coping

We can begin our battle to prevent future shock at the most personal level. It is clear, whether we know it or not, that much of our daily behavior is, in fact, an attempt to ward off future shock. We employ a variety of tactics to lower the levels of stimulation when they threaten to drive us above our adaptive range. For the most part, however, these techniques are employed unconsciously. We can increase their effectiveness by raising them to consciousness.

We can, for example, introvert periodically to examine our own bodily and psychological reactions to change, briefly tuning out the cxternal environment to evaluate our inner environment. This is not a matter of wallowing in subjectivity, but of coolly appraising our own performance. In the words of Hans Selye, whose work on stress opened new frontiers in biology and psychiatry, the individual can "consciously look for signs of being keyed up too much."

Heart palpitations, tremors, insomnia or unexplained fatigue may well signal overstimulation, just as confusion, unusual irritability, profound lassitude and a panicky sense that things are slipping out of control are psychological indications. By observing ourselves, looking back over the changes in our recent past, we can determine whether we are operating comfortably within our adaptive range or pressing its outer limits. We can, in short, consciously assess our own life pace.

Having done this, we can also begin consciously to influence it—speeding it up or slowing it down—first with respect to small things, the micro-environment, and then in terms of the larger, structural patterns of experience. We can learn how by scrutinizing our own unpremeditated responses to over-stimulation.

We employ a de-stimulating tactic, for example, when we storm into the teen-ager's bedroom and turn off a stereo unit that has been battering our eardrums with unwanted and interruptive sounds. We virtually sigh with relief when the noise level drops. We act to reduce sensory bombardment in other ways, too—when we pull down the blinds to darken a room, or search for silence on a deserted strip of beach. We may flip on an air conditioner not so much to lower the temperature as to mask novel and unpredictable street sounds with a steady, predictable drone.

We close doors, wear sunglasses, avoid smelly places and shy away from touching strange surfaces when we want to decrease novel sensory input. Similarly, when we choose a familiar route home from the office, instead of turning a fresh corner, we opt for sensory non-novelty. In short, we employ "sensory shielding"—a thousand subtle behavioral tricks to "turn off" sensory stimuli when they approach our upper adaptive limit.

We use similar tactics to control the level of cognitive stimulation. Even the best of students periodically gazes out the window, blocking out the teacher, shutting off the flow of new data from that source. Even voracious readers sometimes go through periods when they cannot bear to pick up a book or magazine.

Why, during a gregarious evening at a friend's house, does one person in the group refuse to learn a new card game while others urge her on? Many factors play a part: the self-esteem of the individual, the fear of seeming foolish, and so on. But one overlooked factor affecting willingness to learn may well be the general level of cognitive stimulation in the individual's life at the time. "Don't bother me with new facts!" is a phrase usually uttered in jest. But the joke often disguises a real wish to avoid being pressed too hard by new data.

This accounts in part for our specific choices of entertainment—of leisure-time reading, movies or television programs. Sometimes we seek a high novelty ratio, a rich flow of information. At other moments we actively resist cognitive stimulation and reach for "light" entertainment. The typical detective yarn, for example, provides a trace of unpredictability—whodunnit?—within a carefully structured ritual framework, a set of non-novel, hence easily predictable relationships. In this way, we employ entertainment as a device to raise or lower stimulation, adjusting our intake rates so as not to overload our capacities.

By making more conscious use of such tactics, we can "fine-tune" our micro-environment. We can also cut down on unwanted stimulation by acting to lighten our cognitive burdens. "Trying to remember too many things is certainly one of the major sources of psychologic stress," writes Selye. "I make a conscious effort to forget immediately all that is unimportant and to jot down data of possible value . . . This technique can help anyone to accomplish the greatest simplicity compatible with the degree of complexity of his intellectual life."

We also act to regulate the flow of decisioning. We postpone decisions or delegate them to others when we are suffering from decision overload. Sometimes we "freeze up" decisionally. I have seen a woman sociologist, just returned from a crowded, highly stimulating professional conference, sit down in a restaurant and absolutely refuse to make any decisions whatever about her meal. "What would you like?" her husband asked. "You decide for me," she replied. When pressed to choose between specific alternatives, she still explicitly refused, insisting angrily that she lacked the "energy" to make the decision.

Through such methods we attempt, as best we can, to regulate the flow of sensory, cognitive and decisional stimulation, perhaps also attempting in some complicated and as yet unknown way to balance them with one another. But we have stronger ways of coping with the threat of overstimulation. These involve attempts to control the rates of transience, novelty and diversity in our milieu.

Personal Stability Zones

The rate of turnover in our lives, for example, can be influenced by conscious decisions. We can, for example, cut down on change and stimulation by consciously maintaining longer-term relationships with the various elements of our physical environment. Thus, we can refuse to purchase throw-away products. We can hang onto the old jacket for another season; we can stoutly refuse to follow the latest fashion trend; we can resist when the salesman tells us it's time to trade in our automobile. In this way, we reduce the need to make and break ties with the physical objects around us.

We can use the same tactic with respect to people and the other dimensions of experience. There are times when even the most gregarious person feels anti-social and refuses invitations to parties or other events that call for social interaction. We consciously disconnect. In the same way, we can minimize travel. We can resist pointless reorganizations in our company, church, fraternal or community groups. In making important decisions, we can consciously weigh the hidden costs of change against the benefits.

None of this is to suggest that change can or should be stopped. Nothing is less sensible than the advice of the Duke of Cambridge who is said to have harumphed: "Any change, at any time, for any reason is to be deplored." The theory of the adaptive range suggests that, despite its physical costs, some level of change is as vital to health as too much change is damaging.

Some people, for reasons still not clear, are pitched at a much higher level of stimulus hunger than others. They seem to crave change even when others are reeling from it. A new house, a new car, another trip, another crisis on the job, more house guests, visits, financial adventures and misadventures—they seem to accept all these and more without apparent ill effect.

Yet close analysis of such people often reveals the existence of what might be called "stability zones" in their lives—certain enduring relationships that are carefully maintained despite all kinds of other changes.

One man I know has run through a series of love affairs, a divorce and remarriage—all within a very short span of time. He thrives on change, enjoys travel, new foods, new ideas, new movies, plays and books. He has a high intellect and a low "boring point," is impatient with tradition and restlessly eager for novelty. Ostensibly, he is a walking exemplar of change.

When we look more closely, however, we find that he has stayed on the same job for ten years. He drives a battered, seven-year-old automobile. His clothes are several years out of style. His closest friends are long-time professional associates and even a few old college buddies.

Another case involves a man who has changed jobs at a mind-staggering rate, has moved his family thirteen times in eighteen years, travels extensively, rents cars, uses throw-away products, prides himself on leading the neighborhood in trying out new gadgets, and generally lives in a restless whirl of transience, newness and diversity. Once more, however, a second look reveals significant stability zones in his life: a good, tightly woven relationship with his wife of nineteen years; continuing ties with his parents; old college friends interspersed with the new acquaintances.

A different form of stability zone is the habit pattern that goes with the person wherever he travels, no matter what other changes alter his life. A professor who has moved seven times in ten years, who travels constantly in the United States, South America, Europe and Africa, who has changed jobs repeatedly, pursues the same daily regimen wherever he is. He reads between eight and nine in the morning, takes forty-five minutes for exercise at lunch time, and then catches a half-hour cap-nap before plunging into work that keeps him busy until 10:00 P.M.

The problem is not, therefore, to suppress change, which cannot be done, but to manage it. If we opt for rapid change in certain sectors of life, we can consciously attempt to build stability zones elsewhere. A divorce, perhaps, should not be too closely followed by a job transfer. Since the birth of a child alters all the human ties within a family, it ought not, perhaps, be followed too closely by a relocation which causes tremendous turnover in human ties outside the family. The recent widow should not, perhaps, rush to sell her house.

To design workable stability zones, however, to alter the larger patterns of life, we need far more potent tools. We need, first of all, a radically new orientation toward the future.

Ultimately, to manage change we must anticipate it. However, the notion that one's personal future can be, to some extent, anticipated, flies in the face of persistent folk prejudice. Most people, deep down, believe that the future is a blank. Yet the truth is that we *can* assign probabilities to some of the changes that lie in store for us, especially certain large structural changes, and there are ways to use this knowledge in designing personal stability zones.

We can, for example, predict with certainty that unless death intervenes, we shall grow older; that our children, our relatives and friends will also grow older; and that after a certain point our health will begin to deteriorate. Obvious as this may seem, we can, as a result of this simple statement, infer a great deal about our lives one, five or ten years hence, and about the amount of change we will have to absorb in the interim.

Few individuals or families plan ahead systematically. When they do, it is usually in terms of a budget. Yet we can forecast and influence our expenditure of time and emotion as well as money. Thus it is possible to gain revealing glimpses of one's own future, and to estimate the gross level of change lying ahead, by periodically preparing what might be called a Time and Emotion Forecast. This is an attempt to assess the percentage of time and emotional energy invested in various important aspects of life—and to see how this might change over the years.

One can, for example, list in a column those sectors of life that seem most important to us: Health, Occupation, Leisure, Marital Relations, Parental Relations, Filial Relations, etc. It is then possible to jot down next to each item a "guesstimate" of the amount of time we presently allocate to that sector. By way of illustration: given a nine-to-five job, a half-hour commute, and the usual vacations and holidays, a man employing this method would find that he devotes approximately 25 percent of his time to work. Although it is, of course, much more difficult, he can also make a subjective assessment of the percentage of his emotional energy invested in the job. If he is bored and secure, he may invest very little—there being no necessary correlation between time devoted and emotion invested.

If he performs this exercise for each of the important sectors of his life, forcing himself to write in a percentage even when it is no more than an extremely crude estimate, and toting up the figures to make sure they never exceed 100 percent, he will be rewarded with some surprising insights. For the way he distributes his time and emotional energies is a direct clue to his value system and his personality.

The payoff for engaging in this process really begins, however, when he projects forward, asking himself honestly and in detail how his job, or his marriage, or his relationship with his children or his parents is likely to develop within the years ahead.

If, for example, he is a forty-year-old middle manager with two teen-age sons, two surviving parents or in-laws, and an incipient duodenal ulcer, he can assume that within half a decade his boys will be off to college or living away on their own. Time devoted to parental concerns will probably decline. Similarly, he can anticipate some decline in the emotional energies demanded by his parental role. On the other hand, as his own parents and in-laws grow older, his filial responsibility will probably loom larger. If they are sick, he may have to devote large amounts of time and emotion to their care. If they are statistically likely to die within the period under study, he needs to face this fact. It tells him that he can expect a major change in his commitments. His own health, in the meantime, will not be getting any better. In the same way, he can hazard some guesses about his job—his chances for promotion, the possibility of reorganization, relocation, retraining, etc.

All this is difficult, and it does not yield "knowledge of the future." Rather, it helps him make explicit some of his assumptions about the future. As he moves forward, filling in the forecast for the present year, the next year, the fifth or tenth year, patterns of change will begin to emerge. He will see that in certain years there are bigger shifts and redistributions to be expected than in others. Some years are choppier, more change-filled than others. And he can then, on the strength of these systematic assumptions, decide how to handle major decisions in the present.

Should the family move next year—or will there be enough turmoil and change without that? Should he quit his job? Buy a new car? Take a costly vacation? Put his elderly father-in-law in a nursing home? Have an affair? Can he afford to rock his marriage or change his profession? Should he attempt to maintain certain levels of commitment unchanged?

These techniques are extremely crude tools for personal planning. Perhaps the psychologists and social psychologists can design sharper instruments, more sensitive to differences in probability, more refined and insight-yielding. Yet, if we search for clues rather than certainties, even these primitive devices can help us moderate or channel the flow of change in our lives. For, by helping us identify the zones of rapid change, they also help us identify—or invent—stability zones, patterns of relative constancy in the overwhelming flux. They improve the odds in the personal stuggle to manage change.

Nor is this a purely negative process—a struggle to suppress or limit change. The issue for any individual attempting to cope with rapid change is how to maintain himself within the adaptive range, and beyond that, how to find the exquisite optimum point at which he lives at peak effectiveness. Dr. John L. Fuller, a senior scientist at the Jackson Laboratory, a bio-medical research center in Bar Harbor, Maine, has conducted experiments in the impact of experiential deprivation and overload. "Some people," he says, "achieve a certain sense of serenity, even in the midst of turmoil, not because they are immune to emotion, but because they have found ways to get just the 'right' amount of change in their lives." The search for that optimum may be what much of the "pursuit of happiness" is about.

Trapped, temporarily, with the limited nervous and endocrine systems given us by evolution, we must work out new tactics to help us regulate the stimulation to which we subject ourselves.

Situational Grouping

The trouble is that such personal tactics become less effective with every passing day. As the rate of change climbs, it becomes harder for individuals to create the personal stability zones they need. The costs of non-change escalate.

We may stay in the old house—only to see the neighborhood transformed. We may keep the old car—only to see repair bills mount beyond reach. We may refuse to transfer to a new location—only to lose our job as a result. For while there are steps we can take to reduce the impact of change in our personal lives, the real problem lies outside ourselves.

To create an environment in which change enlivens and enriches the individual, but does not everwhelm him, we must employ not merely personal tactics but social strategies. If we are to carry people through the accelerative period, we must begin now to build "future shock absorbers" into the very fabric of super-industrial society. And this requires a fresh way of thinking about change and non-change in our lives. It even requires a different way of classifying people.

Today we tend to categorize individuals not according to the changes they happen to be undergoing at the moment, but according to their status or position between changes. We consider a union man as someone who has joined a union and not yet quit. Our designation refers not to joining or quitting, but to the "non-change" that happens in between. Welfare recipient, college student, Methodist, executive—all refer to the person's condition between changes, as it were.

There is, however, a radically different way to view people. For example, "one who is moving to a new residence" is a classification into which more than 100,000 Americans fit on any given day, yet they are seldom thought of as a group. The classification "one who is changing his job" or "one who is joining a church," or "one who is getting a divorce" are all based on temporary, transitional conditions, rather than on the more enduring conditions between transitions.

This sudden shift of focus, from thinking about what people "are" to thinking about what they are "becoming," suggests a whole array of new approaches to adaptation.

One of the most imaginative and simplest of these comes from Dr. Herbert Gerjuoy, a psychologist on the staff of the Human Resources Research Organization. He terms it "situational grouping," and like most good ideas, it sounds obvious once it is described. Yet it has never been systematically exploited. Situational grouping may well become one of the key social services of the future.

Dr. Gerjuoy argues that we should provide temporary organizations—"situational groups"—for people who happen to be passing through similar life transitions at the same time. Such situational groups should be established, Gerjuoy contends, "for families caught in the upheaval of relocation, for men and women about to be divorced, for people about to lose a parent or a spouse, for those about to gain a child, for men preparing to switch to a new occupation, for families that have just moved into a community, for those about to marry off their last child, for those facing imminent retirement—for anyone, in other words, who faces an important life change.

"Membership in the group would, of course, be temporary—just long enough to help the person with the transitional difficulties. Some groups might meet for a few months, others might not do more than hold a single meeting."

By bringing together people who are sharing, or are about to share, a common adaptive experience, he argues, we help equip them to cope with it. "A man required to adapt to a new life situation loses some of his bases for self-esteem. He begins to doubt his own abilities. If we bring him together with others who are moving through the same experience, people he can identify with and respect, we strengthen him. The members of the group come to share, even if briefly, some sense of identity. They see their problems more objectively. They trade useful ideas and insights. Most important, they suggest future alternatives for one another."

This emphasis on the future, say Gerjuoy, is critical. Unlike some group therapy sessions, the meetings of situational groups should not be devoted to hashing over the past, or to griping about it, or to soul-searching self-revelation, but to discussing personal objectives, and to planning practical strategies for future use in the new life situation. Members might watch movies of other similar groups wrestling with the same kinds of problems. They might hear from others who are more advanced in the transition than they are. In short, they are given the opportunity to pool their personal experiences and ideas before the moment of change is upon them.

In essence, there is nothing novel about this approach. Even now certain organizations are based on situational principles. A group of Peace Corps volunteers preparing for an overseas mission is, in effect, just such a situational grouping, as are pre- and post-natal classes. Many American towns have a "Newcomer's Club" that invites new residents to casserole dinners or other socials, permitting them to mix with other recent arrivals and compare problems and plans. Perhaps there ought to be an "Outmovers Club" as well. What is new is the suggestion that we systematically honeycomb the society with such "coping classrooms."

Crisis Counseling

Not all help for the individual can, or necessarily should come from groups. In many cases, what the change-pressed person needs most is one-to-one counseling during the crisis of adaptation. In psychiatric jargon a "crisis" is any significant transition. It is roughly synonymous with "major life change."

Today persons in transitional crisis turn to a variety of experts—doctors, marriage counselors, psychiatrists, vocational specialists and others—for individualized advice. Yet for many kinds of crisis there are no appropriate experts. Who helps the family or individual faced with the need to move to a new city for the third time in five years? Who is available to counsel a leader who is up- or down-graded by a reorganization of his or her club or community organization? Who is there to help the secretary just bounced back to the typing pool?

People like these are not sick. They neither need nor should receive psychiatric attention, yet there is, by and large, no counseling machinery available to them.

Not only are there many kinds of present-day life transitions for which no counseling help is provided, but the invasion of novelty will slam individuals up against wholly new kinds of personal crises in the future. And as the society races toward heterogeneity, the variety of problems will increase. In slowly changing societies the types of crises faced by individuals are more uniform and the sources of specialized advice more easily identifiable. The crisis-caught person went to his priest, his witch doctor or his local chief. Today personalized counseling services in the high technology countries have become so specialized that we have developed, in effect, second-layer advice-givers who do nothing but counsel the individual about where to seek advice.

These referral services interpose additional red tape and delay between the individual and the assistance he needs. By the time help reaches him, he may already have made the crucial decision—and done so badly. So long as we assume that advice is something that must come from evermore specialized professionals, we can anticipate ever greater difficulty. Moreover, so long as we base specialties on what people "are" instead of what they are "becoming" we miss many of the real adaptive problems altogether. Conventional social service systems will never be able to keep up.

The answer is a counterpart to the situational grouping system—a counseling set-up that not only draws on full-time professional advice givers, but on multitudes of lay experts as well. We must recognize that what makes a person an expert in one type of crisis is not necessarily formal education, but the very experience of having undergone a similar crisis himself.

To help tide millions of people over the difficult transitions they are likely to face, we shall be forced to "deputize" large numbers of non-professional people in the community—businessmen, students, teachers, workers, and others—to serve as "crisis counselors." Tomorrow's crisis counselors will be experts not in such conventional disciplines as psychology or health, but in specific transitions such as relocation, job promotion, divorce, or subcult-hopping. Armed with their own recent experience, working on a volunteer basis or for minimal pay, they will set aside some small part of their time for listening to other lay people talk out their problems, apprehensions and plans. In return, they will have access to others for similar assistance in the course of their own adaptive development.

Once again, there is nothing new about people seeking advice from one another. What is new is our ability, through the use of computerized systems, to assemble situational groups swiftly, to match up individuals with counselors, and to do both with considerable respect for privacy and anonymity.

We can already see evidence of a move in this direction in the spread of "listening" and "caring" services. In Davenport, Iowa, lonely people can dial a telephone number and be connected with a "listener"—one of a rotating staff of volunteers who man the telephone twenty-four hours a day. The program, initiated by a local commission on the aging, is similar to, but not the same as, the Care-Ring service in New York. Care-Ring charges its subscribers a fee, in return for which they receive two check-in calls each day at designated times. Subscribers provide the service with the names of their doctor, a neighbor, their building superintendent, and a close relative. In the event they fail to respond to a call, the service tries again half an hour later. If they still do not respond, the doctor is notified and a nurse dispatched to the scene. Care-Ring services are now being franchised in other cities. In both these services we see forerunners of the crisis-counseling system of the future.

Under that system, the giving and getting of advice becomes not a "social service" in the usual bureaucratic, impersonal sense, but a highly personalized process that not only helps individuals crest the currents of change in their own lives, but helps cement the entire society together in a kind of "love network"—an integrative system based on the principle of "I need you as much as you need me." Situational grouping and person-to-person crisis counseling are likely to become a significant part of everyone's life as we all move together into the uncertainties of the future.

Half-way Houses

A "future shock absorber" of a quite different type is the "half-way house" idea already employed by progressive prison authorities to ease the convict's way back into normal life. According to criminologist Daniel Glaser, the distinctive feature of the correctional institutions of the future will be the idea of "gradual release."

Instead of taking a man out of the under-stimulating, tightly regimented life of the prison and plunging him violently and without preparation into open society, he is moved first to an intermediate institution which permits him to work in the community by day, while continuing to return to the institution at night. Gradually, restrictions are lifted until he is fully adjusted to the outside world. The same principle has been explored by various mental institutions.

Similarly it has been suggested that the problems of rural populations suddenly shifted to urban centers might be sharply reduced if something like this half-way house principle were employed to ease their entry into the new way of life. What cities need, according to this theory, are reception facilities where newcomers live for a time under conditions half-way between those of the rural society they are leaving behind and the urban society they are seeking to penetrate. If instead of treating city-bound migrants with contempt and leaving them to find their own way, they were first acclimatized, they would adapt far more successfully.

A similar idea is filtering through the specialists who concern themselves with "squatter housing" in major cities in the technologically underdeveloped world. Outside Khartoum in the Sudan, thousands of former nomads have created a concentric ring of settlements. Those furthest from the city live in tents, much like the ones they occupied before migration. The next-closer group lives in mud-walled huts with tent roofs. Those still closer to the city occupy huts with mud walls and tin roofs.

When police set out to tear down the tents, urban planner Constantinos Doxiadis recommended that they not only *not* destroy them, but that certain municipal services be provided to their inhabitants. Instead of seeing these concentric rings in wholly negative terms, he suggested, they might be viewed as a tremendous teaching machine through which individuals and families move, becoming urbanized step by step.

The application of this principle, however, need not be limited to the poor, the insane or the criminal. The basic idea of providing change in controlled, graduated stages, rather than abrupt transitions, is crucial to any society that wishes to cope with rapid social or technological upheaval. The veteran, for example, could be released from service more gradually. The student from a rural community could spend a few weeks at a college in a medium-size city before entering the large urban university. The long-term hospital patient might be encouraged to go home on a trial basis, once or twice, before being discharged.

We are already experimenting with these strategies, but others are possible. Retirement, for example, should not be the abrupt, all-or-nothing, ego-crushing change that it now is for most men. There is no reason why it cannot be gradualized. Military induction, which typically separates a young man from his family in a sudden and almost violent fashion, could be done by stages. Legal separation, which is supposed to serve as a kind of half-way house on the way to divorce, could be made less legally complicated and psychologically costly. Trial marriage could be encouraged, instead of denigrated. In short, wherever a change of status is contemplated, the possibility of gradualizing it should be considered.

Enclaves of the Past

No society racing through the turbulence of the next several decades will be able to do without specialized centers in which the rate of change is artificially depressed. To phrase it differently, we shall need enclaves of the past—communities in which turnover, novelty and choice are deliberately limited.

These may be communities in which history is partially frozen, like the Amish villages of Pennsylvania, or places in which the past artfully simulated, like Williamsburg, Virginia or Mystic, Connecticut. Unlike Williamsburg or Mystic, however, through which visitors stream at a steady and rapid clip, tomorrow's enclaves of the past must be placed where people faced with future shock can escape the pressures of overstimulation for weeks, months, even years, if they choose.

In such slow-paced communities, individuals who need or want a more relaxed, less stimulating existence should be able to find it. The communities must be consciously encapsulated, selectively cut off from the surrounding society. Vehicular access should be limited to avoid traffic. Newspapers should be weeklies instead of dailies. If permitted at all, radio and television should be broadcast only for a few hours a day, instead of round the clock. Only special emergency services—health, for example—should be maintained at the maximum efficiency permitted by advanced technology.

Such communities not only should not be derided, they should be subsidized by the larger society as a form of mental and social insurance. In times of extremely rapid change, it is possible for the larger society to make some irreversible, catastrophic error. Imagine, for instance, the widespread diffusion of a food additive that accidentally turns out to have thalidomide-like effects. One can conceive of accidents capable of sterilizing or even killing whole populations.

By proliferating enclaves of the past, living museums as it were, we increase the chance that someone will be there to pick up the pieces in case of massive calamity. Such communities might also serve as experiential teaching machines. Thus children from the outside world might spend a few months in a simulated feudal village, living and actually working as children did centuries ago. Teenagers might be required to spend some time living in a typical early industrial community and to actually work in its mill or factory. Such living education would give them a historical perspective no book could ever provide. In these communities, the men and women who want a slower life might actually make a career out of "being" Shakespeare or Ben Franklin or Napoleon—not merely acting out their parts on stage, but living, eating, sleeping, as they did. The career of "historical simulant" would attract a great many naturally talented actors.

In short, every society will need sub-societies whose members are committed to staying away from the latest fads. We may even want to pay people *not* to use the latest goods, not to enjoy the most automated and sophisticated conveniences.

Enclaves of the Future

By the same token, just as we make it possible for some people to live at the slower pace of the past, we must also make it possible for individuals to experience aspects of their future in advance. Thus, we shall also have to create enclaves of the future.

In a limited sense, we are already doing this. Astronauts, pilots and other specialists are often trained by placing them in carefully assembled simulations of the environments they will occupy at some date in the future when they actually participate in a mission. By duplicating the interior of a cockpit or a capsule, we allow them to become accustomed, by degrees, to their future environment. Police and espionage agents, as well as commandos and other military specialists, are pre-trained by watching movies of the people they will have to deal with, the factories they are supposed to infiltrate, the terrain they will have to cover. In this way they are prepared to cope with a variety of future contingencies.

There is no reason why the same principle cannot be extended. Before dispatching a worker to a new location, he and his family ought to be shown detailed movies of the neighborhood they will live in, the school their children will attend, the stores in which they will shop, perhaps even of the teachers, shopkeepers, and neighbors they will meet. By preadapting them in this way, we can lower their anxieties about the unknown and prepare them, in advance, to cope with many of the problems they are likely to encounter.

Tomorrow, as the technology of experimental simulation advances, we shall be able to go much further. The pre-adapting individual will be able not merely to see and hear, but to touch, taste and smell the environment he is about to enter. He will be able to interact vicariously with the people in his future, and to undergo carefully contrived experiences designed to improve his coping abilities.

The "psych-corps" of the future will find a fertile market in the design and operation of such preadaptive facilities. Whole families may go to "work-learn-and-play" enclaves which will, in effect, constitute museums of the future, preparing them to cope with their own personal tomorrows.

Global Space Pageants

"Mesmerized as we are by the very idea of change," writes John Gardner in *Self-Renewal*, "we must guard against the notion that continuity is a negligible—if not reprehensible—factor in human history. It is a vitally important ingredient in the life of individuals, organizations and societies."

In the light of theory of the adaptive range, it becomes clear that an insistence on continuity in our experience is not necessarily "reactionary," just as the demand for abrupt or discontinuous change is not necessarily "progressive." In stagnant societies, there is a deep psychological need for novelty and stimulation. In an accelerative society, the need may well be for the preservation of certain continuities.

In the past, ritual provided an important change-buffer. Anthropologists tell us that certain repeated ceremonial forms—rituals surrounding birth, death, puberty, marriage and so on—helped individuals in primitive societies to re-establish equilibrium after some major adaptive event had taken place.

"There is no evidence," writes S. T. Kimball, "that a secularized urban world has lessened the need for ritualized expression . . ." Carleton Coon declares that "Whole societies, whatever their sizes and degrees of complexity, need controls to ensure the maintenance of equilibrium, and control comes in several forms. One is ritual." He points out that ritual survives today in the public appearances of heads of state, in religion, in business.

These, however, represent the merest tip of the ritual iceberg. In Western societies, for example, the sending of Christmas cards is an annual ritual that not only represents continuity in its own right, but which helps individuals prolong their all-too-temporary friendships or acquaintanceships. The celebration of birthdays, holidays or anniversaries are additional examples. The fast-burgeoning greeting-card industry—2,248,000,000 Christmas cards are sold annually in the United States alone—is an economic monument to the society's continuing need for some semblance of ritual.

Repetitive behavior, whatever else its functions, helps give meaning to non-repetitive events, by providing the backdrop against which novelty is silhouetted. Sociologists James Bossard and Eleanor Boll, after examining one hundred published autobiographies, found seventy-three in which the writers described procedures which were "unequivocally classifiable as family rituals." These rituals arising from "some simple or random bits of family interaction, started to set, because they were successful or satisfying to members, and through repetition they 'jelled' into very definite forms."

As the pace of change accelerates, many of these rituals are broken down or denatured. Yet we struggle to maintain them. One non-religious family periodically offers a secular grace at the dinner table, to honor such benefactors of mankind as Johann Sebastian Bach or Martin Luther King. Husbands and wives speak of "our song" and periodically revisit "the place we first met." In the future, we can anticipate greater variety in the kinds of rituals adhered to in family life.

As we accelerate and introduce arhythmic patterns into the pace of change, we need to mark off certain regularities for preservation, exactly the way we now mark off certain forests, historical monuments, or bird sanctuaries for protection. We may even need to manufacture ritual.

No longer at the mercy of the elements as we once were, no longer condemned to darkness at night or frost in the morning, no longer positioned in an unchanging physical environment, we are helped to orient ourselves in space and time by social, as distinct from natural, regularities.

In the United States, the arrival of spring is marked for most urban dwellers not by a sudden greenness—there is little green in Manhattan—but by the opening of the baseball season. The first ball is thrown by the President or some other dignitary, and thereafter millions of citizens follow, day by day, the unfolding of a mass ritual. Similarly, the end of summer is marked as much by the World Series as by any natural symbol.

Even those who ignore sports cannot help but be aware of these large and pleasantly predictable events. Radio and television carry baseball into every home. Newspapers are filled with sports news. Images of baseball form a backdrop, a kind of musical obbligato that enters our awareness. Whatever happens to the stock market, or to world politics, or to family life, the American League and the National League run through their expected motions. Outcomes of individual games vary. The standings of the teams go up and down. But the drama plays itself out within a set of reassuringly rigid and durable rules.

The opening of Congress every January; the appearance of new car models in the fall; seasonal variations in fashion; the April 15 deadline for filing income tax; the arrival of Christmas; the New Year's Eve party; the fixed national holidays. All these punctuate our time predictably, supplying a background of temporal regularity that is necessary (though hardly sufficient) for mental health.

The pressure of change, however, is to "unhitch" these from the calendar, to loosen and irregularize them. Often there are economic benefits for doing so. But there may also be hidden costs through the loss of stable temporal points of reference that today still lend some pattern and continuity to everyday life. Instead of eliminating these wholesale, we may wish to retain some, and, indeed, to introduce certain regularities where they do not exist. (Boxing championship matches are held at irregular, unpredictable times. Perhaps these highly ritualistic events should be held at fixed intervals as the Olympic games are.)

As leisure increases, we have the opportunity to introduce additional stability points and rituals into the society, such as new holidays, pageants and games. Such mechanisms could not only provide a backdrop of continuity in everyday life, but serve to integrate societies, and cushion them somewhat against the fragmenting impact of super-industrialism. We might, for example, create holidays to honor Galileo or Mozart, Einstein or Cézanne. We might create a global pageantry based on man's conquest of outer space.

Even now the succession of space launchings and capsule retrievals is beginning to take on a kind of ritual dramatic pattern. Millions stand transfixed as the countdown begins and the mission works itself out. For at least a fleeting instant, they share a realization of the oneness of humanity and its potential competence in the face of the universe.

By regularizing such events and by greatly adding to the pageantry that surrounds them, we can weave them into the ritual framework of the new society and use them as sanity-preserving points of temporal reference. Certainly, July 20, the day Astronaut Armstrong took "one small step for man, one giant leap for mankind," ought to be made into an annual global celebration of the unity of man.

In this way, by making use of new materials, as well as already existing rituals, by introducing change, wherever possible, in the form of predictable, rather than erratic chains of events, we can help provide elements of continuity even in the midst of social upheaval.

The cultural transformation of the Manus Islanders was simple compared with the one we face. We shall survive it only if we move beyond personal tactics to social strategies—providing new support services for the change-harassed individual, building continuity and change-buffers into the emergent civilization of tomorrow.

All this is aimed at minimizing the human damage wrought by rapid change. But there is another way of attacking the problem too. This is to expand man's adaptive capacities—the central task of education during the Super-industrial Revolution.